Lippincott's Illustrated Q&A Review of

Rubin's Pathology

SECOND EDITION

Bruce A. Fenderson, PhD
Professor of Pathology
Department of Pathology, Anatomy and Cell Biology
Jefferson Medical College
Thomas Jefferson University
Philadelphia, Pennsylvania

David S. Strayer, MD, PhD
Professor of Pathology
Department of Pathology, Anatomy and Cell Biology
Jefferson Medical College
Thomas Jefferson University
Philadelphia, Pennsylvania

Raphael Rubin, MD
Professor of Pathology
Department of Pathology, Anatomy and Cell Biology
Jefferson Medical College
Thomas Jefferson University
Philadelphia, Pennsylvania

Emanuel Rubin, MD
Founder and Consulting Editor, *Rubin's Pathology*
Recipient of the Tom Kent Award for Excellence
 in Pathology Education
Gonzalo E. Aponte Distinguished Professor
Department of Pathology, Anatomy and Cell Biology
Jefferson Medical College
Thomas Jefferson University
Philadelphia, Pennsylvania

 Wolters Kluwer | Lippincott Williams & Wilkins
Health

Philadelphia • Baltimore • New York • London
Buenos Aires • Hong Kong • Sydney • Tokyo

Acquisitions Editor: Susan Rhyner
Product Manager: Catherine Noonan
Vendor Manager: Bridgett Dougherty
Manufacturing Manager: Margie Orzech
Designer: Doug Smock
Compositor: SPi Technologies

Second Edition

Library of Congress Cataloging-in-Publication Data
Lippincott's illustrated Q & A review of Rubin's pathology / Bruce A. Fenderson ... [et al.]. — 2nd ed.
      p. ; cm.
   Other title: Illustrated Q & A review of Rubin's pathology
   Other title: Lipppincott's illustrated Q and A review of Rubin's pathology
   Rev. ed. of: Lippincott's review of pathology / Bruce A. Fenderson, Raphael Rubin, Emanuel Rubin. c2007.
   A learning companion to 5th and 6th ed. of Rubin's pathology.
   Includes index.
   Summary: "Lippincott's Illustrated Review of Rubin's Pathology, Second Edition offers up-to-date, clinically relevant board-style questions-perfect for course review and board prep! Approximately 1,000 multiple-choice questions with detailed answer explanations cover frequently tested topics in general and systemic pathology. The book is heavily illustrated with photos in the question or answer explanation. Online access to the questions and answers provides flexible study options"—Provided by publisher.
   ISBN 978-1-60831-640-3 (pbk.)
   1. Pathology—Examinations, questions, etc. I. Fenderson, Bruce A. II. Fenderson, Bruce A. Lippincott's review of pathology. III. Rubin's pathology. IV. Title: Illustrated Q & A review of Rubin's pathology. V. Title: Lipppincott's illustrated Q and A review of Rubin's pathology.
   [DNLM: 1. Pathology—Examination Questions. QZ 18.2 L765 2011]
   RB31.F46   2011
   616.07076—dc22
                                                                        2010025179

9 8 7 6

Dedication

We dedicate this book to our many teachers and colleagues for generously sharing their time and knowledge, and to all students of medicine for their intellectual stimulation and passion for learning.

Preface

Lippincott's Illustrated Q&A Review of Rubin's Pathology presents the key concepts of modern pathology in the form of clinical vignette-style questions. Using the format of the National Board of Medical Examiners (NBME), the questions address the major topics in general and systemic pathology presented in *Rubin's Pathology: Clinicopathologic Foundations of Medicine.* In addition to being a learning companion to this textbook, these questions will serve as a stand-alone resource for self-assessment and board review.

The questions are prepared at a level appropriate for second-year medical students. They provide a roadmap for students completing their courses in pathology and preparing for the United States Medical Licensing Examination (USMLE). Students in the allied health sciences (e.g., nursing and physical therapy) will also find considerable didactic value in clinical vignette-style questions.

Clinical vignette-style questions strengthen problem-solving skills. Students must integrate clinical and laboratory data, thereby simulating the practice of pathology and medicine in general. Case-based questions probe a level of competency that is expected for success on national licensing examinations. Given below are key features of this text:

- Multiple choice questions follow the USMLE template. Case-based questions include (1) patients' demographics, (2) clinical history, (3) physical examination findings, and (4) results of diagnostic tests and procedures. Each clinical vignette is followed by a question stem that addresses a key concept in pathology.
- Questions frequently involve "two-step" logic—a strategy that probes the student's ability to integrate basic knowledge into a clinical setting. The answer choices appear homogeneous and are listed alphabetically to avoid unintended cueing.
- Over 200 full-color images link clinical and pathologic findings.
- Answers are linked to the clinical vignettes and address key concepts. Incorrect answers are explained in context.
- Normal laboratory reference values are included for key laboratory tests.
- As an additional test-taking practice tool, the questions are also presented in an electronic format on our connection Web site (http://thePoint.lww.com/LIQARpathology2). Questions can be presented in both "quiz" and "test" modes. In quiz mode, students receive instant feedback regarding the correctness of their answer choice, along with a rationale. The test mode helps familiarize the user with the computer-generated USMLE experience.

We hope that this review of pathology will encourage students to think critically and formulate their own questions concerning mechanisms of disease. We are mindful of the words of e. e. Cummings, who wrote "always the beautiful answer who asks a more beautiful question." We wish our students success in their learning adventure. Most importantly, *have fun with pathology*.

Bruce A. Fenderson
Raphael Rubin
David S. Strayer
Emanuel Rubin

Acknowledgments

The contributions of the editors and authors of *Rubin's Pathology: Clinicopathologic Foundations of Medicine,* 5th and 6th editions were invaluable in the preparation of this text. We are particularly indebted to Dr. Ivan Damjanov and Dr. Hector Lopez for their contributions. Finally, we gratefully acknowledge the staff at Lippincott Williams & Wilkins for their expert help with manuscript preparation.

Contents

Chapter 1

Cell Injury

QUESTIONS

Select the single best answer.

1 Bone marrow cells from an organ donor are cultured in vitro at 37°C in the presence of recombinant erythropoietin. A photomicrograph of a typical "burst-forming unit" is shown in the image. This colony, committed to the erythrocyte pathway of differentiation, represents an example of which of the following physiologic adaptations to transmembrane signaling?

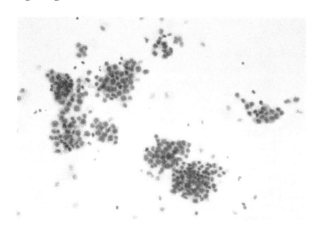

(A) Atrophy
(B) Dysplasia
(C) Hyperplasia
(D) Hypertrophy
(E) Metaplasia

2 A 50-year-old chronic alcoholic presents to the emergency room with 12 hours of severe abdominal pain. The pain radiates to the back and is associated with an urge to vomit. Physical examination discloses exquisite abdominal tenderness. Laboratory studies show elevated serum amylase. Which of the following morphologic changes would be expected in the peripancreatic tissue of this patient?
(A) Coagulative necrosis
(B) Caseous necrosis
(C) Fat necrosis
(D) Fibrinoid necrosis
(E) Liquefactive necrosis

3 A 68-year-old man with a history of gastroesophageal reflux disease suffers a massive stroke and expires. The esophagus at autopsy is shown in the image. Histologic examination of the abnormal tissue shows intestine-like epithelium composed of goblet cells and surface cells similar to those of incompletely intestinalized gastric mucosa. There is no evidence of nuclear atypia. Which of the following terms best describes this morphologic response to persistent injury in the esophagus of this patient?

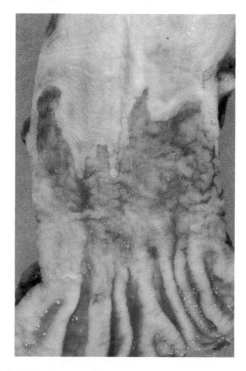

(A) Atypical hyperplasia
(B) Complex hyperplasia
(C) Glandular metaplasia
(D) Simple hyperplasia
(E) Squamous metaplasia

4 A CT scan of a 43-year-old woman with a parathyroid adenoma and hyperparathyroidism reveals extensive calcium deposits in the lungs and kidney parenchyma. These radiologic findings are best explained by which of the following mechanisms of disease?

(A) Arteriosclerosis
(B) Dystrophic calcification
(C) Granulomatous inflammation
(D) Metastatic calcification
(E) Tumor embolism

5 A 75-year-old woman with Alzheimer disease dies of congestive heart failure. The brain at autopsy is shown in the image. This patient's brain exemplifies which of the following responses to chronic injury?

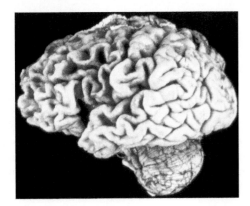

(A) Anaplasia
(B) Atrophy
(C) Dysplasia
(D) Hyperplasia
(E) Hypertrophy

6 A 68-year-old woman with a history of heavy smoking and repeated bouts of pneumonia presents with a 2-week history of fever and productive cough. A chest X-ray reveals a right lower lobe infiltrate. A transbronchial biopsy confirms pneumonia and further demonstrates preneoplastic changes within the bronchial mucosa. Which of the following best characterizes the morphology of this bronchial mucosal lesion?

(A) Abnormal pattern of cellular maturation
(B) Increased numbers of otherwise normal cells
(C) Invasiveness through the basement membrane
(D) Transformation of one differentiated cell type to another
(E) Ulceration and necrosis of epithelial cells

7 A 64-year-old man with long-standing angina pectoris and arterial hypertension dies of spontaneous intracerebral hemorrhage. At autopsy, the heart appears globoid. The left ventricle measures 2.8 cm on cross section (shown in the image). This adaptation to chronic injury was mediated primarily by changes in the intracellular concentration of which of the following components?

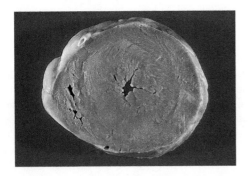

(A) DNA
(B) Glycogen
(C) Lipid
(D) mRNA
(E) Water

8 A 24-year-old woman contracts toxoplasmosis during her pregnancy and delivers a neonate at 37 weeks of gestation with a severe malformation of the central nervous system. MRI studies of the neonate reveal porencephaly and hydrocephalus. An X-ray film of the head shows irregular densities in the basal ganglia. These X-ray findings are best explained by which of the following mechanisms of disease?

(A) Amniotic fluid embolism
(B) Dystrophic calcification
(C) Granulomatous inflammation
(D) Metastatic calcification
(E) Organ immaturity

9 A 30-year-old man with AIDS-dementia complex develops acute pneumonia and dies of respiratory insufficiency. At autopsy, many central nervous system neurons display hydropic degeneration. This manifestation of sublethal neuronal injury was most likely mediated by impairment of which of the following cellular processes?

(A) DNA synthesis
(B) Lipid peroxidation
(C) Mitotic spindle assembly
(D) Plasma membrane sodium transport
(E) Ribosome biosynthesis

10 A 62-year-old man is brought to the emergency room in a disoriented state. Physical examination reveals jaundice, splenomegaly, and ascites. Serum levels of ALT, AST, alkaline phosphatase, and bilirubin are all elevated. A liver biopsy demonstrates alcoholic hepatitis with Mallory bodies. These cytoplasmic structures are composed of interwoven bundles of which of the following proteins?

(A) α_1-Antitrypsin
(B) β-Amyloid (Aβ)
(C) Intermediate filaments
(D) Prion protein (PrP)
(E) α-Synuclein

11 A 65-year-old man suffers a heart attack and expires. Examination of the lungs at autopsy reveals numerous pigmented nodules scattered throughout the parenchyma (shown in the image). What is the appropriate diagnosis?

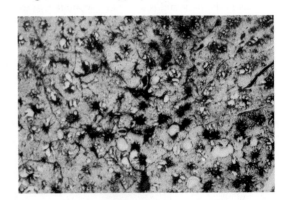

(A) Anthracosis
(B) Asbestosis
(C) Hemosiderosis
(D) Sarcoidosis
(E) Silicosis

12 A 32-year-old woman with poorly controlled diabetes mellitus delivers a healthy boy at 38 weeks of gestation. As a result of maternal hyperglycemia during pregnancy, pancreatic islets in the neonate would be expected to show which of the following morphologic responses to injury?
(A) Atrophy
(B) Dysplasia
(C) Hyperplasia
(D) Metaplasia
(E) Necrosis

13 A 59-year-old female alcoholic is brought to the emergency room with a fever (38.7°C/103°F) and foul-smelling breath. The patient subsequently develops acute bronchopneumonia and dies of respiratory insufficiency. A pulmonary abscess is identified at autopsy (shown in the image). Histologic examination of the wall of this lesion would most likely demonstrate which of the following pathologic changes?

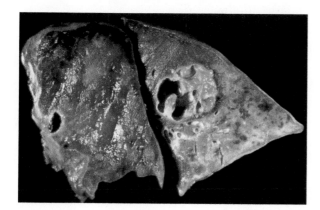

(A) Caseous necrosis
(B) Coagulative necrosis
(C) Fat necrosis
(D) Fibrinoid necrosis
(E) Liquefactive necrosis

14 A 20-year-old man from China is evaluated for persistent cough, night sweats, low-grade fever, and general malaise. A chest X-ray reveals findings "consistent with a Ghon complex." Sputum cultures grow acid-fast bacilli. Examination of hilar lymph nodes in this patient would most likely demonstrate which of the following pathologic changes?
(A) Caseous necrosis
(B) Coagulative necrosis
(C) Fat necrosis
(D) Fibrinoid necrosis
(E) Liquefactive necrosis

15 A 31-year-old woman complains of increased vaginal discharge of 1-month duration. A cervical Pap smear is shown in the image. Superficial epithelial cells are identified with arrows. When compared to cells from the deeper intermediate

layer (top), the nuclei of these superficial cells exhibit which of the following cytologic features?

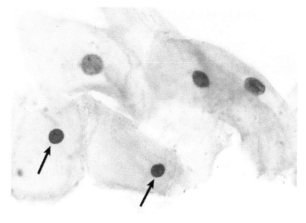

(A) Karyolysis
(B) Karyorrhexis
(C) Pyknosis
(D) Segmentation
(E) Viral inclusion bodies

16 A 30-year-old woman suffers a tonic-clonic seizure and presents with delirium and hydrophobia. The patient states that she was bitten on the hand by a bat about 1 month ago. The patient subsequently dies of respiratory failure. Viral particles are found throughout the brainstem and cerebellum at autopsy. In addition to direct viral cytotoxicity, the necrosis of virally infected neurons in this patient was mediated primarily by which of the following mechanisms?
(A) Histamine release from mast cells
(B) Humoral and cellular immunity
(C) Neutrophil-mediated phagocytosis
(D) Release of oxygen radicals from macrophages
(E) Vasoconstriction and ischemia

17 A 52-year-old woman loses her right kidney following an automobile accident. A CT scan of the abdomen 2 years later shows marked enlargement of the left kidney. The renal enlargement is an example of which of the following adaptations?
(A) Atrophy
(B) Dysplasia
(C) Hyperplasia
(D) Hypertrophy
(E) Metaplasia

18 An 82-year-old man has profound bleeding from a peptic ulcer and dies of hypovolemic shock. The liver at autopsy displays centrilobular necrosis. Compared to viable hepatocytes, the necrotic cells contain higher intracellular concentrations of which of the following?
(A) Calcium
(B) Cobalt
(C) Copper
(D) Iron
(E) Selenium

19 A 28-year-old woman is pinned by falling debris during a hurricane. An X-ray film of the leg reveals a compound fracture of the right tibia. The leg is immobilized in a cast for 6 weeks.

When the cast is removed, the patient notices that her right leg is weak and visibly smaller in circumference than the left leg. Which of the following terms best describes this change in the patient's leg muscle?

(A) Atrophy
(B) Hyperplasia
(C) Metaplasia
(D) Ischemic necrosis
(E) Irreversible cell injury

20 A 70-year-old man is hospitalized after suffering a mild stroke. While in the hospital, he suddenly develops crushing substernal chest pain. Analysis of serum proteins and ECG confirm a diagnosis of acute myocardial infarction. The patient subsequently develops an arrhythmia and expires. A cross section of the left ventricle at autopsy is shown in the image. Histologic examination of the affected heart muscle would demonstrate which of the following morphologic changes?

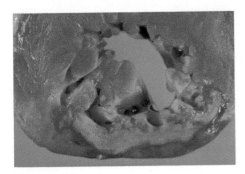

(A) Caseous necrosis
(B) Coagulative necrosis
(C) Fat necrosis
(D) Fibrinoid necrosis
(E) Liquefactive necrosis

21 Which of the following histologic features would provide definitive evidence of necrosis in the myocardium of the patient described in Question 20?

(A) Disaggregation of polyribosomes
(B) Increased intracellular volume
(C) Influx of lymphocytes
(D) Mitochondrial swelling and calcification
(E) Nuclear fragmentation

22 A 90-year-old woman with mild diabetes and Alzheimer disease dies in her sleep. At autopsy, hepatocytes are noted to contain golden cytoplasmic granules that do not stain with Prussian blue. Which of the following best accounts for pigment accumulation in the liver of this patient?

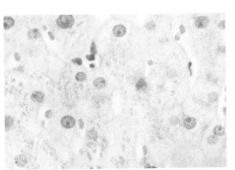

(A) Advanced age
(B) Alzheimer disease
(C) Congestive heart failure
(D) Diabetic ketoacidosis
(E) Hereditary hemochromatosis

23 Which of the following mechanisms of disease best describes the pathogenesis of pigment accumulation in hepatocytes in the patient described in Question 22?

(A) Degradation of melanin pigments
(B) Inhibition of glycogen biosynthesis
(C) Malabsorption and enhanced deposition of iron
(D) Peroxidation of membrane lipids
(E) Progressive oxidation of bilirubin

24 A 45-year-old man presents with increasing abdominal girth and yellow discoloration of his skin and sclera. Physical examination reveals hepatomegaly and jaundice. A Prussian blue stain of a liver biopsy is shown in the image. What is the major intracellular iron storage protein in this patient's hepatocytes?

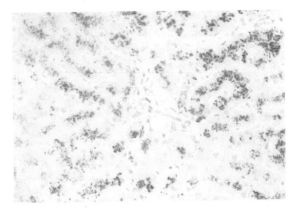

(A) Bilirubin
(B) Haptoglobin
(C) Hemoglobin
(D) Hemosiderin
(E) Transferrin

25 A 60-year-old man with chronic cystitis complains of urinary frequency and pelvic discomfort. Digital rectal examination is unremarkable. Biopsy of the bladder mucosa reveals foci of glandular epithelium and chronic inflammatory cells. No cytologic signs of atypia or malignancy are observed. Which of the following terms best describes the morphologic response to chronic injury in this patient?

(A) Atrophy
(B) Dysplasia
(C) Hyperplasia
(D) Hypertrophy
(E) Metaplasia

26 A 60-year-old man is rushed to the hospital with acute liver failure. He undergoes successful orthotopic liver transplantation; however, the transplanted liver does not produce much bile for the first 3 days. Poor graft function in this patient is thought to be the result of "reperfusion injury." Which of the following substances was the most likely cause of reperfusion injury in this patient's transplanted liver?

(A) Cationic proteins

(B) Free ferric iron

(C) Hydrochlorous acid

(D) Lysosomal acid hydrolases

(E) Reactive oxygen species

27 A 68-year-old woman with a history of hyperlipidemia dies of cardiac arrhythmia following a massive heart attack. Peroxidation of which of the following molecules was primarily responsible for causing the loss of membrane integrity in cardiac myocytes in this patient?

(A) Cholesterol

(B) Glucose transport proteins

(C) Glycosphingolipids

(D) Phospholipids

(E) Sodium-potassium ATPase

28 A 22-year-old construction worker sticks himself with a sharp, rusty nail. Within 24 hours, the wound has enlarged to become a 1-cm sore that drains thick, purulent material. This skin wound illustrates which of the following morphologic types of necrosis?

(A) Caseous necrosis

(B) Coagulative necrosis

(C) Fat necrosis

(D) Fibrinoid necrosis

(E) Liquefactive necrosis

29 A 42-year-old man undergoes liver biopsy for evaluation of the grade and stage of his hepatitis C virus infection. The biopsy reveals swollen (ballooned) hepatocytes and moderate lobular inflammatory activity (shown in the image). The arrow identifies an acidophilic (Councilman) body. Which of the following cellular processes best accounts for the presence of scattered acidophilic bodies in this liver biopsy?

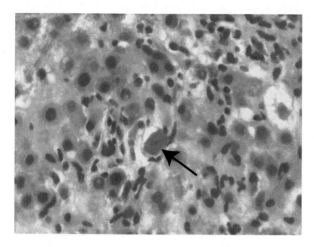

(A) Aggregation of intermediate filament proteins

(B) Apoptotic cell death

(C) Coagulative necrosis

(D) Collagen deposition

(E) Intracellular viral inclusions

30 Which of the following biochemical changes characterizes the formation of acidophilic bodies in the patient described in Question 29?

(A) Fragmentation of DNA

(B) Loss of tumor suppressor protein p53

(C) Mitochondrial swelling

(D) Synthesis of arachidonic acid

(E) Triglyceride accumulation

31 A 56-year-old woman with a history of hyperlipidemia and hypertension develops progressive, right renal artery stenosis. Over time, this patient's right kidney is likely to demonstrate which of the following morphologic adaptations to partial ischemia?

(A) Atrophy

(B) Dysplasia

(C) Hyperplasia

(D) Hypertrophy

(E) Neoplasia

32 A 5-year-old boy suffers blunt trauma to the leg in an automobile accident. Six months later, bone trabeculae have formed within the striated skeletal muscle at the site of tissue injury. This pathologic condition is an example of which of the following morphologic adaptations to injury?

(A) Atrophy

(B) Dysplasia

(C) Metaplasia

(D) Metastatic calcification

(E) Dystrophic calcification

33 A 43-year-old man presents with a scaly, erythematous lesion on the dorsal surface of his left hand. A skin biopsy reveals atypical keratinocytes filling the entire thickness of the epidermis (shown in the image). The arrows point to apoptotic bodies. Which of the following proteins plays the most important role in mediating programmed cell death in this patient's skin cancer?

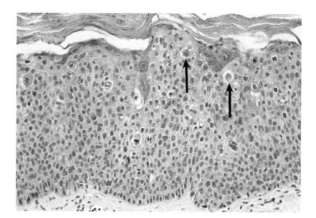

(A) Catalase

(B) Cytochrome *c*

(C) Cytokeratins

(D) Myeloperoxidase

(E) Superoxide dismutase

34 A 16-year-old girl with a history of suicidal depression swallows a commercial solvent. A liver biopsy is performed to assess the degree of damage to the hepatic parenchyma. Histologic examination demonstrates severe swelling of the centrilobular hepatocytes (shown in the image). Which of the following mechanisms of disease best accounts for the reversible changes noted in this liver biopsy?

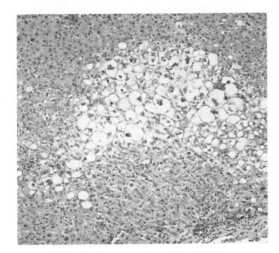

(A) Decreased stores of intracellular ATP
(B) Increased storage of triglycerides and free fatty acids
(C) Intracytoplasmic rupture of lysosomes
(D) Mitochondrial membrane permeability transition
(E) Protein aggregation due to increased cytosolic pH

35 A 40-year-old man is pulled from the ocean after a boating accident and resuscitated. Six hours later, the patient develops acute renal failure. Kidney biopsy reveals evidence of karyorrhexis and karyolysis in renal tubular epithelial cells. Which of the following biochemical events preceded these pathologic changes?
(A) Activation of Na⁺/K⁺ ATPase
(B) Decrease in intracellular calcium
(C) Decrease in intracellular pH
(D) Increase in ATP production
(E) Increase in intracellular pH

36 A 58-year-old man presents with symptoms of acute renal failure. His blood pressure is 220/130 mm Hg (malignant hypertension). While in the emergency room, the patient suffers a stroke and expires. Microscopic examination of the kidney at autopsy is shown in the image. Which of the following morphologic changes accounts for the red material in the wall of the artery?

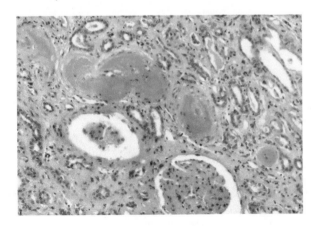

(A) Apoptosis
(B) Caseous necrosis
(C) Fat necrosis
(D) Fibrinoid necrosis
(E) Liquefactive necrosis

37 A 10-year-old girl presents with advanced features of progeria (patient shown in the image). This child has inherited mutations in the gene that encodes which of the following types of intracellular proteins?

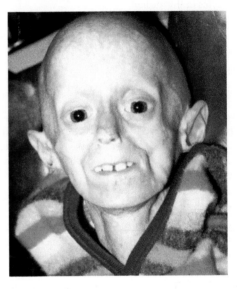

(A) Helicase
(B) Lamin
(C) Oxidase
(D) Polymerase
(E) Topoisomerase

38 A 32-year-old woman develops an Addisonian crisis (acute adrenal insufficiency) 3 months after suffering massive hemorrhage during the delivery of her baby. A CT scan of the abdomen shows small adrenal glands. Which of the following mechanisms of disease best accounts for adrenal atrophy in this patient?
(A) Chronic inflammation
(B) Chronic ischemia
(C) Hemorrhagic necrosis
(D) Lack of trophic signals
(E) Tuberculosis

39 A 47-year-old man with a history of heavy smoking complains of chronic cough. A "coin lesion" is discovered in his right upper lobe on chest X-ray. Bronchoscopy and biopsy fail to identify a mass, but the bronchial mucosa displays squamous metaplasia. What is the most likely outcome of this morphologic adaptation if the patient stops smoking?
(A) Atrophy
(B) Malignant transformation
(C) Necrosis and scarring
(D) Persistence throughout life
(E) Reversion to normal

40 A 60-year-old farmer presents with multiple patches of discoloration on his face. Biopsy of lesional skin reveals actinic keratosis. Which of the following terms best describes this response of the skin to chronic sunlight exposure?
(A) Atrophy
(B) Dysplasia
(C) Hyperplasia
(D) Hypertrophy
(E) Metaplasia

41 A 59-year-old woman smoker complains of intermittent blood in her urine. Urinalysis confirms 4+ hematuria. A CBC reveals increased red cell mass (hematocrit). A CT scan demonstrates a 3-cm renal mass, and a CT-guided biopsy displays renal cell carcinoma. Which of the following cellular adaptations in the bone marrow best explains the increased hematocrit in this patient?
(A) Atrophy
(B) Dysplasia
(C) Hyperplasia
(D) Hypertrophy
(E) Metaplasia

42 A 33-year-old woman has an abnormal cervical Pap smear. A cervical biopsy reveals that the epithelium lacks normal polarity (shown in the image). Individual cells display hyperchromatic nuclei, a larger nucleus-to-cytoplasm ratio, and disorderly tissue arrangement. Which of the following adaptations to chronic injury best describes these changes in the patient's cervical epithelium?

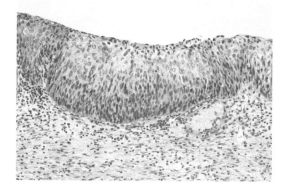

(A) Atrophy
(B) Dysplasia
(C) Hyperplasia
(D) Hypertrophy
(E) Metaplasia

43 A 24-year-old woman accidentally ingests carbon tetrachloride (CCl_4) in the laboratory and develops acute liver failure. Which of the following cellular proteins was directly involved in the development of hepatotoxicity in this patient?
(A) Acetaldehyde dehydrogenase
(B) Alcohol dehydrogenase
(C) Glucose-6-phosphate dehydrogenase
(D) Mixed function oxygenase
(E) Superoxide dismutase

44 A 30-year-old woman presents with a 2-month history of fatigue, mild fever, and an erythematous scaling rash. She also notes joint pain and swelling, primarily involving the small bones of her fingers. Physical examination reveals erythematous plaques with adherent silvery scales that induce punctate bleeding points when removed. Biopsy of lesional skin reveals markedly increased thickness of the epidermis (shown in the image). Which of the following terms best describes this adaptation to chronic injury in this patient with psoriasis?

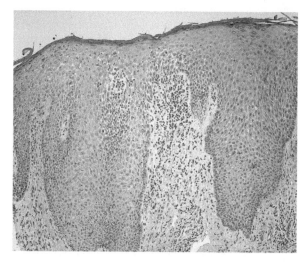

(A) Atrophy
(B) Dysplasia
(C) Hyperplasia
(D) Hypertrophy
(E) Metaplasia

45 A 24-year-old woman with chronic depression ingests a bottle of acetaminophen tablets. Two days later, she is jaundiced (elevated serum bilirubin) and displays symptoms of encephalopathy, including impairment in spatial perception. In the liver, toxic metabolites of acetaminophen are generated by which of the following organelles?
(A) Golgi apparatus
(B) Mitochondria
(C) Nucleus
(D) Peroxisomes
(E) Smooth endoplasmic reticulum

46 A 45-year-old woman presents with a 2-month history of fatigue and recurrent fever. She also complains of tenderness below the right costal margin and dark urine. Physical examination reveals jaundice and mild hepatomegaly. The serum is positive for hepatitis B virus antigen. Which of the following best describes the mechanism of indirect virus-mediated hepatocyte cell death in this patient?
(A) Accumulation of abnormal cytoplasmic proteins
(B) Immune recognition of viral antigens on the cell surface
(C) Generation of cytoplasmic free radicals
(D) Impaired plasma membrane Na^+/K^+ ATPase activity
(E) Interference with cellular energy generation

47 You are asked to present a grand rounds seminar on the role of abnormal proteins in disease. In this connection, intracellular accumulation of an abnormally folded protein plays a role in the pathogenesis of which of the following diseases?

(A) AA amyloidosis
(B) AL amyloidosis
(C) α_1-Antitrypsin deficiency
(D) Gaucher disease
(E) Tay-Sachs disease

48 A 38-year-old woman shows evidence of early cataracts, hair loss, atrophy of skin, osteoporosis, and accelerated atherosclerosis. This patient has most likely inherited mutations in both alleles of a gene that encodes which of the following types of intracellular proteins?

(A) Deaminase
(B) Helicase
(C) Oxidase
(D) Polymerase
(E) Topoisomerase

49 A 28-year-old man with a history of radiation/bone marrow transplantation for leukemia presents with severe diarrhea. He subsequently develops septic shock and expires. Microscopic examination of the colon epithelium at autopsy reveals numerous acidophilic bodies and small cells with pyknotic nuclei. Which of the following proteins most likely played a key role in triggering radiation-induced cell death in this patient's colonic mucosa?

(A) Cytochrome P450
(B) β-Catenin
(C) E-Cadherin
(D) P-Selectin
(E) p53

ANSWERS

1 **The answer is C: Hyperplasia.** Hyperplasia is defined as an increase in the number of cells in an organ or tissue. Like hypertrophy (choice D), it is often a response to trophic signals or increased functional demand and is commonly a normal process. Erythroid hyperplasia is typically seen in people living at high altitude. Low oxygen tension evokes the production of erythropoietin, which promotes the survival and proliferation of erythroid precursors in the bone marrow. The cellular and molecular mechanisms that are responsible for hyperplasia clearly relate to the control of cell proliferation (i.e., cell cycle). None of the other choices describe increased numbers of cells.
Diagnosis: Erythropoiesis, hyperplasia

2 **The answer is C: Fat necrosis.** Saponification of fat derived from peripancreatic fat cells exposed to pancreatic enzymes is a typical feature of fat necrosis. Lipase, released from pancreatic acinar cells during an attack of acute pancreatitis, hydrolyzes fat into fatty acids and glycerol. Free fatty acids bind with calcium to form soaps, which is a process known as saponification. Entry of calcium ions into the injured tissue reduces the level of calcium in blood. Hypocalcemia is, therefore, a typical finding in patients who had a recent bout of

acute pancreatitis. Patients with acute pancreatitis experience sudden-onset abdominal pain, distention, and vomiting. The other choices are not typically seen in peripancreatic tissue following acute pancreatitis, although liquefactive necrosis (choice E) may be observed.
Diagnosis: Acute pancreatitis

3 **The answer is C: Glandular metaplasia.** The major adaptive responses of cells to sublethal injury are atrophy, hypertrophy, hyperplasia, metaplasia, dysplasia, and intracellular storage. Metaplasia is defined as the conversion of one differentiated cell pathway to another. In this case, the esophageal squamous epithelium is replaced by columnar epithelium as a result of chronic gastroesophageal reflux. The lesion is characterized histologically by intestine-like epithelium composed of goblet cells and cells similar to those of incompletely intestinalized gastric mucosa. Squamous metaplasia (choice E) occurs in the bronchial epithelium of smokers, among other examples. Choices A, B, and D are preneoplastic changes that are most often described in the uterine endometrium of postmenopausal women.
Diagnosis: Barrett esophagus, metaplasia

4 **The answer is D: Metastatic calcification.** Metastatic calcification is associated with an increased serum calcium concentration (hypercalcemia). Almost any disorder that increases serum calcium levels can lead to calcification in the alveolar septa of the lung, renal tubules, and blood vessels. The patient in this case had a parathyroid adenoma that produced large quantities of parathyroid hormone. Other examples of metastatic calcification include multiple opacities in the cornea of a child given large amounts of vitamin D and partially calcified alveolar septa in the lungs of a patient with breast cancer metastatic to bone. Breast cancer metastases to bone are often osteolytic and, therefore, accompanied by hypercalcemia. Dystrophic calcification (choice B) has its origin in direct cell injury. Arteriosclerosis (choice A) is an example of dystrophic calcification.
Diagnosis: Hyperparathyroidism, metastatic calcification

5 **The answer is B: Atrophy.** Clinically, atrophy is recognized as diminution in the size or function of an organ. It is often seen in areas of vascular insufficiency or chronic inflammation and may result from disuse. Atrophy may be thought of as an adaptive response to stress, in which the cell shuts down its differentiated functions. Reduction in the size of an organ may reflect reversible cell atrophy or may be caused by irreversible loss of cells. For example, atrophy of the brain in this patient with Alzheimer disease is secondary to extensive cell death, and the size of the organ cannot be restored. This patient's brain shows marked atrophy of the frontal lobe. The gyri are thinned, and sulci are widened. Anaplasia (choice A) represents lack of differentiated features in a neoplasm.
Diagnosis: Alzheimer disease, atrophy

6 **The answer is A: Abnormal pattern of cellular maturation.** Cells that compose an epithelium exhibit uniformity of size and shape, and they undergo maturation in an orderly fashion (e.g., from plump basal cells to flat superficial cells in a squamous epithelium). When we speak of dysplasia, we mean that this regular appearance is disturbed by (1) variations in the size and shape of the cells; (2) enlargement, irregularity, and hyperchromatism of the nuclei; and (3) disorderly arrangement of the cells within the epithelium. Dysplasia of the bronchial epithelium is a reaction of respiratory epithelium to carcinogens in tobacco smoke. It is potentially reversible if the patient stops smoking but is considered preneoplastic and may progress to carcinoma. Choices B, D, and E are not preneoplastic changes. Invasiveness (choice C) connotes malignant behavior.

Diagnosis: Pneumonia, dysplasia

7 The answer is D: mRNA. Hypertrophic cardiac myocytes have more cytoplasm and larger nuclei than normal cells. Although the elucidation of the cellular and molecular mechanisms underlying the hypertrophic response is still actively pursued, it is clear that the final steps include increases in mRNA, rRNA, and protein. Hypertrophy results from transcriptional regulation. Aneuploidy (choice A) is not a feature of myofiber hypertrophy. Water influx (choice E), which is typical of hydropic swelling in acute injury, is not a common feature of hypertrophy.

Diagnosis: Hypertrophic heart disease, hypertrophy

8 The answer is B: Dystrophic calcification. Dystrophic calcification reflects underlying cell injury. Serum levels of calcium are normal, and the calcium deposits are located in previously damaged tissue. Intrauterine *Toxoplasma* infection affects approximately 0.1% of all pregnancies. Acute encephalitis in the fetus afflicted with TORCH syndrome may be associated with foci of necrosis that become calcified. Microcephaly, hydrocephalus, and microgyria are frequent complications of these intrauterine infections. Metastatic calcification (choice D) reflects an underlying disorder in calcium metabolism.

Diagnosis: Dystrophic calcification

9 The answer is D: Plasma membrane sodium transport. Hydropic swelling reflects acute, reversible (sublethal) cell injury. It results from impairment of cellular volume regulation, a process that controls ionic concentrations in the cytoplasm. This regulation, particularly for sodium, involves (1) the plasma membrane, (2) the plasma membrane sodium pump, and (3) the supply of ATP. Injurious agents may interfere with these membrane-regulated processes. Accumulation of sodium in the cell leads to an increase in water content to maintain isosmotic conditions, and the cell then swells. Lipid peroxidation (choice B) is often a feature of irreversible cell injury. The other choices are unrelated to volume control.

Diagnosis: Acute reversible injury

10 The answer is C: Intermediate filaments. Hyaline is a term that refers to any material that exhibits a reddish, homogeneous appearance when stained with hematoxylin and eosin (H&E). Standard terminology includes hyaline arteriolosclerosis, alcoholic hyaline in the liver, hyaline membranes in the lung, and hyaline droplets in various cells. Alcoholic (Mallory) hyaline is composed of cytoskeletal intermediate filaments (cytokeratins), whereas pulmonary hyaline membranes consist of plasma proteins deposited in alveoli. Structurally abnormal α_1-antitrypsin molecules (choice A) accumulate in

the liver of patients with α_1-antitrypsin deficiency. α-Synuclein (choice E) accumulates in neurons in the substantia nigra of patients with Parkinson disease.

Diagnosis: Alcoholic liver disease

11 The answer is A: Anthracosis. Anthracosis refers to the storage of carbon particles in the lung and regional lymph nodes. These particles accumulate in alveolar macrophages and are also transported to hilar and mediastinal lymph nodes, where the indigestible material is stored indefinitely within tissue macrophages. Although the gross appearance of the lungs of persons with anthracosis may be alarming, the condition is innocuous. Workers who mine hard coal (anthracite) develop pulmonary fibrosis, owing to the presence of toxic/fibrogenic dusts such as silica. This type of pneumoconiosis is more properly classified as anthracosilicosis. Hemosiderosis (choice C) represents intracellular storage of iron (hemosiderin). The other choices are not associated with dark pigmentation in the lung.

Diagnosis: Pneumoconiosis, anthracosis

12 The answer is C: Hyperplasia. Infants of diabetic mothers show a 5% to 10% incidence of major developmental abnormalities, including anomalies of the heart and great vessels and neural tube defects. The frequency of these lesions relates to the control of maternal diabetes during early gestation. During fetal development, the islet cells of the pancreas have proliferative capacity and respond to increased demand for insulin by undergoing physiologic hyperplasia. Fetuses exposed to hyperglycemia in utero may develop hyperplasia of the pancreatic β cells, which may secrete insulin autonomously and cause hypoglycemia at birth. Metaplasia (choice D) is defined as the conversion of one differentiated cell pathway to another.

Diagnosis: Diabetes mellitus

13 The answer is E: Liquefactive necrosis. When the rate of dissolution of the necrotic cells is faster than the rate of repair, the resulting morphologic appearance is termed liquefactive necrosis. The polymorphonuclear leukocytes of the acute inflammatory reaction are endowed with potent hydrolases that are capable of digesting dead cells. A sharply localized collection of these acute inflammatory cells in response to a bacterial infection produces rapid death and dissolution of tissue. The result is often an abscess defined as a cavity formed by liquefactive necrosis in a solid tissue. Caseous necrosis (choice A) is seen in necrotizing granulomas. In coagulative necrosis (choice B), the outline of the cell is retained. Fat (choice C) is not present in the lung parenchyma. Fibrinoid necrosis (choice D) is seen in patients with necrotizing vasculitis.

Diagnosis: Pulmonary abscess, liquefactive necrosis

14 The answer is A: Caseous necrosis. Caseous necrosis is a characteristic of primary tuberculosis, in which the necrotic cells fail to retain their cellular outlines. They do not disappear by lysis, as in liquefactive necrosis (choice E), but persist indefinitely as amorphous, coarsely granular, eosinophilic debris. Grossly, this debris resembles clumpy cheese, hence the name caseous necrosis. Primary tuberculosis is often asymptomatic or presents with nonspecific symptoms, such as low-grade fever, loss of appetite, and occasional spells of coughing. The

Ghon complex includes parenchymal consolidation and ipsilateral enlargement of hilar lymph nodes and is often accompanied by a pleural effusion. Fibrinoid necrosis (choice D) is seen in patients with necrotizing vasculitis.

Diagnosis: Tuberculosis, *Mycobacterium tuberculosis*

15   The answer is C: Pyknosis.   Coagulative necrosis refers to light microscopic alterations in dying cells. When stained with the usual combination of hematoxylin and eosin, the cytoplasm of a necrotic cell is eosinophilic. The nucleus displays an initial clumping of chromatin followed by its redistribution along the nuclear membrane. In pyknosis, the nucleus becomes smaller and stains deeply basophilic as chromatin clumping continues. Karyorrhexis (choice B) and karyolysis (choice A) represent further steps in the fragmentation and dissolution of the nucleus. These steps are not evident in the necrotic cells shown in this Pap smear.

Diagnosis: Cervical intraepithelial neoplasia, pyknosis

16   The answer is B: Humoral and cellular immunity.   Both humoral and cellular arms of the immune system protect against the harmful effects of viral infections. Thus, the presentation of viral proteins to the immune system immunizes the body against the invader and elicits both killer cells and the production of antiviral antibodies. These arms of the immune system eliminate virus-infected cells by either inducing apoptosis or directing complement-mediated cytolysis. In this patient, the rabies virus entered a peripheral nerve and was transported by retrograde axoplasmic flow to the spinal cord and brain. The inflammation is centered in the brainstem and spills into the cerebellum and hypothalamus. The other choices are seen in acute inflammation, but they do not represent antigen-specific responses to viral infections.

Diagnosis: Rabies

17   The answer is D: Hypertrophy.   Hypertrophy is a response to trophic signals or increased functional demand and is commonly a normal process. For example, if one kidney is rendered inoperative because of vascular occlusion, the contralateral kidney hypertrophies to accommodate increased demand. The molecular basis of hypertrophy reflects increased expression of growth-promoting genes (protooncogenes) such as *myc*, *fos*, and *ras*. Hyperplasia (choice C) of renal tubular cells may occur, but enlargement of the kidney in this patient is best referred to as hypertrophy (i.e., increased organ size and function).

Diagnosis: Hypertrophy

18   The answer is A: Calcium.   Coagulative necrosis is characterized by a massive influx of calcium into the cell. Under normal circumstances, the plasma membrane maintains a steep gradient of calcium ions, whose concentration in interstitial fluids is 10,000 times higher than that inside the cell. Irreversible cell injury damages the plasma membrane, which then fails to maintain this gradient, allowing the influx of calcium into the cell. The other choices would most likely be released upon cell death.

Diagnosis: Coagulative necrosis

19   The answer is A: Atrophy.   The most common form of atrophy follows reduced functional demand. For example, after immobilization of a limb in a cast as treatment for a bone fracture, muscle cells atrophy, and muscular strength is reduced. The expression of differentiation genes is repressed. On restoration of normal conditions, atrophic cells are fully capable of resuming their differentiated functions; size increases to normal, and specialized functions, such as protein synthesis or contractile force, return to their original levels. Ischemic necrosis (choice D) is typically a complication of vascular insufficiency. Irreversible injury to skeletal muscle (choice E) would be an unlikely complication of bone fracture.

Diagnosis: Atrophy, bone fracture

20   The answer is B: Coagulative necrosis.   Ischemic necrosis of cardiac myocytes is the leading cause of death in the Western world. In brief, the interruption of blood supply to the heart decreases the delivery of O_2 and glucose. Lack of O_2 impairs mitochondrial electron transport, thereby decreasing ATP synthesis and facilitating the production of reactive oxygen species. Mitochondrial damage promotes the release of cytochrome *c* to the cytosol, and the cell dies. The morphologic appearance of the necrotic cell has traditionally been termed coagulative necrosis because of its similarity to the coagulation of proteins that occurs upon heating.

Diagnosis: Myocardial infarction, coagulative necrosis

21   The answer is E: Nuclear fragmentation.   Nuclear fragmentation (karyorrhexis and karyolysis) is a hallmark of coagulative necrosis. Choices A, B, and D are incorrect because they are features of both reversibly and irreversibly injured cells. Lymphocytes (choice C) are a hallmark of chronic inflammation.

Diagnosis: Myocardial infarction

22   The answer is A: Advanced age.   Substances that cannot be metabolized accumulate in cells. Examples include (1) endogenous substrates that are not processed because a key enzyme is missing (lysosomal storage diseases), (2) insoluble endogenous pigments (lipofuscin and melanin), and (3) exogenous particulates (silica and carbon). Lipofuscin is a "wear and tear" pigment of aging that accumulates in organs such as the brain, heart, and liver. None of the other choices are associated with lipofuscin accumulation.

Diagnosis: Aging, lipofuscin

23   The answer is D: Peroxidation of membrane lipids.   Lipofuscin is found in lysosomes and contains peroxidation products of unsaturated fatty acids. The presence of this pigment is thought to reflect continuing lipid peroxidation of cellular membranes as a result of inadequate defenses against activated oxygen radicals. None of the other mechanisms of disease leads to the formation and accumulation of lipofuscin granules.

Diagnosis: Lipofuscin, intracellular storage disorder

24   The answer is D: Hemosiderin.   Hemosiderin is a partially denatured form of ferritin that aggregates easily and is recognized microscopically as yellow-brown granules in the cytoplasm, which turn blue with the Prussian blue reaction. In hereditary hemochromatosis, a genetic abnormality of iron absorption in the small intestine, excess iron is stored mostly in the form of hemosiderin, primarily in the liver. Hemoglobin (choice C) is the iron-containing pigment of RBCs. Bilirubin (choice A) is a product of heme catabolism that may accumulate in liver cells but does not stain with Prussian blue. Transferrin (choice E) binds serum iron.

Diagnosis: Hereditary hemochromatosis

25 The answer is E: Metaplasia. Metaplasia of transitional epithelium to glandular epithelium is seen in patients with chronic inflammation of the bladder (cystitis glandularis). Metaplasia is considered to be a protective mechanism, but it is not necessarily a harmless process. For example, squamous metaplasia in a bronchus may protect against injury produced by tobacco smoke, but it also impairs the production of mucus and ciliary clearance of debris. Furthermore, neoplastic transformation may occur in metaplastic epithelium. Lack of cytologic evidence for atypia and neoplasia rules out dysplasia (choice B).

Diagnosis: Chronic cystitis, metaplasia

26 The answer is E: Reactive oxygen species. Ischemia/reperfusion (I/R) injury is a common clinical problem that arises in the setting of occlusive cardiovascular disease, infection, transplantation, shock, and many other circumstances. The genesis of I/R injury relates to the interplay between transient ischemia and the re-establishment of blood flow (reperfusion). Initially, ischemia produces a type of cellular damage that leads to the generation of free radical species. Subsequently, reperfusion provides abundant molecular oxygen (O_2) to combine with free radicals to form reactive oxygen species. Oxygen radicals are formed inside cells through the xanthine oxidase pathway and released from activated neutrophils.

Diagnosis: Myocardial infarction

27 The answer is D: Phospholipids. During lipid peroxidation, hydroxyl radicals remove a hydrogen atom from the unsaturated fatty acids of membrane phospholipids. The lipid radicals so formed react with molecular oxygen and form a lipid peroxide radical. A chain reaction is initiated. Lipid peroxides are unstable and break down into smaller molecules. The destruction of the unsaturated fatty acids of phospholipids results in a loss of membrane integrity. The other choices represent targets for reactive oxygen species, but protein cross-linking (choices B and E) does not lead to rapid loss of membrane integrity in patients with myocardial infarction.

Diagnosis: Myocardial infarction

28 The answer is E: Liquefactive necrosis. Polymorphonuclear leukocytes (segmented neutrophils) rapidly accumulate at sites of injury. They are loaded with acid hydrolases and are capable of digesting dead cells. A localized collection of these inflammatory cells may create an abscess with central liquefaction (pus). Liquefactive necrosis is also commonly seen in the brain. Caseous necrosis (choice A) is seen in necrotizing granulomas. Fat necrosis (choice C) is typically encountered in patients with acute pancreatitis. Fibrinoid necrosis (choice D) is seen in patients with necrotizing vasculitis.

Diagnosis: Abscess, acute inflammation

29 The answer is B: Apoptotic cell death. Apoptosis is a programmed pathway of cell death that is triggered by a variety of extracellular and intracellular signals. It is often a self-

defense mechanism, destroying cells that have been infected with pathogens or those in which genomic alterations have occurred. After staining with hematoxylin and eosin, apoptotic cells are visible under the light microscope as acidophilic (Councilman) bodies. These deeply eosinophilic structures represent membrane-bound cellular remnants that are extruded into the hepatic sinusoids. The other choices do not appear as acidophilic bodies.

Diagnosis: Viral hepatitis

30 The answer is A: Fragmentation of DNA. Fragmentation of DNA is a hallmark of cells undergoing both necrosis and apoptosis, but apoptotic cells can be detected by demonstrating nucleosomal "laddering." This pattern of DNA degradation is characteristic of apoptotic cell death. It results from the cleavage of chromosomal DNA at nucleosomes by endonucleases. Since nucleosomes are regularly spaced along the genome, a pattern of regular bands can be seen when fragments of cellular DNA are separated by electrophoresis. The other choices are associated with cell injury, but they do not serve as distinctive markers of programmed cell death.

Diagnosis: Viral hepatitis

31 The answer is A: Atrophy. Interference with blood supply to tissues is known as ischemia. Total ischemia results in cell death. Partial ischemia occurs after incomplete occlusion of a blood vessel or in areas of inadequate collateral circulation. This results in a chronically reduced oxygen supply, a condition often compatible with continued cell viability. Under such circumstances, cell atrophy is common. For example, it is frequently seen around the inadequately perfused margins of infarcts in the heart, brain, and kidneys. None of the other choices describe decreased organ size and function.

Diagnosis: Renal artery stenosis

32 The answer is C: Metaplasia. Myositis ossificans is a disease characterized by formation of bony trabeculae within striated muscle. It represents a form of osseous metaplasia (i.e., replacement of one differentiated tissue with another type of normal differentiated tissue). Although dystrophic calcification (choice E) frequently occurs at sites of prior injury, it does not lead to the formation of bone trabeculae.

Diagnosis: Myositis ossificans, metaplasia

33 The answer is B: Cytochrome c. The mitochondrial membrane is a key regulator of apoptosis. When mitochondrial pores open, cytochrome *c* leaks out and activates Apaf-1, which converts procaspase-9 to caspase-9, resulting in the activation of downstream caspases (cysteine proteases). These effector caspases cleave target proteins, including endonucleases nuclear proteins, and cytoskeletal proteins to mediate the varied morphological and biochemical changes that accompany apoptosis. Reactive oxygen species (related to choices A, D, and E) are triggers of apoptosis, but they do not mediate programmed cell death.

Diagnosis: Apoptosis, squamous cell carcinoma of skin

34 The answer is A: Decreased stores of intracellular ATP. Hydropic swelling may result from many causes, including chemical and biologic toxins, infections, and ischemia. Injurious agents cause hydropic swelling by (1) increasing the permeability of the plasma membrane to sodium; (2) damaging the membrane sodium-potassium ATPase (pump); or (3) interfering with the synthesis of ATP, thereby depriving the pump of its fuel. The other choices are incorrect because they do not regulate concentrations of intracellular sodium.

Diagnosis: Hydropic swelling, hepatotoxicity

35 **The answer is C: Decrease in intracellular pH.** During periods of ischemia, anaerobic glycolysis leads to the overproduction of lactate and a decrease in intracellular pH. Lack of O_2 during myocardial ischemia blocks the production of ATP. Pyruvate is reduced to lactate in the cytosol and lowers intracellular pH. The acidification of the cytosol initiates a downward spiral of events that propels the cell toward necrosis. The other choices point to changes in the opposite direction of what would be expected in irreversible cell injury.

Diagnosis: Acute tubular necrosis

36 **The answer is D: Fibrinoid necrosis.** Fibrinoid necrosis is an alteration of injured blood vessels, in which the insudation and accumulation of plasma proteins cause the wall to stain intensely with eosin. The other choices are not typically associated directly with vascular injury.

Diagnosis: Malignant hypertension, fibrinoid necrosis

37 **The answer is B: Lamin.** Hutchinson-Gilford progeria is a rare genetic disease characterized by early cataracts, hair loss, atrophy of the skin, osteoporosis, and atherosclerosis. This phenotype gives the impression of premature aging in children. Progeria is one of many diseases caused by mutations in the human lamin A gene (*LMNA*). Lamins are intermediate filament proteins that form a fibrous meshwork beneath the nuclear envelope. Defective lamin A is thought to make the nucleus unstable, leading to cell injury and death. Mutations in the other genes are not linked to Hutchinson-Gilford progeria syndrome.

Diagnosis: Progeria

38 **The answer is D: Lack of trophic signals.** Atrophy of an organ may be caused by interruption of key trophic signals. Postpartum infarction of the anterior pituitary in this patient resulted in decreased production of adrenocorticotropic hormone (ACTH, also termed corticotropin). Lack of corticotropin results in atrophy of the adrenal cortex, which leads to adrenal insufficiency. Symptoms of acute adrenal insufficiency (Addisonian crisis) include hypotension and shock, as well as weakness, vomiting, abdominal pain, and lethargy. The other choices are unlikely causes of postpartum adrenal insufficiency.

Diagnosis: Sheehan syndrome, adrenal insufficiency

39 **The answer is E: Reversion to normal.** Metaplasia is almost invariably a response to persistent injury and can be thought of as an adaptive mechanism. Prolonged exposure of the bronchi to tobacco smoke leads to squamous metaplasia of the bronchial epithelium. Unlike malignancy (choice B) and necrosis with scarring (choice C), metaplasia is usually fully reversible. If the source of injury in this patient is removed

(the patient stops smoking), then the metaplastic epithelium will eventually return to normal.

Diagnosis: Chronic bronchitis, metaplasia

40 **The answer is B: Dysplasia.** Actinic keratosis is a form of dysplasia in sun-exposed skin. Histologically, such lesions are composed of atypical squamous cells, which vary in size and shape. They show no signs of regular maturation as the cells move from the basal layer of the epidermis to the surface. Dysplasia is a preneoplastic lesion, in the sense that it is a necessary stage in the multistep evolution to cancer. However, unlike cancer cells, dysplastic cells are not entirely autonomous, and the histologic appearance of the tissue may still revert to normal. None of the other choices represent preneoplastic changes in sun-exposed skin.

Diagnosis: Actinic keratosis, dysplasia

41 **The answer is C: Hyperplasia.** Renal cell carcinomas often secrete erythropoietin. This hormone stimulates the growth of erythrocyte precursors in the bone marrow by inhibiting programmed cell death. Increased hematocrit in this patient is the result of bone marrow hyperplasia affecting the erythroid lineage. The other choices do not represent physiologic responses to erythropoietin.

Diagnosis: Renal cell carcinoma, hyperplasia

42 **The answer is B: Dysplasia.** The distinction between severe dysplasia and early cancer of the cervix is a common diagnostic problem for the pathologist. Both are associated with disordered growth and maturation of the tissue. Similar to the development of cancer, dysplasia is believed to result from mutations in a proliferating cell population. When a particular mutation confers a growth or survival advantage, the progeny of the affected cell will tend to predominate. In turn, their continued proliferation provides the opportunity for further mutations. The accumulation of such mutations progressively distances the cell from normal regulatory constraints and may lead to neoplasia. None of the other choices are associated with lack of normal tissue polarity.

Diagnosis: Cervical intraepithelial neoplasia, dysplasia

43 **The answer is D: Mixed function oxygenase.** The metabolism of CCl_4 is a model system for toxicologic studies. CCl_4 is first metabolized via the mixed function oxygenase system (P450) of the liver to a chloride ion and a highly reactive trichloromethyl free radical. Like the hydroxyl radical, this radical is a potent initiator of lipid peroxidation, which damages the plasma membrane and leads to cell death. The other choices are not involved in the formation of the trichloromethyl free radical in liver cells.

Diagnosis: Hepatic failure, hepatotoxicity

44 **The answer is C: Hyperplasia.** Psoriasis is a disease of the dermis and epidermis that is characterized by persistent epidermal hyperplasia. It is a chronic, frequently familial disorder that features large, erythematous, scaly plaques, commonly on the dorsal extensor cutaneous surfaces. There is evidence to suggest that deregulation of epidermal proliferation and an abnormality in the microcirculation of the dermis are responsible for the development of psoriatic lesions. Abnormal proliferation of keratinocytes is thought to be related to defective epidermal cell surface receptors and altered intracellular signaling. The other choices do not describe increased numbers of otherwise normal epidermal cells.

Diagnosis: Psoriasis, hyperplasia

---

45 The answer is E: Smooth endoplasmic reticulum. Carbon tetrachloride and acetaminophen are well-studied hepatotoxins. Each is metabolized by cytochrome P450 of the mixed-function oxidase system, located in the smooth endoplasmic reticulum. These hepatotoxins are metabolized differently, and it is possible to relate the subsequent evolution of lethal cell injury to the specific features of this metabolism. Acetaminophen, an important constituent of many analgesics, is innocuous in recommended doses, but when consumed to excess it is highly toxic to the liver. The metabolism of acetaminophen to yield highly reactive quinones is accelerated by alcohol consumption, an effect mediated by an ethanol-induced increase in cytochrome P450.

Diagnosis: Hepatotoxicity, necrosis

---

46 The answer is B: Immune recognition of viral antigens on the cell surface. Viral cytotoxicity is either direct or indirect (immunologically mediated). Viruses may injure cells directly by subverting cellular enzymes and depleting the cell's nutrients, thereby disrupting the normal homeostatic mechanisms. Some viruses also encode proteins that induce apoptosis once daughter virions are mature. Viruses may also injure cells indirectly through activation of the immune system. Both humoral and cellular arms of the immune system protect against the harmful effects of viral infections by eliminating infected cells. In brief, the presentation of viral proteins to the immune system in the context of a self major histocompatibility complex on the cell surface immunizes the body against the invader and elicits both killer cells and antiviral antibodies. These arms of the immune system eliminate virus-infected cells by inducing apoptosis or by lysing the virally infected target cell with complement. None of the other choices describe mechanisms of indirect viral cytotoxicity.

Diagnosis: Hepatitis, viral

---

47 The answer is C: α₁-Antitrypsin deficiency. Several acquired and inherited diseases are characterized by intracellular accumulation of abnormal proteins. The deviant tertiary structure of the protein may result from an inherited mutation that alters the normal primary amino acid sequence, or may reflect an acquired defect in protein folding. α_1-Antitrypsin deficiency is a heritable disorder in which mutations in the gene for α_1-antitrypsin yield an insoluble protein. The mutant

protein is not easily exported. It accumulates in liver cells, causing cell injury and cirrhosis. Pulmonary emphysema is another complication of α_1-antitrypsin deficiency. Choices A and B are amyloidoses that represent extracellular deposits of fibrillar proteins arranged in β-pleated sheet. Choices D and E are lysosomal storage diseases that represent intracellular deposits of unmetabolized sphingolipids.

Diagnosis: α_1-Antitrypsin deficiency

---

48 The answer is B: Helicase. Werner syndrome is a rare autosomal recessive disease characterized by early cataracts, hair loss, atrophy of the skin, osteoporosis, and accelerated atherosclerosis. Affected persons are also at risk for development of a variety of cancers. Unlike Hutchinson-Gilford progeria, patients with Werner syndrome typically die in the fifth decade from either cancer or cardiovascular disease. Werner syndrome is caused by mutations in the *WRN* gene, which encodes a protein with multiple DNA-dependent enzymatic functions, including proteins with ATPase, helicase, and exonuclease activity. Hutchinson-Gilford progeria is caused by mutations in the human lamin A gene, which encodes an intermediate filament protein that form a fibrous meshwork beneath the nuclear envelope. Mutations in the other choices are not associated with Werner syndrome.

Diagnosis: Werner syndrome

---

49 The answer is E: p53. Apoptosis detects and destroys cells that harbor dangerous mutations, thereby maintaining genetic consistency and preventing the development of cancer. There are several means, the most important of which is probably p53, by which the cell recognizes genomic abnormalities and "assesses" whether they can be repaired. If the damage to DNA is so severe that it cannot be repaired, the cascade of events leading to apoptosis is activated, and the cell dies. This process protects an organism from the consequences of a nonfunctional cell or one that cannot control its own proliferation (e.g., a cancer cell). After it binds to areas of DNA damage, p53 activates proteins that arrest the cell in G1 of the cell cycle, allowing time for DNA repair to proceed. It also directs DNA repair enzymes to the site of injury. If the DNA damage cannot be repaired, p53 activates mechanisms that terminate in apoptosis. There are several pathways by which p53 induce apoptosis. This molecule downregulates transcription of the antiapoptotic protein Bcl-2, while it upregulates transcription of the proapoptotic genes bax and bak. Cytochrome P450 (choice A) is a member of the mixed function oxidase system. β-Catenin (choice B) is a membrane protein associated with cell adhesion molecules. Selectins (choices C and D) are cell adhesion molecules involved in leukocyte recirculation.

Diagnosis: Apoptosis

Chapter 2

Inflammation

QUESTIONS

Select the single best answer.

1 A 22-year-old woman nursing her newborn develops a tender erythematous area around the nipple of her left breast. A thick, yellow fluid is observed to drain from an open fissure. Examination of this breast fluid under the light microscope will most likely reveal an abundance of which of the following inflammatory cells?
(A) B lymphocytes
(B) Eosinophils
(C) Mast cells
(D) Neutrophils
(E) Plasma cells

2 Which of the following mediators of inflammation facilitates chemotaxis, cytolysis, and opsonization at the site of inflammation in the patient described in Question 1?
(A) Complement proteins
(B) Defensins
(C) Kallikrein
(D) Kinins
(E) Prostaglandins

3 A 63-year-old man becomes febrile and begins expectorating large amounts of mucopurulent sputum. Sputum cultures are positive for Gram-positive diplococci. Which of the following mediators of inflammation provides potent chemotactic factors for the directed migration of inflammatory cells into the alveolar air spaces of this patient?
(A) Bradykinin
(B) Histamine
(C) Myeloperoxidase
(D) N-formylated peptides
(E) Plasmin

4 A 59-year-old man suffers a massive heart attack and expires 24 hours later due to ventricular arrhythmia. Histologic examination of the affected heart muscle at autopsy would show an abundance of which of the following inflammatory cells?

(A) Fibroblasts
(B) Lymphocytes
(C) Macrophages
(D) Neutrophils
(E) Plasma cells

5 A 5-year-old boy punctures his thumb with a rusty nail. Four hours later, the thumb appears red and swollen. Initial swelling of the boy's thumb is primarily due to which of the following mechanisms?
(A) Decreased intravascular hydrostatic pressure
(B) Decreased intravascular oncotic pressure
(C) Increased capillary permeability
(D) Increased intravascular oncotic pressure
(E) Vasoconstriction of arterioles

6 Which of the following serum proteins activates the complement, coagulation, and fibrinolytic systems at the site of injury in the patient described in Question 5?
(A) Bradykinin
(B) Hageman factor
(C) Kallikrein
(D) Plasmin
(E) Thrombin

7 An 80-year-old woman presents with a 4-hour history of fever, shaking chills, and disorientation. Her blood pressure is 80/40 mm Hg. Physical examination shows diffuse purpura on her upper arms and chest. Blood cultures are positive for Gram-negative organisms. Which of the following cytokines is primarily involved in the pathogenesis of direct vascular injury in this patient with septic shock?
(A) Interferon-γ
(B) Interleukin-1
(C) Platelet-derived growth factor
(D) Transforming growth factor-β
(E) Tumor necrosis factor-α

8 A 24-year-old intravenous drug abuser develops a 2-day history of severe headache and fever. His temperature is 38.7°C (103°F). Blood cultures are positive for Gram-positive cocci.

The patient is given intravenous antibiotics, but he deteriorates rapidly and dies. A cross section of the brain at autopsy (shown in the image) reveals two encapsulated cavities. Which of the following terms best characterizes this pathologic finding?

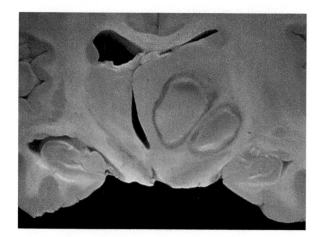

(A) Chronic inflammation
(B) Fibrinoid necrosis
(C) Granulomatous inflammation
(D) Reactive gliosis
(E) Suppurative inflammation

9 A 36-year-old woman with pneumococcal pneumonia develops a right pleural effusion. The pleural fluid displays a high specific gravity and contains large numbers of polymorphonuclear (PMN) leukocytes. Which of the following best characterizes this pleural effusion?
(A) Fibrinous exudate
(B) Lymphedema
(C) Purulent exudate
(D) Serosanguineous exudate
(E) Transudate

10 A 33-year-old man presents with a 5-week history of calf pain and swelling and low-grade fever. Serum levels of creatine kinase are elevated. A muscle biopsy reveals numerous eosinophils. What is the most likely etiology of this patient's myalgia?
(A) Autoimmune disease
(B) Bacterial infection
(C) Muscular dystrophy
(D) Parasitic infection
(E) Viral infection

11 A 10-year-old boy with a history of recurrent bacterial infections presents with fever and a productive cough. Biochemical analysis of his neutrophils demonstrates that he has an impaired ability to generate reactive oxygen species. This patient most likely has inherited mutations in the gene that encodes which of the following proteins?
(A) Catalase
(B) Cytochrome P450
(C) Myeloperoxidase
(D) NADPH oxidase
(E) Superoxide dismutase

12 A 25-year-old woman presents with a history of recurrent shortness of breath and severe wheezing. Laboratory studies demonstrate that she has a deficiency of C1 inhibitor, an esterase inhibitor that regulates the activation of the classical complement pathway. What is the diagnosis?
(A) Chronic granulomatous disease
(B) Hereditary angioedema
(C) Myeloperoxidase deficiency
(D) Selective IgA deficiency
(E) Wiskott-Aldrich syndrome

13 A 40-year-old man complains of a 2-week history of increasing abdominal pain and yellow discoloration of his sclera. Physical examination reveals right upper quadrant pain. Laboratory studies show elevated serum levels of alkaline phosphatase (520 U/dL) and bilirubin (3.0 mg/dL). A liver biopsy shows portal fibrosis, with scattered foreign bodies consistent with schistosome eggs. Which of the following inflammatory cells is most likely to predominate in the portal tracts in the liver of this patient?
(A) Basophils
(B) Eosinophils
(C) Macrophages
(D) Monocytes
(E) Plasma cells

14 A 41-year-old woman complains of excessive menstrual bleeding and pelvic pain of 4 months. She uses an intrauterine device for contraception. Endometrial biopsy (shown in the image) reveals an excess of plasma cells (arrows) and macrophages within the stroma. The presence of these cells and scattered lymphoid follicles within the endometrial stroma is evidence of which of the following conditions?

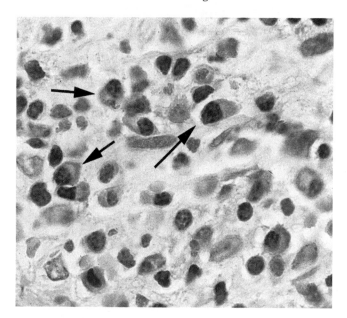

(A) Acute inflammation
(B) Chronic inflammation
(C) Granulation tissue
(D) Granulomatous inflammation
(E) Menstruation

15 A 62-year-old woman undergoing chemotherapy for breast cancer presents with a 3-day history of fever and chest pain. Cardiac catheterization reveals a markedly reduced ejection fraction with normal coronary blood flow. A myocardial biopsy is obtained, and a PCR test for coxsackievirus is positive. Histologic examination of this patient's myocardium will most likely reveal an abundance of which of the following inflammatory cells?

(A) Eosinophils
(B) Lymphocytes
(C) Macrophages
(D) Mast cells
(E) Neutrophils

16 A 58-year-old woman with long-standing diabetes and hypertension develops end-stage renal disease and dies in uremia. A shaggy fibrin-rich exudate is noted on the visceral pericardium at autopsy (shown in the image). Which of the following best explains the pathogenesis of this fibrinous exudate?

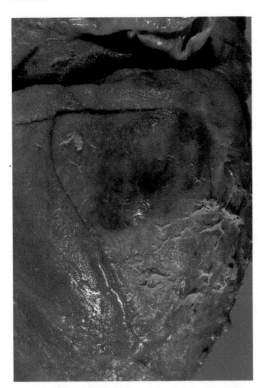

(A) Antibody binding and complement activation
(B) Chronic passive congestion
(C) Injury and increased vascular permeability
(D) Margination of segmented neutrophils
(E) Thrombosis of penetrating coronary arteries

17 A 68-year-old man presents with fever, shaking chills, and shortness of breath. Physical examination shows rales and decreased breath sounds over both lung fields. The patient exhibits grunting respirations, 30 to 35 breaths per minute, with flaring of the nares. The sputum is rusty yellow and displays numerous polymorphonuclear leukocytes. Which of the following mediators of inflammation is chiefly responsible for the development of fever in this patient?

(A) Arachidonic acid
(B) Interleukin-1
(C) Leukotriene B$_4$
(D) Prostacyclin (PGI$_2$)
(E) Thromboxane A$_2$

18 Sputum cultures obtained from the patient described in Question 17 are positive for *Streptococcus pneumoniae*. Removal of bacteria from the alveolar air spaces in this patient involves opsonization by complement, an important step in mediating which of the following leukocyte functions?

(A) Chemotaxis
(B) Diapedesis
(C) Haptotaxis
(D) Margination
(E) Phagocytosis

19 Which of the following mediators of inflammation is primarily responsible for secondary injury to alveolar basement membranes and lung parenchyma in the patient described in Questions 17 and 18?

(A) Complement proteins
(B) Fibrin split products
(C) Immunoglobulins
(D) Interleukin-1
(E) Lysosomal enzymes

20 Which of the following proteins inhibits fibrinolysis, activation of the complement system, and protease-mediated damage in the lungs of the patient described in the previous questions?

(A) Acid phosphatase
(B) Lactoferrin
(C) Lysozyme
(D) α_2-Macroglobulin
(E) Myeloperoxidase

21 A 35-year-old woman presents with a 5-day history of a painful sore on her back. Physical examination reveals a 1-cm abscess over her left shoulder. Biopsy of the lesion shows vasodilation and leukocyte margination (shown in the image). What glycoprotein mediates initial tethering of segmented neutrophils to endothelial cells in this skin lesion?

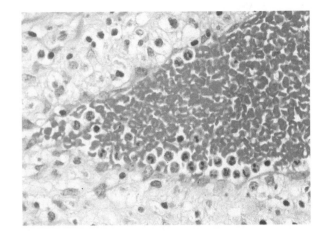

(A) Cadherin
(B) Entactin
(C) Integrin
(D) Laminin
(E) Selectin

22 A 14-year-old boy receives a laceration on his forehead during an ice hockey game. When he is first attended to by the medic, there is blanching of the skin around the wound. Which of the following mechanisms accounts for this transient reaction to neurogenic and chemical stimuli at the site of injury?
(A) Constriction of postcapillary venules
(B) Constriction of precapillary arterioles
(C) Dilation of postcapillary venules
(D) Dilation of precapillary arterioles
(E) Ischemic necrosis

23 An 8-year-old girl with asthma presents with respiratory distress. She has a history of allergies and upper respiratory tract infections. She also has history of wheezes associated with exercise. Which of the following mediators of inflammation is the most powerful stimulator of bronchoconstriction and vasoconstriction in this patient?
(A) Bradykinin
(B) Complement proteins
(C) Interleukin-1
(D) Leukotrienes
(E) Tumor necrosis factor-α

24 Which of the following preformed substances is released from mast cells and platelets, resulting in increased vascular permeability in the lungs of the patient described in Question 23?
(A) Bradykinin
(B) Hageman factor
(C) Histamine
(D) Leukotrienes (SRS-A)
(E) Thromboxane A_2

25 A 75-year-old woman complains of recent onset of chest pain, fever, and productive cough with rust-colored sputum. A chest X-ray reveals an infiltrate in the right middle lobe. Sputum cultures are positive for *Streptococcus pneumoniae*. Phagocytic cells in this patient's affected lung tissue generate bacteriocidal hypochlorous acid using which of the following enzymes?
(A) Catalase
(B) Cyclooxygenase
(C) Myeloperoxidase
(D) NADPH oxidase
(E) Superoxide dismutase

26 A 28-year-old woman cuts her hand while dicing vegetables in the kitchen. The wound is cleaned and sutured. Five days later, the site of injury contains an abundance of chronic inflammatory cells that actively secrete interleukin-1, tumor necrosis factor-α, interferon-α, numerous arachidonic acid derivatives, and various enzymes. Name these cells.
(A) B lymphocytes
(B) Macrophages
(C) Plasma cells
(D) Smooth muscle cells
(E) T lymphocytes

27 A 68-year-old man with prostate cancer and bone metastases presents with shaking chills and fever. The peripheral WBC count is 1,000/μL (normal = 4,000 to 11,000/μL). Which of the following terms best describes this hematologic finding?
(A) Leukocytosis
(B) Leukopenia
(C) Neutrophilia
(D) Pancytopenia
(E) Leukemoid reaction

28 A 25-year-old machinist is injured by a metal sliver in his left hand. Over the next few days, the wounded area becomes reddened, tender, swollen, and feels warm to the touch. Redness at the site of injury in this patient is caused primarily by which of the following mechanisms?
(A) Hemorrhage
(B) Hemostasis
(C) Neutrophil margination
(D) Vasoconstriction
(E) Vasodilation

29 The patient described in Question 28 goes to the emergency room to have the sliver removed. Which of the following mediators of inflammation plays the most important role in stimulating platelet aggregation at the site of injury following this minor surgical procedure?
(A) Leukotriene C_4
(B) Leukotriene D_4
(C) Prostaglandin E_2
(D) Prostaglandin I_2
(E) Thromboxane A_2

30 Twenty-four hours later, endothelial cells at the site of injury in the patient described in Questions 28 and 29 release a chemical mediator that inhibits further platelet aggregation. Name this mediator of inflammation.
(A) Plasmin
(B) Prostaglandin (PGI_2)
(C) Serotonin
(D) Thrombin
(E) Thromboxane A_2

31 A 37-year-old man with AIDS is admitted to the hospital with a 3-week history of chest pain and shortness of breath. An X-ray film of the chest shows bilateral nodularities of the lungs. A CT-guided lung biopsy is shown in the image. The multinucleated cell in the center of this field is most likely derived from which of the following inflammatory cells?

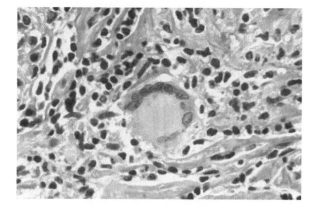

(A) Basophils
(B) Capillary endothelial cells
(C) Macrophages
(D) Myofibroblasts
(E) Smooth muscle cells

32 A 45-year-old woman with autoimmune hemolytic anemia presents with increasing fatigue. Which of the following mediators of inflammation is primarily responsible for antibody-mediated hemolysis in this patient?
(A) Arachidonic acid metabolites
(B) Coagulation proteins
(C) Complement proteins
(D) Kallikrein and kinins
(E) Lysophospholipids

33 A 59-year-old alcoholic man is brought to the emergency room with a fever (38.7°C/103°F) and foul-smelling breath. A chest X-ray reveals a pulmonary abscess in the right lower lobe. The patient subsequently develops acute bronchopneumonia and dies. Microscopic examination of the lungs at autopsy is shown in the image. Activation of phospholipase A_2 in these intra-alveolar cells resulted in the formation of which of the following mediators of inflammation?

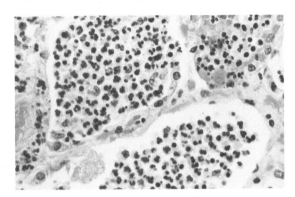

(A) Arachidonic acid
(B) cAMP
(C) cGMP
(D) Diacylglycerol
(E) Inositol trisphosphate

34 A 10-year-old girl presents with a 2-week history of puffiness around her eyes and swelling of the legs and ankles. Laboratory studies show hypoalbuminemia and proteinuria. The urinary sediment contains no inflammatory cells or red blood cells. Which of the following terms describes this patient's peripheral edema?
(A) Effusion
(B) Exudate
(C) Hydropic change
(D) Lymphedema
(E) Transudate

35 A 25-year-old woman develops a sore, red, hot, swollen left knee. She has no history of trauma and no familial history of joint disease. Fluid aspirated from the joint space shows an abundance of segmented neutrophils. Transendothelial migration of acute inflammatory cells into this patient's joint space was mediated primarily by which of the following families of proteins?

(A) Entactins
(B) Fibrillins
(C) Fibronectins
(D) Integrins
(E) Laminins

36 Aspirin is effective in relieving symptoms of acute inflammation in the patient described in Question 35 because it inhibits which of the following enzymes?
(A) Cyclooxygenase
(B) Myeloperoxidase
(C) Phospholipase A_2
(D) Protein kinase C
(E) Superoxide dismutase

37 A 50-year-old woman is discovered to have metastatic breast cancer. One week after receiving her first dose of chemotherapy, she develops bacterial pneumonia. Which of the following best explains this patient's susceptibility to bacterial infection?
(A) Depletion of serum complement
(B) Impaired neutrophil respiratory burst
(C) Inhibition of clotting factor activation
(D) Lymphocytosis
(E) Neutropenia

38 A 53-year-old man develops weakness, malaise, cough with bloody sputum, and night sweats. A chest X-ray reveals numerous apical densities bilaterally. Exposure to *Mycobacterium tuberculosis* was documented 20 years ago, and *M. tuberculosis* is identified in the sputum. The patient subsequently dies of respiratory insufficiency. The lungs are examined at autopsy (shown in the image). Which of the following best characterizes the histopathologic features of this pulmonary lesion?

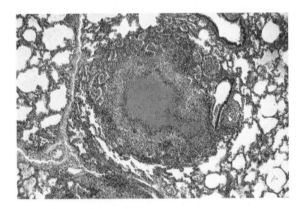

(A) Acute suppurative inflammation
(B) Chronic inflammation
(C) Fat necrosis
(D) Fibrinoid necrosis
(E) Granulomatous inflammation

39 A 59-year-old man experiences acute chest pain and is rushed to the emergency room. Laboratory studies and ECG demonstrate an acute myocardial infarction; however, coronary artery angiography performed 2 hours later does not show evidence of thrombosis. Intravascular thrombolysis that occurred in this patient was mediated by plasminogen activators that were released by which of the following cells?

(A) Cardiac myocytes

(B) Endothelial cells

(C) Macrophages

(D) Segmented neutrophils

(E) Vascular smooth muscle cells

40 Which of the following mediators of inflammation causes relaxation of vascular smooth muscle cells and vasodilation of arterioles at the site of myocardial infarction in the patient described in Question 39?

(A) Bradykinin

(B) Histamine

(C) Leukotrienes

(D) Nitric oxide

(E) Thromboxane A$_2$

41 A 68-year-old coal miner with a history of smoking and emphysema develops severe air-flow obstruction and expires. Autopsy reveals a "black lung," with coal-dust nodules scattered throughout the parenchyma and a central area of dense fibrosis. The coal dust entrapped within this miner's lung was sequestered primarily by which of the following cells?

(A) Endothelial cells

(B) Fibroblasts

(C) Lymphocytes

(D) Macrophages

(E) Plasma cells

42 A 40-year-old man presents with 5 days of productive cough and fever. *Pseudomonas aeruginosa* is isolated from a pulmonary abscess. The CBC shows an acute effect characterized by marked leukocytosis (50,000 WBC/µL), and the differential count reveals numerous immature cells (band forms). Which of the following terms best describes these hematologic findings?

(A) Leukemoid reaction

(B) Leukopenia

(C) Myeloid metaplasia

(D) Myeloproliferative disease

(E) Neutrophilia

43 A 19-year-old woman presents with 5 days of fever (38°C/101°F) and sore throat. She reports that she has felt fatigued for the past week and has difficulty swallowing. A physical examination reveals generalized lymphadenopathy. If this patient has a viral infection, a CBC will most likely show which of the following hematologic findings?

(A) Eosinophilia

(B) Leukopenia

(C) Lymphocytosis

(D) Neutrophilia

(E) Thrombocythemia

44 A 40-year-old woman presents with an 8-month history of progressive generalized itching, weight loss, fatigue, and yellow sclerae. Physical examination reveals mild jaundice. The antimitochondrial antibody test is positive. A liver biopsy discloses periductal inflammation and bile duct injury (shown in the image). Which of the following inflammatory cells is the principal mediator of destructive cholangitis in this patient?

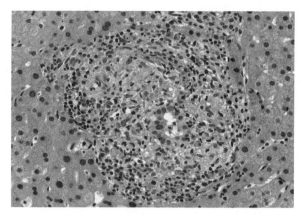

(A) Eosinophils

(B) B lymphocytes

(C) T lymphocytes

(D) Mast cells

(E) Neutrophils

45 A 25-year-old woman presents with a 2-week history of febrile illness and chest pain. She has an erythematous, macular facial rash and tender joints, particularly in her left wrist and elbow. A CBC shows mild anemia and thrombocytopenia. Corticosteroids are prescribed for the patient. This medication induces the synthesis of an inhibitor of which of the following enzymes in inflammatory cells?

(A) Lipoxygenase

(B) Myeloperoxidase

(C) Phospholipase A$_2$

(D) Phospholipase C

(E) Superoxide dismutase

46 The patient described in Question 45 is noted to have increased serum levels of ceruloplasmin, fibrinogen, α$_2$-macroglobulin, serum amyloid A protein, and C-reactive protein. Together, these markers belong to which of the following families of proteins?

(A) Acute phase proteins

(B) Anaphylatoxins

(C) Inhibitors of platelet activation

(D) Protease inhibitors

(E) Regulators of coagulation

ANSWERS

1 **The answer is D: Neutrophils.** The thick, yellow fluid draining from the breast fissure in this patient represents a purulent exudate. Purulent exudates and effusions are associated with pathologic conditions such as pyogenic bacterial infections, in which the predominant cell type is the segmented neutrophil (polymorphonuclear leukocyte). Mast cells (choice C) are granulated cells that contain receptors for IgE on their cell surface. They are additional cellular sources of vasoactive mediators, particularly in response to allergens. B lymphocytes (choice A) and plasma cells (choice E) are mediators of chronic inflammation and provide antigen-specific immunity to infectious diseases.

Diagnosis: Acute mastitis

2 **The answer is A: Complement proteins.** Complement proteins act upon one another in a cascade, generating biologically active fragments (e.g., C5a, C3b) or complexes (e.g., C567). These products of complement activation cause local edema by increasing the permeability of blood vessels. They also promote chemotaxis of leukocytes and lyse cells (membrane attack complex) and act as opsonins by coating bacteria. Although the other choices are mediators of inflammation, they have a more restricted set of functions. Kinins (choice D) are formed following tissue trauma and mediate pain transmission. None of the other choices are involved in opsonization or cytolysis.
Diagnosis: Acute mastitis

3 **The answer is D: *N*-formylated peptides.** The most potent chemotactic factors for leukocytes at the site of injury are (1) complement proteins (e.g., C5a); (2) bacterial and mitochondrial products, particularly low molecular weight N-formylated peptides; (3) products of arachidonic acid metabolism (especially LTB4); and (4) chemokines (e.g., interleukin-1 and interferon-γ). Plasmin (choice E) is a fibrinolytic enzyme generated by activated Hageman factor (clotting factor XII). Histamine (choice B) is one of the primary mediators of increased vascular permeability. None of the other choices are chemotactic agents.
Diagnosis: Pneumonia

4 **The answer is D: Neutrophils.** During acute inflammation, neutrophils (PMNs) adhere to the vascular endothelium. They flatten and migrate from the vasculature, through the endothelial cell layer, and into the surrounding tissue. About 24 hours after the onset of infarction, PMNs are observed to infiltrate necrotic tissue at the periphery of the infarct. Their function is to clear debris and begin the process of wound healing. Lymphocytes (choice B) and plasma cells (choice E) are mediators of chronic inflammation and provide antigen-specific immunity to infectious diseases. Fibroblasts (choice A) and macrophages (choice C) regulate scar tissue formation at the site of infarction.
Diagnosis: Acute myocardial infarction

5 **The answer is C: Increased capillary permeability.** Forces that regulate the balance of vascular and tissue fluids include (1) hydrostatic pressure, (2) oncotic pressure, (3) osmotic pressure, and (4) lymph flow. During inflammation, an increase in the permeability of the endothelial cell barrier results in local edema. Vasodilation of arterioles exacerbates fluid leakage, and vasoconstriction of postcapillary venules increases the hydrostatic pressure in the capillary bed (thus, not choice A), potentiating the formation of edema. Vasodilation of venules decreases capillary hydrostatic pressure and inhibits the movement of fluid into the extravascular spaces. Acute inflammation is not associated with changes in plasma oncotic pressure (choices B and D).
Diagnosis: Inflammatory edema

6 **The answer is B: Hageman factor.** Hageman factor (clotting factor XII) provides a key source of vasoactive mediators. Activation of this plasma protein at the site of tissue injury stimulates (1) conversion of plasminogen to plasmin, which induces fibrinolysis; (2) conversion of prekallikrein to kallikrein, which generates vasoactive peptides of low molecular weight referred to as kinins; (3) activation of the alternative complement pathway; and (4) activation of the coagulation system. Although the other choices are mediators of inflammation, they have a more restricted set of functions.
Diagnosis: Inflammation

7 **The answer is E: Tumor necrosis factor-α (TNF-α).** Septicemia (bacteremia) denotes the clinical condition in which bacteria are found in the circulation. It can be suspected clinically, but the final diagnosis is made by culturing the organisms from the blood. In patients with endotoxic shock, lipopolysaccharide released from Gram-negative bacteria stimulates monocytes/macrophages to secrete large quantities of TNF-α. This glycoprotein causes direct cytotoxic damage to capillary endothelial cells. The other choices do not cause direct vascular injury.
Diagnosis: Septic shock

8 **The answer is E: Suppurative inflammation.** Suppurative inflammation describes a condition in which a purulent exudate is accompanied by significant liquefactive necrosis. It is the equivalent of pus. The photograph shows two encapsulated cavities in the brain. These abscesses are composed of a central cavity filled with pus, surrounded by a layer of granulation tissue. Chronic inflammation (choice A) is nonsuppurative. Fibrinoid necrosis (choice B) is observed in areas of necrotizing vasculitis. Granulomatous inflammation (choice C) is seen in patients with tuberculosis. Reactive gliosis (choice D) is a normal response of the brain to injury and infection but is not visible on the cut surface of the brain at autopsy.
Diagnosis: Cerebral abscess

9 **The answer is C: Purulent exudate.** The pleural effusion encountered in this patient represents excess fluid in a body cavity. A transudate denotes edema fluid with low protein content, whereas an exudate denotes edema fluid with high protein content. A purulent exudate or effusion contains a prominent cellular component (PMNs). A serous exudate or effusion is characterized by the absence of a prominent cellular response and has a yellow, strawlike color. Fibrinous exudate (choice A) does not contain leukocytes. Serosanguineous exudate (choice D) contains RBCs and has a red tinge.
Diagnosis: Bacterial pneumonia, pleural effusion

10 **The answer is D: Parasitic infection.** Eosinophils are particularly evident during allergic-type reactions and parasitic infestations. Infections with *Trichinella* are accompanied by eosinophilia, and skeletal muscle is typically infiltrated by eosinophils. Patients with muscular dystrophy (choice C) show elevated serum levels of creatine kinase, but eosinophils are not seen on muscle biopsy. Bacterial infections (choice B) are associated with neutrophilia, and affected tissues are infiltrated with PMNs. Viral infections (choice E) are associated with lymphocytosis, and affected tissues are infiltrated with B and T lymphocytes. Polymyositis, an autoimmune disease (choice A), does not feature eosinophils.
Diagnosis: Trichinosis

11 The answer is D: NAPDH oxidase. The importance of oxygen-dependent mechanisms in the bacterial killing by phagocytic cells is exemplified in chronic granulomatous disease of childhood. Children with this disease suffer from a hereditary deficiency of NADPH oxidase, resulting in a failure to produce superoxide anion and hydrogen peroxide during phagocytosis. Persons with this disorder are susceptible to recurrent bacterial infections. Patients deficient in myeloperoxidase (choice C) cannot produce hypochlorous acid (HOCl) and experience an increased susceptibility to infections with the fungal pathogen *Candida*. Catalase (choice A) converts hydrogen peroxide to water and molecular oxygen.
Diagnosis: Chronic granulomatous disease

12 The answer is B: Hereditary angioedema. Deficiency of C1 inhibitor, with excessive cleavage of C4 and C2 by C1s, is associated with the syndrome of hereditary angioedema. This disease is characterized by episodic, painless, nonpitting edema of soft tissues. It is the result of chronic complement activation, with the generation of a vasoactive peptide from C2, and may be life threatening because of the occurrence of laryngeal edema. Chronic granulomatous disease (choice A) is due to a hereditary deficiency of NADPH oxidase. Myeloperoxidase deficiency (choice C) increases susceptibility to infections with *Candida*. Selective IgA deficiency (choice D) and Wiskott-Aldrich syndrome (choice E) are congenital immunodeficiency disorders associated with defects in lymphocyte function.
Diagnosis: Hereditary angioedema

13 The answer is B: Eosinophils. Eosinophils are recruited in parasitic infestations and would be expected to predominate in the portal tracts of the liver in patients with schistosomiasis. Eosinophils contain leukotrienes and platelet-activating factor, as well as acid phosphatase and eosinophil major basic protein. Plasma cells (choice E) are differentiated B lymphocytes that secrete large amounts of monospecific immunoglobulin.
Diagnosis: Schistosomiasis, eosinophils

14 The answer is B: Chronic inflammation. Inflammation has historically been referred to as either acute or chronic, depending on the persistence of the injury, clinical symptoms, and the nature of the inflammatory response. The cellular components of chronic inflammation are lymphocytes, antibody-producing plasma cells (see arrows on photomicrograph), and macrophages. The chronic inflammatory response is often prolonged and may be associated with aberrant repair (i.e., fibrosis). Neutrophils are featured in acute inflammation (choice A) and menstruation (choice E). Choices C and D do not exhibit the histopathology shown in the image.
Diagnosis: Chronic endometritis

15 The answer is B: Lymphocytes. This patient with viral myocarditis will show an accumulation of lymphocytes in the affected heart muscle. Naïve lymphocytes encounter antigen-presenting cells (macrophages and dendritic cells) in the secondary lymphoid organs. In response to this cell-cell interaction, they become activated, circulate in the vascular system, and are recruited to peripheral tissues (e.g., heart). The other choices are not characteristic responders to viral infections, although acute inflammation may be observed in lytic infections.
Diagnosis: Viral myocarditis

16 The answer is C: Injury and increased vascular permeability. Binding of vasoactive mediators to specific receptors on endothelial cells results in contraction and gap formation. This break in the endothelial barrier leads to the leakage of intravascular fluid into the extravascular space. Direct injury to endothelial cells also leads to leakage of intravascular fluid. A fibrinous exudate contains large amounts of fibrin as a result of activation of the coagulation system. When a fibrinous exudate occurs on a serosal surface, such as the pleura or pericardium, it is referred to as fibrinous pleuritis or fibrinous pericarditis. Although the other choices describe aspects of inflammation, they do not address the pathogenesis of edema formation with activation of the coagulation system.
Diagnosis: End-stage kidney disease, fibrinous pericarditis

17 The answer is B: Interleukin-1. Release of exogenous pyrogens by bacteria, viruses, or injured cells stimulates the production of endogenous pyrogens such as IL-1α, IL-1β, and TNF-α. IL-1 is a 15-kDa protein that stimulates prostaglandin synthesis in the hypothalamic thermoregulatory centers, thereby altering the "thermostat" that controls body temperature. Inhibitors of cyclooxygenase (e.g., aspirin) block the fever response by inhibiting PGE$_2$ synthesis in the hypothalamus. Chills, rigor (profound chills with shivering and piloerection), and sweats (to allow heat dissipation) are symptoms associated with fever. The other choices are mediators of inflammation, but they do not directly control body temperature.
Diagnosis: Bacterial pneumonia

18 The answer is E: Phagocytosis. Many inflammatory cells are able to recognize, internalize, and digest foreign materials, microorganisms, and cellular debris. This process is termed phagocytosis, and the effector cells are known as phagocytes. Phagocytosis of most biologic agents is enhanced by their coating with specific plasma components (opsonins), particularly immunoglobulins or the C3b fragment of complement. The other functions are not enhanced by opsonization.
Diagnosis: Bacterial pneumonia

19 The answer is E: Lysosomal enzymes. The primary role of neutrophils in inflammation is host defense and débridement of damaged tissue. However, when the response is extensive or unregulated, the chemical mediators of inflammation may prolong tissue damage. Thus, the same neutrophil-derived lysosomal enzymes that are beneficial when active intracellularly can be harmful when released to the extracellular environment. The other choices are less likely to cause direct injury to the lung in a patient with pneumonia.
Diagnosis: Bacterial pneumonia

20 The answer is D: α_2-Macroglobulin. Proteolytic enzymes that are released by phagocytic cells during inflammation are regulated by a family of protease inhibitors, including α_1-antitrypsin and α_2-macroglobulin. These plasma-derived proteins inhibit plasmin-activated fibrinolysis and activation of the complement system and help protect against nonspecific tissue injury during acute inflammation. Lysozyme (choice C) is a glycosidase that degrades the peptidoglycans of Gram-positive bacterial cell walls. Myeloperoxidase (choice E) is contained within neutrophil granules.
Diagnosis: Bacterial pneumonia

21 The answer is E: Selectin. Selectins are sugar-binding glycoproteins that mediate the initial adhesion of leukocytes to endothelial cells at sites of inflammation. E-selectins are found on endothelial cells, P-selectins are found on platelets, and L-selectins are found on leukocytes. E-selectins are stored in Weibel-Palade bodies of resting endothelial cells. Upon activation, E-selectins are redistributed along the luminal surface of the endothelial cells, where they mediate the initial adhesion (tethering) and rolling of leukocytes. After leukocytes have come to a rest, integrins (choice C) mediate transendothelial cell migration and chemotaxis. Cadherins (choice A) mediate cell-cell adhesion, but they are not involved in neutrophil adhesion to vascular endothelium. Entactin (choice B) and laminin (choice D) are basement membrane proteins.

Diagnosis: Carbuncle

22 The answer is B: Constriction of precapillary arterioles. The initial response of arterioles to neurogenic and chemical stimuli is transient vasoconstriction. However, shortly thereafter, vasodilation (choice D) occurs, with an increase in blood flow to the inflamed area. This process is referred to as active hyperemia. None of the other choices cause transient skin blanching.

Diagnosis: Laceration

23 The answer is D: Leukotrienes. Asthma is a chronic lung disease caused by increased responsiveness of the airways to a variety of stimuli. Chemical mediators released by chronic inflammatory cells in the lungs of these patients stimulate bronchial mucus production and bronchoconstriction. Among these mediators are leukotrienes, also known as slow-reacting substances of anaphylaxis. They are derived from arachidonic acid through the lipoxygenase pathway. Leukotrienes stimulate contraction of smooth muscle and enhance vascular permeability. They are responsible for the development of many of the clinical symptoms associated with asthma and other allergic reactions. Although the other choices are important mediators of inflammation, they do not play a leading role in the development of bronchoconstriction in patients with bronchial asthma.

Diagnosis: Asthma

24 The answer is C: Histamine. When IgE-sensitized mast cells are stimulated by antigen, preformed mediators of inflammation are secreted into the extracellular tissues. Histamine binds to specific H_1 receptors in the vascular wall, inducing endothelial cell contraction, gap formation, and edema. Massive release of histamine may cause circulatory collapse (anaphylactic shock). Bradykinin (choice A) and Hageman factor (choice B) are plasma-derived mediators. The other choices are not preformed molecules but are synthesized de novo following cell activation.

Diagnosis: Asthma

25 The answer is C: Myeloperoxidase. Myeloperoxidase catalyzes the conversion of H_2O_2, in the presence of a halide (e.g., chloride ion), to form hypochlorous acid. This powerful oxidant is a major bactericidal agent produced by phagocytic cells. Patients deficient in myeloperoxidase cannot produce hypochlorous acid and have an increased susceptibility to recurrent infections. Catalase (choice A) catabolizes H_2O_2. Cyclooxygenase (choice B) mediates the conversion of arachidonic acid to prostaglandins. NADPH oxidase (choice D) is involved in oxygen-free radical formation during the neutrophil respiratory burst. Superoxide dismutase (choice E) reduces the superoxide radical to H_2O_2.

Diagnosis: Bacterial pneumonia

26 The answer is B: Macrophages. The macrophage is the pivotal cell in regulating chronic inflammation. Macrophages, which are derived from circulating monocytes, regulate lymphocyte responses to antigens and secrete a variety of mediators that modulate the proliferation and function of fibroblasts and endothelial cells. None of the other cells have this wide spectrum of regulatory functions.

Diagnosis: Laceration, wound healing

27 The answer is B: Leukopenia. Leukopenia is defined as an absolute decrease in the circulating WBC count. It is occasionally encountered under conditions of chronic inflammation, especially in patients who are malnourished or who suffer from a chronic debilitating disease. Leukopenia may also be caused by typhoid fever and certain viral and rickettsial infections. Leukocytosis (choice A) is defined as an absolute increase in the circulating WBC count. Neutrophilia (choice C) is defined as an absolute increase in the circulating neutrophil count. Pancytopenia (choice D) refers to decreased circulating levels of all formed elements in the blood.

Diagnosis: Prostate cancer

28 The answer is E: Vasodilation. Vasodilation of precapillary arterioles increases blood flow at the site of tissue injury. This condition (active hyperemia) is caused by the release of specific mediators. Vasodilation and hyperemia are primarily responsible for the redness and warmth (rubor and calor) at sites of injury. The other choices do not regulate active hyperemia.

Diagnosis: Acute inflammation

29 The answer is E: Thromboxane A_2. Platelet adherence, aggregation, and degranulation occur when platelets come in contact with fibrillar collagen or thrombin (after activation of the coagulation system). Platelet degranulation is associated with the release of serotonin, which directly increases vascular permeability. In addition, the arachidonic acid metabolite thromboxane A_2 plays a key role in the second wave of platelet aggregation and mediates smooth muscle constriction. Prostaglandins E_2 and I_2 (choices C and D) inhibit inflammatory cell functions. Leukotrienes C_4 and D_4 (choices A and B) induce smooth muscle contraction.

Diagnosis: Acute inflammation

30 The answer is B: Prostaglandin (PGI_2). PGI_2 is a derivative of arachidonic acid that is formed in the cyclooxygenase enzyme pathway. It promotes vasodilation and bronchodilation and also inhibits platelet aggregation. It activates adenylyl cyclase and increases intracellular levels of cAMP. Its action is diametrically opposite to that of thromboxane A_2 (choice E), which activates guanylyl cyclase and increases intracellular levels of cGMP. Plasmin (choice A) degrades fibrin. Serotonin (choice C) is a vasoactive amine. Thrombin (choice D) is a protease that mediates the conversion of fibrinogen to fibrin.

Diagnosis: Acute inflammation

31 **The answer is C: Macrophages.** Granulomas are collections of epithelioid cells and multinucleated giant cells that are formed by cytoplasmic fusion of macrophages. When the nuclei are arranged around the periphery of the cell in a horseshoe pattern (see photomicrograph), the cell is termed a Langhans giant cell. Frequently, a foreign pathogenic agent is identified within the cytoplasm of a multinucleated giant cell, in which case the label foreign body giant cell is used. The other cells do not form multinucleated giant cells in granulomas.
Diagnosis: AIDS, granulomatous inflammation

32 **The answer is C: Complement proteins.** Activation of the complement cascade by the classical or alternative pathway leads to the cleavage of complement fragments and the formation of biologically active complexes. The C5b fragment aggregates with complement proteins C6, C7, C8, and C9, resulting in the polymerization of the membrane attack complex (MAC). MAC lyses cells by inserting into the lipid bilayer, forming a pore, and destroying the permeability barrier of the plasma membrane. Kallikrein and kinins (choice D) are formed following tissue trauma and mediate pain transmission. None of the other choices mediate hemolysis.
Diagnosis: Hemolytic anemia, autoimmune disease

33 **The answer is A: Arachidonic acid.** Cellular sources of vasoactive mediators are (1) derived from the metabolism of arachidonic acid (prostaglandins, thromboxanes, leukotrienes, and platelet-activating factor), (2) preformed and stored in cytoplasmic granules (histamine, serotonin, and lysosomal hydrolases), or (3) generated as normal regulators of vascular function (nitric oxide and neurokinins). The photomicrograph shows polymorphonuclear leukocytes responding to a bacterial pneumonia. Free arachidonic acid in these acute inflammatory cells is derived from membrane phospholipids (primarily phosphatidylcholine) by stimulus-induced activation of phospholipase A$_2$. Phospholipase A$_2$ activation does not generate the other inflammatory mediators listed.
Diagnosis: Bacterial pneumonia

34 **The answer is E: Transudate.** According to the Starling principle, the interchange of fluid between vascular and extravascular compartments results from a balance of forces that draw fluid into the vascular space or out into tissues. These forces include (1) hydrostatic pressure, (2) oncotic pressure (reflects plasma protein concentration), (3) osmotic pressure, and (4) lymph flow. When the balance of these forces is altered, the net result is fluid accumulation in the interstitial spaces (i.e., edema). Although edema accompanies acute inflammation, a variety of noninflammatory conditions also lead to the formation of edema. For example, obstruction of venous outflow or decreased right ventricular function results in a back pressure in the vasculature, thereby increasing hydrostatic pressure. Loss of albumin (kidney disorders, this case) or decreased synthesis of plasma proteins (liver disease, malnutrition) reduces plasma oncotic pressure. Noninflammatory edema is referred to as a transudate. A transudate is edema fluid with a low protein content. An exudate (choice B) is edema fluid with a high protein and lipid concentration that frequently contains inflammatory cells. An effusion (choice A) represents excess fluid in a body cavity such as the peritoneum or pleura.

Lymphedema (choice D) is usually associated with obstruction of lymphatic flow (e.g., surgery or infection).
Diagnosis: Nephrotic syndrome, noninflammatory edema

35 **The answer is D: Integrins.** Chemokines and other proinflammatory molecules activate a family of cell adhesion molecules, namely the integrins. Molecules in this family participate in cell-cell and cell-substrate adhesions and cell signaling. Integrins are involved in leukocyte recruitment to sites of injury in acute inflammation. The other choices are extracellular matrix molecules that maintain tissue architecture and facilitate wound healing.
Diagnosis: Gonococcal arthritis

36 **The answer is A: Cyclooxygenase.** Arachidonic acid is metabolized by cyclooxygenases (COX-1, COX-2) and lipoxygenases (5-LOX) to generate prostanoids and leukotrienes, respectively. The early inflammatory prostanoid response is COX-1 dependent. COX-2 becomes the major source of prostanoids as inflammation progresses. Inhibition of COX is one mechanism by which nonsteroidal anti-inflammatory drugs (NSAIDs), including aspirin, indomethacin, and ibuprofen, exert their potent analgesic and anti-inflammatory effects. NSAIDs block COX-2–induced formation of prostaglandins, thereby mitigating pain and inflammation. Myeloperoxidase (choice B) catalyzes the conversion of H$_2$O$_2$, in the presence of a halide (e.g., chloride ion) to form hypochlorous acid. This powerful oxidant is a major bactericidal agent produced by phagocytic cells. Superoxide dismutase (choice E) reduces the superoxide radical to H$_2$O$_2$.
Diagnosis: Gonococcal arthritis

37 **The answer is E: Neutropenia.** The importance of protection afforded by acute inflammatory cells is emphasized by the frequency and severity of infections in persons with defective phagocytic cells. The most common defect is iatrogenic neutropenia secondary to cancer chemotherapy. Chemotherapy would not be expected to deplete serum levels of complement (choice A) or alter the respiratory burst within activated neutrophils (choice B).
Diagnosis: Bacterial pneumonia

38 **The answer is E: Granulomatous inflammation.** The photograph shows a necrotizing granuloma due to *M. tuberculosis*. The necrotic center is surrounded by histiocytes, giant cells, and fibrous tissue. Granulomatous inflammation is elicited by fungal infections, tuberculosis, leprosy, schistosomiasis, and the presence of foreign material. It is characteristically associated with caseous necrosis produced by *M. tuberculosis*. The other choices may be seen as secondary features in granulomatous inflammation.
Diagnosis: Pulmonary tuberculosis

39 **The answer is B: Endothelial cells.** The vascular endothelium has the ability to promote or inhibit tissue perfusion and inflammatory cell influx through multiple mechanisms. For example, endothelial cells in the vicinity of the thrombus produce tissue-type plasminogen activators, which activate plasmin and initiate thrombolysis (fibrinolysis). None of the other cells produce significant quantities of plasminogen activators.
Diagnosis: Myocardial infarction, hemostasis

40 The answer is D: Nitric oxide. Nitric oxide (NO), which was previously known as endothelium-derived relaxing factor, leads to relaxation of vascular smooth muscle cells and vasodilation of arterioles. NO also inhibits platelet aggregation and mediates the killing of bacteria and tumor cells by macrophages. Histamine (choice B), leukotrienes (choice C), and thromboxane A_2 (choice E) stimulate the contraction of smooth muscle cells.

Diagnosis: Acute myocardial infarction

41 The answer is D: Macrophages. Coal workers' pneumoconiosis reflects the inhalation of carbon particles. The characteristic pulmonary lesions of simple coal worker's pneumoconiosis include nonpalpable coal-dust macules and palpable coal-dust nodules, both of which are typically multiple and scattered throughout the lung as 1- to 4-mm black foci. Nodules consist of dust-laden macrophages associated with a fibrotic stroma. Nodules occur when coal is admixed with fibrogenic dusts such as silica and are more properly classified as anthracosilicosis. Coal-dust macules and nodules appear on a chest radiograph as small nodular densities. The other choices are not phagocytic cells.

Diagnosis: Anthracosilicosis, coal workers' pneumoconiosis

42 The answer is A: Leukemoid reaction. Circulating levels of leukocytes and their precursors may occasionally reach very high levels (>50,000 WBC/μL). Such a situation, referred to as a leukemoid reaction, is sometimes difficult to differentiate from leukemia. In contrast to bacterial infections, viral infections (including infectious mononucleosis) are characterized by lymphocytosis, an absolute increase in the number of circulating lymphocytes. Parasitic infestations and certain allergic reactions cause eosinophilia, an increase in the number of circulating eosinophils. Leukopenia is defined as an absolute decrease in the circulating WBC count. Myeloid metaplasia (choice C) and myeloproliferative disease (choice D) are chronic disorders of the hematopoietic system. Although technically correct, neutrophilia (choice E) by itself does not demonstrate immature cells (band forms) and usually refers to lower levels of increased neutrophils.

Diagnosis: Pulmonary abscess

43 The answer is C: Lymphocytosis. Peripheral blood lymphocytosis is defined as an increase in the absolute peripheral blood lymphocyte count above the normal range (<4,000/μL in children and 9,000/μL in infants). The principal causes of absolute peripheral blood lymphocytosis are (1) acute viral infections (infectious mononucleosis, whooping cough, and acute infection lymphocytosis), (2) chronic bacterial infections (tuberculosis, brucellosis), and (3) lymphoproliferative diseases. The other choices are not features of acute viral infections.

Diagnosis: Infectious mononucleosis

44 The answer is C: T lymphocytes. Primary biliary cirrhosis (PBC) is a chronic progressive cholestatic liver disease characterized by destruction of intrahepatic bile ducts (nonsuppurative destructive cholangitis). PBC occurs principally in middle-aged women and is an autoimmune disease. Most patients with PBC have at least one other disease usually classed as autoimmune (e.g., thyroiditis, rheumatoid arthritis, scleroderma, Sjögren syndrome, or systemic lupus erythematosus). More than 95% of patients with PBC have circulating antimitochondrial antibodies. The cells surrounding and infiltrating the sites of bile duct damage are predominantly suppressor/cytotoxic (CD8$^+$) T lymphocytes, suggesting that they mediate the destruction of the ductal epithelium. Macrophages and B lymphocytes (choice B) are associated with periductal inflammation but do not mediate epithelial cytotoxicity. Eosinophils (choice A) have no role in primary immune-related mechanisms. The other inflammatory cells (choices D and E) do not participate in the pathogenesis of PBC.

Diagnosis: Primary biliary cirrhosis, chronic inflammation

45 The answer is C: Phospholipase A$_2$. Corticosteroids are widely used to suppress the tissue destruction associated with many chronic inflammatory diseases, including rheumatoid arthritis and systemic lupus erythematosus. Corticosteroids induce the synthesis of an inhibitor of phospholipase A$_2$ and block the release of arachidonic acid from the plasma membranes of inflammatory cells. Although corticosteroids are widely used to suppress inflammatory responses, the prolonged administration of these compounds can have deleterious effects, including atrophy of the adrenal glands. Myeloperoxidase (choice B) catalyzes the conversion of H_2O_2, in the presence of a halide (e.g., chloride ion) to form hypochlorous acid. This powerful oxidant is a major bactericidal agent produced by phagocytic cells. Superoxide dismutase (choice E) reduces the superoxide radical to H_2O_2.

Diagnosis: Systemic lupus erythematosus

46 The answer is A: Acute phase proteins. These proteins are synthesized primarily by the liver and are released into the circulation in response to an acute inflammatory challenge. Changes in the plasma levels of acute phase proteins are mediated primarily by cytokines (IL-1, IL-6, and TNF-α). Increased plasma levels of some acute phase proteins are reflected in an accelerated erythrocyte sedimentation rate, which is an index used clinically to monitor the activity of many inflammatory diseases. None of the other choices describe the set of serum markers listed in this question.

Diagnosis: Systemic lupus erythematosus

Chapter 3

Repair, Regeneration, and Fibrosis

QUESTIONS

Select the single best answer.

1 A 74-year-old woman presents with acute chest pain and shortness of breath. Cardiac catheterization demonstrates occlusion of the left anterior descending coronary artery. Laboratory studies and ECG are consistent with acute myocardial infarction. Which of the following is the most likely pathologic finding in the affected heart muscle 4 weeks later?
(A) Capillary-rich granulation tissue
(B) Collagen-rich scar tissue
(C) Granulomatous inflammation
(D) Neutrophils and necrotic debris
(E) Vascular congestion and edema

2 A 4-year-old boy falls on a rusty nail and punctures his skin. The wound is cleaned and covered with sterile gauze. Which of the following is the initial event in the healing process?
(A) Accumulation of acute inflammatory cells
(B) Deposition of proteoglycans and collagen
(C) Differentiation and migration of myofibroblasts
(D) Formation of a fibrin clot
(E) Macrophage-mediated phagocytosis of cellular debris

3 An 82-year-old man dies 4 years after developing congestive heart failure. He had a history of multiple myocardial infarcts over the past 10 years. A trichrome stain of heart muscle at autopsy is shown in the image. What is the predominant type of collagen found in this mature scar tissue?

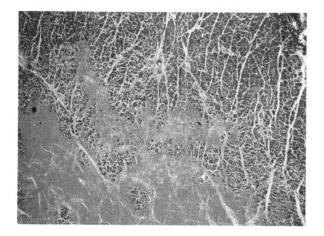

(A) Type I
(B) Type II
(C) Type IV
(D) Type V
(E) Type VI

4 A 25-year-old woman sustains a deep, open laceration over her right forearm in a motorcycle accident. The wound is cleaned and sutured. Which of the following cell types mediates contraction of the wound to facilitate healing?
(A) Endothelial cells
(B) Fibroblasts
(C) Macrophages
(D) Myofibroblasts
(E) Smooth muscle cells

5 During the next 3 months, the wound heals with formation of a linear scar. Which of the following nutritional factors is required for proper collagen assembly in the scar tissue of the patient described in Question 4?
(A) Folic acid
(B) Thiamine
(C) Vitamin A
(D) Vitamin C
(E) Vitamin E

6 A 70-year-old woman with diabetes develops an ulcer on her right leg (shown in the image). The ulcer bed is covered with granulation tissue. Which of the following are the principle cellular components found in the bed of this wound?

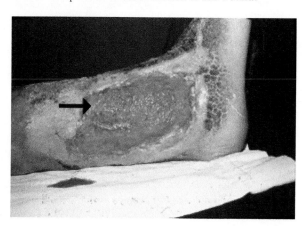

25

(A) Fibroblasts and endothelial cells
(B) Myofibroblasts and eosinophils
(C) Neutrophils and lymphocytes
(D) Plasma cells and macrophages
(E) Smooth muscle cells and Merkel cells

7 Which of the following proteins helps stimulate healing and angiogenesis in the wound of the patient described in Question 6?
(A) α_1-Antitrypsin
(B) Caspase-9
(C) Lysozyme
(D) α_2-Macroglobulin
(E) Metalloproteinase

8 A 68-year-old man presents for repair of an abdominal aortic aneurysm. Severe complicated atherosclerosis is noted at surgery, prompting concern for embolism of atheromatous material to the kidneys and other organs. If the patient were to develop a renal cortical infarct as a result of surgery, which of the following would be the most likely outcome?
(A) Chronic inflammation
(B) Granulomatous inflammation
(C) Hemangioma formation
(D) Repair and regeneration
(E) Scar formation

9 A 40-year-old woman presents with a painless lesion on her right ear lobe (shown in the image). She reports that her ears were pierced 4 months ago. Which of the following best explains the pathogenesis of this lesion?

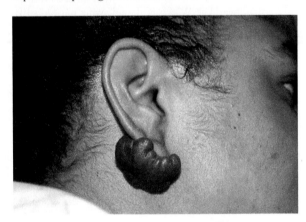

(A) Clonal expansion of smooth muscle cells
(B) Exuberant formation of granulation tissue
(C) Increased growth of capillary endothelial cells
(D) Increased turnover of extracellular matrix proteoglycans
(E) Maturation arrest of collagen assembly

10 A 58-year-old woman undergoes lumpectomy for breast cancer. One month following surgery, she notices a firm 0.3-cm nodule along one edge of the surgical incision. Biopsy of this nodule reveals chronic inflammatory cells, multinucleated giant cells, and extensive fibrosis. The multinucleated cells in this nodule most likely formed in response to which of the following pathogenic stimuli?

(A) Bacterial infection
(B) Foreign material
(C) Lymphatic obstruction
(D) Neoplastic cells
(E) Viral infection

11 A 57-year-old man with a history of alcoholism presents with yellow discoloration of his skin and sclerae. Laboratory studies show elevated serum levels of liver enzymes (AST and ALT). A trichrome stain of a liver biopsy is shown in the image. A similar pattern of regeneration and fibrosis would be expected in the liver of a patient with which of the following conditions?

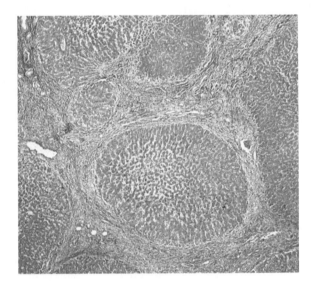

(A) Acute toxic liver injury
(B) Chronic viral hepatitis
(C) Fulminant hepatic necrosis
(D) Hepatocellular carcinoma
(E) Thrombosis of the portal vein

12 A 10-year-old boy trips at school and scrapes the palms of his hands. The wounds are cleaned and covered with sterile gauze. Which of the following terms best characterizes the healing of these superficial abrasions?
(A) Fibrosis
(B) Granulation tissue
(C) Primary intention
(D) Regeneration
(E) Secondary intention

13 Which of the following cellular processes helps restore normal epithelial structure and function in the patient described in Question 12?
(A) Collagen and fibronectin-rich extracellular matrix deposition
(B) Contact inhibition of epithelial cell growth and motility
(C) Myofibroblast differentiation and syncytia formation
(D) Platelet activation and intravascular coagulation
(E) Proliferation of capillary endothelial cells (angiogenesis)

14 A 34-year-old woman has a benign nevus removed from her back under local anesthesia. Which of the following families of cell adhesion molecules is the principal component of the "provisional matrix" that forms during early wound healing?

(A) Cadherins
(B) Fibronectins
(C) Integrins
(D) Laminins
(E) Selectins

15 Which of the following families of glycoproteins plays the most important role in regulating the migration and differentiation of leukocytes and connective tissue cells during wound healing in the patient described in Question 14?

(A) Cadherins
(B) Fibrillins
(C) Integrins
(D) Laminins
(E) Selectins

16 A 29-year-old carpenter receives a traumatic laceration to her left arm. Which of the following is the most important factor that determines whether this wound will heal by primary or secondary intention?

(A) Apposition of edges
(B) Depth of wound
(C) Metabolic status
(D) Skin site affected
(E) Vascular supply

17 Activated fibroblasts, myofibroblasts, and capillary sprouts are most abundant in the wound of the patient described in Question 16 at which of the following times after injury?

(A) 3 to 6 hours
(B) 12 to 24 hours
(C) 3 to 5 days
(D) 8 to 10 days
(E) 2 weeks

18 A 9-year-old boy receives a deep laceration over his right eyebrow playing ice hockey. The wound is cleaned and sutured. Which of the following describes the principal function of macrophages that are present in the wound 24 to 48 hours after injury?

(A) Antibody production
(B) Deposition of collagen
(C) Histamine release
(D) Phagocytosis
(E) Wound contraction

19 Which of the following collagens is deposited first during wound healing in the patient described in Question 18?

(A) Type I
(B) Type II
(C) Type III
(D) Type IV
(E) Type V

20 A 16-year-old boy suffers a concussion during an ice hockey game and is rushed to the emergency room. A CT scan of the brain reveals a cerebral contusion of the left frontal lobe. The boy lies comatose for 3 days but eventually regains consciousness. Which of the following cells is the principal mediator of scar formation in the central nervous system of this patient?

(A) Fibroblasts
(B) Glial cells
(C) Neurons
(D) Oligodendrocytes
(E) Schwann cells

21 A 30-year-old firefighter suffers extensive third-degree burns over his arms and hands. This patient is at high risk for developing which of the following complications of wound healing?

(A) Contracture
(B) Dehiscence
(C) Incisional hernia
(D) Keloid
(E) Traumatic neuroma

22 A 23-year-old man suffers a crush injury of his foot, which becomes secondarily infected. He undergoes a below-the-knee amputation. Six months later, the patient complains of chronic pain at the site of amputation. A firm nodule is identified at the scar site. A biopsy of the nodule demonstrates haphazard growth of nerves (shown in the image). Which of the following is the most likely diagnosis?

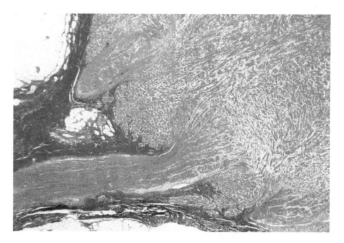

(A) Ganglioma
(B) Ganglioneuroma
(C) Hamartoma
(D) Neural nevus
(E) Neuroma

23 A 34-year-old man presents with a 5-day history of a painful sore on his hand. Physical examination reveals a 0.5-cm abscess on the extensor surface of the left hand that drains a thick, purulent material. Diapedesis of leukocytes into and around this patient's infected wound occurs primarily at which of the following anatomic locations?

(A) Lymphatic capillaries
(B) Postcapillary venules
(C) Precapillary arterioles
(D) Small dermal arteries
(E) Small dermal veins

24   A 35-year-old pregnant woman with a history of chronic gastritis presents to the emergency room complaining of acute abdominal pain. Physical examination reveals hepatomegaly, ascites, and mild jaundice. The patient subsequently develops acute hepatic failure and expires. Autopsy reveals thrombosis of the hepatic veins (Budd-Chiari syndrome). During the autopsy, a lesion is identified in the distal stomach and examined by light microscopy (shown in the image). Which of the following best describes this incidental finding at autopsy?

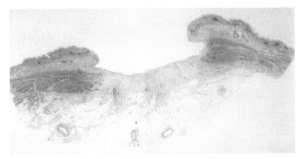

(A) Carcinoma
(B) Contracture
(C) Diverticulum
(D) Granuloma
(E) Ulcer

ANSWERS

1   **The answer is B: Collagen-rich scar tissue.**   Pathologic findings in congestive heart failure include microscopic signs of coagulative necrosis approximately 24 hours after the onset of vascular occlusion. Polymorphonuclear leukocytes and macrophages predominate during the next 2 to 5 days (choice D). Toward the end of the first week, the infarct is invaded by capillary-rich granulation tissue (choice A). Ultimately, the necrotic myocardium is replaced by collagen-rich scar tissue (weeks to months). Granulomatous inflammation (choice C) does not occur after an ischemic myocardial infarct. Vascular congestion and edema (choice E) are features of acute inflammation.
Diagnosis: Myocardial infarction

2   **The answer is D: Formation of a fibrin clot.**   The initial phase of the repair reaction, which typically begins with hemorrhage, involves the formation of a fibrin clot that fills the gap created by the wound. A thrombus (clot), referred to as a scab after drying out, forms on the wounded skin as a barrier to invading microorganisms. It also prevents the loss of plasma and tissue fluid. Formed primarily from plasma fibrin, the thrombus is rich in fibronectin. The thrombus also contains contracting platelets, which are an initial source of growth factors. Much later, the thrombus undergoes proteolysis, after which it is penetrated by regenerating epithelium. The scab then detaches. Accumulation of acute inflammatory cells (choice

A) might occur after formation of the initial fibrin clot. Collagen formation (choice B) and macrophage activity (choice E) occur much later. Myofibroblasts (choice C) begin to accumulate in the wound around the 3rd day.
Diagnosis: Wound healing

3   **The answer is A: Type I collagen.**   A mature scar is composed primarily of type I collagen. By contrast, the early matrix of granulation tissue contains proteoglycans, glycoproteins, and type III collagen. Eventually, the temporary matrix is removed by a combination of extracellular and intracellular digestion, and the definitive matrix is deposited. Extracellular cross-linking of the newly synthesized type I collagen progressively increases wound strength. Collagen type II (choice B) is found in cartilage. Collagen type IV (choice C) is found in basement membranes. Collagen types V and VI (choices D and E) are found in various organs.
Diagnosis: Myocardial infarction

4   **The answer is D: Myofibroblasts.**   The myofibroblast is the cell responsible for wound contraction as well as the deforming pathologic process termed wound contracture. These cells express α-smooth muscle actin, desmin, and vimentin, and they respond to pharmacologic agents that cause smooth muscle to contract or relax. Myofibroblasts exert their contractile effects by forming syncytia, in which the myofibroblasts are bound together by tight junctions. By contrast, fibroblasts (choice B) tend to be solitary cells, surrounded by collagen fibers. Endothelial cells (choice A) respond to growth factors and form capillaries, which are necessary for the delivery of nutrients and inflammatory cells. Neither macrophages (choice C) nor smooth muscle cells (choice E) mediate wound contraction.
Diagnosis: Wound contraction

5   **The answer is D: Vitamin C.**   Vitamin C (ascorbic acid) is a powerful, biologic reducing agent that is necessary for the hydroxylation of proline residues in collagen. Most of the clinical features associated with vitamin C deficiency (scurvy) are caused by the formation of an abnormal collagen that lacks tensile strength. Patients with vitamin C deficiency exhibit poor wound healing. Dehiscence (bursting open) of previously healed wounds may also occur. None of the other choices are required for collagen assembly.
Diagnosis: Wound healing

6   **The answer is A: Fibroblasts and endothelial cells.**   Granulation tissue has two major components: cells and proliferating capillaries. The cells are mostly fibroblasts, myofibroblasts, and macrophages. Fibroblasts and myofibroblasts derive from mesenchymal stem cells. Capillaries arise from adjacent blood vessels by division of endothelial cells in a process termed angiogenesis. Macrophages are a principal source of growth factors and are recognized for their phagocytic functions. Granulation tissue is fluid laden, and its cellular constituents supply antibacterial antibodies and growth factors. Once repair has been achieved, most of the newly formed capillaries are obliterated and then reabsorbed, leaving a pale avascular scar. Although the other inflammatory cells listed may be found in this healing wound, they do not constitute the principal components of granulation tissue.
Diagnosis: Diabetic ulcer, granulation tissue

7 The answer is E: Metalloproteinase. Matrix metalloproteinases (MMPs) are crucial components in wound healing because they enable cells to migrate by degrading matrix proteins. Members of this protein family include collagenase, stromelysin, and gelatinase. In addition to enhancing cell migration, MMPs can disrupt cell-cell adhesions and release bioactive molecules stored in the matrix. MMP activity can be minimized by binding to specific proteinase inhibitors such as α_1-antitrypsin (choice A) and α_2-macroglobulin (choice D). Lysozyme (choice C) is a secretory product of neutrophils that degrades bacterial cell walls.
Diagnosis: Diabetes mellitus

8 The answer is E: Scar formation. A large infarct of the kidney will heal by fibrosis (scar formation). In most renal diseases, there is destruction of the extracellular matrix framework. Repair and regeneration (choice D) is then incomplete, and scar formation is the expected outcome. The regenerative capacity of renal tissue is maximal in cortical tubules, less in medullary tubules, and *nonexistent* in glomeruli. Recent data suggest that renal tubule repair occurs due to the proliferation of endogenous renal progenitor (stem) cells. Chronic inflammation (choice A) precedes scar formation. Granulomatous inflammation (choice B) is not a complication of renal cortical infarction. Hemangiomas (choice C) are common benign tumors of endothelial cells that usually occur in the skin.
Diagnosis: Infarction; embolism, atheroembolus

9 The answer is E: Maturation arrest of collagen assembly. Keloid is an exuberant scar that tends to progress beyond the site of initial injury and recurs after excision. Dark-skinned persons are more frequently affected by keloids than light-skinned people. Keloids are characterized by changes in the ratio of type III to type I collagen, suggesting a "maturation arrest" in the healing process. Further support for maturation arrest as an explanation for keloids and hypertrophic scars is the overexpression of fibronectin in these lesions. Keloids are unsightly, and attempts at surgical repair are always problematic. The other choices do not address the pathogenesis of keloids.
Diagnosis: Keloid

10 The answer is B: Foreign material. Granulomatous inflammation is a subtype of chronic inflammation, which develops when acute inflammatory cells are unable to digest the injurious agent (e.g., suture or talc). Fusion of macrophages within the lesion results in the formation of multinucleated giant cells. None of the other choices elicit this type of granulomatous reaction.
Diagnosis: Granulomatous inflammation

11 The answer is B: Chronic viral hepatitis. Chronic liver injury (e.g., chronic viral hepatitis) is associated with the development of broad collagenous scars within the hepatic parenchyma. This is termed cirrhosis. Hepatocytes form regenerative nodules that lack central veins and expand to obstruct blood vessels and bile flow. Portal hypertension and jaundice ensue, despite adequate numbers of regenerated but disconnected hepatocytes. Acute toxic liver injury (choice A) is generally reversible. Fulminant hepatic necrosis (choice C), if the patient survives, usually regenerates. Hepatocellular carcinoma (choice D) may be associated with tumor fibrosis but not with regeneration. Portal vein thrombosis (choice E) does not cause hepatic fibrosis but may be a complication of embolism.
Diagnosis: Alcoholic liver disease, cirrhosis

12 The answer is D: Regeneration. Superficial abrasions of the skin heal by a process of regeneration. It is mediated by stem cells or stabile cells that are able to progress through the cell cycle and fully restore normal tissue organization and function. Cellular migration is the predominant means by which the wound surface is reepithelialized. Fibrosis (choice A) refers to aberrant healing with deposition of collagen-rich scar tissue. Granulation tissue (choice B) forms during the repair of deep wounds. Primary and secondary intentions (choices C and E) are features of healing in deeper wounds.
Diagnosis: Superficial abrasion

13 The answer is B: Contact inhibition of epithelial growth and motility. Maturation of the epidermis requires an intact layer of basal cells that are in direct contact with one another. If this contact is disrupted, basal epithelial cells at the wound margin become activated and eventually reestablish contact with other basal cells through extensive cell migration and mitosis. When epithelial continuity is reestablished, migration and cell division cease, and the epidermis resumes its normal cycle of maturation and shedding. This process of epithelial growth regulation is referred to as "contact inhibition of growth and motility." The other choices describe responses to deep wound healing.
Diagnosis: Superficial abrasion, regeneration

14 The answer is B: Fibronectins. Fibronectins are adhesive glycoproteins that are widely distributed in stromal connective tissue and deposited at the site of tissue injury. During the initial phase of healing, fibronectin in the extravasated plasma is cross-linked to fibrin, collagen, and other extracellular matrix components by the action of transglutaminases. This cross-linking provides a provisional stabilization of the wound during the first several hours. Fibronectin, cell debris, and bacterial products are chemoattractants for a variety of cells that are recruited to the wound site over the next several days. Selectins (choice E) are sugar-binding glycoproteins that mediate the initial adhesion of leukocytes to endothelial cells at sites of inflammation. They are found at the cell surface and are not part of the extracellular matrix. Cadherins (choice A) and integrins (choice C) are cell adhesion molecules. Like the selectin family of cell adhesion proteins, they are found at the cell surface and are not part of the extracellular matrix.
Diagnosis: Wound healing

15 The answer is C: Integrins. The locomotion of leukocytes is powered by membrane extensions called lamellipodia. Slower moving cells, such as fibroblasts, extend fingerlike membrane protrusions called filopodia. The leading edge of the cell membrane adheres to the extracellular matrix through transmembrane adhesion receptors termed integrins. These cell surface glycoproteins transmit mechanical and chemical signals, thereby regulating cellular survival, proliferation, differentiation, and migration. The motility of epithelial cells is also regulated by integrin receptors. Cadherins (choice A) are cell-cell adhesion molecules. Fibrillins (choice B) are structural molecules that interact with elastic fibrils. Laminins (choice D) are basement membrane glycoproteins. Selectins (choice E) mediate the recruitment of neutrophils in acute inflammation but do not mediate directed cell migration at the site of tissue injury.

Diagnosis: Wound healing

16 The answer is A: Apposition of edges. Healing by primary intention occurs in wounds with closely apposed edges and minimal tissue loss. Such a wound requires only minimal cell proliferation and neovascularization to heal, and the result is a small scar. Healing by secondary intention occurs in a gouged wound, in which the edges are far apart and in which there is substantial tissue loss. This wound requires wound contraction, extensive cell proliferation, and neovascularization (granulation tissue) to heal. Granulation tissue is eventually resorbed and replaced by a large scar that is functionally and esthetically unsatisfactory. The other choices are important determinants of the outcome of wound healing, but they do not provide a point of distinction between primary and secondary intentions healing.

Diagnosis: Healing by primary intention

17 The answer is C: 3 to 5 days. Activated fibroblasts, myofibroblasts, and capillary sprouts are abundant in healing wounds 3 to 5 days following injury. Activated fibroblasts change shape from oval to bipolar as they begin to form collagen and synthesize a variety of extracellular matrix proteins. Neutrophils accumulate in the wound 12 to 24 hours after injury (choice B). Mature scar tissue would be visible 2 weeks following injury (choice E).

Diagnosis: Healing by primary intention

18 The answer is D: Phagocytosis. Macrophages arrive at the site of injury shortly after neutrophils, but they persist in the wound for days longer. Macrophages remove debris and orchestrate the formation of granulation tissue by releasing cytokines and chemoattractants. None of the other choices are functions of tissue macrophages. For example, plasma cells produce antibodies (choice A), and myofibroblasts mediate wound contraction (choice E).

Diagnosis: Laceration

19 The answer is C: Type III. Concurrent with fibrinolysis, a temporary matrix composed of proteoglycans, glycoproteins, and type III collagen is deposited. The secretion of type III collagen is a forerunner to the formation of type I collagen (choice A), which will impart greater tensile strength to the wound. TGF-β enhances the synthesis of collagen and fibronectin and decreases metalloproteinase transcription and matrix degradation. Extracellular cross-linking of newly synthesized collagen further increases the mechanical strength of the wound. Type II collagen (choice B) is found in cartilage. Type IV collagen (choice D) is found in basement membranes.

Diagnosis: Laceration

20 The answer is B: Glial cells. Damage to the brain or spinal cord is followed by growth of capillaries and gliosis (i.e., the proliferation of astrocytes and microglia). Gliosis in the central nervous system is the equivalent of scar formation elsewhere; once established, it remains permanently. In spinal cord injuries, axonal regeneration can be seen up to 2 weeks after injury. After 2 weeks, gliosis has taken place and attempts at axonal regeneration end. In the central nervous system, axonal regeneration occurs only in the hypothalamohypophysial region, where glial and capillary barriers do not interfere with axonal regeneration. Axonal regeneration seems to require contact with extracellular fluid containing plasma proteins. The other cells listed do not proliferate significantly in response to brain or spinal cord injury.

Diagnosis: Cerebral contusion, gliosis

21 The answer is A: Contracture. A mechanical reduction in the size of a wound depends on the presence of myofibroblasts and sustained cell contraction. An exaggeration of these processes is termed contracture and results in severe deformity of the wound and surrounding tissues. Contractures are particularly conspicuous in the healing of serious burns and can be severe enough to compromise the movement of joints.

Diagnosis: Contracture

22 The answer is E: Neuroma. Neurons in the peripheral nervous system can regenerate their axons, and under ideal circumstances, interruption in the continuity of a peripheral nerve results in complete functional recovery. However, if the cut ends are not in perfect alignment or are prevented from establishing continuity by inflammation, a traumatic neuroma results. This bulbous lesion consists of disorganized axons and proliferating Schwann cells and fibroblasts. In this patient's biopsy, the original nerve (lower left) enters the neuroma. The nerve is surrounded by dense collagenous tissue, which appears dark blue in this trichrome stain. Ganglioma (choice A), ganglioneuroma (choice B), and hamartoma (choice C) are benign neoplasms.

Diagnosis: Traumatic neuroma

23 The answer is B: Postcapillary venules. One of the earliest responses following tissue injury occurs within the microvasculature at the level of the capillary and postcapillary venule. Within this vascular network are the major components of the inflammatory response, including plasma, platelets, erythrocytes, and circulating leukocytes. Following injury, changes in the structure of the vascular wall lead to activation of endothelial cells, loss of vascular integrity, leakage of fluid and plasma components from the intravascular compartment, and emigration of erythrocytes and leukocytes from the vascular space into the extravascular tissue (diapedesis). Leukocyte recruitment in the postcapillary venule is initiated by interaction of leukocytes with endothelial cell surface selectin molecules. Leukocytes do not typically undergo diapedesis at the other anatomic locations listed.

Diagnosis: Carbuncle, margination

24 The answer is E: Ulcer. Incidental findings are frequently encountered at autopsy. In this case, a peptic ulcer is identified in the distal stomach. Histologic examination shows focal destruction of the mucosa and full-thickness replacement of the muscularis with collagen-rich connective tissue (see photomicrograph). Gastric ulcers are usually single and less than 2 cm in diameter. Ulcers on the lesser curvature are commonly associated with chronic gastritis (this patient), whereas those on the greater curvature are often related to NSAIDs. Grossly, chronic peptic ulcers may closely resemble gastric carcinoma (choice A). Thus, the endoscopist must take multiple biopsies from the edges and bed of any gastric ulcer.

Although contraction and scarring of gastric ulcers (choice B) may occur and may cause pyloric stenosis, the histopathologic findings do not suggest this complication. Diverticula of the stomach (choice C) are rare and, if present, are usually lined by a normal gastric mucosa. Granuloma (choice D) features inflammatory cells that are not observed.

Diagnosis: Gastric ulcer, peptic ulcer disease

Chapter 4

Immunopathology

QUESTIONS

Select the single best answer.

1 A 35-year-old man asks for advice regarding seasonal eye itching and runny nose. Recurrent conjunctivitis in this patient is most likely caused by which of the following mechanisms of disease?
(A) Autoimmunity
(B) Bacterial infection
(C) Chemical toxicity
(D) Hypersensitivity
(E) Viral infection

2 An 8-year-old boy presents with periorbital edema and throbbing headaches. His parents report that the boy had a "strep throat" 2 weeks ago. Urinalysis shows 3+ hematuria. A renal biopsy shows hypercellular glomeruli, and electron microscopic examination of glomeruli discloses subepithelial "humps." Which of the following best explains the pathogenesis of glomerulonephritis in this patient?
(A) Antineutrophil cytoplasmic autoantibodies
(B) Deposition of circulating immune complexes
(C) Directly cytotoxic IgG and IgM antibodies
(D) IgE-mediated mast cell degranulation
(E) T cell–mediated delayed hypersensitivity reaction

3 A 21-year-old woman presents with a 3-month history of malaise, joint pain, weight loss, and sporadic fever. The patient appears agitated. Her temperature is 38°C (101°F). Other physical findings include malar rash, erythematous-pink plaques with telangiectatic vessels, oral ulcers, and nonblanching purpuric papules on her legs. Laboratory studies show elevated levels of blood urea nitrogen and creatinine. Antibodies directed to which of the following antigens would be expected in the serum of this patient?
(A) C-ANCA (anti-proteinase-3)
(B) Double-stranded DNA
(C) P-ANCA (anti-myeloperoxidase)
(D) Rheumatoid factor
(E) Scl-70 (anti-topoisomerase I)

4 Serum levels of complement proteins may be reduced during the active phase of disease in the patient described in Question 3 due to which of the following mechanisms of disease?

(A) Binding of complement to immune complexes
(B) Decreased complement protein biosynthesis
(C) Defective activation of the complement cascade
(D) Increased urinary excretion of immunoglobulins
(E) Stimulation of the acute phase response

5 A 45-year-old woman complains of severe headaches and difficulty swallowing. Over the past 6 months, she has noticed small, red lesions around her mouth as well as thickening of her skin. The patient has "stone facies" on physical examination. Which of the following antigens is the most common and most specific target of autoantibody in patients with this disease?
(A) C-ANCA (anti-proteinase-3)
(B) Double-stranded DNA
(C) P-ANCA (anti-myeloperoxidase)
(D) Scl-70 (anti-topoisomerase I)
(E) SS-A/SS-B

6 A skin biopsy in the patient described in Question 5 would most likely show a perivascular accumulation of which of the following extracellular matrix proteins?
(A) Collagen
(B) Elastin
(C) Entactin
(D) Fibronectin
(E) Laminin

7 During the physical examination of a 22-year-old man, a purified protein derivative isolated from *Mycobacterium tuberculosis* is injected into the skin. Three days later, the injection site appears raised and indurated. Which of the following glycoproteins was directly involved in antigen presentation during the initiation phase of delayed hypersensitivity in this patient?
(A) CD4
(B) CD8
(C) Class I HLA molecules
(D) Class II HLA molecules
(E) GlyCAM-1

8 A 54-year-old woman is involved in an automobile accident and requires a blood transfusion. Five hours later, she becomes febrile and has severe back pain. Laboratory studies show evidence of intravascular hemolysis. It is discovered that type A Rh+ blood was given by mistake to this type B Rh+ patient. Which of the following best explains the development of intravascular hemolysis in this patient?

(A) Antibody-dependent cellular cytotoxicity
(B) Antibody-mediated complement fixation
(C) Delayed-type hypersensitivity
(D) Immune complex disease
(E) Immediate hypersensitivity

9 A 40-year-old man complains of having yellow skin and sclerae, abdominal tenderness, and dark urine. Physical examination reveals jaundice and mild hepatomegaly. Laboratory studies demonstrate elevated serum bilirubin (3.1 mg/dL), decreased serum albumin (2.5 g/dL), and prolonged prothrombin time (17 seconds). Serologic tests reveal antibodies to hepatitis B core antigen (IgG anti-HBcAg). The serum is also positive for HBsAg and HBeAg. Which of the following glycoproteins serves as the principal cell surface receptor for viral antigens on B lymphocytes in this patient?

(A) CD4
(B) CD8
(C) HLA class I molecules
(D) HLA class II molecules
(E) Membrane immunoglobulin

10 What glycoprotein on virally infected hepatocytes provides a target for cell-mediated cytotoxicity in the patient described in Question 9?

(A) CD4
(B) CD8
(C) Class I HLA molecules
(D) Class II HLA molecules
(E) GlyCAM-1

11 A 45-year-old woman presents with a 1-year history of dry mouth and eyes. A biopsy of a minor salivary gland reveals infiltrates of lymphocytes forming focal germinal centers. Which of the following cellular organelles is a target for autoantibodies in this patient?

(A) Centromere
(B) Lysosome
(C) Nucleus
(D) Peroxisome
(E) Plasma membrane

12 An 8-month-old boy with a history of recurrent pneumonia is found to have almost no circulating IgG. Cellular immunity is normal. His brother had this same disease and died of echovirus encephalitis. His parents and sisters have normal serum levels of IgG. What is the appropriate diagnosis?

(A) DiGeorge syndrome
(B) Isolated IgA deficiency
(C) Severe combined immunodeficiency
(D) Wiskott-Aldrich syndrome
(E) X-linked agammaglobulinemia of Bruton

13 A 52-year-old woman with a history of systemic hypertension and chronic renal failure undergoes kidney transplantation, but the graft fails to produce urine. A renal biopsy is diagnosed as "hyperacute transplant rejection." Graft rejection in this patient is caused primarily by which of the following mediators of immunity and inflammation?

(A) Cytotoxic T lymphocytes
(B) Helper T lymphocytes
(C) Mononuclear phagocytes
(D) Natural killer cells
(E) Preformed antibodies

14 A 30-year-old woman complains of impaired speech and frequent aspiration of food. Physical examination reveals diplopia and drooping eyelids. A mediastinal mass is removed and diagnosed as thymoma. The symptoms of muscle weakness in this patient are caused by antibodies directed against which of the following cellular components?

(A) Acetylcholine receptor
(B) Calcium channel
(C) Desmoglein-3
(D) Rheumatoid factor
(E) Thyroid-stimulating hormone (TSH) receptor

15 A 31-year-old man with AIDS complains of difficulty swallowing. Examination of his oral cavity demonstrates whitish membranes covering much of his tongue and palate. Endoscopy also reveals several whitish, ulcerated lesions in the esophagus. These pathologic findings are fundamentally caused by loss of which of the following immune cells in this patient?

(A) B lymphocytes
(B) Helper T lymphocytes
(C) Killer T lymphocytes
(D) Monocytes/macrophages
(E) Natural killer (NK) cells

16 Which of the following enzymes converts the HIV genome into double-stranded DNA in host cells in the patient described in Question 15?

(A) DNA polymerase (Pol-1)
(B) DNA polymerase (Pol-2)
(C) Integrase
(D) Reverse transcriptase
(E) Topoisomerase

17 A 20-year-old woman with a history of asthma and allergies undergoes skin testing to identify potential allergens in her environment. A positive skin reaction to ragweed in this patient would be mediated by which of the following classes of immunoglobulin?

(A) IgA
(B) IgD
(C) IgE
(D) IgG
(E) IgM

18 A 53-year-old woman complains of progressive weight loss, nervousness, and sweating (patient shown in the image). Physical examination reveals tachycardia and exophthalmos. Her thyroid is diffusely enlarged and warm on palpation. Serum levels of thyroid-stimulating hormone (TSH) are low, and levels of thyroid hormones (T_3 and T_4) are markedly elevated. Which of the following mechanisms of disease best explains the pathogenesis of this patient's thyroid condition?

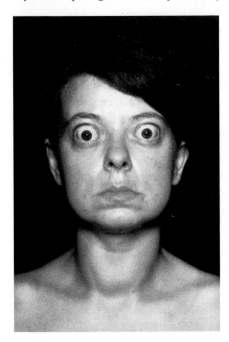

(A) Antibody-dependent cellular cytotoxicity
(B) Cytopathic autoantibodies
(C) Delayed-type hypersensitivity
(D) Immediate hypersensitivity
(E) Immune complex disease

19 A 12-month-old infant with a history of recurrent infections, eczema, generalized edema, and easy bruising is diagnosed with an X-linked, recessive, congenital immunodeficiency. The CBC shows thrombocytopenia. What is the most likely diagnosis?
(A) DiGeorge syndrome
(B) Isolated IgA deficiency
(C) Severe combined immunodeficiency
(D) Wiskott-Aldrich syndrome
(E) X-linked agammaglobulinemia of Bruton

20 A 24-year-old woman with leukemia receives an allogeneic bone marrow transplant. Three weeks later, she develops a skin rash and diarrhea. Liver function tests show elevated serum levels of AST and ALT. A skin biopsy discloses a sparse lymphocytic infiltrate in the dermis and epidermis, as well as apoptotic cells in the epidermal basal cell layer. Skin rash and diarrhea in this patient are caused primarily by which of the following cells?
(A) Donor lymphocytes
(B) Donor plasma cells
(C) Fixed tissue macrophages
(D) Recipient lymphocytes
(E) Recipient plasma cells

21 A 20-year-old gardener presents to his family physician for treatment of what he describes as "poison ivy." The patient's hands and arms appear red and are covered with oozing blisters and crusts. Which of the following best describes the pathogenesis of these skin lesions?
(A) Cytotoxic antibody production
(B) Delayed-type hypersensitivity
(C) Deposition of antigluten antibodies
(D) Deposition of circulating immune complexes
(E) IgE-mediated mast cell degranulation

22 A 9-month-old girl with a history of recurrent pulmonary infections is found to have a congenital deficiency of adenosine deaminase, which is associated with a virtual absence of lymphocytes in her peripheral lymphoid organs. What is the appropriate diagnosis?
(A) Bruton X-linked agammaglobulinemia
(B) DiGeorge syndrome
(C) Isolated IgA deficiency
(D) Severe combined immunodeficiency
(E) Wiskott-Aldrich syndrome

23 A 50-year-old man complains of fever, weight loss, abdominal pain, and bloody urine. Physical examination reveals red-purple discoloration of the skin. Serologic findings are inconclusive, but a positive P-ANCA test suggests an autoimmune disease. Biopsy of lesional skin discloses fibrinoid necrosis of a small muscular artery (shown in the image). Which of the following immune responses best explains the pathogenesis of inflammation and necrotizing vasculitis in this patient?

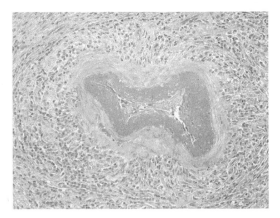

(A) Antibody-dependent cellular cytotoxicity
(B) Cytopathic autoantibodies
(C) Delayed-type hypersensitivity
(D) Immediate hypersensitivity
(E) Immune complex disease

24 A neonate develops spastic contractions on the second postpartum day. Laboratory studies show hypocalcemia. MRI studies demonstrate aplasia of the thymus and parathyroid glands. What is the appropriate diagnosis?
(A) Adenosine deaminase deficiency
(B) Common variable immunodeficiency
(C) DiGeorge syndrome
(D) Transient hypogammaglobulinemia of infancy
(E) Wiskott-Aldrich syndrome

25 A 50-year-old woman complains of intermittent tingling and pain in the tips of her fingers. She also reports joint and muscle pain. Physical examination reveals lymphadenopathy. Laboratory studies show hypergammaglobulinemia. The antinuclear antibody test is positive, but there is no evidence of antibodies against double-stranded DNA. Urinalysis is normal. The patient responds well to steroids. Which of the following is the most likely diagnosis?

(A) Graves disease
(B) Mixed connective tissue disease
(C) Myasthenia gravis
(D) Scleroderma
(E) Sjögren syndrome

26 A 25-year-old woman complains of low-grade fever, fatigue, and persistent rash over her nose and upper chest. She also notes pain in her knees and elbows. A skin biopsy shows dermal inflammation and granular deposits of IgG and C3 complement along the basement membrane at the epidermal/dermal junction. Urinalysis reveals microscopic hematuria and proteinuria. The antinuclear antibody test is positive. The development of thromboembolic complications (e.g., deep venous thrombosis) in this patient is commonly associated with elevated serum levels of antibodies to which of the following antigens?

(A) ABO blood group antigens
(B) Class II HLA molecules
(C) Clotting factors
(D) Fibrinolytic enzymes
(E) Phospholipids

27 A 30-year-old woman is found to have a congenital immunodeficiency that has remained largely asymptomatic throughout her life. Which of the following is the most likely diagnosis?

(A) Adenosine deaminase deficiency
(B) Chronic mucocutaneous candidiasis
(C) Purine nucleoside phosphorylase deficiency
(D) Selective IgA deficiency
(E) Wiskott-Aldrich syndrome

28 A 60-year-old woman with type 2 diabetes and end-stage renal disease receives a kidney transplant. Three weeks later, the patient presents with azotemia and oliguria. If this patient has developed acute renal failure, which of the following pathologic findings would be expected on renal biopsy?

(A) Arterial intimal thickening and vascular stenosis
(B) Glomerulosclerosis
(C) Interstitial infiltrates of lymphocytes and macrophages
(D) Neutrophilic vasculitis and fibrinoid necrosis
(E) Tubular atrophy and interstitial fibrosis

29 A 12-year-old boy presents with a 5-day history of sore throat. His temperature is 38.7°C (103°F). Physical examination reveals inflamed tonsils and swollen cervical lymph nodes. Trafficking and recirculation of blood-borne lymphocytes through the cervical lymph nodes in this patient occurs primarily at which of the following locations?

(A) Afferent lymphatic vessel
(B) Efferent lymphatic vessel
(C) Hassall corpuscles
(D) High endothelial venules
(E) Peyer patches

30 A 28-year-old woman with a history of drug abuse presents with an infectious mononucleosis-like syndrome and lymphadenopathy. Blood tests subsequently indicate that she is HIV-positive. Which of the following lymphocyte-associated proteins mediates the entry of HIV into host cells in this patient?

(A) CD4
(B) CD8
(C) GP41
(D) GP120
(E) LFA-1

ANSWERS

1 **The answer is D: Hypersensitivity.** Although the incorrect choices may cause eye irritation, seasonal conjunctivitis is typically caused by allergies to pollens that are released during a particular time of the year. Allergic rhinitis (hay fever) is the most common type I hypersensitivity disease in adults. It may be caused by pollen, house dust, animal dandruff, and many other allergens. Antigens inhaled react with the IgE attached to basophils in the nasal mucosa, thereby triggering the release of vasoactive substances stored in cytoplasmic granules. Histamine, the main mediator released from mast cells, increases the permeability of mucosal vessels, causing edema and sneezing.
Diagnosis: Conjunctivitis, hypersensitivity reaction

2 **The answer is B: Deposition of circulating immune complexes.** Type III hypersensitivity reactions are characterized by immune complex deposition, complement fixation, and localized inflammation. Antibody directed against either a circulating antigen or an antigen that is deposited in a tissue can give rise to a type III response. Diseases that seem to be most clearly attributable to the deposition of immune complexes are systemic lupus erythematosus, rheumatoid arthritis, and varieties of glomerulonephritis. Streptoccocal infection in this case led to the deposition of antigens and antibodies in glomerular basement membranes, resulting in clinical features of nephritic syndrome (e.g., hematuria, oliguria, and hypertension). Post-streptococcal illnesses do not include any of the other choices.
Diagnosis: Postinfectious glomerulonephritis

3 **The answer is B: Double-stranded DNA.** Systemic lupus erythematosus (SLE) is an autoimmune, inflammatory disease that may involve almost any organ but characteristically affects the kidneys, joints, serous membranes, and skin. Autoantibodies are formed against a variety of self-antigens. The most important diagnostic autoantibodies are those against nuclear antigens—in particular, antibody to double-stranded DNA and to a soluble nuclear antigen complex that is part of the spliceosome and is termed Sm (Smith) antigen. High titers of these two autoantibodies (termed antinuclear antibodies) are nearly pathognomonic for SLE. Antibodies to rheumatoid factor (choice D) are seen in patients with rheumatoid arthritis. Antineutrophil cytoplasmic antibodies (choices A and C) are seen in patients with small vessel vasculitis (e.g., Wegener granulomatosis).
Diagnosis: Systemic lupus erythematosus

4 **The answer is A: Binding of complement to immune complexes.** Acquired deficiencies of early complement components occur in patients with autoimmune diseases, especially those associated with circulating immune complexes (e.g., systemic lupus erythematosus [SLE]). Antigen-antibody complexes formed in the circulation during the active stage of these diseases lead to a marked reduction in circulating levels of complement proteins (hypocomplementemia). None of the other choices mediates hypocomplementemia in patients with SLE.

Diagnosis: Systemic lupus erythematosus

5 The answer is D: Scl-70 (anti-topoisomerase I). Scleroderma is an autoimmune disease of connective tissue. Circulating male fetal cells have been demonstrated in blood and blood vessel walls of many women with scleroderma who bore male children many years before the disease began. Accordingly, it has been suggested that scleroderma in these patients is similar to graft-versus-host disease. Antinuclear antibodies are common but are usually present in a lower titer than in patients with SLE. Antibodies virtually specific for scleroderma include (1) nucleolar autoantibodies (primarily against RNA polymerase); (2) antibodies to Scl-70, a nonhistone nuclear protein topoisomerase; and (3) anticentromere antibodies, which are associated with the "CREST" variant of the disease. The Scl-70 autoantibody is most common and specific for the diffuse form of scleroderma and is seen in 70% of patients. Autoantibodies to double-stranded DNA (choice B) are seen in patients with SLE. Autoantibodies to SS-A/SS-B (choice E) are seen in patients with Sjögren syndrome.

Diagnosis: Scleroderma

6 The answer is A: Collagen. Scleroderma is characterized by vasculopathy and excessive collagen deposition in the skin and internal organs, such as the lung, gastrointestinal tract, heart, and kidney. The disease occurs four times as often in women as in men and mostly in persons aged 25 to 50 years. Progressive systemic sclerosis is characterized by widespread excessive collagen deposition. There is emerging evidence for the expansion of fibrogenic clones of fibroblasts. These clones display augmented procollagen synthesis, including increased circulating levels of type III collagen aminopropeptide. Tissue levels of the other proteins are not significantly altered in patients with scleroderma.

Diagnosis: Scleroderma

7 The answer is D: Class II HLA molecules. Delayed-type hypersensitivity is defined as a tissue reaction involving lymphocytes and mononuclear phagocytes, which occurs in response to a soluble protein antigen and reaches greatest intensity 24 to 48 hours after initiation. In the initial phase, foreign protein antigens or chemical ligands interact with accessory cells bearing class II HLA molecules. Protein antigens are actively processed into short peptides within phagolysosomes and are presented on the cell surface in conjunction with the class II HLA molecules. The latter are recognized by CD4+ T cells (choice A), which become activated to synthesize an array of cytokines. The cytokines recruit and activate lymphocytes, monocytes, fibroblasts, and other inflammatory cells. Suppressor T cells are CD8+ (choice B). Class I HLA molecules (choice C) provide targets for cell-mediated cytotoxicity. GlyCAM-1 (choice E) is a cell adhesion molecule involved in lymphocyte trafficking.

Diagnosis: Delayed-type hypersensitivity

8 The answer is B: Antibody-mediated complement fixation. Type II hypersensitivity reactions are mediated by antibodies directed against fixed antigens. In this case, preformed antibodies in the patient's blood attached to foreign antigens (oligosaccharides) on the membranes of the transfused erythrocytes. At sufficient density, bound immunoglobulins fix complement. Once activated, the complement cascade leads to the destruction of the target cell through formation of a membrane attack complex. This type of complement-mediated cell lysis occurs in autoimmune hemolytic anemia. Antibody-dependent cell-mediated cytotoxicity (ADCC, choice A) involves cytolytic leukocytes that attack antibody-coated target cells. ADCC may be involved in the pathogenesis of some autoimmune diseases (e.g., autoimmune thyroiditis). Delayed-type hypersensitivity (choice C) occurs over a period of days and does not involve preformed antibodies.

Diagnosis: Hemolytic anemia, jaundice

9 The answer is E: Membrane immunoglobulin (mIg). The clinicopathologic findings presented here indicate that this patient is a chronic HBV carrier with active hepatitis. Humoral immune responses to specific viral antigens in this patient involve the activation and differentiation of B lymphocytes into antibody-secreting plasma cells. Analogous to T cells, B cells express an antigen-binding receptor, namely mIg. This immunoglobulin bears the same antigen specificity as the soluble immunoglobulin that is ultimately secreted. Class I HLA molecules (choice C) provide targets for CD8+ T cells in cell-mediated cytotoxicity. Class II HLA molecules (choice D) are recognized by CD4+ T cells, which become activated to synthesize an array of cytokines.

Diagnosis: Humoral immunity, chronic hepatitis

10 The answer is C: Class I HLA molecules. Class I molecules of the major histocompatibility complex present foreign peptides and are recognized by cytotoxic T lymphocytes during graft rejection or during cell-mediated killing of virus-infected cells. All tissues express class I molecules, whereas class II molecules (choice D) are displayed primarily on macrophages and B lymphocytes. CD4 and CD8 (choices A and B) are cell surface markers of helper and killer T lymphocytes, respectively. GlyCAM-1 (choice E) facilitates lymphocyte recirculation by providing a receptor for leukocyte attachment to high endothelial venules.

Diagnosis: Chronic hepatitis B

11 The answer is C: Nucleus. Sjögren syndrome (SS) is an autoimmune disorder characterized by keratoconjunctivitis sicca and xerostomia in the absence of other connective tissue disease. The production of autoantibodies, particularly antinuclear antibodies directed against DNA or nonhistone proteins, typically occurs in patients with SS. Autoantibodies to soluble nuclear nonhistone proteins, especially the antigens SS-A and SS-B, are found in half of patients with primary SS and are associated with more severe glandular and extraglandular manifestations. Autoantibodies to DNA or histones are rare. Organ-specific autoantibodies, such as those directed against salivary gland antigens, are distinctly uncommon. Autoantibodies to centromere proteins (choice A) are seen in the CREST variant of progressive systemic sclerosis.

Diagnosis: Sjögren syndrome

12 The answer is E: X-linked agammaglobulinemia of Bruton. The congenital disorder Bruton X-linked agammaglobulinemia appears in male infants at 5 to 8 months of age, the period during which maternal antibody levels begin to decline. The infant suffers from recurrent pyogenic infections and severe hypogammaglobulinemia. There is an absence of both mature B cells in peripheral blood and plasma cells in lymphoid tissues. The genetic defect, located on the long arm of the X chromosome, is an inactivating mutation of the gene for B-cell tyrosine kinase, an enzyme critical to B-lymphocyte maturation. Wiskott-Aldrich syndrome (choice D) is also an X-linked genetic disease but is characterized by defects in both B-cell and T-cell functions (i.e., humeral and cellular immunity). DiGeorge syndrome (choice A) is a developmental disorder characterized by thymic and parathyroid aplasia.

Diagnosis: X-linked agammaglobulinemia of Bruton

13 **The answer is E: Preformed antibodies.** Hyperacute rejection occurs within minutes to hours after transplantation. It is manifested clinically as a sudden cessation of urine output, along with fever and pain in the area of the graft site. This immediate rejection is mediated by preformed antibodies and complement activation products. Lymphocytes and macrophages (choices A, B, and C) are associated with acute and chronic graft rejection.

Diagnosis: Hyperacute graft rejection

14 **The answer is A: Acetylcholine receptor.** Myasthenia gravis is a type II hypersensitivity disorder caused by antibodies that bind to the acetylcholine receptor. These antibodies interfere with the transmission of neural impulses at the neuromuscular junction, causing muscle weakness and easy fatigability. External ocular and eyelid muscles are most often affected, but the disease is often progressive and may cause death by respiratory muscle paralysis. Autoantibodies to desmoglein-3 (choice C) are found in patients with pemphigus vulgaris, an autoimmune blistering skin disorder. Antibodies to the TSH receptor (choice E) are seen in patients with Graves hyperthyroidism. Antibodies to calcium channels (choice B) are found in patients with Eaton-Lambert syndrome. This paraneoplastic syndrome also manifests as muscle weakness but is usually associated with small cell carcinoma of the lung. Rheumatoid factor (choice D) represents multiple antibodies directed against the Fc portion of IgG and is seen in patients with rheumatoid arthritis and many other collagen vascular diseases.

Diagnosis: Myasthenia gravis, thymoma

15 **The answer is B: Helper T lymphocytes.** The relentless progression of HIV infection is now recognized as a continuum that extends from an initial asymptomatic state to the immune depletion that characterizes patients with overt AIDS. The fundamental lesion is infection of CD4⁺ (helper) T lymphocytes, which leads to the depletion of this cell population and impaired immune function. As a result, patients with AIDS usually die of opportunistic infections. HIV does infect the monocyte/macrophage lineage (choice D), but infected cells exhibit little if any cytotoxicity. NK cell activity (choice E) is also decreased in AIDS. This defect may contribute to the appearance of malignant tumors and the viral infections that plague these patients. The suppression of NK cell activity has been related to a decrease in the number of NK cells and to a reduction in IL-2 levels due to the loss of CD4⁺ cells.

Diagnosis: AIDS

16 **The answer is D: Reverse transcriptase.** The primary etiologic agent of AIDS is HIV-1, an enveloped RNA retrovirus that contains a reverse transcriptase (RNA-dependent DNA polymerase). After it enters into the cytoplasm of a T lymphocyte, the virus is uncoated, and its RNA is copied into double-stranded DNA by retroviral reverse transcriptase. The DNA derived from the virus is integrated into the host genome by the viral integrase protein (choice C), thereby producing the latent proviral form of HIV-1. Viral genes are replicated along with host chromosomes and, therefore, persist for the life of the cell.

Diagnosis: AIDS

17 **The answer is C: IgE.** Immediate-type hypersensitivity is manifested by a localized or generalized reaction that occurs within minutes after exposure to an antigen or "allergen" to which the person has previously been sensitized. In its generalized and most severe form, immediate hypersensitivity reactions are associated with bronchoconstriction, airway obstruction, and circulatory collapse, as seen in anaphylactic shock. Type I hypersensitivity reactions feature the formation of IgE antibodies that bind avidly to Fc-epsilon (Fc-ε) receptors on mast cells and basophils. The high-avidity binding of IgE accounts for the term cytophilic antibody. Once exposed to a specific allergen that has resulted in the formation of IgE, a person is sensitized. Subsequent responses to the allergen induce an immediate release of a cascade of proinflammatory mediators. These mediators are responsible for smooth muscle contraction, edema formation, and the recruitment of eosinophils. None of the other immunoglobulin classes mediates immediate hypersensitivity.

Diagnosis: Asthma

18 **The answer is B: Cytopathic autoantibodies.** Graves disease is a type II hypersensitivity disorder caused by antibodies to the TSH receptor on follicular cells of the thyroid. Antibody binding to the TSH receptor stimulates a release of tetraiodothyronine (T₄) and triiodothyronine (T₃) from the thyroid into the circulation. Circulating T₄ and T₃ suppress TSH production in the pituitary. Sweating, weight loss, and tachycardia are evidence of the hypermetabolism typical of hyperthyroidism. Graves disease also causes exophthalmos. Delayed-type hypersensitivity (choice C) is seen in patients with poison ivy and graft rejection. Immune complex disease (choice E) is caused by deposition of immune complexes and complement activation.

Diagnosis: Graves disease

19 **The answer is D: Wiskott-Aldrich syndrome.** This rare syndrome is characterized by (1) recurrent infections, (2) hemorrhages secondary to thrombocytopenia, and (3) eczema. It typically manifests in boys within the first few months of life as petechiae and recurrent infections (e.g., diarrhea). It is caused by numerous distinct mutations in a gene on the X chromosome that encodes a protein called WASP (Wiskott-Aldrich syndrome protein), which is expressed at high levels in lymphocytes and megakaryocytes. WASP binds members of the Rho family of GTPases. WASP itself controls the assembly of actin filaments that are required to form microvesicles. X-linked agammaglobulinemia of Bruton (choice E) is not associated with thrombocytopenia and eczema. Choices A, B, and C are not X-linked genetic diseases.

Diagnosis: Wiskott-Aldrich syndrome

20 The answer is A: Donor lymphocytes. The advent of transplantation of bone marrow into patients whose immune system has been ablated or into otherwise immunodeficient patients has resulted in the complication of graft-versus-host disease (GVHD). GVHD occurs when lymphocytes in the grafted tissue recognize and react to the recipient. GVHD can also occur when an immunodeficient patient is transfused with blood containing HLA-incompatible lymphocytes. The major organs affected in GVHD include the skin, gastrointestinal tract, and liver. Clinically, GVHD manifests as rash, diarrhea, abdominal cramps, anemia, and liver dysfunction. None of the other cells mediates GVHD.
Diagnosis: Graft-versus-host disease

21 The answer is B: Delayed-type hypersensitivity. "Poison ivy" is a type IV hypersensitivity reaction to plants of the *Rhus* genus. This T-lymphocyte–mediated allergic contact dermatitis presents as urticaria and bullous eruption. Blisters rupture and heal with crusts, usually without scarring. Deposition of antigluten antibodies (choice C) occurs in patients with dermatitis herpetiformis. IgE-mediated mast cell degranulation (choice E) is part of the response to poison ivy (hypersensitivity reactions overlap), but this immediate response does not explain the pathogenesis of delayed hypersensitivity in this patient.
Diagnosis: Allergic contact dermatitis

22 The answer is D: Severe combined immunodeficiency (SCID). SCID is a group of disorders of T and B lymphocytes that are characterized by recurrent viral, bacterial, fungal, and protozoal infections. Many infants with SCID have severely reduced volumes of lymphoid tissue and an immature thymus that lacks lymphocytes. In some patients, lymphocytes fail to develop beyond pre-B cells and pre-T cells. About one half of these severely immunodeficient children lack adenosine deaminase (ADA). ADA deficiency causes the accumulation of intermediate products that are toxic to lymphocytes. These children cannot survive beyond early infancy unless they are raised in a sterile environment ("bubble children"). None of the other choices are associated with ADA deficiency.
Diagnosis: Severe combined immunodeficiency

23 The answer is E: Immune complex disease. Immune complex (type III) hypersensitivity reactions cause vasculitis. Antigen-antibody complexes are either formed in the circulation and deposited in the tissues or formed in situ. Immune complexes induce a localized inflammatory response by fixing complement, which leads to the recruitment of neutrophils and monocytes. The vasculitis in patients with polyarteritis nodosa involves small to medium-sized muscular arteries. The diagnosis is usually made by biopsy of the skin, muscle, peripheral nerves, or the most affected internal organ (the kidney in this case). The most prominent morphologic feature of the affected artery is an area of fibrinoid necrosis (see photomicrograph). Other examples of type III hypersensitivity reactions include Henoch-Schönlein purpura (vascular IgA deposits) and vasculitis associated with hepatitis C infection. The other choices are uncommon mediators of vasculitis in patients with polyarteritis nodosa.
Diagnosis: Polyarteritis nodosa

24 The answer is C: DiGeorge syndrome. DiGeorge syndrome is a chromosomal defect that results in developmental anomalies of the branchial (pharyngeal) pouches and organs that develop from these embryonic structures (thymus, parathyroids, and aortic arch). These children present with tetany caused by hypoparathyroidism and deficiency of cellular immunity. They also have characteristic facial features ("angry look"). In the absence of a thymus, T-cell maturation is interrupted at the pre-T stage. DiGeorge syndrome has been corrected by transplanting thymic tissue. None of the other choices are associated with thymic aplasia.
Diagnosis: DiGeorge syndrome

25 The answer is B: Mixed connective tissue disease (MCTD). MCTD has features of other common autoimmune diseases (e.g., SLE and scleroderma) but appears to be distinct. Patients typically have autoantibodies to ribonucleoproteins, but unlike SLE, they do not have antibodies to Sm antigen or double-stranded DNA. Some patients with MCTD develop symptoms of scleroderma or rheumatoid arthritis, suggesting that MCTD may be an intermediate stage in a genetically determined progression. Whether MCTD represents a distinct entity or simply an overlap of symptoms in patients with other types of collagen vascular diseases remains an open question. Intermittent episodes of ischemia of the fingers, marked by pallor, paresthesias, and pain, are referred to as Raynaud phenomenon. None of the other choices feature this constellation of signs and symptoms.
Diagnosis: Mixed connective tissue disease

26 The answer is E: Phospholipids. One third of patients with systemic lupus erythematosus (SLE) possess elevated concentrations of antiphospholipid antibodies. This phenomenon predisposes these patients to thromboembolic complications, including stroke, pulmonary embolism, deep venous thrombosis, and portal vein thrombosis. The clinical course of SLE is highly variable and typically exhibits exacerbations and remissions. With the recognition of mild forms of the disease, improved antihypertensive medications, and the use of immunosuppressive agents, the overall 10-year survival rate approaches 90%. Antibodies against clotting factors (choice C) or fibrinolytic enzymes (choice D) are not involved in the clotting tendency associated with SLE.
Diagnosis: Systemic lupus erythematosus

27 The answer is D: Selective IgA deficiency. Selective IgA deficiency is the most common primary immunodeficiency syndrome, with an incidence of 1:700 among Europeans. Although patients are often asymptomatic, they occasionally present with respiratory or gastrointestinal infections of varying severity. They also display a strong predilection for allergies and collagen vascular diseases. Patients with IgA deficiency have normal numbers of IgA-bearing B cells, and their varied defects result in an inability to synthesize and secrete IgA subclasses. Patients with chronic mucocutaneous candidiasis (choice B) show an increased susceptibility to *Candida* infections and also may exhibit various endocrine disorders (e.g., hypoparathyroidism and Addison disease). The other choices are associated with severe immunodeficiency.
Diagnosis: Selective IgA deficiency

28 The answer is C: Interstitial infiltrates of lymphocytes and macrophages. Transplant rejection reactions have been traditionally categorized into hyperacute, acute, and chronic rejection based on the clinical tempo of the response and on the mechanisms involved. Acute rejection is characterized by an abrupt onset of azotemia and oliguria, which may be associated with fever and graft tenderness. A needle biopsy would be expected to show (1) interstitial infiltrates of lymphocytes and macrophages, (2) edema, (3) lymphocytic tubulitis, and (4) tubular necrosis. Neutrophilic vasculitis and fibrinoid necrosis (choice D) are seen in hyperacute rejection. Arterial intimal thickening (choice A), glomerulosclerosis (choice B), and tubular atrophy (choice E) are seen in chronic graft rejection.

Diagnosis: Acute graft rejection

29 **The answer is D: High endothelial venules (HEVs).** B and T lymphocytes circulate via the vascular system to secondary lymphoid organs and tissues. Included among these tissues are lymph nodes, mucosa-associated lymphoid tissues, and spleen. In the case of lymph nodes, lymphocyte trafficking occurs through specialized postcapillary venules termed high endothelial venules (HEVs). HEVs express an array of specific cell adhesion molecules (e.g., CD31) that allow lymphocyte binding and diapedesis. The cuboidal shape of HEV cells reduces flow-mediated shear forces and specialized intercellular connections facilitate egress of lymphocytes out of the vascular space. Afferent and efferent lymphatic channels (choices A and B) do not possess HEVs. Hassall corpuscles (choice C) are found in the medulla of the thymus. Peyer patches (choice E) are organized lymphoid tissues found in the small intestine.

Diagnosis: Lymphadenopathy, streptococcal pharyngitis

30 **The answer is A: CD4.** The HIV-1 genome consists of two identical 9.7-kb single strands of RNA enclosed within a core of viral proteins. The core is enveloped by a phospholipid bilayer derived from the host cell membrane, in which are found virally encoded glycoproteins (gp120 and gp41). In addition to the *gag*, *pol*, and *env* genes—characteristic of all replication-competent RNA viruses—HIV-1 contains six other genes that code for proteins involved in replication. The specific target cells for HIV-1 are CD4+ helper T lymphocytes and mononuclear phagocytes, although infection of other cells occurs. The HIV envelope glycoprotein gp120 (either on the free virus or on the surface of an infected cell) binds CD4 on the surface of helper T lymphocytes. The binding of gp120 to CD4 allows gp41 to insert into the cell membrane of the lymphocyte, thereby promoting fusion of the viral envelope with the lymphocyte. Entry of HIV-1 into a target cell in vivo also requires viral binding to a coreceptor, β-chemokine receptor 5 (CCR-5). Choices C and D (gp41 and gp120) are involved in viral replication, but they are present on the viral envelope. Choice E (LFA-1) is a member of the leukocyte integrin family that is involved in cell-cell adhesion.

Diagnosis: Acquired immunodeficiency

Chapter 5

Neoplasia

QUESTIONS

Select the single best answer.

1 A 25-year-old man presents 1 week after discovering that his left testicle is twice the normal size. Physical examination reveals a nontender, testicular mass that cannot be transilluminated. Serum levels of alpha-fetoprotein and human chorionic gonadotropin are normal. A hemiorchiectomy is performed, and histologic examination of the surgical specimen shows embryonal carcinoma. Compared to normal adult somatic cells, this germ cell neoplasm would most likely show high levels of expression of which of the following proteins?

(A) Desmin
(B) Dystrophin
(C) Cytochrome *c*
(D) P selectin
(E) Telomerase

2 A 25-year-old woman presents for a gynecologic examination. The cervical Pap smear shows "koilocytic atypia" characterized by perinuclear halos and wrinkled nuclei (shown in the image). A cervical biopsy reveals invasive squamous cell carcinoma. Molecular tests for human papillomavirus (HPV) in the tumor cells are positive. Which of the following mechanisms of disease best explains the role of HPV in the pathogenesis of neoplasia in this patient?

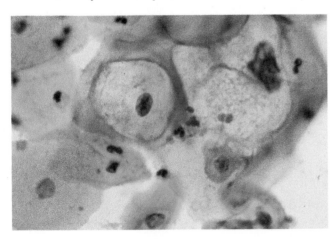

(A) Activation of cellular oncogenes
(B) Enhanced transcription of telomerase gene
(C) Episomal viral replication
(D) Inactivation of tumor suppressor proteins
(E) Insertional mutagenesis

3 The patient described in Question 2 undergoes a hysterectomy. In addition to a focus of invasive carcinoma, the pathologist identifies dysplastic squamous cells occupying the entire thickness of the cervical epithelium, with no evidence of epithelial maturation. The basal membrane in these areas appears intact. Which of the following terms best describes this cervical lesion?

(A) Atypical hyperplasia
(B) Carcinoma in situ
(C) Carcinomatosis
(D) Complex hyperplasia
(E) Koilocytic atypia

4 A 62-year-old woman presents with a breast lump that she discovered 6 days ago. A breast biopsy shows lobular carcinoma in situ. Compared to normal epithelial cells of the breast lobule, these malignant cells would most likely show decreased expression of which of the following proteins?

(A) Desmin
(B) E-cadherin
(C) Lysyl hydroxylase
(D) P selectin
(E) Telomerase

5 An 80-year-old man complains of lower abdominal pain, increasing weakness, and fatigue. He has lost 16 lb (7.3 kg) in the past 6 months. The prostate-specific antigen test is elevated (8.5 ng/mL). Rectal examination reveals an enlarged and nodular prostate. A needle biopsy of the prostate discloses invasive prostatic adenocarcinoma. Histologic grading of this patient's carcinoma is based primarily on which of the following criteria?

(A) Capsular involvement
(B) Extent of regional lymph nodes involvement
(C) Pulmonary metastases
(D) Resemblance to normal tissue of origin
(E) Volume of prostate involved by tumor

6 A 50-year-old woman presents with a lump in her breast. A 4-cm firm and fixed mass is noted on breast examination. Excisional biopsy reveals malignant cells that form gland-like structures and solid nests, surrounded by a dense collagenous stroma. A connective tissue stain (trichrome) of the biopsy is shown in the image. Which of the following descriptive terms best describes the blue areas observed in this specimen?

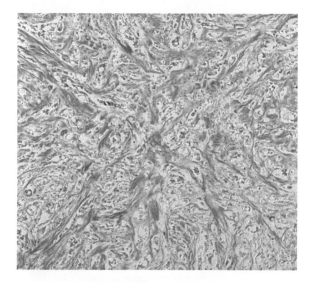

(A) Colloid carcinoma
(B) Comedocarcinoma
(C) Desmoplastic change
(D) Medullary carcinoma
(E) Papillomatosis

7 A 65-year-old man complains of muscle weakness and a dry cough for 4 months. He has smoked two packs of cigarettes daily for 45 years. A chest X-ray shows a 4-cm central, left lung mass. Laboratory studies reveal hyperglycemia and hypertension. A transbronchial biopsy is diagnosed as small cell carcinoma. Metastases to the liver are detected by CT scan. Which of the following might account for the development of hyperglycemia and hypertension in this patient?

(A) Adrenal metastases
(B) Paraneoplastic syndrome
(C) Pituitary adenoma
(D) Pituitary metastases
(E) Thrombosis of the renal artery

8 A 60-year-old man presents with a 4-month history of increasing weight loss, wheezing, and shortness of breath. He has smoked two packs of cigarettes a day for 40 years. His past medical history is significant for emphysema and chronic bronchitis. A chest X-ray shows a 10-cm mass in the left lung. Bronchoscopy discloses obstruction of the left main stem bronchus. A biopsy is obtained (shown in the image). Immunohistochemical studies of this biopsy specimen would most likely show strong expression of which of the following tumor markers?

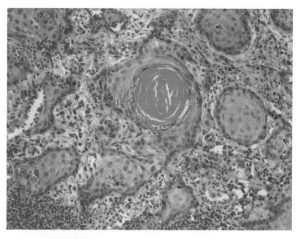

(A) Alpha-fetoprotein
(B) Calretinin
(C) Carcinoembryonic antigen
(D) Cytokeratins
(E) Synaptophysin

9 Which of the following potent carcinogens was most likely involved in the pathogenesis of lung cancer in the patient described in Question 8?

(A) Aflatoxin B_1
(B) Asbestos
(C) Azo dyes
(D) Polycyclic aromatic hydrocarbons
(E) Vinyl chloride

10 A 33-year-old woman discovers a lump in her left breast on self-examination. Her mother and sister both had breast cancer. A mammogram demonstrates an ill-defined density in the outer quadrant of the left breast, with microcalcifications. Needle aspiration reveals the presence of malignant, ductal epithelial cells. Genetic screening identifies a mutation in *BRCA1*. In addition to cell cycle control, BRCA1 protein promotes which of the following cellular functions?

(A) Apoptosis
(B) Cell adhesion
(C) DNA repair
(D) Gene transcription
(E) Transmembrane signaling

11 A 60-year-old man who worked for 30 years in a chemical factory complains of blood in his urine. Urine cytology discloses dysplastic cells. A bladder biopsy demonstrates transitional cell carcinoma. Which of the following carcinogens was most likely involved in the pathogenesis of bladder cancer in this patient?

(A) Aniline dyes
(B) Arsenic
(C) Benzene
(D) Cisplatinum
(E) Vinyl chloride

12 A 60-year-old man presents with an ulcerated, encrusted, and infiltrating lesion on the sun-exposed dorsal aspect of a finger (shown in the image). A biopsy reveals squamous cell carcinoma. The metastatic potential of this neoplasm would be enhanced by upregulation of the gene for which of the following proteins?

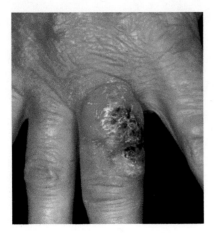

(A) Collagen type IV
(B) Desmin
(C) E-cadherin
(D) Glutathione peroxidase
(E) Plasminogen activator

13 A 45-year-old man presents with a 9-month history of a reddish nodule on his foot. Biopsy of the nodule discloses a poorly demarcated lesion composed of fibroblasts and endothelial-like cells lining vascular spaces. Further work-up identifies similar lesions in the lymph nodes and liver. The tumor cells contain sequences of human herpesvirus-8 (HHV-8). This patient most likely has which of the following diseases?
(A) Acquired immunodeficiency
(B) Ataxia telangiectasia
(C) Li-Fraumeni syndrome
(D) Neurofibromatosis type I
(E) Xeroderma pigmentosum

14 During a routine checkup, a 50-year-old man is found to have blood in his urine. He is otherwise in excellent health. An abdominal CT scan reveals a 2-cm right renal mass. You inform the patient that staging of this tumor is key to selecting treatment and evaluating prognosis. Which of the following is the most important staging factor for this patient?
(A) Histologic grade of the tumor
(B) Metastases to regional lymph nodes
(C) Proliferative capacity of the tumor cells
(D) Somatic mutations in the *p53* tumor suppressor gene
(E) Tumor cell karyotype (aneuploidy)

15 A 68-year-old man who has worked in a shipyard and manufacturing plant all his adult life complains of a 4-month history of chest discomfort, malaise, fever, night sweats, and weight loss. A chest X-ray reveals a large pleural effusion. The patient dies 5 months later of cardiorespiratory failure. The lung at autopsy is shown in the image. This malignant neoplasm is associated with environmental exposure to which of the following carcinogens?

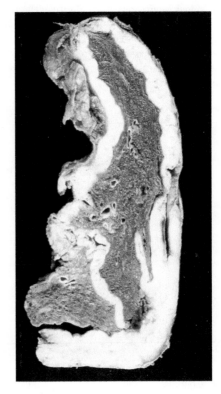

(A) Aflatoxin B_1
(B) Asbestos
(C) Beryllium
(D) Ionizing radiation
(E) Silica

16 A 58-year-old woman with colon cancer presents with 3 months of increasing shortness of breath. A chest X-ray reveals numerous, bilateral, round masses in both lungs. Histologic examination of an open-lung biopsy discloses malignant gland-like structures, which are nearly identical to the colon primary. Which of the following changes in cell behavior was the first step in the process leading to tumor metastasis from the colon to the lung in this patient?
(A) Arrest within the circulating blood or lymph
(B) Exit from the circulation into a new tissue
(C) Invasion of the underlying basement membrane
(D) Penetration of vascular or lymphatic channels
(E) Stimulation of angiogenesis within the pulmonary metastases

17 A 68-year-old man complains of recent changes in bowel habits and blood-tinged stools. Colonoscopy reveals a 3-cm mass in the sigmoid colon. Biopsy of the mass shows infiltrating malignant glands. These neoplastic cells have most likely acquired a set of mutations that cause which of the following changes in cell behavior?
(A) Decreased cellular motility
(B) Enhanced stem cell differentiation
(C) Increased cell-cell adhesion
(D) Increased susceptibility to apoptosis
(E) Loss of cell cycle restriction point control

18 A 35-year-old woman complains of nipple discharge and irregular menses of 5 months duration. Physical examination reveals a milky discharge from both nipples. MRI shows an enlargement of the anterior pituitary. Which of the following is the most likely histologic diagnosis of this patient's pituitary tumor?

(A) Adenoma

(B) Choristoma

(C) Hamartoma

(D) Papilloma

(E) Teratoma

19 A 52-year-old woman presents with a 1-year history of upper truncal obesity and moderate depression. Physical examination shows hirsutism and moon facies. A CT scan of the thorax displays a hilar mass. A transbronchial lung biopsy discloses small cell carcinoma. Electron microscopy of this patient's lung tumor will most likely reveal which of the following cytologic features?

(A) Councilman bodies

(B) Hyperplasia of endoplasmic reticulum

(C) Mitochondrial calcification

(D) Myelin figures in lysosomes

(E) Neuroendocrine granules

20 Cytogenetic studies in a 40-year-old woman with follicular lymphoma demonstrate a t(14;18) chromosomal translocation involving the *bcl-2* gene. Constitutive expression of the protein encoded by the *bcl-2* gene inhibits which of the following processes in this patient's transformed lymphocytes?

(A) Apoptosis

(B) DNA excision repair

(C) G1-to-S cell cycle progression

(D) Oxidative phosphorylation

(E) Protein (*N*-linked) glycosylation

21 A 60-year-old man presents with a 6-month history of increasing weight loss and fatigue. Physical examination reveals conspicuous hepatomegaly. An abdominal CT scan reveals multiple "canon ball" nodules in the liver (shown in the image). A CT-guided biopsy reveals a mucous-secreting adenocarcinoma. This patient's metastatic liver cancer most likely originated in which of the following anatomic locations?

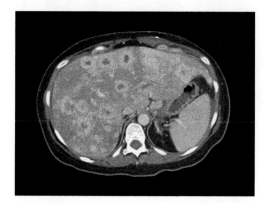

(A) Adrenal medulla

(B) Bone marrow

(C) Brain

(D) Pancreas

(E) Urinary bladder

22 A 59-year-old woman presents with increasing pigmentation of the skin. Physical examination shows hyperkeratosis and hyperpigmentation of the axilla, neck, flexures, and anogenital region. Endocrinologic studies reveal normal serum levels of adrenal corticosteroids and glucocorticoids. If this patient's skin pigmentation represents a paraneoplastic syndrome, the primary tumor would most likely be found in which of the following anatomic locations?

(A) Bladder

(B) Cervix

(C) Esophagus

(D) Pleura

(E) Stomach

23 A 65-year-old man dies after a protracted battle with metastatic colon carcinoma. At autopsy, the liver is filled with multiple nodules of cancer, many of which display central necrosis (umbilication). Which of the following best explains the pathogenesis of tumor umbilication in this patient?

(A) Biphasic tumor

(B) Chronic inflammation

(C) Granulomatous inflammation

(D) Ischemia and infarction

(E) Stimulation of angiogenesis

24 A 59-year-old man complains of progressive weakness. He reports that his stools are very dark. Physical examination demonstrates fullness in the right lower quadrant. Laboratory studies show iron deficiency anemia, with a serum hemoglobin level of 7.4 g/dL. Stool specimens are positive for occult blood. Colonoscopy discloses an ulcerating lesion of the cecum. Which of the following serum tumor markers is most likely to be useful for following this patient after surgery?

(A) Alpha-fetoprotein

(B) Carcinoembryonic antigen

(C) Chorionic gonadotropin

(D) Chromogranin

(E) Coagulation factor VIII

25 Laboratory studies of the surgical specimen obtained from the patient described in Question 24 demonstrate hypermethylation of the *p53* gene. Which of the following best characterizes this biochemical change in the neoplastic cells?

(A) Epigenetic modification

(B) Gene amplification

(C) Insertional mutagenesis

(D) Nonreciprocal translocation

(E) Protooncogene mutation

26 A 20-year-old woman has an ovarian tumor removed. The surgical specimen is 10 cm in diameter and cystic. The cystic cavity is found to contain black hair and sebaceous material. Histologic examination of the cyst wall reveals a variety of benign differentiated tissues, including skin, cartilage, brain, and mucinous glandular epithelium. What is the diagnosis?

(A) Adenoma

(B) Chondroma

(C) Hamartoma

(D) Teratocarcinoma

(E) Teratoma

27 A 42-year-old man presents with upper gastrointestinal bleeding. Upper endoscopy and biopsy reveal gastric adenocarcinoma. Which country of the world has the highest incidence of this malignant neoplasm?
(A) Argentina
(B) Canada
(C) Japan
(D) Mexico
(E) United States

28 An 8-year-old girl with numerous hypopigmented, ulcerated, and crusted patches on her face and forearms develops an indurated, crater-like, skin nodule on the back of her left hand. Biopsy of this skin nodule discloses a squamous cell carcinoma. Molecular biology studies reveal that this patient has germline mutations in the gene encoding a nucleotide excision repair enzyme. What is the appropriate diagnosis?
(A) Ataxia telangiectasia
(B) Hereditary albinism
(C) Li-Fraumeni syndrome
(D) Neurofibromatosis, type I
(E) Xeroderma pigmentosum

29 A 59-year-old woman complains of "feeling light-headed" and losing 5 kg (11 lb) in the last month. A CBC reveals a normocytic, normochromic anemia. The patient subsequently dies of metastatic cancer. Based on current epidemiologic data for cancer-associated mortality in women, which of the following is the most likely primary site for this patient's malignant neoplasm?
(A) Brain
(B) Breast
(C) Colon
(D) Lung
(E) Urinary bladder

30 The parents of a 6-month-old girl palpate a mass on the left side of the child's abdomen. Urinalysis shows high levels of vanillylmandelic acid. A CT scan reveals an abdominal tumor and bony metastases. The primary tumor is surgically resected. Histologic examination of the surgical specimen discloses neuroblastoma. Evaluation of the N-*myc* protooncogene in this child's tumor will most likely demonstrate which of the following genetic changes?
(A) Chromosomal translocation
(B) Exon deletion
(C) Expansion of a trinucleotide repeat
(D) Frameshift mutation
(E) Gene amplification

31 An 8-year-old African boy presents with swelling in his jaw and massive facial disfiguration. Biopsy reveals a tumor invading the bone marrow of the jaw. The pathogenesis of this malignant neoplasm is associated with a virus that exhibits a tropism for which of the following cells?

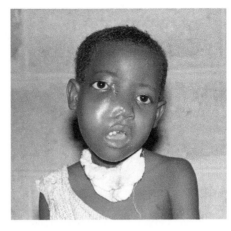

(A) Chondrocytes
(B) Fibroblasts
(C) Lymphocytes
(D) Macrophages
(E) Osteocytes

32 A 58-year-old woman undergoes routine colonoscopy. A 2-cm submucosal nodule is identified in the appendix. Biopsy of the nodule shows nests of cells with round, uniform nuclei. Electron microscopy reveals numerous neuroendocrine granules in the cytoplasm. This patient's neoplastic disease is associated with which of the following clinical features?
(A) Congestive heart failure
(B) Flushing and wheezing
(C) Muscular dystrophy
(D) Progressive systemic sclerosis
(E) Pulmonary embolism

33 A 55-year-old woman presents with increasing weight loss and fatigue and subsequently dies of metastatic cancer. The vertebral column at autopsy is shown in the image. What is the diagnosis?

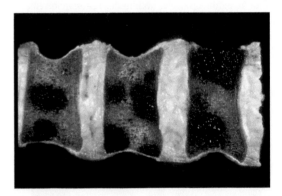

(A) Chondrosarcoma
(B) Melanoma
(C) Multiple myeloma
(D) Osteosarcoma
(E) Rhabdomyosarcoma

34 A 45-year-old woman presents with abdominal pain and vaginal bleeding. A hysterectomy is performed and shows a benign tumor of the uterus derived from a smooth muscle cell. What is the appropriate diagnosis?
(A) Angiomyolipoma
(B) Leiomyoma
(C) Leiomyosarcoma
(D) Myxoma
(E) Rhabdomyoma

35 Cytogenetic studies in a 70-year-old woman with chronic myelogenous leukemia (CML) demonstrate a t(9;22) chromosomal translocation. Which of the following best explains the role of this translocation in the pathogenesis of leukemia in this patient?
(A) Altered DNA methylation status
(B) Enhanced expression of telomerase gene
(C) Expansion of a trinucleotide repeat
(D) Inactivation of tumor suppressor protein
(E) Protooncogene activation

36 A 33-year-old woman presents with a diffuse scaly skin rash of 4 weeks duration. Biopsy of lesional skin reveals a cutaneous T-cell lymphoma (mycosis fungoides). Which of the following immunohistochemical markers would be most useful for identifying malignant cells in the skin of this patient?
(A) Calcitonin
(B) CD4
(C) Desmin
(D) HMB-45
(E) S-100

37 A 63-year-old woman with chronic bronchitis presents with shortness of breath. A chest X-ray reveals a 2-cm "coin lesion" in the upper lobe of the left lung. A CT-guided lung biopsy is obtained. Which of the following describes the histologic features of this lesion if the diagnosis is hamartoma?
(A) Benign neoplasm of epithelial origin
(B) Disorganized normal tissue
(C) Ectopic islands of normal tissue
(D) Granulation tissue
(E) Granulomatous inflammation

38 A 67-year-old woman presents with a massively swollen abdomen. The patient was diagnosed with papillary, serous cystadenocarcinoma of the ovary 3 years ago. She dies in a hospice 1 month later. At autopsy, the peritoneum is studded with small tumors (shown in the image), and there are 4 L of ascites. Which of the following routes of tumor metastasis accounts for these autopsy findings?

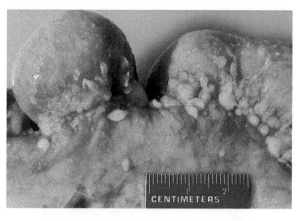

(A) Direct tumor extension
(B) Hematogenous spread
(C) Lymphatic spread
(D) Seeding of body cavity
(E) Venous spread

39 A 2-year-old boy is found to have bilateral retinal tumors. Molecular studies demonstrate a germline mutation in one allele of the *Rb* gene. Which of the following genetic events best explains the mechanism of carcinogenesis in this patient?
(A) Balanced translocation
(B) Expansion of trinucleotide repeat
(C) Gene amplification
(D) Loss of heterozygosity
(E) Maternal nondisjunction

40 A 48-year-old nulliparous woman complains that her menstrual blood flow is more abundant than usual. An ultrasound examination reveals a polypoid mass in the uterine fundus. The patient subsequently, undergoes a hysterectomy, which reveals a poorly differentiated endometrial adenocarcinoma. The development of this neoplasm was preceded by which of the following histopathologic changes in the glandular epithelium?
(A) Atrophy
(B) Hydropic swelling
(C) Hyperplasia
(D) Hypertrophy
(E) Metaplasia

41 A 53-year-old woman with a longstanding history of ulcerative colitis presents with increasing chest pain and shortness of breath of 2 months duration. She reports four recent episodes of hemoptysis. The patient subsequently develops overwhelming sepsis and expires. A section through the right lung is examined at autopsy (shown in the image). What is the appropriate diagnosis?

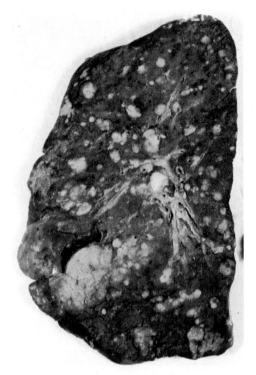

(A) Carcinoid tumor of the lung
(B) Primary adenocarcinoma of the lung
(C) Metastatic carcinoma of the lung
(D) Miliary tuberculosis
(E) Sarcoidosis

42 A 50-year-old woman presents with a 2-year history of upper truncal obesity and depression. Serum levels of glucose and cortisol are elevated. A CT scan of the abdomen reveals a 2-cm suprarenal mass. The surgical specimen is shown in the image. If this neoplasm is benign, which of the following is the most appropriate diagnosis?

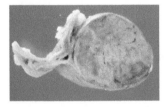

(A) Adenoma
(B) Chondroma
(C) Lipoma
(D) Papilloma
(E) Teratoma

43 A 65-year-old man presents with a pearly papule on his upper lip (patient shown in the image). A biopsy reveals buds of atypical, deeply basophilic keratinocytes extending from the overlying epidermis into the papillary dermis. Which of the following carcinogenic stimuli was the most important risk factor for development of this patient's skin cancer?

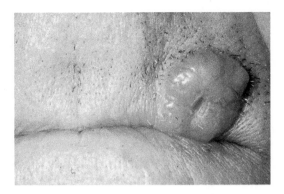

(A) Aflatoxin B_1
(B) Divalent metal cations
(C) Aromatic amines and azo dyes
(D) Vinyl chloride
(E) Sunlight

44 A 28-year-old man with a familial disease affecting the gastrointestinal tract undergoes a colectomy. The surgical specimen is shown in the image. Molecular studies demonstrate a germline mutation in the *APC* gene. The normal product of this gene (protooncogene) primarily regulates which of the following cell behaviors?

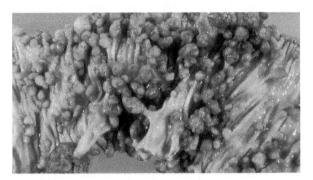

(A) Apoptosis
(B) Autophagy
(C) Cell cycle
(D) Differentiation
(E) Motility

ANSWERS

1 **The answer is E: Telomerase.** Somatic cells do not normally express telomerase, which is an enzyme that adds repetitive sequences to maintain the length of the telomere. Thus, with each round of somatic cell replication, the telomere shortens. The length of telomeres may act as a "molecular clock" and govern the lifespan of replicating cells. Because cancer cells and embryonic cells express high levels of telomerase, the reactivation of this enzyme may be important for maintaining stem cell proliferation. Most human cancers show activation of the gene for the catalytic subunit of telomerase: human telomerase reverse transcriptase. P selectin (choice D) is a cell adhesion molecule that mediates the margination of neutrophils during acute inflammation. The other choices are not involved in malignant transformation.

Diagnosis: Embryonal carcinoma

2 The answer is D: Inactivation of tumor suppressor proteins. Unlike RNA tumor viruses, whose oncogenes have normal cellular counterparts, the transforming genes of DNA viruses are not homologous with any cellular genes. This conundrum was resolved with the discovery that the gene products of oncogenic DNA viruses inactivate tumor suppressor proteins. For example, proteins encoded by the *E6* and *E7* genes of HPV16 bind p53 and pRb. The other choices are involved in the pathogenesis of neoplasia, but they are not specific for HPV.

Diagnosis: Cervical intraepithelial neoplasia, HPV infection

3 The answer is B: Carcinoma in situ. Most carcinomas begin as localized growths confined to the epithelium in which they arise. As long as these early cancers do not penetrate the basement membrane on which the epithelium rests, such tumors are labeled carcinoma in situ. When the in situ tumor acquires invasive potential and extends directly through the underlying basement membrane, it is in a position to compromise neighboring tissues and metastasize. Carcinomatosis (choice C) is a clinical term used to describe widespread dissemination of cancer. Koilocytosis (choice E) implies the presence of squamous cells with perinuclear halos and nuclear changes. It is indicative of human papillomavirus infection and carries an increased risk of carcinoma. Atypical and complex hyperplasia (choices A and D) refer to proliferative lesions of the glands within the uterine endometrium.

Diagnosis: Cervical carcinoma, carcinoma in situ

4 The answer is B: E-cadherin. Cadherins are Ca^{2+}-dependent transmembrane glycoproteins that mediated cell–cell adhesion. E-cadherin is expressed on the surface of all epithelia and mediates cell adhesion by "zipper-like" interactions. Overall, cadherins suppress invasion and metastasis. Thus, it is perhaps not surprising that the expression of E-cadherin is reduced in most carcinomas. Desmin (choice A) is an intermediate filament protein found in cells of mesenchymal origin. Lysyl hydroxylase (choice C) is involved in the posttranslational modification of collagen. P selectin is a cell adhesion molecule that mediates the margination of neutrophils during acute inflammation. Telomerase (choice E) is increased in certain malignancies.

Diagnosis: Breast cancer

5 The answer is D: Resemblance to normal tissue of origin. To establish criteria for therapy, many cancers are classified according to histologic grading schemes or by staging protocols that describe the extent of spread. Cancer grading reflects cellular characteristics. Low-grade tumors are well differentiated, whereas high-grade tumors lack differentiated features (anaplasia). The general correlation between cytologic grade and the behavior of a neoplasm is not invariable. Indeed, there are many examples of tumors of low cytologic grades that exhibit substantial malignant properties. The other choices pertain to cancer staging.

Diagnosis: Prostate cancer

6 The answer is C: Desmoplastic change. Secondary descriptors are used to refer to a tumor's morphologic and functional characteristics. Papillomatosis (choice E) describes frond-like structures. Medullary (choice D) signifies a soft cellular tumor, whereas scirrhous or desmoplastic implies dense fibrous stroma. Colloid carcinomas (choice A) secrete abundant mucus. Comedocarcinoma (choice B) is an intraductal neoplasm in which necrotic material can be expressed from the ducts.

Diagnosis: Breast cancer

7 The answer is B: Paraneoplastic syndrome. Cancers may produce remote effects, collectively termed paraneoplastic syndromes. For example, the secretion of corticotropin (ACTH) by a tumor leads to clinical features of Cushing syndrome, including hyperglycemia and hypertension. Corticotropin production is most commonly seen with cancers of the lung, particularly small cell carcinoma. Adrenal and pituitary metastases (choices A and D) would lead to loss of adrenal function (Addison disease). Although pituitary adenoma (choice C) is a possible cause of Cushing syndrome, this choice would be unlikely in a patient with lung cancer.

Diagnosis: Small cell carcinoma of lung, paraneoplastic syndrome

8 The answer is D: Cytokeratins. Tumor markers are products of malignant neoplasms that can be detected in cells or body fluids. Useful tumor markers include immunoglobulins, fetal proteins, enzymes, hormones, and cytoskeletal proteins. Carcinomas uniformly express cytokeratins, which are intermediate filaments. Alpha-fetoprotein (choice A) is a marker for yolk sac carcinoma and hepatocellular carcinoma. Calretinin (choice B) provides a marker for mesothelioma. Carcinoembryonic antigen (choice C) is a marker for colon carcinoma and many other malignancies. Synaptophysin (choice E) is a marker for neuroendocrine tumors, including small cell carcinoma of the lung.

Diagnosis: Squamous cell carcinoma of lung

9 The answer is D: Polycyclic aromatic hydrocarbons. Polycyclic aromatic hydrocarbons, originally derived from coal tar, are among the most extensively studied carcinogens. These compounds produce cancers at the site of application. Since polycyclic hydrocarbons have been identified in cigarette smoke, it has been suggested (but not proved) that they are involved in the pathogenesis of lung cancer. Aflatoxin B_1 (choice A), a natural product of the fungus *Aspergillus flavus*, is among the most potent liver carcinogens. Asbestos (choice B), a mineral, is associated with mesothelioma and adenocarcinoma of lung. Industrial workers exposed to high levels of vinyl chloride (choice E) in the ambient atmosphere developed angiosarcomas of the liver.

Diagnosis: Squamous cell carcinoma of lung

10 The answer is C: DNA repair. Breast (BR) cancer (CA) susceptibility genes (*BRCA1* and *BRCA2*) encode tumor suppressor proteins involved in checkpoint functions related to progression of the cell cycle into S phase. BRCA1 and BRCA2 proteins also promote DNA repair by binding to RAD51, a molecule that mediates DNA double-strand repair breaks. The other choices may be abnormal in neoplasia, but they are not primarily affected by BRCA1.

Diagnosis: Breast cancer

11 **The answer is A: Aniline dyes.** Transitional cell carcinoma is the most common malignant tumor of the urinary bladder, and the incidence of bladder cancer is increased in aniline dye workers. These azo dyes are converted to water-soluble carcinogens in the liver. They are excreted in the urine, where they primarily affect the transitional epithelium of the bladder. Benzene exposure (choice C) is associated with leukemia. Vinyl chloride exposure (choice E) has been associated with hepatic angiosarcomas.
Diagnosis: Transitional cell carcinoma of bladder

12 **The answer is E: Plasminogen activator.** Malignant cells and stromal cells associated with cancers elaborate a variety of proteases that degrade basement membrane components. Such enzymes include the urokinase-type plasminogen activator (u-PA) and matrix metalloproteinases. u-PA converts serum plasminogen to plasmin, a serine protease that degrades laminin and activates type IV procollagenase. Changes in the expression of u-PA, the u-PA receptor, and PA inhibitors have been reported in different cancers. Metastatic cells would be expected to show reduced expression of collagens (choice A) and cadherins (choice C). Desmin (choice B) is found in cells of mesenchymal origin.
Diagnosis: Squamous cell carcinoma of skin

13 **The answer is A: Acquired immunodeficiency.** Kaposi sarcoma is the most common neoplasm associated with acquired immunodeficiency syndrome (AIDS). The neoplastic cells contain sequences of a novel virus, HHV-8, which is also known as Kaposi sarcoma–associated herpesvirus. In addition to infecting the spindle cells of Kaposi sarcoma, HHV-8 is lymphotropic and has been implicated in two uncommon B-cell lymphoid malignancies, namely, primary effusion lymphoma and multicentric Castleman disease. Like other DNA viruses, the HHV-8 genome encodes proteins that interfere with the p53 and pRb tumor suppressor pathways. The other choices are hereditary conditions associated with cancer; however, these patients do not typically acquire Kaposi sarcoma. The predominant malignancy seen in patients with ataxia telangiectasia (choice B) is lymphoma/leukemia.
Diagnosis: Kaposi sarcoma, AIDS

14 **The answer is B: Metastases to regional lymph nodes.** The choice of surgical approach or treatment modalities is influenced more by the stage of a cancer than by its cytologic grade. The significant criteria used for staging vary with different organs. Commonly used criteria include (1) tumor size, (2) extent of local growth, (3) presence of lymph node metastases, and (4) presence of distant metastases. The other choices reflect grade of the tumor.
Diagnosis: Renal cell carcinoma

15 **The answer is B: Asbestos.** The characteristic tumor associated with asbestos exposure is mesothelioma of the pleural and peritoneal cavities. This cancer has been reported to occur in 2% to 3% of heavily exposed workers. The pipe fitters in shipyards were the most exposed workers. Many of these workers developed mesotheliomas 20 to 40 years after exposure. It is reasonable to surmise that mesotheliomas of both the pleura and the peritoneum reflect the close contact of these membranes with asbestos fibers transported to them by lymphatic channels. Like the polycyclic aromatic hydrocarbons, aflatoxin B_1 (choice A) can bind covalently to DNA and is among the most potent liver carcinogens recognized. Beryllium (choice C) and silica (choice E) cause lung disease, but they are not carcinogenic.
Diagnosis: Mesothelioma

16 **The answer is C: Invasion of the underlying basement membrane.** The first event in tumor cell invasion is breach of the basement membrane that separates an epithelium from the underlying mesenchyme. After invading the interstitial tissue, malignant cells penetrate lymphatic or vascular channels (choice D). In the lymph nodes, communications between the lymphatics and venous tributaries allow malignant cells access to the systemic circulation. The other choices are important for tumor metastases, but they occur later than basement membrane invasion.
Diagnosis: Adenocarcinoma of colon

17 **The answer is E: Loss of cell cycle restriction point control.** Cancer cells often display loss of cell cycle restriction point control through mechanisms such as overexpression of cyclin D1, loss of Cdk inhibitors, or inactivation of the pRb or p53 proteins. The *p53* gene is deleted or mutated in 75% of cases of colorectal cancer and frequently mutated in numerous other tumors. The p53 protein is a negative regulator of cell division. Inactivating mutations of *p53* cause loss of cell cycle restriction point control and allow cells with damaged DNA to progress through the cell cycle. Malignant cells have increased cellular motility (see choice A), reduced stem cell differentiation (see choice B), decreased cell adhesion (see choice C), and decreased susceptibility to apoptosis (see choice D).
Diagnosis: Adenocarcinoma of colon

18 **The answer is A: Adenoma.** Benign tumors arising from a glandular epithelium are termed adenomas. Patients with a prolactin-secreting pituitary adenoma present with amenorrhea and galactorrhea. Ectopic islands of normal tissue are called choristomas (choice B). Localized, disordered differentiation during development results in a hamartoma (choice C). Papillomas (choice D) do not occur in the pituitary. Benign tumors that arise from germ cells and contain all three germ layers are termed teratomas (choice E).
Diagnosis: Pituitary adenoma, prolactinoma

19 **The answer is E: Neuroendocrine granules.** Neuroendocrine tumors may synthesize a number of hormones. The presence of small, membrane-bound granules with a dense core is a feature of these neoplasms. Dense granules are visible by electron microscopy. In this way, electron microscopy may aid in the diagnosis of poorly differentiated cancers, whose classification is problematic by light microscopy. Carcinomas often exhibit desmosomes and specialized junctional complexes, which are structures that are not typical of sarcomas or lymphomas. Myelin figures (choice D) are seen in patients with inherited lysosomal storage disease. Councilman bodies (choice A) are apoptotic hepatocytes (acidophilic bodies).
Diagnosis: Small cell carcinoma of lung, paraneoplastic syndrome

20 The answer is A: Apoptosis. Many human cancers show abnormalities in the control of apoptosis. For example, follicular B-cell lymphomas display a characteristic chromosomal translocation in which the *bcl-2* gene is brought under the transcriptional control of the immunoglobulin light-chain gene promoter, thereby causing overexpression of *bcl-2*. As a result of the antiapoptotic properties of *bcl-2*, the neoplastic clone accumulates in lymph nodes. Since its demonstration in follicular lymphomas, *bcl-2* expression has been observed in a variety of other human cancers. None of the other choices describes the function of *bcl-2*.
Diagnosis: Follicular lymphoma

21 The answer is D: Pancreas. Radiologic evidence of "canon ball" lesions in the liver or lung suggests metastatic cancer. The liver is involved in a third of all metastatic cancers, including half of those of the gastrointestinal tract, breast, and lung. Other tumors that characteristically metastasize to the liver are pancreatic carcinoma and malignant melanoma. Liver metastases are the most common cause of massive hepatomegaly. Visible secretions of tumor cells, such as mucin or serous fluid, provide important clues for tumor diagnosis. Mucin-secreting glandular epithelium and mucin-secreting adenocarcinoma are expected in the pancreas. None of the other organs are composed of glandular epithelial cells or produce mucin.
Diagnosis: Metastatic cancer

22 The answer is E: Stomach. Acanthosis nigricans is a cutaneous disorder marked by hyperkeratosis and pigmentation of the axilla, neck, flexures, and anogenital region. It is of particular interest because more than half of patients with acanthosis nigricans have cancer. Over 90% of cases occur in association with gastrointestinal carcinomas (primarily stomach cancer). The other tumors are uncommon causes of acanthosis nigricans.
Diagnosis: Paraneoplastic syndrome, acanthosis nigricans

23 The answer is D: Ischemia and infarction. Angiogenesis is a requirement for the continued growth of cancers, whether primary or metastatic. In the absence of new vessels to supply the nutrients and remove waste products, malignant tumors do not grow larger than 1 to 2 mm in diameter. In general, causes of tumor cell death in situ include (1) programmed cell death (apoptosis); (2) inadequate blood supply, with consequent ischemia; (3) a paucity of nutrients; and (4) vulnerability to specific and nonspecific host defenses. The CT scan provided for Question 21 shows central necrosis (umbilication) in most of the metastatic tumor nodules. None of the other choices are likely causes of tumor necrosis.
Diagnosis: Metastatic cancer

24 The answer is B: Carcinoembryonic antigen (CEA). Colorectal cancer is asymptomatic in its initial stages. As the tumor grows, the most common sign is occult blood in feces, especially when the tumor is in the proximal portion of the colon. Chronic, asymptomatic bleeding typically causes iron-deficiency anemia. Adenocarcinomas of the colon usually express CEA, a glycoprotein that is released into the circulation and serves as a serologic marker for these tumors.

CEA is also found in association with malignant tumors of the pancreas, lung, and ovary. AFP (choice A) is expressed by hepatocellular carcinoma and yolk sac tumors. Chromogranin (choice D) is expressed by neuroendocrine tumors. Chorionic gonadotropin (choice C) is secreted by choriocarcinoma.
Diagnosis: Colon cancer

25 The answer is A: Epigenetic modification. Hypermethylation of many tumor suppressor and DNA repair genes has been demonstrated in human tumors. The pathways controlled by these genes are, therefore, suppressed. For example, the normal *p53* gene can be inactivated by hypermethylation. Thus, aberrant methylation of tumor suppressor genes may be an epigenetic mechanism for a "second hit," leading to loss of heterozygosity. Unlike genetic changes in cancer, epigenetic changes are reversible, and a search for drugs that influence DNA methylation is under way. The other choices are unrelated to DNA methylation.
Diagnosis: Colon cancer

26 The answer is E: Teratoma. Teratomas are benign tumors composed of tissues derived from all three primary germ layers: ectoderm, mesoderm, and endoderm. They are most common in the ovary but also occur in the testis and extragonadal sites. Teratocarcinomas (choice D) are malignant tumors that harbor embryonal carcinoma stem cells. Adenoma (choice A) is a benign tumor of epithelial origin. Chondroma (choice B) is a benign cartilaginous tumor. Hamartoma (choice C) is disorganized normal tissue.
Diagnosis: Mature teratoma

27 The answer is C: Japan. The highest incidence of stomach cancer occurs in Japan, where the disease is almost ten times as frequent as it is among American whites. A study of Japanese residents of Hawaii found that emigrants from Japanese regions with the highest risk of stomach cancer continued to exhibit an excess risk in Hawaii. By contrast, their offspring who were born in Hawaii had the same incidence of this cancer as American whites. The highest incidence of colorectal cancer is found in the United States (choice E).
Diagnosis: Gastric cancer

28 The answer is E: Xeroderma pigmentosum. Xeroderma pigmentosum is an autosomal recessive disease in which increased sensitivity to sunlight is accompanied by a high incidence of skin cancers, including basal cell carcinoma, squamous cell carcinoma, and malignant melanoma. Several xeroderma pigmentosum genes are involved in nucleotide excision of ultraviolet-damaged DNA. Li-Fraumeni syndrome (choice C) refers to an inherited predisposition to develop cancers in many organs due to germline mutations of *p53*. Ataxia telangiectasia (choice A) features cerebellar degeneration, immunologic abnormalities, and a predisposition to cancer. The mutated gene codes for a nuclear phosphoprotein involved in regulation of the cell cycle and DNA repair. Patients with hereditary albinism (choice B) are also at high risk for development of squamous cell carcinoma of the skin, but they do not have a defect in DNA excision repair. Patients with neurofibromatosis (choice D) develop benign cutaneous neurofibromas.
Diagnosis: Xeroderma pigmentosum

29 The answer is D: Lung. Lung carcinoma is the cause of most cancer-related deaths in the United States and Western Europe in men and women. The second most common cause of death from cancer in women is breast cancer (choice B). One of the most common findings in patients with cancer is anemia, but the mechanism for this paraneoplastic syndrome is not clear. The anemia is usually normocytic and normochromic, although iron deficiency anemia is common in cancers that bleed into the gastrointestinal tract.
Diagnosis: Lung cancer

30 The answer is E: Gene amplification. Chromosomal alterations that result in an increased number of copies of a gene have been found primarily in solid tumors. Such aberrations are recognized as (1) homogeneous staining regions (HSRs); (2) abnormal banding regions on chromosomes; or (3) double minutes, which are visualized as small, paired cytoplasmic bodies. In some cases, gene amplification has been shown to involve protooncogenes. For example, HSRs may be seen in neuroblastomas and are all derived from the N-*myc* protooncogene. The presence of N-*myc* HSRs is associated with up to 700-fold amplification of this gene and is a marker of advanced disease with a poor prognosis. Although the other choices are mechanisms for protooncogene activation, they do not cause upregulation of N-*myc* in patients with neuroblastoma.
Diagnosis: Neuroblastoma

31 The answer is C: Lymphocytes. Four DNA viruses (human papillomavirus, Epstein-Barr virus [EBV], hepatitis B virus, and herpesvirus-8) are incriminated in the development of human cancers. EBV was the first virus to be unequivocally linked to the development of a human tumor. In 1958, Burkitt described a form of childhood lymphoma in a geographical belt across equatorial Africa, which he suggested might have a viral etiology. A few years later, Epstein and Barr discovered viral particles in cell lines cultured from patients with Burkitt lymphoma. African Burkitt lymphoma is a B-cell tumor, in which the neoplastic lymphocytes invariably contain EBV in their DNA and manifest EBV-related antigens. EBV does not infect the other choices.
Diagnosis: Burkitt lymphoma, EBV

32 The answer is B: Flushing and wheezing. Carcinoid syndrome is a systemic paraneoplastic disease caused by the release of hormones from carcinoid tumors (via neuroendocrine granules) into venous blood. Symptoms of flushing, bronchial wheezing, watery diarrhea, and abdominal colic are caused by the release of serotonin, bradykinin, and histamine. Carcinoids are neuroendocrine tumors of low malignancy that are most commonly located in the submucosa of the intestines (e.g., appendix, terminal ileum, and rectum). The other choices are not associated with this paraneoplastic syndrome.
Diagnosis: Carcinoid tumor, paraneoplastic syndrome

33 The answer is B: Melanoma. The photograph shows pigmented cells in the vertebral bodies of a person who died of malignant melanoma. This autopsy finding illustrates the point that accurate tumor identification depends on morphologic resemblance to normal tissue. Tumor emboli in this case probably reached bone after surviving passage through the pulmonary microcirculation. None of the other tumors show pigmentation.
Diagnosis: Melanoma

34 The answer is B: Leiomyoma. Leiomyoma is the most common benign tumor of the uterus, usually arising in women of reproductive age. It originates from smooth muscle cells of the myometrium. None of the other choices are benign tumors of smooth muscle.
Diagnosis: Leiomyoma of uterus

35 The answer is E: Protooncogene activation. The best-known example of an acquired chromosomal translocation in a human cancer is the Philadelphia chromosome, which is found in 95% of patients with CML. The c-*abl* protooncogene on chromosome 9 is translocated to chromosome 22, it is placed in juxtaposition to the breakpoint cluster region (*bcr*). The c-*abl* gene and *bcr* region unite to produce a hybrid oncogene that codes for an aberrant protein with very high levels of tyrosine kinase activity, which generates mitogenic and antiapoptotic signals.
Diagnosis: Chronic myelogenous leukemia, Philadelphia chromosome

36 The answer is B: CD4. CD4 is a cluster-differentiation antigen of helper T lymphocytes. HMB-45 and S-100 (choices D and E) are markers for malignant melanoma, among other tumors. Calcitonin (choice A) is a peptide hormone. Desmin (choice C) is an intermediate filament protein found in cells of mesenchymal origin.
Diagnosis: Mycosis fungoides

37 The answer is B: Disorganized normal tissue. Localized, disordered differentiation during embryonic development results in a hamartoma, a disorganized caricature of normal tissue components. Such tumors, which are not strictly neoplasms, contain varying combinations of cartilage, ducts or bronchi, connective tissue, blood vessels, and lymphoid tissue. Ectopic islands of normal tissue (choice C), called choristoma, may also be mistaken for true neoplasms. These small lesions are represented by pancreatic tissue in the wall of the stomach or intestine, adrenal rests under the renal capsule, and nodules of splenic tissue in the peritoneal cavity.
Diagnosis: Hamartoma

38 The answer is D: Seeding of body cavity. The photograph shows a loop of small bowel and mesentery studded with small nodules of metastatic cancer. Malignant tumors that arise in organs adjacent to body cavities (e.g., ovaries, gastrointestinal tract, or lung) may shed malignant cells into these spaces. Such body cavities include principally the peritoneal and pleural cavities, although occasional seeding of the pericardial cavity, joint space, and subarachnoid space are observed. Tumor cells in these sites grow in masses and often produce fluid (e.g., ascites or pleural fluid), sometimes in massive quantities. Although the other choices provide routes for tumor metastasis, they do not lead to peritoneal carcinomatosis in patients with ovarian cancer.
Diagnosis: Ovarian cancer, carcinomatosis

39 **The answer is D: Loss of heterozygosity.** Retinoblastomas are malignant ocular tumors of young children. In cases of hereditary retinoblastoma, an affected child inherits one defective *Rb* allele together with one normal gene. This heterozygous state is not associated with any observable changes in the retina because 50% of the *Rb* gene product is sufficient to prevent the development of retinoblastoma. However, if the remaining normal *Rb* allele is inactivated by deletion or mutation, the loss of its suppressor function leads to the appearance of a neoplasm. This genetic process is referred to as loss of heterozygosity. The other choices have not been associated with the loss of tumor suppressor genes in somatic cells.

Diagnosis: Retinoblastoma

40 **The answer is C: Hyperplasia.** The cellular and molecular mechanisms of hyperplasia are related to the control of cell proliferation and provide a basis for further genetic changes that can lead to neoplasia. Endometrial hyperplasia refers to a spectrum that ranges from simple glandular crowding to conspicuous proliferation of atypical glands. These changes are often difficult to distinguish from carcinoma. The risk of developing endometrial cancer increases with higher degrees of endometrial hyperplasia. Estrogen exposure is thought to be a risk factor for both endometrial hyperplasia and endometrial carcinoma. Neoplastic transformation may occur in the setting of a metaplastic epithelium (e.g., cancers of the lung, cervix, stomach, and bladder); however, metaplasia (choice E) does not precede the development of uterine adenocarcinoma. The other choices do not represent risk factors for cancer.

Diagnosis: Endometrial adenocarcinoma

41 **The answer is C: Metastatic carcinoma of the lung.** This patient's lung shows numerous nodules of metastatic carcinoma corresponding to "cannon ball" metastases seen radiologically. Pulmonary metastases are more common than primary lung tumors, and the histologic appearance of most metastases resembles that of the primary tumor. Persons with ulcerative colitis (such as this patient) have a higher risk of colorectal cancer than the general population. The risk is related to the extent of colorectal involvement and the duration of the inflammatory disease. Carcinoid tumor of the lung (choice A) and primary lung cancer (choice B) would not typically show multiple, circumscribed nodules. Miliary tubercu-

losis (choice D) and sarcoidosis (choice E) feature mm-sized inflammatory nodules (minute granulomas).

Diagnosis: Metastatic cancer, metastatic carcinoma of the lung

42 **The answer is A: Adenoma.** The patient shows signs and symptoms of Cushing syndrome (upper truncal obesity and hypercortisolism). The surgical specimen reveals a circumscribed tumor of the adrenal cortex that produces cortisol. Histologic examination of this tumor reveals nests of clear, lipid-laden epithelial cells. None of the other choices describe a benign tumor of glandular epithelial origin.

Diagnosis: Adrenal adenoma, Cushing syndrome

43 **The answer is E: Sunlight.** Basal cell carcinoma (BCC) is the most common malignant tumor in persons with pale skin. BCC usually develops on the sun-damaged skin of people with fair skin and freckles. There is a direct correlation between total exposure to sunlight and the incidence of BCC, as well as squamous cell carcinoma and melanoma. The deleterious effects of sunlight (UV radiation) include enzyme inactivation, mutagenesis, and cell death. Divalent metal cations such as nickel, lead, cadmium, cobalt, and beryllium (choice B) can react with biomolecules and induce cancer. Most metal-induced cancers occur in an occupational setting; however the carcinogenic mechanisms are unknown.

Diagnosis: Basal cell carcinoma

44 **The answer is C: Cell cycle.** The surgical specimen reveals thousands of small adenomatous polyps on the mucosal surface of the colon. Patients with adenomatous polyposis coli have mutations in the *APC* tumor suppressor gene. Most cases are familial, but 30% to 50% represent new mutations. The mean age for occurrence of symptoms is 36 years. Without the *APC* protooncogene, cells are unable to downregulate signals from E-cadherin to β-catenin to nuclear transcription factors (myc and cyclin D) that regulate cell cycle progression. Autophagy (choice B) is a normal catabolic process in which cellular components and organelles are degraded in lysosomes. Autophagy is often a response to cell injury. It is also believed to protect cells from intracellular pathogens and slow the progression of various chronic diseases, including cancer.

Diagnosis: Adenomatous polyposis coli

Chapter 6

Developmental and Genetic Diseases

QUESTIONS

Select the single best answer.

1 A 4-year-old girl presents for a preschool physical examination. The child has a small head circumference, thin upper lip, and low-bridge nose. She shows evidence of mild mental retardation. Her parents state that she is often "emotional." Which of the following maternal causes of birth defects most likely accounts for these clinicopathologic findings?
(A) Alcohol abuse
(B) Cigarette smoking
(C) Congenital syphilis
(D) Inadequate nutrition
(E) Poorly controlled diabetes mellitus

2 A 12-month-old boy is brought to the emergency room for examination of his right arm following a tumble at home. Radiologic examination of the limb reveals a recent fracture of the right ulna and evidence of additional healing fractures. The child is noted to have blue sclerae. This patient most likely carries a mutation in a gene that encodes which of the following proteins?
(A) Collagen
(B) Fibrillin
(C) Keratin
(D) Myosin
(E) Tubulin

3 A 28-year-old woman gives birth to a stillborn with a severe neural tube defect (neonate shown in the image). This birth defect was caused by an error of morphogenesis that occurred at which of the following stages of development after fertilization?

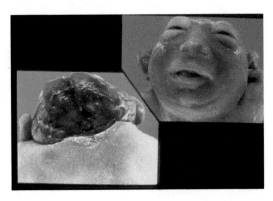

(A) 1 to 10 days
(B) 20 to 40 days
(C) 90 to 120 days
(D) 6 to 9 months
(E) Birth trauma

4 A 20-year-old man is examined by a new family physician who discovers numerous pigmented patches and pedunculated skin tumors on his chest. Biopsy of a tumor discloses a benign neoplasm derived from Schwann cells. Neither the patient's father nor mother shows signs of this disease. This patient most likely carries a mutation in a gene that encodes which of the following proteins?
(A) Epidermal growth factor receptor
(B) GTPase activating protein
(C) NF-κB transcription factor
(D) Protein kinase C
(E) Ras protein p21

5 The patient described in Question 4 is at increased risk of developing which of the following malignant neoplasms?
(A) Ganglioneuroma
(B) Glioblastoma multiforme
(C) Neurofibrosarcoma
(D) Serous cystadenocarcinoma
(E) Squamous cell carcinoma

6 A 25-year-old pregnant woman, at 16 weeks of gestation, visits her obstetrician. A screening test suggests the possibility of a neural tube defect in her fetus. An ultrasound examination shows a 3-cm neural tube defect in the thoracic spine. The screening test that was administered to the mother measured serum levels of which of the following proteins?
(A) Albumin
(B) Alpha-fetoprotein
(C) Bilirubin
(D) Chromogranin
(E) Human chorionic gonadotropin

7 A 25-year-old man presents for a routine physical examination. The patient is tall (6 ft, 5 in) and has long fingers (shown in the image). One year later, he suffers a dissecting aortic aneurysm. This patient most likely carries a mutation in a gene that encodes which of the following proteins?

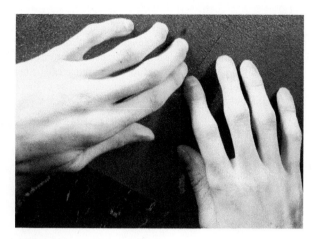

(A) Collagen
(B) Dystrophin
(C) Elastin
(D) Fibrillin
(E) Myosin

8 The genetic disease encountered in the patient described in Question 7 follows which of the following patterns of inheritance?
(A) Autosomal dominant
(B) Autosomal recessive
(C) Multifactorial
(D) X-linked dominant
(E) X-linked recessive

9 A 12-month-old boy shows progressive weakness, mental deterioration, and loss of vision. Laboratory studies demonstrate decreased activity of hexosaminidase A. The child eventually becomes blind and dies at 3 years of age. Which of the following best describes the pathogenesis of neuronal degeneration in this patient?
(A) Accumulation of unmetabolized substrate
(B) Decreased utilization of metabolic end-product
(C) Formation of an abnormal metabolic end-product
(D) Opening of mitochondrial membrane pore
(E) Synthesis of a novel glycosphingolipid

10 If the parents of the child described in Question 9 have a total of four sons and two daughters, then, on average, how many of their children may be expected to be asymptomatic (i.e., silent) carriers of this gene mutation?
(A) One child
(B) Two children
(C) Three children
(D) Four children
(E) Five children

11 A 4-year-old boy is admitted to the hospital with pneumonia and respiratory distress. The nurses report that the child's bowel movements are greasy and have a pungent odor. A sweat-chloride test is positive. Which of the following mechanisms of disease is the most likely cause of steatorrhea in this child?

(A) Abnormal dietary intake
(B) Bacterial overgrowth
(C) Hyperbilirubinemia with kernicterus
(D) Lack of pancreatic enzyme secretion
(E) Obstruction caused by meconium ileus

12 The patient described in Question 11 carries mutations in the gene that encodes which of the following types of protein?
(A) Membrane ion channel
(B) Mitochondrial transport protein
(C) Na⁺/K⁺ ATPase
(D) Nuclear transport protein
(E) Receptor tyrosine kinase

13 A 10-year-old child presents with xanthomas on the extensor surfaces of his forearms. Laboratory studies demonstrate a total serum cholesterol of 820 mg/dL. The child's mother and maternal grandfather also have elevated serum cholesterol. This patient most likely has mutations in the gene that encodes which of the following proteins involved in lipid metabolism?
(A) ApoE4
(B) Cholesterol hydroxylase
(C) Chylomicron transport protein
(D) High-density lipoprotein receptor
(E) Low-density lipoprotein receptor

14 A 10-month-old boy who was adopted from an orphanage in Eastern Europe presents for a physical examination. His parents believe that he is failing to meet developmental milestones. The child is fair skinned and has blond hair. On physical examination, the patient is noted to have a "mousy" odor. Laboratory studies demonstrate an inborn error of amino acid metabolism. To prevent mental retardation, this patient should be placed on a special diet that lacks which of the following essential amino acids?
(A) Isoleucine
(B) Methionine
(C) Phenylalanine
(D) Threonine
(E) Tryptophan

15 Which of the following best describes the pathogenesis of mental retardation in the patient described in Question 14?
(A) Accumulation of unmetabolized substrate
(B) Decreased utilization of metabolic end-product
(C) Formation of an abnormal metabolic end-product
(D) Increased utilization of metabolic end-product
(E) Opening of mitochondrial membrane pore

16 A 4-year-old boy is found to have extremely pliable skin. His parents note that he bruises easily. His joints can be hyperextended. Biochemical studies demonstrate a deficiency of lysyl hydroxylase. Ultrastructural examination of a skin biopsy of this patient would most likely reveal abnormalities associated with which of the following cell/tissue components?

(A) Actin-myosin filaments
(B) Collagen fibers
(C) Glycocalyx
(D) Intermediate filaments
(E) Mitochondria

17 A 25-year-old woman complains of recurrent bone pain and increasing abdominal girth. Physical examination reveals massive hepatosplenomegaly. Radiologic studies reveal several radiolucent bone defects. A bone marrow biopsy discloses enlarged cells with a fibrillar appearance reminiscent of "wrinkled tissue paper." Microscopic examination of a splenectomy specimen is shown. This patient most likely carries mutations in the gene that encodes which of the following types of hydrolytic enzymes?

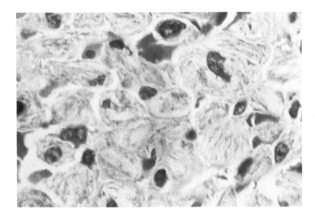

(A) Galactosidase
(B) Glucosidase
(C) Hexokinase
(D) N-acetylgalactosaminidase
(E) Neuraminidase

18 Which of the following best describes the pathogenesis of hepatosplenomegaly and bone pain in the patient described in Question 17?
(A) Accumulation of unmetabolized substrate
(B) Decreased utilization of metabolic end-product
(C) Formation of an abnormal metabolic end-product
(D) Increased utilization of metabolic end-product
(E) Opening of mitochondrial membrane pore

19 A neonate is born with severe motor dysfunction involving the lower extremities. Radiologic studies show that vertebral bodies in the lumbar region lack posterior arches. The vertebral defects are covered by a thin membrane. The space underneath the membrane contains a mass of tissue that is composed of meninges and spinal cord. The parents ask for information regarding risks for similar birth defects in their future offspring. You mention that dietary supplementation of the maternal diet has been shown to reduce the incidence of neural tube defects. What is this substance?
(A) Folic acid
(B) Niacin
(C) Thiamine
(D) Vitamin B_6
(E) Vitamin B_{12}

20 The parents of an infant with cleft lip and palate (infant shown in the image) visit a genetic counselor to discuss the chance that a similar birth defect will occur in their future offspring. In addition to teratogen exposure and multifactorial inheritance, which of the following is an important cause of this error of morphogenesis?

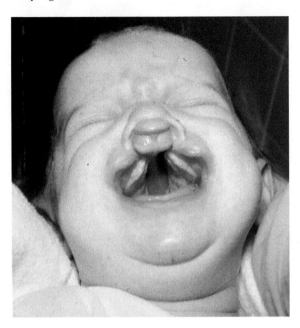

(A) Down syndrome
(B) First pregnancy before 25 years of age
(C) Maternal-fetal Rh incompatibility
(D) Structural chromosomal abnormality
(E) Turner syndrome

21 A 4-year-old boy is brought to the physician by his parents because he tires easily. Physical examination reveals weakness in the pelvic and shoulder girdles and enlargement of the child's calf muscle. Serum levels of creatine kinase are elevated. A biopsy of calf muscle shows marked variation in size and shape of muscle fibers. There are foci of muscle fiber necrosis, with myophagocytosis, regenerating fibers, and fibrosis. Molecular diagnostic assays would most likely show alterations in the length of the primary transcript for which of the following muscle-associated proteins?
(A) Actin
(B) Desmin
(C) Dystrophin
(D) Glycogen phosphorylase
(E) Myosin

22 What will be the likely cause of death in the patient described in Question 21?
(A) Cardiomyopathy
(B) Cerebrovascular disease
(C) End-stage renal disease
(D) Pulmonary saddle embolism
(E) Respiratory insufficiency

23 A 22-year-old man complains about his inability to conceive a child. On physical examination, the patient is noted to be tall

(6 ft, 5 in) and exhibits gynecomastia and testicular atrophy. Laboratory studies demonstrate increased serum levels of follicle-stimulating hormone. Cytogenetic studies reveal a chromosomal abnormality. What is the most common cause of this patient's chromosomal abnormality?

(A) Expansion of a trinucleotide repeat
(B) Isochromosome formation
(C) Meiotic nondisjunction
(D) Nonreciprocal translocation
(E) Ring chromosome formation

24 A 35-year-old pregnant woman delivers a baby prematurely at 28 weeks of gestation. Shortly after birth, the neonate becomes short of breath, with intercostal retraction and nasal flaring during respiration. The neonate is placed on a ventilator, but dies of respiratory insufficiency and intraventricular hemorrhage. Microscopic examination of the lungs at autopsy is shown. The eosinophilic material lining the air spaces represents an accumulation of which of the following proteins?

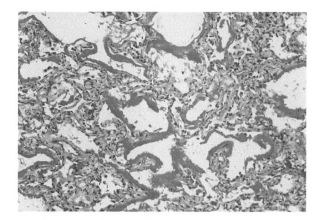

(A) Collagen
(B) Dystrophin
(C) Fibrin
(D) Fibronectin
(E) Laminin

25 If the neonate described in Question 24 had survived, which of the following would be the most likely complication related to anoxia and acidosis?

(A) Bilirubin encephalopathy (kernicterus)
(B) Erythroblastosis fetalis
(C) Necrotizing enterocolitis
(D) Pulmonary embolism
(E) Ventricular septal defect

26 A 16-year-old girl complains that she has not started menstruating like other girls her age. The patient is short (4 ft, 11 in) and has a thick-webbed neck. Physical examination reveals widely spaced nipples and poor breast development. If this patient's genetic disease was caused by nondisjunction during mitosis of a somatic cell in the early stages of embryogenesis, which of the following is the patient's most likely karyotype?

(A) 45,X
(B) 45,X/46,XX
(C) 45,X/46,XY
(D) 47,XX,+21
(E) 47,XXY

27 A 34-year-old woman in her second pregnancy delivers a female neonate with severe generalized edema and jaundice. A CBC of the neonate shows hemolytic anemia. Subsequent workup of the mother and the newborn reveal an Rh-incompatibility. Transplacental passage of which of the following proteins is the principal cause of anasarca and jaundice in this neonate?

(A) Complement C3
(B) Complement C4
(C) IgG
(D) IgM
(E) Interferon-α

28 The parents of a 2-year-old boy with hyposadias (urethra opens on the ventral aspect of the penis) visit a genetic counselor to discuss the chances that a similar birth defect will occur in their future offspring. This birth defect shows which of the following patterns of inheritance?

(A) Autosomal recessive
(B) Autosomal dominant
(C) Multifactorial
(D) X-linked dominant
(E) X-linked recessive

29 A 42-year-old woman gives birth to a neonate with multiple congenital abnormalities. Physical findings included a flat facial profile, slanted eyes, epicanthal folds, Brushfield spots, short nose, short neck, dysplastic ears, clinodactyly, a large protruding tongue, and a pronounced heart murmur. What is the most common cause of this developmental birth disease?

(A) Chromosomal deletion
(B) Chromosomal translocation
(C) Expansion of trinucleotide repeat
(D) Frameshift point mutation
(E) Nondisjunction

30 As an adult, the brain of the patient described in Question 29 will show histopathologic changes that are seen in patients with which of the following neurologic diseases?

(A) Alzheimer disease
(B) Huntington disease
(C) Krabbe disease
(D) Multiple sclerosis
(E) Parkinson disease

31 A 50-year-old man with a history of type 2 diabetes mellitus asks about the chances that his children will inherit this metabolic disorder. The patient is told that he has a genetic disease that shows which of the following patterns of inheritance?

(A) Autosomal dominant
(B) Autosomal recessive
(C) Multifactorial
(D) X-linked dominant
(E) X-linked recessive

32   A 25-year-old man with a history of autism and mental retardation is seen by a genetic counselor. The man has coarse facial features, an increased head circumference, and macro-orchidism. His maternal uncle is similarly affected. After further evaluation, a diagnosis of fragile X syndrome is rendered. What is the most likely underlying cause of this patient's genetic disease?
(A) Chromosomal nondisjunction
(B) Chromosome inversion
(C) Expansion of trinucleotide repeat
(D) Frame-shift mutation
(E) Nonreciprocal translocation

33   A 28-year-old man presents to the emergency room 1 hour after experiencing crushing substernal chest pain. Laboratory studies and ECG confirm the diagnosis of acute myocardial infarction. The patient dies 24 hours later of cardiac arrhythmia. This patient most likely had which of the following genetic diseases?
(A) Adult-onset (type 2) diabetes
(B) α_1-Antitrypsin deficiency
(C) Familial hypercholesterolemia
(D) Marfan syndrome
(E) Niemann-Pick disease

34   A 5-year-old boy presents with a maculopapular rash. On physical examination, the rash affects the palms and soles. Cracks and fissures are noted around the mouth and anus. There is funduscopic evidence of interstitial keratitis. Mild hepatosplenomegaly is present. The anterior tibial bones exhibit an outward curvature. What is the most likely etiology of these clinicopathologic findings?
(A) AIDS
(B) Cytomegalovirus
(C) Herpes
(D) Syphilis
(E) Toxoplasmosis

35   A 3-year-old boy dies in an automobile accident. At autopsy, the right lung is markedly shrunken. Dissection shows that the right main stem bronchus ends blindly in nondescript tissue composed of rudimentary ducts and connective tissue. This finding represents an example of which of the following errors of morphogenesis?
(A) Aplasia
(B) Atresia
(C) Dysraphic anomaly
(D) Hypoplasia
(E) Involution failure

36   The mother of a newborn boy is alarmed that her baby regurgitates at every feeding. An endoscopic examination reveals that the child's esophagus is almost completely occluded. This finding represents an example of which of the following errors of morphogenesis?
(A) Aplasia
(B) Atresia
(C) Dysplasia
(D) Dysraphic anomaly
(E) Ectopia

37   An 87-year-old woman dies peacefully in her sleep. At autopsy, a rest of pancreatic tissue is identified in the wall of the lower esophagus. This finding represents an example of which of the following congenital tumor-like conditions?
(A) Choristoma
(B) Hamartoma
(C) Hemangioma
(D) Papilloma
(E) Teratoma

38   A 30-year-old pregnant woman visits her obstetrician for prenatal care and eventual delivery. The patient volunteers that two of her three children had "yellow jaundice" at birth. Her youngest girl had been severely jaundiced and had been given two blood transfusions. Prenatal laboratory tests indicate that the mother is blood type O, Rh negative, whereas her husband is blood type A, Rh positive. The obstetrician samples amniotic fluid at 36 weeks of gestation to ascertain whether the fetus is mature enough for preterm delivery. Quantitative analysis of which of the following was most likely used as an indicator of fetal lung maturity?
(A) Absorbance at 450 nm
(B) Alpha-fetoprotein
(C) Creatinine
(D) Lecithin
(E) Total protein

39   The patient described in Question 38 delivers a female at 37 weeks of gestation with evidence of severe generalized edema (neonate shown in the image). The baby is given exchange transfusions with Rh-negative cells but subsequently dies. Which of the following best describes the pathogenesis of anasarca in this baby?

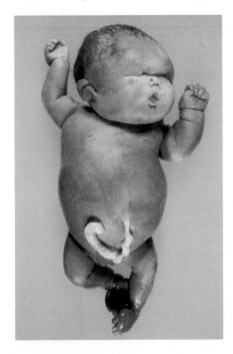

(A) Bilirubin encephalopathy
(B) Congestive heart failure
(C) Nephrotic syndrome
(D) Respiratory distress syndrome
(E) Rupture of the liver

40 An 18-year-old woman delivers a male neonate following a difficult labor and delivery (dystocia). The baby appears vigorous at birth (Apgar score = 9), but a cephalohematoma is apparent 2 hours later. A CT scan of the baby's head shows subperiosteal hemorrhage over one of the calvarial bones. What is the most likely outcome of this complication of labor and delivery?

(A) Facial nerve palsy
(B) Kernicterius
(C) Respiratory distress syndrome
(D) Spontaneous resolution
(E) Subarachnoid hemorrhage

41 A 42-year-old woman in her third pregnancy delivers a female neonate at 30 weeks of gestation. The baby develops jaundice within 2 days. The unconjugated serum bilirubin is 15 mg/dL. Which of the following is the most serious complication of untreated hyperbilirubinemia in this neonate?

(A) Acute pancreatitis
(B) Bronchopulmonary dysplasia
(C) Encephalopathy
(D) Gallstones
(E) Hemolytic anemia

42 A 27-year-old woman presents for a pregnancy test. She recalls drinking heavily during the week in which she may have conceived. What is the most likely consequence of toxic exposure to the conceptus during early (preimplantation) development?

(A) Conjoined twins
(B) Embryonic lethality
(C) Placenta accreta
(D) Neural tube defect
(E) Ventricular-septal defect

ANSWERS

1 **The answer is A: Alcohol abuse.** Fetal alcohol syndrome refers to a complex of abnormalities induced by the maternal consumption of alcoholic beverages while pregnant that includes (1) growth retardation, (2) dysfunction of the central nervous system, and (3) characteristic facial dysmorphology (e.g., small head circumference and thin upper lip). One fifth of children with fetal alcohol syndrome have IQs below 70, and 40% have IQs between 70 and 85. Even with a normal IQ, these children tend to have short memory spans, impulsiveness, and emotional instability. The children of mothers who smoke (choice B) or who have inadequate nutrition (choice D) may also exhibit deficiencies in physical growth and intellectual development; however, there is no association with the pattern of facial dysmorphology and emotional instability seen in this case. Congenital syphilis (choice C) may also cause mental retardation, but it would show protean manifestations not illustrated in this case. Gestational diabetes (choice E) does not cause mental retardation.
Diagnosis: Fetal alcohol syndrome

2 **The answer is A: Collagen.** Osteogenesis imperfecta (OI), or brittle bone disease, is a group of inherited disorders

expressed principally as fragility of bone. The genetic defects in the four types of OI are heterogeneous, but all affect the synthesis of type I collagen. Type I OI is characterized by a normal appearance at birth, but fractures of many bones occur during infancy and at the time the child learns to walk. Such patients have been described as being as "fragile as a China doll." Children with type I OI typically have blue sclerae as a result of the deficiency in collagen fibers, which imparts translucence to the sclera. A high incidence of hearing loss occurs because fractures and fusion of bones of the middle ear restrict their mobility. Fibrillin gene mutations (choice B) are found in patients with Marfan syndrome. Keratin gene mutations (choice C) are found in patients with epidermolytic hyperkeratosis.
Diagnosis: Osteogenesis imperfecta

3 **The answer is B: 20 to 40 days.** Anencephaly refers to the congenital absence of the cranial vault, with cerebral hemispheres either missing or reduced to small masses. It is a dysraphic anomaly of neural tube closure that results from an injury to the fetus between the 23rd and 26th day of gestation. During fetal development, the neural plate is transformed into the neural tube by fusion of the posterior surfaces. Failure of the neural tube to close results in the lack of closure of the overlying bony structures of the cranium and an absence of the calvarium, skin, and subcutaneous tissues of this region. The exposed brain is incompletely formed or absent. Blastocyst formation and implantation occur on days 1 to 10 after fertilization (choice A).
Diagnosis: Acrania, neural tube defect

4 **The answer is B: GTPase activating protein.** Neurofibromatosis type 1 (NF1) is characterized by (1) disfiguring neurofibromas, (2) areas of dark pigmentation of the skin (café au lait spots), and (3) pigmented lesions of the iris (Lisch nodules). It is one of the more common autosomal dominant disorders. The *NF1* gene has a high rate of mutation, and half of cases are sporadic rather than familial. The protein product, termed neurofibromin, is expressed in many tissues and belongs to a family of GTPase-activating proteins (GAPs), which inactivate ras protein (choice E). Thus, *NF1* is a classic tumor suppressor gene. Loss of GAP activity (in cells acquiring a second hit mutation) permits uncontrolled ras p21 activation, an effect that predisposes to the formation of benign neurofibromas. None of the other choices (A, C, and D) are associated with the pathogenesis of neurofibromatosis.
Diagnosis: Neurofibromatosis, type 1

5 **The answer is C: Neurofibrosarcoma.** One of the major complications of neurofibromatosis type 1 (NF1), occurring in 3% to 5% of patients, is the appearance of a neurofibrosarcoma in a neurofibroma. NF1 is also associated with an increased incidence of other neurogenic tumors, including meningioma, optic glioma, and pheochromocytoma. The other tumors listed are not associated with NF1.
Diagnosis: Neurofibromatosis, type 1

6 **The answer is B: Alpha-fetoprotein (AFP).** Screening of pregnant women for serum AFP and examination by ultrasonography allow detection of virtually all anencephalic fetuses.

Levels of the other proteins are not significantly affected by a neural tube defect in the fetus.

Diagnosis: Neural tube defect, spina bifida

7 **The answer is D: Fibrillin.** The cause of Marfan syndrome has been established as missense mutations in the gene coding for fibrillin-1 (*FBN1*). Fibrillin is a family of connective tissue proteins analogous to the collagens. It is widely distributed in many tissues in the form of a fiber system termed microfibrils. For example, the deposition of elastin on microfibrillar fibers produces the concentric rings of elastin in the aortic wall. Collagen gene mutations (choice A) are found in patients with Ehlers-Danlos syndrome and osteogenesis imperfecta. Dystrophin gene mutations (choice B) are found in patients with muscular dystrophy.

Diagnosis: Marfan syndrome

8 **The answer is A: Autosomal dominant.** Marfan syndrome is an autosomal dominant, inherited disorder of connective tissue characterized by a variety of abnormalities in many organs, including the heart, aorta, skeleton, eyes, and skin. One third of cases represent sporadic mutations. The incidence in the United States is 1 per 10,000.

Diagnosis: Marfan syndrome

9 **The answer is A: Accumulation of unmetabolized substrate.** Tay-Sachs disease is the catastrophic infantile variant of a class of lysosomal storage diseases known as GM_2 gangliosidoses. This ganglioside is deposited in neurons of the central nervous system due to a failure of lysosomal degradation and accumulation of an unmetabolized substrate. Gangliosides are glycosphingolipids that are present in the outer leaflet of the plasma membrane, particularly in neurons. The lysosomal catabolism of ganglioside GM_2 is accomplished through the activity of the β-hexosaminidases (A and B), which are composed of α and β subunits and require the participation of the GM_2-activator protein. A deficiency in any of these components results in clinical disease. None of the other choices explains the pathogenesis of this disease.

Diagnosis: Tay-Sachs disease

10 **The answer is C: Three children.** Tay-Sachs disease is inherited as an autosomal recessive trait and is predominantly a disorder of Ashkenazi Jews, in whom the carrier rate is 1 in 30, and the natural incidence of homozygotes is 1 in 4,000 live newborns. In autosomal recessive diseases, on average, half of the offspring are expected to be heterozygotes and silent carriers of the gene mutation.

Diagnosis: Tay-Sachs disease

11 **The answer is D: Lack of pancreatic enzyme secretion.** Cystic fibrosis (CF) is an autosomal recessive disorder affecting children, which is characterized by (1) chronic pulmonary disease, (2) deficient exocrine pancreatic function, and (3) other complications of inspissated mucus in a number of organs, including the small intestine, the liver, and the reproductive tract. The diagnosis of CF is most reliably made by the demonstration of increased concentrations of electrolytes in the sweat. The decreased chloride conductance characteristic of CF results in a failure of chloride reabsorption by the cells of the sweat gland ducts and, hence, to the accumulation of sodium chloride in the sweat. All of the pathologic consequences of CF can be attributed to the presence of abnormally thick mucus. Lack of pancreatic enzyme secretion in patients with CF causes malabsorption and foul-smelling fatty stools (steatorrhea). The other choices do not address the underlying cause of malabsorption in patients with CF.

Diagnosis: Cystic fibrosis

12 **The answer is A: Membrane ion channel.** The gene responsible for cystic fibrosis (CF) encodes a large protein termed the cystic fibrosis transmembrane conductance regulator (CFTR). CFTR is a member of the ATP-binding family of membrane transporter proteins that constitutes a chloride channel in most epithelia. The secretion of chloride anions by mucous-secreting epithelial cells controls the parallel secretion of fluid and, consequently, the viscosity of the mucus. It is estimated that 1 in 25 whites is a heterozygous carrier of the CF gene, and the incidence is 1 in 2,500 newborns. The most common cause of morbidity and mortality in patients with CF is pulmonary disease, secondary to chronic infections. Receptor tyrosine kinase gene mutations often lead to uncontrolled cell growth.

Diagnosis: Cystic fibrosis

13 **The answer is E: Low-density lipoprotein (LDL) receptor.** Familial hypercholesterolemia is an autosomal dominant disorder characterized by high levels of LDLs in the blood, accompanied by the deposition of cholesterol in arteries, tendons, and skin. It is one of the most common autosomal dominant disorders, and in its heterozygous form, it affects at least 1 in 500 adults in the United States. Only 1 in 1 million persons is homozygous for the disease. Familial hypercholesterolemia results from abnormalities in the gene that encodes the cell surface receptor that removes LDLs from the blood. Mutations in the other genes do not cause hypercholesterolemia.

Diagnosis: Familial hypercholesterolemia

14 **The answer is C: Phenylalanine.** Phenylketonuria (PKU, hyperphenylalaninemia) is an autosomal recessive disorder characterized by progressive mental deterioration in the first few years of life due to high levels of circulating phenylalanine, secondary to a deficiency of phenylalanine hydroxylase. The disorder is based on a genetic defect, but its expression depends on the provision of a dietary constituent. The affected infant appears normal at birth, but mental retardation is evident within a few months. Infants with PKU tend to have fair skin, blond hair, and blue eyes because the inability to convert phenylalanine to tyrosine leads to reduced melanin synthesis. These patients exude a "mousy" odor due to the formation of phenylacetic acid. The treatment of PKU involves the restriction of phenylalanine in the diet. None of the other essential amino acids accumulates in patients with PKU.

Diagnosis: Phenylketonuria

15 **The answer is A: Accumulation of unmetabolized substrate.** Phenylalanine is an essential amino acid that is derived exclusively from the diet and is oxidized in the liver to tyrosine by phenylalanine hydroxylase (PAH). A deficiency in PAH results in both hyperphenylalaninemia and the formation of phenylketones from the transamination of phenylalanine. The excretion in the urine of phenylpyruvic acid and its derivatives accounts for the original name of phenylketonuria. However, it is now established that phenylalanine itself, rather than its metabolites, is responsible for the neurologic damage central to this disease. Thus, the term hyperphenylalaninemia is actually a more appropriate designation than PKU. None of the other choices explains the accumulation of phenylalanine in these patients.

Diagnosis: Phenylketonuria

16 **The answer is B: Collagen fibers.** Ehlers-Danlos syndromes (EDS) are a group of rare, autosomal dominant, inherited disorders of connective tissue that feature remarkable hyperelasticity and fragility of the skin, joint hypermobility, and often a bleeding diathesis. The common feature of most types of EDS is a generalized defect in collagen, including abnormalities in its molecular structure, synthesis, secretion, and degradation. Patients typically can stretch the skin many centimeters, and trivial injuries can lead to serious wounds. Because sutures do not hold well, dehiscence of surgical incisions is common. Hypermobility of the joints allows unusual extension and flexion. Abnormalities would not be expected in the other cell/tissue components listed.

Diagnosis: Ehlers-Danlos syndrome

17 **The answer is B: Glucosidase.** Gaucher disease is characterized by the accumulation of glucosylceramide, primarily in the lysosomes of macrophages. The underlying abnormality in Gaucher disease is a deficiency in glucocerebrosidase, a type of lysosomal acid β-glucosidase. The hallmark of this disorder is the presence of Gaucher cells, which are lipid-laden macrophages that are characteristically present in the red pulp of the spleen, liver sinusoids, lymph nodes, lungs, and bone marrow. These cells are derived from the resident macrophages in the respective organs (e.g., Kupffer cells in the liver and alveolar macrophages in the lung). Galactosidase gene mutations (choice A) are found in patients with Fabry disease. N-acetylgalactosaminidase gene mutations (choice D) are found in patients with Tay-Sachs disease.

Diagnosis: Gaucher disease

18 **The answer is A: Accumulation of unmetabolized substrate.** Glucosylceramide is a common core structure for membrane glycosphingolipids. The glucosylceramide that accumulates in Gaucher cells in the spleen, liver, bone marrow, and lymph nodes derives principally from the catabolism of senescent leukocytes. The membranes of these cells are rich in the cerebrosides, and when their degradation is blocked by the deficiency of glucocerebrosidase, the intermediate metabolite, glucosylceramide, accumulates. The other biochemical pathways listed do not cause sphingolipid accumulation in patients with lysosomal storage diseases.

Diagnosis: Gaucher disease

19 **The answer is A: Folic acid.** Spina bifida is a congenital defect in the closure of the spinal canal. Like other dysraphic disorders (anencephaly, meningocele, and meningomyelocele), spina bifida is of polygenic origin. Folic acid supplied in the periconceptional period lowers the incidence of neural tube defects. In 1998, the United States Food and Drug Administration began requiring manufacturers of enriched

flour, bread, and some other products to supplement these foods with folate. This mandate has been associated with a significant decrease in the incidence of neural tube defects. Folic acid deficiency can result in elevated serum levels of homocysteine, a maternal risk factor for neural tube defects. Thiamine deficiency (choice C) causes beri-beri (polyneuropathy, edema, and heart failure). Vitamin B_{12} deficiency (choice E) causes megaloblastic anemia but not neural tube defects.

Diagnosis: Spina bifida

20 **The answer is D: Structural chromosomal abnormality.** Cleft lip and cleft palate exemplify multifactorial inheritance in which multiple genes interact with various environmental factors to produce disease. On the 35th day of gestation, the frontal prominence fuses with the maxillary process to form the upper lip. Disturbances in gene expression at this time (hereditary or environmental) lead to interference with proper fusion and result in cleft lip, with or without cleft palate. In addition to multifactorial inheritance, this developmental anomaly may be part of a malformation syndrome caused by teratogens (e.g., rubella and anticonvulsants). It is also often encountered in children with chromosomal abnormalities (correct answer). The incidence of cleft lip, with or without cleft palate, is 1 in 1,000, and the incidence of cleft palate alone is 1 in 2,500. If one child is born with a cleft lip, the chances are 4% that the second child will exhibit the same defect. If the first two children are affected, the risk of cleft lip increases to 9% for the third child. The more severe the anatomical defect, the greater the probability of transmitting cleft lip will be. Whereas 75% of cases of cleft lip occur in boys, the sons of women with cleft lip have a four times higher risk of acquiring the defect than the sons of affected fathers. None of the other choices are associated with a significantly increased risk of cleft lip.

Diagnosis: Cleft lip, multifactorial inheritance

21 **The answer is C: Dystrophin.** Duchenne muscular dystrophy (DMD) is a severe, X-linked condition characterized by progressive degeneration of muscles, particularly those of the pelvic and shoulder girdles. A milder form of the disease is known as Becker muscular dystrophy (BMD). Both DMD and BMD are caused by a deficiency of dystrophin, a member of the family of membrane cytoskeletal proteins, which includes α-actinin and spectrin. The protein is located on the cytoplasmic face of the plasma membrane of muscle cells and is linked to it by integral membrane glycoproteins (dystrophin-associated glycoprotein complex), which in turn, are bound to extracellular laminin. It has been proposed that the absence of dystrophin leads to a defective membrane that is damaged during contraction, an effect that predisposes to death of the myocyte. Serum levels of creatine kinase are increased. Glycogen phosphorylase gene mutations (choice D) are found in patients with McArdle disease.

Diagnosis: Duchenne muscular dystrophy

22 **The answer is A: Cardiomyopathy.** The symptoms of Duchenne muscular dystrophy (DMD) progress with age. During the first year of life, the infants appear normal, but more than half fail to walk by 18 months of age. More than 90% of afflicted boys are wheelchair bound by the age of 11 years.

In advanced disease, cardiac symptoms are almost universal, and cardiomyopathy is a common cause of death. The mean age at death in boys with DMD is 17 years. The other choices are unrelated to DMD.

Diagnosis: Duchenne muscular dystrophy

23   The answer is C: Meiotic nondisjunction. Klinefelter syndrome, or testicular dysgenesis, is related to the presence of one or more X chromosomes in excess of the normal male XY complement. Most persons with Klinefelter syndrome (80%) have one extra X chromosome (47,XXY karyotype). The additional X chromosome(s) arises as a result of nondisjunction during gametogenesis. In half of cases, nondisjunction occurs during paternal meiosis I, leading to a sperm containing both an X and a Y chromosome. Fertilization of a normal oocyte by such a sperm gives a zygote with a 47,XXY complement of chromosomes. Klinefelter syndrome occurs in 1 per 1,000 male newborns, which is roughly comparable to the incidence of Down syndrome. None of the other choices are associated with trisomy.

Diagnosis: Klinefelter syndrome

24   The answer is C: Fibrin. The pathogenesis of respiratory distress syndrome (RDS) of the newborn is intimately linked to a deficiency of surfactant. Collapse of the alveoli (atelectasis) secondary to surfactant deficiency results in perfused but not ventilated alveoli, a situation that leads to hypoxia and acidosis. The leak of fibrin-rich fluid into the alveoli from the injured vascular bed contributes to the typical clinical and pathologic features of RDS. On gross examination, the lungs are dark red and airless. The alveolar ducts are lined by conspicuous, eosinophilic, fibrin-rich, amorphous structures, termed hyaline membranes. Although collagen (choice A), fibronectin (choice D), and laminin (choice E) are found in most tissues, they do not represent the major protein found in hyaline membranes.

Diagnosis: Respiratory distress syndrome of the neonate

25   The answer is C: Necrotizing enterocolitis. The first symptom of RDS (usually appearing within an hour of birth) is increased respiratory effort, with forceful intercostal retraction and the use of accessory neck muscles. Despite advances in neonatal intensive care, the overall mortality of RDS is about 15%. Necrotizing enterocolitis is the most common acquired gastrointestinal emergency in newborns and is thought to be related to ischemia of the intestinal mucosa. This injury is followed by bacterial colonization, usually with *Clostridium difficile*. The lesions vary from those of typical pseudomembranous enterocolitis to gangrene and perforation of the bowel. None of the other choices are related to respiratory insufficiency.

Diagnosis: Respiratory distress syndrome of the neonate, enterocolitis

26   The answer is B: 45,X/46,XX. Mitotic nondisjunction may involve embryonic cells during early stages of development and result in chromosomal aberrations. This condition in which the body contains two or more karyotypically different cell lines is called mosaicism. Mosaicism involving sex chromosomes is found in patients with Turner and Klinefelter syndromes. Turner syndrome refers to the spectrum of abnormalities that result from the presence of complete or partial monosomy of the X chromosome in a phenotypic female. Half of women with Turner syndrome lack an entire X chromosome (monosomy X, choice A). The remainder of women with Turner syndrome are mosaics or display structural aberrations of the X chromosome. Mosaics characterized by a 45,X/46,XX karyotype (15%; choice B) tend to have milder phenotypic manifestations. In about 5% of patients, the mosaic karyotype is 45,X/46,XY (choice C). A patient with the 47,XX,+21 karyotype (choice D) is a female with Down syndrome. The 47,XXY karyotype (choice E) is a feature of Klinefelter syndrome.

Diagnosis: Turner syndrome

27   The answer is C: IgG. Erythroblastosis fetalis is an antibody-mediated hemolytic disease that affects the fetus in utero. It is usually caused by transplacental passage of maternal antibodies to antigens expressed on fetal RBCs. The introduction of Rh-positive fetal erythrocytes (>1 mL) into the circulation of an Rh-negative mother at the time of delivery sensitizes her to the D antigen. When the antigen-sensitized mother again bears an Rh-positive fetus, much smaller quantities of fetal D antigen elicit an increase in antibody titer. In contrast to IgM (choice D), IgG antibodies are small enough to cross the placenta and thus produce hemolysis in the fetus. This cycle is exaggerated in multiparous women, and the severity of erythroblastosis tends to increase progressively with each succeeding pregnancy.

Diagnosis: Hemolytic anemia of the neonate, erythroblastosis fetalis

28   The answer is C: Multifactorial. The inheritance of a number of birth defects is multifactorial. Most normal human traits are inherited neither as dominant nor as recessive mendelian attributes, but rather in a more complex manner. For example, multifactorial inheritance determines intelligence, height, skin color, body habitus, and even emotional disposition. Similarly, most of the common chronic disorders of adults represent multifactorial genetic diseases and are well known to "run in families." Such maladies include diabetes, atherosclerosis, and many forms of cancer and arthritis, and hypertension. The inheritance of a number of birth defects is also multifactorial (e.g., cleft lip and palate, pyloric stenosis, hypospadias, and congenital heart disease). The concept of multifactorial inheritance is based on the notion that multiple genes interact with various environmental factors to produce disease in an individual patient. Such inheritance leads to familial aggregation that does not obey simple mendelian rules (see choices A, B, D, and E). As a consequence, the inheritance of polygenic diseases is studied by the methods of population genetics, rather than by the analysis of individual family pedigrees.

Diagnosis: Hypospadias, multifactorial inheritance

29   The answer is E: Nondisjunction. Nondisjunction during the first meiotic division of gametogenesis accounts for most (92% to 95%) patients with Down syndrome who have trisomy 21. The extra chromosome 21 is of maternal origin in about 95% of Down syndrome children. Translocation of an extra long arm of chromosome 21 to another acrocentric chromosome (choice B) causes about 5% of cases of Down syndrome. The other choices are unrelated to trisomy 21.

Diagnosis: Down syndrome, trisomy 21

30 **The answer is A: Alzheimer disease.** One of the most intriguing neurologic features of Down syndrome is its association with Alzheimer disease. The morphologic lesions characteristic of Alzheimer disease progress in all patients with Down syndrome and are universally demonstrable by age 35 years. These changes in the brain include (1) granulovacuolar degeneration, (2) neurofibrillary tangles, (3) senile plaques, and (4) loss of neurons. The senile plaques and cerebral blood vessels of both Alzheimer disease and Down syndrome always contain an amyloid composed of the same fibrillar protein (β-amyloid protein). The other choices are unrelated to Down syndrome.
Diagnosis: Down syndrome

31 **The answer is C: Multifactorial.** Most of the common chronic disorders of adults represent multifactorial genetic diseases that tend to "run in families." Such maladies include diabetes, atherosclerosis, and many forms of cancer, arthritis, and hypertension. Fragile X syndrome and Duchenne-Becker muscular dystrophy are examples of X-linked recessive genetic diseases.
Diagnosis: Diabetes mellitus

32 **The answer is C: Expansion of trinucleotide repeat.** Fragile X syndrome, the most common cause of inherited mental retardation, is caused by expansion of a CGG trinucleotide repeat in a noncoding region immediately adjacent to the *FMR1* gene on the X chromosome. In a poorly understood manner, the expanded CGG repeat silences the *FMR1* gene by methylation of its promoter. The abnormal repeat is associated with an inducible "fragile site" on the X chromosome, which appears in cytogenetic studies as a nonstaining gap or chromosomal break. The male newborn afflicted with the fragile X syndrome appears normal, but during childhood, characteristic features appear, including an increased head circumference, facial coarsening, joint hyperextensibility, enlarged testes, and abnormalities of the cardiac valves. Mental retardation is profound, with IQ scores varying from 20 to 60. A significant proportion of autistic male children carry a fragile X chromosome. The other choices do not cause fragile X syndrome.
Diagnosis: Fragile X syndrome

33 **The answer is C: Familial hypercholesterolemia.** Familial hypercholesterolemia is an autosomal dominant disorder caused by mutations of the gene encoding the LDL receptor. It is one of the most common autosomal dominant disorders, affecting 1 in 500 adults in the United States. The gene defect affects the uptake of LDL in the liver, causing hypercholesterolemia. Clinically, the disease presents as severe atherosclerosis, which usually becomes symptomatic at an early age. Diabetes mellitus (choice A) also causes accelerated atherosclerosis but rarely at this age. Marfan syndrome (choice D) is associated with dissecting aortic aneurysm. Niemann-Pick disease (choice E) is a hereditary lysosomal storage disease.
Diagnosis: Familial hypercholesterolemia

34 **The answer is D: Syphilis.** The acronym TORCH refers to a complex of similar signs and symptoms produced by fetal or neonatal infection with a variety of microorganisms, including *Toxoplasma* (T), Rubella (R), *Cytomegalovirus* (C), and Herpes (H). The letter "O" represents "others" including congenital syphilis. The acronym was coined to alert pediatricians to the fact that infections in the fetus and newborn by TORCH agents are usually indistinguishable from each other and that testing for one of the four major TORCH agents should include testing for the other three and others as well. The organism that causes syphilis, *Treponema pallidum*, is transmitted to the fetus by a mother who has acquired syphilis during pregnancy. A maculopapular rash is a common early finding in congenital syphilis. The most common osseous lesion in congenital syphilis is periostitis and outward curving of the anterior tibia (saber shins). Flat raised plaques (condylomata lata) around the anus and female genitalia may develop early or after a few years. The diagnosis of congenital syphilis is suggested by clinical findings and a history of maternal infection. None of the other pathogens cause these clinicopathologic findings.
Diagnosis: TORCH syndrome, syphilis

35 **The answer is A: Aplasia.** Aplasia is the absence of an organ coupled with persistence of the organ anlage or a rudiment. Thus, aplasia of the lung refers to a condition in which the main bronchus ends blindly in nondescript tissue composed of rudimentary ducts and connective tissue. Dysraphic anomalies (choice C) are defects caused by the failure of apposed structures to fuse. Hypoplasia (choice D) refers to reduced size owing to the incomplete development of all or part of an organ. Examples include microphthalmia and microcephaly. Involution failures (choice E) reflect the persistence of embryonic or fetal structures that should involute at certain stages of development. A persistent thyroglossal duct is the result of incomplete involution of the tract that connects the base of the tongue with the thyroid.
Diagnosis: Pulmonary aplasia

36 **The answer is B: Atresia.** Atresia refers to defects caused by the incomplete formation of a lumen. Many hollow organs originate as strands and cords of cells whose centers are programmed to die, thus forming a central cavity or lumen. Atresia of the esophagus is characterized by partial occlusion of the lumen, which was not fully established in embryogenesis. Dysplasia (choice C) is caused by abnormal organization of cells into tissues, which is a situation that results in abnormal histogenesis. Tuberous sclerosis is a striking example of dysplasia, in which the brain contains aggregates of normally developed cells arranged into grossly visible "tubers." Ectopia (choice E) is an anomaly in which an organ is outside its normal anatomic site.
Diagnosis: Esophageal atresia

37 **The answer is A: Choristoma.** Choristomas are minute or microscopic aggregates of normal tissue in aberrant locations. Choristomas are represented by rests of pancreatic tissue in the wall of the gastrointestinal tract or of adrenal tissue in the renal cortex. By contrast, hamartomas (choice B) represent focal, benign overgrowths of one or more of the mature cellular elements of a normal tissue, often with one element predominating. Hemangiomas (choice C) are the most frequently encountered tumors in childhood.
Diagnosis: Choristoma

38 **The answer is D: Lecithin.** Immaturity of the lungs poses one of the most common and immediate threats to the viability of the low birth weight infant because the lining cells of the fetal alveoli do not differentiate until late pregnancy. Alveoli are maintained in the expanded state, in part, by the presence of pulmonary surfactant. This material, which is produced by type II pneumocytes, is a complex mixture of several phospholipids, 75% phosphatidylcholine (lecithin) and 10% phosphatidylglycerol. The concentration of lecithin increases rapidly at the beginning of the third trimester and, thereafter, rises rapidly to reach a peak near term. Maturity of the fetal lung can be assessed by measuring pulmonary surfactant released into the amniotic fluid. A lecithin-to-sphingomyelin ratio above 2:1 implies that the fetus will survive without developing respiratory distress syndrome. Alpha-fetoprotein (choice B) is used to monitor for anencephaly.
Diagnosis: Erythroblastosis fetalis

39 **The answer is B: Congestive heart failure.** Erythroblastosis fetalis is a hemolytic disease of the newborn caused by maternal antibodies against fetal erythrocytes. Erythroblastosis fetalis does not ordinarily occur during the first pregnancy, because the quantity of fetal blood necessary to sensitize the mother is introduced into her circulation only at the time of delivery, too late to affect the fetus. However, when the sensitized mother again bears an Rh-positive fetus, much smaller quantities of fetal D antigen can elicit an increase in IgG antibody titer. This cycle is exaggerated in multiparous women, and the severity of erythroblastosis tends to increase progressively with each succeeding pregnancy. However, even after multiple pregnancies, only 5% of Rh-negative women are ever delivered of infants with erythroblastosis fetalis. The severity of erythroblastosis fetalis varies from a mild hemolysis to fatal anemia, and the pathological findings are determined by the extent of the hemolytic disease. Hydrops fetalis refers to the most serious form of erythroblastosis fetalis, and is characterized by severe edema secondary to congestive heart failure caused by severe anemia. The other choices do not cause of anasarca in erythroblastosis fetalis.
Diagnosis: Erythroblastosis fetalis, hydrops fetalis

40 **The answer is D: Spontaneous resolution.** Birth injury spans the spectrum from mechanical trauma to anoxic damage. Some birth injuries relate to poor obstetric manipulation, whereas many are unavoidable sequelae of routine delivery. Birth injuries occur in about 5 per 1,000 live births. Factors that predispose to birth injury include cephalopelvic disproportion, dystocia (difficult labor), prematurity, and breech presentation. Cephalohematoma is defined as a subperiosteal hemorrhage that is confined to a single cranial bone and becomes apparent within the first few hours after birth. It may or may not be associated with a linear fracture of the underlying bone. Most cephalohematomas resolve without complication and require no treatment.
Diagnosis: Cephalohematoma

41 **The answer is C: Encephalopathy.** Kernicterus, also termed bilirubin encephalopathy, is defined as a neurological condition associated with severe jaundice and characterized by bile staining of the brain, particularly of the basal ganglia, pontine nuclei, and dentate nuclei in the cerebellum. Kernicterus (German: *kern*, nucleus) is essentially confined to newborns with severe unconjugated hyperbilirubinemia, usually related to erythroblastosis fetalis. The bilirubin derived from the destruction of erythrocytes and the catabolism of the released heme is not easily conjugated by the immature liver, which is deficient in glucuronyl transferase. The development of kernicterus is directly related to the level of unconjugated bilirubin and is rare in term infants when serum bilirubin levels are below 20 mg/dL. Premature infants are more vulnerable to hyperbilirubinemia and may develop kernicterus at levels as low as 12 mg/dL. Bilirubin is thought to injure the cells of the brain by interfering with mitochondrial function. Severe kernicterus leads initially to loss of the startle reflex and athetoid movements, which in 75% progresses to lethargy and death. Most surviving infants have severe choreoathetosis and mental retardation; a minority have varying degrees of intellectual and motor retardation. Exchange transfusions may keep the maximum serum bilirubin at an acceptable level. However, phototherapy, which converts the toxic unconjugated bilirubin into isomers that are nontoxic and excreted in the urine, has greatly reduced the need for exchange transfusions. The other choices are not complications of untreated hyperbilirubinemia in newborns.
Diagnosis: Kernicterus, physiological jaundice

42 **The answer is B: Embryonic lethality.** If a conceptus is exposed to harmful exogenous influences, the noxious agent exerts the same effect on all blastomeres and also causes death. Thus, either a conceptus dies or development proceeds uninterrupted, since the interchangeable blastomeres replace the loss. As a rule, exogenous toxins acting on preimplantation-stage embryos do not produce errors of morphogenesis and do not cause malformations. The most common consequence of toxic exposure at the preimplantation stage is death of the embryo, which often passes unnoticed or is perceived as heavy, albeit delayed, menstrual bleeding. Approximately 30% of fertilized ova are aborted spontaneously, without the woman being aware that pregnancy had occurred. Placenta accreta (choice C) is an abnormal adherence of the placenta to the underlying uterine wall. The other choices are errors of morphogenesis that manifest at later stages of development.
Diagnosis: Spontaneous abortion

Chapter 7

Hemodynamic Disorders

QUESTIONS

Select the single best answer.

1 A 60-year-old man with a history of multiple myocardial infarcts is hospitalized for shortness of breath. Physical examination reveals marked jugular distension, hepatomegaly, ascites, and pitting edema. A chest X-ray reveals cardiomegaly. The patient subsequently dies of cardiorespiratory failure. Examination of the lungs at autopsy would most likely disclose which of the following pathologic changes?
(A) Diffuse alveolar damage with hyaline membranes
(B) Intra-alveolar purulent exudate
(C) Lymphocytic interstitial pneumonitis
(D) Pulmonary arteriopathy with plexiform lesions
(E) Vascular congestion and hemosiderin-laden macrophages

2 A 92-year-old woman is brought unconscious to the emergency room from a nursing home. Her blood pressure is 70/30 mm Hg. She is febrile (38°C/100.5°F) and tachypneic. Laboratory studies demonstrate a WBC count of 22,000/μL with 92% neutrophils. Urinalysis reveals numerous Gram-negative organisms. Which of the following most likely accounts for this patient's signs and symptoms?
(A) Anaphylactic shock
(B) Cardiogenic shock
(C) Hypovolemic shock
(D) Neurogenic shock
(E) Septic shock

3 A 21-year-old pregnant woman experiences abruptio placentae at 37 weeks of gestation and develops severe vaginal bleeding that is difficult to control. Five months later, the patient presents with profound lethargy, pallor, muscle weakness, failure of lactation, and amenorrhea. Which of the following best explains the pathogenesis of pituitary insufficiency in this patient?
(A) Abscess
(B) Embolism
(C) Infarction
(D) Passive hyperemia
(E) Thrombosis

4 A 62-year-old man with a history of hypertension is rushed to the emergency room with severe "tearing pain" of the anterior chest. His blood pressure is 80/50 mm Hg. Physical examination shows pallor, diaphoresis, and a murmur of aortic regurgitation. Laboratory studies and ECG show no evidence of acute myocardial infarction. Four hours later, the patient goes into cardiac arrest. An ECG reveals electromechanical dissociation. Which of the following best explains the pathogenesis of cardiac tamponade in this patient?
(A) Disseminated intravascular coagulation
(B) Embolism
(C) Hemorrhage
(D) Passive hyperemia
(E) Thrombosis

5 A 58-year-old woman is brought to the emergency department 4 hours after vomiting blood and experiencing bloody stools. The patient was diagnosed with alcoholic cirrhosis 2 years ago. Endoscopy reveals large esophageal varices, one of which is actively bleeding. Which of the following best explains the pathogenesis of dilated esophageal veins in this patient?
(A) Decreased intravascular oncotic pressure
(B) Increased capillary permeability
(C) Increased intravascular hydrostatic pressure
(D) Vasoconstriction of arterioles
(E) Vasodilatation of capillaries

6 A 69-year-old retired man is brought to the emergency department because of the sudden onset of left-sided chest pain, which is exacerbated upon inspiration. Physical examination reveals dyspnea and hemoptysis. His temperature is 38°C (101°F), pulse 110 per minute, respirations 35 per minute, and blood pressure 158/100 mm Hg. A lateral chest wall friction rub is present on auscultation. The left leg is markedly edematous with a positive Homans' sign. A chest X-ray reveals a left pleural effusion. What is the most likely cause of this patient's pulmonary condition?
(A) Congestive heart failure
(B) Cor pulmonale
(C) Mitral stenosis
(D) Subacute endocarditis
(E) Thromboembolism

7 A 22-year-old construction worker falls 30 ft and fractures several bones, including his femoral shafts. Six hours later, the patient develops shortness of breath and cyanosis. Which of the following hemodynamic disorders best explains the pathogenesis of shock in this patient?

(A) Acute myocardial infarction
(B) Deep venous thrombosis
(C) Fat embolism
(D) Paradoxical embolism
(E) Septic shock

8 A 20-year-old woman presents to the emergency room complaining of having had a severe headache for 4 hours. Physical examination reveals numerous small red spots on the extremities and a stiff neck. Her temperature is 38.7°C (103°F). Lumbar puncture returns purulent fluid, with segmented neutrophils and Gram-negative organisms resembling meningococci. A few hours later, the patient goes into shock and becomes comatose. Severe endothelial injury in this patient is primarily mediated by which of the following proteins?

(A) α-Fetoprotein
(B) IgG
(C) Interferon-γ
(D) Transforming growth factor-β
(E) Tumor necrosis factor-α

9 A 69-year-old man is brought to the emergency room complaining of visual difficulty and weakness. On physical examination, the patient is aphasic with a right-sided hemiplegia. Retinal hemorrhages are seen bilaterally. You suspect that a thromboembolus coursed to the left middle cerebral artery and smaller emboli traveled to the retinal arteries. Which of the following anatomic sites is the most likely source for these emboli in this patient?

(A) Adrenals
(B) Deep leg veins
(C) Heart
(D) Liver
(E) Lungs

10 The body of a 28-year-old homeless man is brought to the coroner's office. Histologic examination of the lungs under polarized light is shown. Which of the following is the most likely cause of the birefringence observed in this pulmonary lesion?

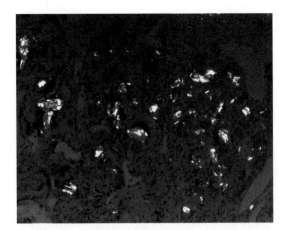

(A) Alcoholism
(B) Aspiration of mineral oil
(C) Bacterial pneumonia
(D) Cocaine abuse
(E) Intravenous drug use

11 A 25-year-old woman delivers a healthy baby at 39 weeks of gestation. Six hours later, the mother develops severe shortness of breath and appears cyanotic. Despite resuscitation, she dies 2 hours later. A section of lung at autopsy is shown in the image. These pathologic findings are associated with which of the following mechanisms of disease?

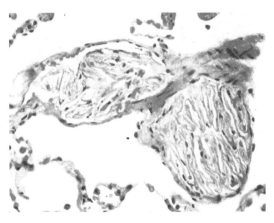

(A) Amniotic fluid embolism
(B) Cardiogenic shock
(C) Maternal-fetal histoincompatibility
(D) Metastatic squamous cell carcinoma
(E) Pulmonary thromboembolism

12 If the patient described in Question 11 had survived the acute episode of cyanosis and shock, she would have been at risk for developing which of the following life-threatening complications?

(A) Bacterial endocarditis
(B) Disseminated intravascular coagulation
(C) Fat embolism
(D) Neurogenic shock
(E) Septic shock

13 A 68-year-old man with ischemic heart disease and a history of smoking complains of increasing shortness of breath. On physical examination, the patient has swollen legs, an enlarged liver, and fluid in the pleural spaces (bubbly rales are heard on oscultation). Which of the following hemodynamic disorders explains the pathogenesis of hepatomegaly in this patient?

(A) Arterial thromboembolism
(B) Chronic passive congestion
(C) Deep venous thrombosis
(D) Multiple hepatic infarcts
(E) Thrombosis of the hepatic vein

14 The patient described in Question 13 suffers a massive heart attack and expires. Microscopic examination of the liver at autopsy would most likely reveal which of the following histopathologic changes?

(A) Diffuse hydropic degeneration
(B) Large iron deposits within hepatocytes
(C) Massive hepatic necrosis
(D) Regenerating hepatic nodules surrounded by fibrous bands
(E) Sinusoids dilated with blood

15 A 33-year-old woman presents with black stools. Laboratory studies demonstrate a hypochromic, microcytic anemia. Upper GI endoscopy reveals a duodenal ulcer. Which of the following best describes the stools in this patient with peptic ulcer disease?

(A) Hematemesis
(B) Hematobilia
(C) Hematochezia
(D) Melena
(E) Steatorrhea

16 A 53-year-old man is hospitalized after injuring his neck in an automobile accident. He is placed in cervical traction. One week later, the patient develops painful swelling and erythema of his left calf. Doppler imaging discloses deep venous thrombosis. Which of the following is the most likely cause for the development of thrombosis in this patient?

(A) Age
(B) Endothelial damage
(C) Hypercoagulability
(D) Infection
(E) Stasis

17 A 23-year-old man with hemophilia is recently wheelchair bound. Which of the following best accounts for this development?

(A) Hemarthrosis
(B) Hematemesis
(C) Hematocephalus
(D) Hematochezia
(E) Hemoptysis

18 A 50-year-old fire fighter emerges from a burning house with third-degree burns over 70% of his body. The patient expires 24 hours later. Which of the following was the most likely cause of death?

(A) Congestive heart failure
(B) Disseminated intravascular coagulation
(C) Hypovolemic shock
(D) Pulmonary saddle embolism
(E) Toxic shock syndrome

19 A 23-year-old woman complains of a recent onset of yellowing of her skin and increasing abdominal girth. Physical examination reveals jaundice and ascites. Ultrasound examination of her abdomen demonstrates thrombosis of the hepatic veins. A liver biopsy discloses severe sinusoidal dilation within the centrilobular regions. This pathologic finding is caused by which of the following hemodynamic disorders?

(A) Active hyperemia
(B) Arterial embolism
(C) Hematoma
(D) Hemorrhage
(E) Passive hyperemia

20 A 42-year-old woman undergoes a face lift. Two days later, she presents for follow-up care with confluent bluish hemorrhages in the skin around her eyes ("black eyes"). Which of the following best describes this pattern of superficial skin hemorrhage?

(A) Ecchymosis
(B) Hematocephalus
(C) Maculopapular rash
(D) Petechiae
(E) Purpura

21 A 19-year-old woman complains of swelling of her eyelids, abdomen, and ankles. At bedtime, there are depressions in her legs at the location of the elastic in her socks. A chest X-ray shows bilateral pleural effusions. Urine protein electrophoresis demonstrates 4+ proteinuria. A percutaneous needle biopsy of the kidney establishes the diagnosis of minimal change nephrotic syndrome. Soft tissue edema in this patient is most likely caused by which of the following mechanisms of disease?

(A) Active hyperemia
(B) Chronic passive congestion
(C) Decreased intravascular oncotic pressure
(D) Hyperalbuminemia
(E) Increased capillary permeability

22 A 50-year-old alcoholic is rushed to the hospital with bleeding esophageal varices and expires. At autopsy, the patient's protruding abdomen is found to contain a large volume of serous fluid. What is the appropriate term used to describe this fluid?

(A) Ascites
(B) Exudate
(C) Hemorrhage
(D) Hydrothorax
(E) Lymphedema

23 A 1-year-old girl is brought to the emergency room by her parents who report she has had a fever and diarrhea for 3 days. Her temperature is 38°C (101°F). The CBC shows a normal WBC count and increased hematocrit (48 g/dL). Which of the following is the most likely cause of increased hematocrit in this patient?

(A) Acute phase response
(B) Dehydration
(C) Diabetes insipidus
(D) Malabsorption
(E) Septic shock

24 A 40-year-old man with a history of bacterial endocarditis notices numerous pinpoint hemorrhages around the orbit of his eyes (shown in the image; see arrows). What is the appropriate term used to describe this form of superficial hemorrhage?

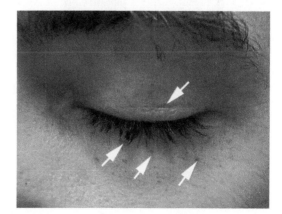

(A) Ecchymosis
(B) Erythema
(C) Hyperemia
(D) Petechia
(E) Purpura

25 A 67-year-old man presents with sudden left leg pain, absence of pulses, and a cold limb. His past medical history is significant for coronary artery disease and a small aortic aneurysm. Which of the following is most likely responsible for development of a cold limb in this patient?
(A) Acute myocardial infarction
(B) Arterial thromboembolism
(C) Cardiogenic shock
(D) Deep venous thrombosis
(E) Ruptured aortic aneurysm

26 A 78-year-old woman dies in her sleep. A Prussian blue stain of the lungs at autopsy is shown in the image. Which of the following is the most likely cause of these histopathologic findings?

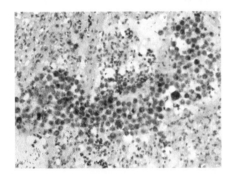

(A) Acute myocardial infarction
(B) Congestive heart failure
(C) Diffuse alveolar damage
(D) Hereditary hemochromatosis
(E) Pulmonary infarction

27 A 60-year-old man who is recovering from surgery to correct an abdominal aneurysm suddenly develops acute chest pain and dies. A thromboembolus at the bifurcation of the left and right pulmonary arteries is noted at autopsy (shown in the image). Which of the following is the most likely cause of this patient's pulmonary embolus?

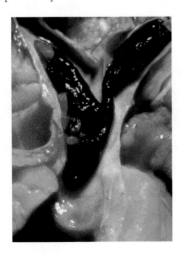

(A) Bacterial endocarditis
(B) Complicated atherosclerotic plaque
(C) Deep venous thrombosis
(D) Paradoxical embolization
(E) Right ventricular mural thrombus

28 A 20-year-old man is brought to the emergency room after rupturing his spleen in a motorcycle accident. His blood pressure on admission is 80/60 mm Hg. Analysis of arterial blood gasses demonstrates metabolic acidosis. This patient is most likely suffering from which of the following conditions?
(A) Acute pancreatitis
(B) Cardiogenic shock
(C) Hypersplenism
(D) Hypovolemic shock
(E) Septic shock

29 A 72-year-old man is dead on arrival after collapsing at home. Renal cortical infarcts are noted at autopsy. A section through the arcuate artery is shown. Which of the following is the most likely source of the atheroembolus occluding this artery?

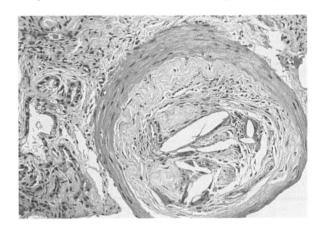

(A) Abdominal aorta
(B) Common carotid artery
(C) Inferior vena cava
(D) Left ventricle
(E) Mesenteric artery

30 A 72-year-old woman complains of shortness of breath on exertion. She states that she also becomes short of breath at night unless she uses three pillows (orthopnea). Physical examination reveals mild obesity, bilateral pitting leg edema, an enlarged liver and spleen, and fine crackling sounds on inspiration (rales). A chest X-ray shows cardiomegaly. What is the most likely cause of orthopnea in this patient?
(A) Asthma
(B) Cardiac tamponade
(C) Emphysema
(D) Hypovolemic shock
(E) Pulmonary edema

31 A 63-year-old man suffers a massive stroke and expires. At autopsy, the pathologist finds a laminated thrombus adherent to the wall of the left ventricle (shown in the image). Which of the following is the most likely cause of this autopsy finding?

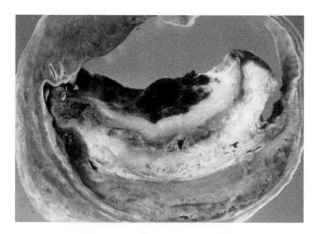

(A) Atrial fibrillation
(B) Bacterial endocarditis
(C) Marantic endocarditis
(D) Myocardial infarction
(E) Viral myocarditis

32 Histologic examination of the heart in the patient described in Question 31 shows extensive growth of fibroblasts and deposition of collagen in the mural thrombus. Which of the following terms describes this outcome of thrombosis?
(A) Canalization
(B) Hyalinization
(C) Organization
(D) Propagation
(E) Regeneration

33 A 50-year-old woman presents with fatigue and shortness of breath. Physical examination shows evidence of pulmonary edema, enlargement of the left atrium, and calcification of the mitral valve. A CT scan demonstrates a large obstructing mass in the left atrium. Before open heart surgery can be performed to remove the tumor, the patient suffers a stroke and expires. Which of the following hemodynamic disorders best explains the pathogenesis of stroke in this patient?
(A) Arterial embolism
(B) Atherosclerosis
(C) Cardiogenic shock
(D) Hypertensive hemorrhage
(E) Septic shock

34 A 50-year-old woman appears at your office. She was subjected to radical mastectomy and axillary node dissection for breast cancer a year ago. She now notices that her arm becomes swollen by the end of the day. What is the appropriate name for this fluid accumulation?
(A) Chylothorax
(B) Hydrothorax
(C) Lymphedema
(D) Purulent exudate
(E) Fibrinous exudate

35 A 68-year-old man develops sudden, severe substernal chest pain. Laboratory studies and ECG confirm an acute myocardial infarct. Despite vigorous therapy, the patient cannot maintain his blood pressure and expires 24 hours later. A cross

section of the left ventricle is examined at autopsy (shown in the image). The arrows point to a soft, yellow area of necrosis. Which of the following was the most likely cause of death?

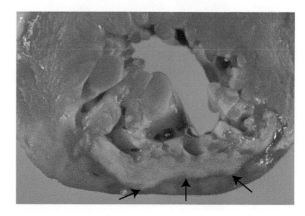

(A) Cardiogenic shock
(B) Hypovolemic shock
(C) Neurogenic shock
(D) Septic shock
(E) Pulmonary edema

36 An 80-year-old woman with a history of hypertension is rushed to the emergency room complaining of chest pain of 1-hour duration. Physical examination discloses bilateral pitting leg edema, hepatosplenomegaly, and rales at the bases of both lungs. The patient is apprehensive and sweating. The patient loses consciousness and dies of a cardiac arrhythmia. Microscopic examination of the lungs at autopsy is shown. Which of the following hemodynamic processes best explains this pathologic finding?

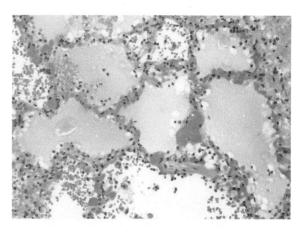

(A) Decreased capillary permeability
(B) Decreased intravascular oncotic pressure
(C) Increased intravascular hydrostatic pressure
(D) Increased intravascular oncotic pressure
(E) Vasoconstriction of precapillary arterioles

37 A 9-month-old infant is brought to the emergency room with a 3-hour history of intense abdominal pain and bloody diarrhea. Physical examination reveals a tender abdomen without ascites. The child dies 24 hours later, and torsion (volvulus) of the small bowel is discovered at autopsy. The small bowel appears dilated and hemorrhagic (shown in the image). Which of the following best describes these pathologic findings?

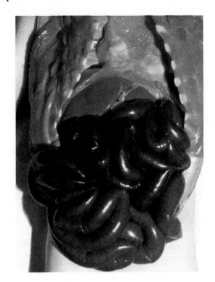

(A) Ecchymosis
(B) Infarct
(C) Petechia
(D) Purpura
(E) Ulcer

38 An autopsy of a 70-year-old woman reveals a subendocardial, circumferential infarct of the left ventricle. This type of infarct is most commonly associated with which of the following?
(A) Deep venous thrombosis
(B) Hypotensive shock
(C) Pericardial tamponade
(D) Thrombotic occlusion of the right coronary artery
(E) Thrombotic occlusion of the circumflex artery

39 A 76-year-old woman is brought to the emergency department because of the sudden onset of two episodes of hemoptysis and left-sided chest pain, which is exacerbated upon inspiration. Her temperature is 38°C (101°F), pulse 110 per minute, respirations 35 per minute, and blood pressure 158/100 mm Hg. The patient is admitted, but suffers a massive stroke and expires 48 hours later. Autopsy reveals a pulmonary infarct in upper segments of the lower lobe (shown in the image). Which of the following best explains the color of this patient's pulmonary infarct?

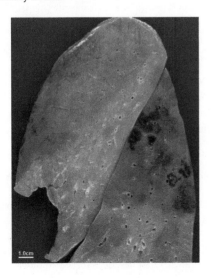

(A) Accumulation of hemosiderin-laden macrophages
(B) Development of bronchopneumonia
(C) Hemorrhage from bronchial arteries
(D) Organization of a pulmonary thromboembolus
(E) Passive congestion of bronchopulmonary segments

40 A 22-year-old woman delivers a baby at 29 weeks of gestation. Shortly after birth, the neonate becomes short of breath. The neonate is placed on a ventilator, but dies of respiratory insufficiency. The brain at autopsy is shown. Which of the following mechanisms of disease best explains this complication of respiratory distress syndrome (RDS) of the neonate?

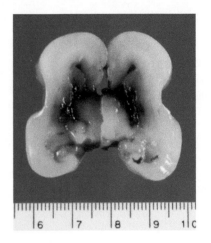

(A) Anoxic injury
(B) Birth trauma
(C) Chronic passive congestion
(D) Hemolytic anemia
(E) Hypertension

ANSWERS

1 **The answer is E: Vascular congestion and hemosiderin-laden macrophages.** Left ventricular failure leads to chronic passive congestion of the lungs. Blood leaks from the congested pulmonary capillaries into the alveoli. Alveolar macrophages degrade RBCs and accumulate hemosiderin. These hemosiderin-laden macrophages are called heart failure cells. Diffuse alveolar damage with hyaline membranes (choice A) is a feature of adult respiratory distress syndrome. Purulent exudate (choice B) is observed in bacterial pneumonia. Lymphocytic interstitial pneumonitis (choice C) is characteristic of viral pneumonitis. Plexiform lesions (choice D) are typically seen in patients with pulmonary hypertension.
Diagnosis: Congestive heart failure, pulmonary edema

2 **The answer is E: Septic shock.** Septic shock results from a systemic inflammatory response syndrome that leads to multiple organ dysfunction and hypotension. Clinical features include two or more signs of systemic inflammation (e.g., fever, tachycardia, tachypnea, leukocytosis, or leukopenia) in the setting of a known cause of inflammation. These processes often progress to multiple organ dysfunction syndrome in critically ill patients. Septicemia with Gram-negative organisms is the most common cause of septic shock. Anaphylactic shock (choice A) occurs as a consequence of a systemic type I hypersensitivity reaction. Neurogenic shock (choice D) can follow acute injury to the brain or spinal cord, which impairs the neural control of vasomotor tone, leading to generalized vasodilation. Cardiogenic shock (choice B) is a feature of advanced heart failure. Hypovolemic shock (choice C) occurs following blood loss.

Diagnosis: Septic shock

3 **The answer is C: Infarction.** Hypotension caused by postpartum bleeding can, in rare cases, lead to infarction of the pituitary. The pituitary is particularly susceptible at this time because its enlargement during pregnancy renders it vulnerable to a reduction in blood flow. None of the other choices cause clinical features of pan-hypopituitarism.

Diagnosis: Sheehan syndrome, pituitary infarction

4 **The answer is C: Hemorrhage.** Pericardial fluid may accumulate rapidly, particularly with hemorrhage caused by a ruptured myocardial infarct, dissecting aortic aneurysm (seen in this patient), or trauma. In these circumstances, the pressure in the pericardial cavity exceeds the filling pressure of the heart, a condition termed cardiac tamponade. The term "electromechanical dissociation" refers to a heart rhythm that should produce a pulse, but does not. The most common cause of this condition is hypovolemia. The resulting precipitous decline in cardiac output is often fatal. The pathogenesis of dissecting aortic aneurysm in most instances can be traced to a weakening of the aortic media (cystic medial necrosis). Most patients have a history of hypertension. Disseminated intravascular coagulation (choice A) refers to widespread ischemic changes secondary to microvascular thrombi. Passive hyperemia (choice D) refers to the engorgement of an organ with venous blood.

Diagnosis: Dissecting aortic aneurysm

5 **The answer is C: Increased intravascular hydrostatic pressure.** This patient with alcoholic cirrhosis has portal hypertension (increased hydrostatic pressure) and bleeding esophageal varices. Massive hematemesis is a frequent cause of death in patients with esophageal varices. Decreased intravascular oncotic pressure (choice A) contributes to the development of ascites in patients with cirrhosis but not to the development of esophageal varices.

Diagnosis: Esophageal varices, hematemesis

6 **The answer is E: Thromboembolism.** This patient with mild congestive heart failure developed pulmonary embolism. Small pulmonary emboli rarely cause infarctions because of the dual blood supply to the lungs and because oxygen can diffuse from the alveoli into lung tissue. Symptoms depend upon the extent of blockage of the pulmonary arterial tree, whether there is already cardiopulmonary disease, and whether pulmonary infarction occurs. The other choices do not induce these pleural signs and symptoms.

Diagnosis: Pulmonary thromboembolism

7 **The answer is C: Fat embolism.** Fat emboli originate from adipose tissue in the medulla of fractured long bones. Fat carried by venous blood reaches the lungs, filters through the pulmonary circulation, enters arterial blood, and is disseminated throughout the body. The occlusion of cerebral capillaries is accompanied by petechial hemorrhages in the brain and is the most important complication of fat embolism.

Acute myocardial infarction (choice A) would be unlikely in a 22-year-old patient. Deep venous thrombosis (choice B) and septic shock (choice E) would be unlikely within this time frame. Paradoxical embolism (choice D) refers to emboli that arise in the venous circulation and bypass the lungs by traveling through an incompletely closed foramen ovale, subsequently entering the arterial circulation.

Diagnosis: Fat embolism

8 **The answer is E: Tumor necrosis factor-α (TNF-α).** Septicemia with Gram-negative organisms is the most common cause of septic shock. The invading bacteria are responsible for the release of endotoxin, a lipopolysaccharide (LPS). On entry into the circulation, LPS binds to the surface of monocytes/macrophages. The CD14 recognition complex mediates signaling through activation of nuclear transcription factor-kappa B (NF-κB) and upregulates the expression of TNF-α. In septic shock, this protein is released in great excess, resulting in effects that are often lethal. None of the other mediators cause severe injury to vascular endothelium in patients with septic shock.

Diagnosis: Meningitis, septic shock

9 **The answer is C: Heart.** The heart is the most common source of arterial thromboemboli, which usually arise from mural thrombi or diseased valves. These emboli tend to lodge at points where the vessel lumen narrows abruptly (e.g., at bifurcations or in the area of an atherosclerotic plaque). The viability of the tissue supplied by the vessel depends on the availability of collateral circulation and on the fate of the embolus itself. Paradoxical emboli from the right side of the circulation are exceedingly rare.

Diagnosis: Cerebral embolism, stroke

10 **The answer is E: Intravenous drug use.** Embolism is the passage through the venous or arterial circulations of any material capable of lodging in a blood vessel and, thereby, obstructing its lumen. Intravenous drug abusers who use talc as a carrier for illicit drugs may introduce it into the lung via the bloodstream (i.e., venous embolism). None of the other choices exhibit birefringence under polarized light.

Diagnosis: Pulmonary embolism, talc embolism

11 **The answer is A: Amniotic fluid embolism.** Amniotic fluid embolism refers to the entry of amniotic fluid containing fetal cells and debris into the maternal circulation through open uterine and cervical veins. It is a rare maternal complication of childbirth, but when it occurs, it is often catastrophic. This disorder usually occurs at the end of labor when the pulmonary emboli are composed of the epithelial constituents (squamae) contained in the amniotic fluid. None of the other choices show these pathologic findings.

Diagnosis: Amniotic fluid embolism

12 **The answer is B: Disseminated intravascular coagulation (DIC).** The clinical presentation of amniotic fluid embolism can be dramatic, with the sudden onset of cyanosis and shock, followed by coma and death. If the mother survives the acute episode, she may die of DIC. Should she overcome this complication, she is at risk of developing acute respiratory distress syndrome. DIC is a thrombotic microangiopathy. Fibrin thrombi form in small blood vessels because of uncontrollable coagulopathy, which consumes fibrin and other coagulation

factors. Once coagulation factors are depleted, uncontrollable hemorrhage ensues. None of the other choices are complications of amniotic fluid embolism.
Diagnosis: Amniotic fluid embolism

13 **The answer is B: Chronic passive congestion.**   A generalized increase in venous pressure, typically from chronic heart failure, results in an increase in the volume of blood in many organs (e.g., liver, spleen, and kidneys). The liver is particularly vulnerable to chronic passive congestion because the hepatic veins empty into the vena cava immediately inferior to the heart. Budd-Chiari syndrome (thrombosis of the hepatic vein; choice E) may cause hepatomegaly, but it is not a complication of congestive heart failure.
Diagnosis: Congestive heart failure, nutmeg liver

14 **The answer is E: Sinusoids dilated with blood.**   In patients with chronic passive congestion of the liver, the central veins of the hepatic lobule become dilated. The increased venous pressure leads to dilation of the sinusoids and pressure atrophy of the centrilobular hepatocytes. Grossly, the cut surface of the chronically congested liver exhibits dark foci of centrilobular congestion surrounded by paler zones of unaffected peripheral portions of the lobules. The result resembles a cross section of a nutmeg and is appropriately called nutmeg liver. Longstanding passive congestion leads to bridging fibrosis; however, only in the most extreme cases is the fibrosis sufficiently severe to justify the label cardiac cirrhosis (choice D). None of the other choices are associated with congestive heart failure.
Diagnosis: Congestive heart failure, nutmeg liver

15 **The answer is D: Melena.**   Melena (black stool) is a symptom of upper gastrointestinal bleeding. Blood from ruptured esophageal varices or a peptic ulcer is partially digested by hydrochloric acid. Hemoglobin is transformed into a black pigment (hematin), which imparts a typical "coffee-grounds" color to the stool. Hematemesis (choice A) is vomiting of blood. Hematobilia (choice B) is bleeding into the biliary passages, as a complication of trauma or neoplasia. Hematochezia (choice C) is passage of bloody stools caused by lower gastrointestinal hemorrhage. Steatorrhea (choice E) is passage of fatty stools caused by pancreatic disease and malabsorption.
Diagnosis: Peptic ulcer disease

16 **The answer is E: Stasis.**   Venous thrombosis is caused by the same factors that predispose to arterial thrombosis, namely endothelial injury, stasis, and a hypercoagulable state. Although all of the choices are risk factors for deep venous thrombosis, the most likely choice, given the patients' immobilization, is stasis. Most venous thromboses occur in the deep veins of the legs.
Diagnosis: Deep venous thrombosis

17 **The answer is A: Hemarthrosis.**   Hemarthrosis refers to bleeding into the joint cavity. It is associated with joint swelling and is a crippling complication of hemophilia. Repeated bleeding may cause deformities and may limit the mobility of the joints. Hematemesis (choice B) is vomiting blood. Hematocephalus (choice C) is an intracranial infusion of blood. Hematochezia (choice D) is passage of blood caused by lower gastrointestinal hemorrhage. Hemoptysis (choice E) is coughing up blood.
Diagnosis: Hemophilia, hemarthrosis

18 **The answer is C: Hypovolemic shock.**   Hypovolemic shock may be caused by hemorrhage, fluid loss from severe burns, diarrhea, excessive urine formation, perspiration, or trauma. In the case of burns or trauma, direct damage to the microcirculation increases vascular permeability. Persons with third-degree burns weep large amounts of plasma. The other choices are unlikely causes of death in an acute burn victim.
Diagnosis: Hyperthermia, hypovolemic shock

19 **The answer is E: Passive hyperemia.**   Passive hyperemia (chronic passive congestion) may be confined to a limb or an organ as a result of localized obstruction to venous drainage. Examples include deep venous thrombosis of the leg veins, with resulting edema of the lower extremity, and thrombosis of the hepatic veins (Budd-Chiari syndrome, this patient) with secondary chronic passive congestion of the liver. Active hyperemia (choice A) is an augmented supply of blood to an organ, usually as a physiologic response to an increased functional demand. The most striking active hyperemia occurs in association with inflammation. Arterial embolism (choice B) typically causes infarction. Hematoma (choice C) and hemorrhage (choice D) represent extravascular accumulation of blood.
Diagnosis: Budd-Chiari syndrome

20 **The answer is A: Ecchymosis.**   Ecchymosis is a larger superficial hemorrhage in the skin. Following hemorrhage, the initially purple discoloration of the skin turns green and then yellow before resolving. This sequence of events reflects the progressive oxidation of bilirubin released from the hemoglobin of degraded erythrocytes. A "black eye" is a good example of an ecchymosis. Petechiae (choice D) are pinpoint hemorrhages, usually in the skin or conjunctiva. Purpura (choice E) is a diffuse superficial hemorrhage in the skin up to 1 cm in diameter.
Diagnosis: Ecchymosis

21 **The answer is C: Decreased intravascular oncotic pressure.**   The pressure differential between the intravascular and the interstitial compartments is largely determined by the concentration of plasma proteins, especially albumin. Any condition that lowers plasma albumin levels, whether from albuminuria in nephrotic syndrome or reduced albumin synthesis in chronic liver disease, tends to promote generalized edema.
Diagnosis: Minimal change nephrotic syndrome

22 **The answer is A: Ascites.**   A protruding belly and fluid accumulation in patients with cirrhosis represents ascites (i.e., accumulation of serous fluid in the abdominal cavity). It is primarily a consequence of portal hypertension and hypoalbuminemia. None of the other choices describe serous fluid accumulation in the abdomen.
Diagnosis: Cirrhosis, portal hypertension

23 **The answer is B: Dehydration.**   Increased hematocrit in this patient reflects hemoconcentration caused by dehydration, secondary to diarrhea. This hematologic condition, termed relative polycythemia, is characterized by decreased plasma volume with a normal red cell mass. When patients suffer from burns, vomiting, excessive sweating, or diarrhea, they not only lose fluid but also suffer electrolyte disturbances. Systemic blood pressure falls with continuous dehydration, and declining perfusion eventually leads to death. Diabetes insipidus (choice C) may cause dehydration but is an unlikely choice because the patient has a history of diarrhea. None of the other choices cause relative polycythemia.

Diagnosis: Dehydration, relative polycythemia

24 The answer is D: Petechia. Petechiae are pinpoint hemorrhages, usually in the skin or conjunctiva. This lesion represents the rupture of a capillary or arteriole and occurs in conjunction with vasculitis and coagulopathy. Petechiae may also be produced by microemboli from infected heart valves (bacterial endocarditis). Hyperemia (choice C) refers to increased blood in a tissue or organ. Erythema (choice B) is inflammatory redness of the skin. Ecchymosis (choice A) is a larger superficial hemorrhage in the skin. Purpura (choice E) is a diffuse superficial hemorrhage in the skin up to 1 cm in diameter.

Diagnosis: Endocarditis, petechia

25 The answer is B: Arterial thromboembolism. Embolism of an artery of the leg leads to sudden pain, absence of pulses, and a cold limb. In some cases, the limb must be amputated. None of the other choices would cause this clinical presentation. Ruptured aortic aneurysm (choice E) presents with pain, shock, and a pulsatile mass in the abdomen.

Diagnosis: Arterial thromboembolism

26 The answer is B: Congestive heart failure. Chronic failure of the left ventricle constitutes an impediment to the exit of blood from the lungs and leads to chronic passive congestion of the lungs. The pressure in the alveolar capillaries increases, and the vessels become engorged with blood. Microhemorrhages release erythrocytes into the alveolar spaces, where they are degraded by alveolar macrophages. The released iron, in the form of hemosiderin, remains in the macrophages, which are then labeled "heart failure cells." None of the other choices are consistent with chronic microhemorrhages in the lung.

Diagnosis: Congestive heart failure

27 The answer is C: Deep venous thrombosis. One of the most tragic calamities complicating hospitalization is the sudden death of a patient who appeared to be on the way to recovery. The cause of this catastrophe is often massive pulmonary embolism. A large pulmonary embolus may lodge at the bifurcation of the main pulmonary artery (saddle embolus), obstructing blood flow to both lungs. With acute obstruction of more than half of the pulmonary arterial tree, the patient experiences severe hypotension and may die within minutes. The other choices are causes of arterial embolism.

Diagnosis: Pulmonary thromboembolism

28 The answer is D: Hypovolemic shock. Hypovolemic shock is secondary to a pronounced decrease in blood or plasma volume, caused by the loss of fluid from the vascular compartment. Hemorrhage, fluid loss from severe burns, diarrhea, excessive urine formation, perspiration, and trauma are major mechanisms of fluid loss that can lead to hypovolemic shock. Cardiogenic shock (choice B) is caused by myocardial pump failure. Septic shock (choice E) is improbable in this setting.

Diagnosis: Hypovolemic shock

29 The answer is A: Abdominal aorta. In patients with severe aortic atherosclerosis, embolization of atheromatous debris into the renal arteries and vascular tree may cause acute renal failure. Cholesterol clefts are observed in the photomicrograph shown. None of the other choices are sources of renal atheroemboli.

Diagnosis: Renal infarct, arterial embolism

30 The answer is E: Pulmonary edema. Patients in left-sided congestive heart failure complain of shortness of breath (dyspnea) on exertion and when recumbent (orthopnea). They may be awakened from sleep by sudden episodes of shortness of breath (paroxysmal nocturnal dyspnea). Physical examination usually reveals distended jugular veins. Persons with right-sided failure have pitting edema of the lower extremities and an enlarged and tender liver. Patients in congestive heart failure with pulmonary edema have crackling breath sounds (rales) caused by the expansion of fluid-filled alveoli. Cardiac tamponade (choice B) occurs when the pressure in the pericardial cavity rises to exceed the filling pressure of the heart. Orthopnea is not a feature of the other choices.

Diagnosis: Congestive heart failure

31 The answer is D: Myocardial infarction. Myocardial infarction is the most common cause of mural thrombi in the left ventricle. These mural thrombi are a common source of arterial thromboemboli. Such emboli may occlude cerebral arteries and cause cerebral infarcts, known clinically as strokes. Atrial fibrillation (choice A) predisposes to the formation of mural thrombi in that location.

Diagnosis: Mural thrombus

32 The answer is C: Organization. Once formed, arterial thrombi may undergo (1) lysis, (2) propagation, (3) organization, (4) canalization, or (5) embolization. Organization refers to the invasion of connective tissue elements, which causes a thrombus to become firm and appear grayish white. Canalization (choice A) is the process by which new lumina lined by endothelial cells form within an organized thrombus. Propagation (choice D) implies an increase in size.

Diagnosis: Mural thrombus

33 The answer is A: Arterial embolism. Cardiac myxoma is the most common primary tumor of the heart. One third of patients with a left atrial or left ventricular myxoma die from tumor embolization to the brain. Less likely causes of stroke in this patient with a cardiac myxoma include atherosclerosis (choice B) and hypertensive hemorrhage (choice D).

Diagnosis: Cardiac myxoma

34 The answer is C: Lymphedema. Obstruction of lymphatic flow may occur in a number of clinical settings, but is most common because of surgical removal of lymph nodes or tumor obstruction. For example, the lymphatic system may be obstructed after axillary lymph node dissection for breast cancer. Prolonged lymphatic obstruction in the patient's shoulder causes edema, progressive dilation of lymphatic vessels (lymphangiectasia), and overgrowth of fibrous tissue. Lymphangiosarcoma has also been described. Chylothorax (choice A) represents an accumulation of lymphedema in the pleural space. Exudates (choices D and E) are associated with acute inflammation.

Diagnosis: Lymphedema, breast cancer

35 The answer is A: Cardiogenic shock. Cardiogenic shock is caused by myocardial pump failure. This condition usually arises as a result of a large myocardial infarction, but myocarditis may also be responsible. Conditions that prevent left or right heart filling reduce cardiac output, resulting in obstructive shock. Such conditions include pulmonary embolism, cardiac tamponade, and (rarely) atrial myxoma. The other choices do not reflect a loss of cardiac output secondary to the loss of myocardial tissue owing to ischemia.

Diagnosis: Acute myocardial infarction

36 The answer is C: Increased intravascular hydrostatic pressure. In patients with congestive heart failure, venous engorgement of the lung leads to accumulation of a transudate in the alveoli. Chronic left ventricle failure impedes blood flow out of the lungs and leads to passive pulmonary congestion. As a result, pressure in the alveolar capillaries increase (increased hydrostatic pressure) and these vessels become engorged with blood. Increased pressure forces fluid from the blood into the alveolar spaces, resulting in pulmonary edema, which interferes with gas exchange. The photomicrograph shows pink staining fluid in the alveoli. None of the other choices cause pulmonary edema in patients with congestive heart failure.

Diagnosis: Pulmonary edema, congestive heart failure

37 The answer is B: Infarct. Volvulus is an example of intestinal obstruction in which a segment of gut twists on its mesentery, thereby kinking the bowel and usually interrupting the blood supply. Ischemia leads to infarction and intestinal gangrene (this case). Volvulus is virtually always a consequence of an underlying congenital abnormality. Defective intestinal rotation in fetal life leads to abnormal positions of the small intestine and colon, anomalous attachments, and bands. The clinical importance of such rotational anomalies lies in their propensity to cause catastrophic volvulus of the small and large intestine and incarceration of the bowel in an internal hernia. Malrotation of the bowel permits undue mobility of the bowel loops and predisposes to midgut volvulus. When the cecum or right colon is invested with a mesentery rather than being retroperitoneal, the result may be cecal volvulus. An unusually long sigmoid colon, which occurs sometimes in patients with idiopathic constipation, permits the development of sigmoid volvulus. Meconium ileus in babies with cystic fibrosis may be complicated by volvulus and intestinal atresia. Ecchymosis (choice A), petechia (choice C), and purpura (choice D) represent hemorrhages of various sizes in the skin.

Diagnosis: Volvulus, ischemic colitis

38 The answer is B: Hypotensive shock. Myocardial infarcts are described as transmural (through the entire wall) or subendocardial. A transmural infarct results from complete occlusion of a major extramural coronary artery. Subendocardial infarction reflects prolonged ischemia caused by partially occluding lesions of the coronary arteries when the requirement for oxygen exceeds the supply. Such a situation prevails in disorders such as shock, anoxia, or severe tachycardia. Thrombotic occlusion (choices D and E) is more likely to cause transmural myocardial infarcts.

Diagnosis: Myocardial infarction

39 The answer is C: Hemorrhage from bronchial arteries. The gross and microscopic appearance of an infarct depends on its location and age. Pale infarcts are typically seen in the heart, kidneys, and spleen. Red infarcts may result from either arterial or venous occlusion. They are distinguished from pale infarcts by bleeding into the necrotic area from adjacent arteries and veins. Red infarcts occur principally in organs with a dual blood supply, such as the lung, or those with extensive collateral circulation, such as the small intestine and brain. In the heart, a red infarct occurs when the infarcted area is reperfused, as may occur following spontaneous or therapeutically induced lysis of the occluding thrombus. Grossly, red infarcts are sharply circumscribed, firm, and dark red to purple. Over a period of several days, acute inflammatory cells infiltrate the necrotic area from the viable border. The cellular debris is phagocytosed and digested by polymorphonuclear leukocytes and later by macrophages. Granulation tissue eventually forms, to be replaced ultimately by a scar. None of the other choices would cause hemorrhage into an infarct.

Diagnosis: Pulmonary infarction, pulmonary thromboembolism

40 The answer is A: Anoxic injury. The pathogenesis of RDS of the newborn is intimately linked to a deficiency of surfactant. This material lowers the surface tension of the alveoli at low lung volumes and thereby prevents collapse (atelectasis) of the alveoli during expiration. Atelectasis secondary to surfactant deficiency results in perfused but not ventilated alveoli, a situation that leads to hypoxia and acidosis. Intraventricular cerebral hemorrhage is a major complication of RDS. The periventricular germinal matrix in the newborn brain is particularly vulnerable to hemorrhage because the dilated, thin-walled veins in this area rupture easily (see photograph). The pathogenesis of this complication is believed to reflect anoxic injury to the periventricular capillaries, venous sludging and thrombosis, and impaired vascular autoregulation. Despite advances in neonatal intensive care, the overall mortality of RDS is about 15%, and one third of infants born before 30 weeks of gestational age die of this disorder. Although the other choices are associated with bleeding, they are unlikely causes of periventricular hemorrhage in a baby with RDS.

Diagnosis: Respiratory distress syndrome of the neonate

Chapter 8

Environmental and Nutritional Pathology

QUESTIONS

Select the single best answer.

1 A 65-year-old woman with a history of smoking presents with a 3-week history of chest pain and bloody sputum. An X-ray film of the chest reveals a hilar lung mass. The surgical specimen reveals a squamous cell carcinoma growing within the lumen of a bronchus (shown in the image). Which of the following chemical agents may be associated with the pathogenesis of the cancer in this patient?

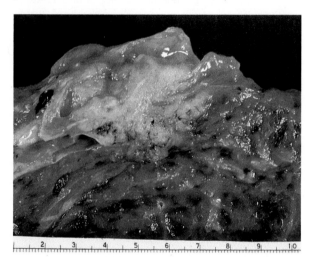

(A) Aflatoxins
(B) Aromatic hydrocarbons
(C) Benzene
(D) Branched chain amino acids
(E) Carbohydrate polymers

2 A 75-year-old man who had worked in a shipyard for 25 years dies of a thoracic tumor. Autopsy reveals a pleural tumor that encases the lung. Interstitial pulmonary fibrosis and multiple pleural plaques are noted. Numerous, brown, beaded ferruginous bodies are also found in the lungs (shown in the image). Which of the following agents is most likely associated with the pathogenesis of the cancer in this patient?

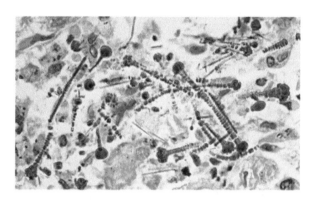

(A) Asbestos
(B) Beryllium
(C) Carbon
(D) Silica
(E) Tobacco

3 A 47-year-old man presents with a 6-week history of increasing fatigue and dark-colored stools. Complete blood count shows hemoglobin of 8.6 g/dL and microcytic, hypochromic RBCs. Upper gastrointestinal endoscopy reveals a peptic ulcer along the lesser curvature of the stomach. This patient's anemia is most likely caused by deficiency of which of the following?
(A) Folic acid
(B) Iron
(C) Thiamine
(D) Vitamin B_{12}
(E) Zinc

4 A 49-year-old woman presents with a 2-month history of yellow discoloration of her eyes, abdominal pain, weight loss, and low-grade fever (38.4°C, 101°F). Physical examination shows a distended abdomen, right upper quadrant tenderness, and a palpable liver 2 cm below the costal margin. A liver biopsy reveals alcoholic hepatitis. The patient recovers and is strongly advised to abstain from alcohol. However, she subsequently imbibes some antifreeze containing ethylene glycol and develops acute failure of which organ?

73

(A) Brain
(B) Heart
(C) Kidney
(D) Liver
(E) Pancreas

5   A neonate was noted to have mild growth retardation and facial dysmorphology. The mother was a known abuser of several substances. This infant's problem most likely resulted from maternal intake of which of the following?
(A) Alcohol
(B) Cocaine
(C) Ethylene glycol
(D) Heroin
(E) Marijuana

6   A 10-year-old boy presents with irritability and ataxia. He is subsequently found to have anemia, basophilic stippling of erythrocytes, and dark-gray pigmentation of the gums. Exposure to which of the following chemical agents is most likely associated with this disease?
(A) Arsenic
(B) Copper
(C) Lead
(D) Mercury
(E) Nickel

7   A 50-year-old man presents for a routine physical examination, which demonstrates an enlarged liver. During the visit, he describes memos from his supervisor at work regarding chronic exposure to vinyl chloride. The patient has an elevated risk for which of the following tumors?
(A) Angiosarcoma of the liver
(B) Carcinoid tumor
(C) Hepatic adenoma
(D) Lymphoma
(E) Metastatic colon cancer

8   A severely depressed 32-year-old man commits suicide by running his car motor in his closed garage for several hours. The mechanism of death in this case of carbon monoxide (CO) poisoning is through which of the following mechanisms?
(A) Displacement of oxygen on hemoglobin by CO
(B) Hepatocellular necrosis
(C) Inhibition of protein synthesis
(D) Inhibition of the respiratory chain enzymes
(E) Myocardial infarction

9   A Japanese fisherman who lives in the vicinity of a plastics factory develops severe neurologic symptoms, including constriction of visual fields, paresthesias, ataxia, dysarthria, and hearing loss. Public health authorities find a number of similar cases in the local village. Exposure to which of the following chemical agents is most likely associated with the pathogenesis of this man's neurologic disease?
(A) Arsenic
(B) Copper
(C) Lead
(D) Mercury
(E) Nickel

10   A 12-year-old boy is rescued 2 days after becoming lost in the Canadian woods in February. Physical examination shows he has gangrene of his fingers and toes. Which of the following mechanisms of cell injury played the most important role in mediating necrosis in the fingers and toes of this patient?
(A) Activation of proapoptotic proteins
(B) Generation of activated oxygen species
(C) Lipid peroxidation
(D) Membrane disruption by water crystals
(E) Protein and DNA crosslinking

11   A 35-year-old man is hospitalized with third-degree burns after being rescued from a house fire. Initially, he suffers from shock and oliguria, but his renal function returns to normal within a few days. Which of the following would be the most likely cause of death if complications were to arise?
(A) Ascites
(B) Curling ulcers with hemorrhage
(C) Cushing ulcers
(D) Pseudomembranous colitis
(E) Sepsis

12   A healthy adult runs a marathon in the summer and develops hot dry skin, cessation of sweating, lactic acidosis, hypocalcemia, and muscle necrosis (rhabdomyolysis). Which of the following is the appropriate diagnosis?
(A) Dysautonomia
(B) Heat stroke
(C) Malignant hyperthermia
(D) Myotonic dystrophy
(E) Polymyositis

13   A 26-year-old electrician is found unconscious in his backyard beside a metal ladder and an exposed electrical wire, suffering from a deep burn on his right hand. Resuscitation attempts are unsuccessful. Which of the following was the most likely cause of death?
(A) Cardiac arrhythmia
(B) Disseminated intravascular coagulation
(C) Myocardial infarction
(D) Rupture of the ascending aorta
(E) Uncoupling of oxidative phosphorylation

14   A sailor on a nuclear-powered submarine is seen by a physician after a breach in the reactor containment system. Physical examination is unremarkable, but the patient subsequently develops profound pancytopenia. Hemoglobin is 7.8 g/dL, WBC count is 900/μL, and platelets are 20,000/μL. How many rads of acute total-body radiation did this patient most likely receive?
(A) 1
(B) 3
(C) 30
(D) 300
(E) 3,000

15   Another sailor on the submarine (see Question 14) dies 10 days after the accident as a result of severe diarrhea and dehydration. Which of the following doses (in rads) of acute total-body radiation did this sailor most likely receive?

(A) 1

(B) 3

(C) 100

(D) 300

(E) 1,000

16 A 66-year-old woman presents with a 6-month history of scaling and abnormal pigmentation of the skin. Her past medical history is significant for the treatment of thyroid cancer 1 year ago. Biopsy of lesional skin shows atrophy of the epidermis and dense fibrosis of the dermis, which displays dilated superficial blood vessels. These pathologic findings are most likely caused by previous exposure to which of the following?

(A) Chemotherapy

(B) Corticosteroids

(C) Organic iodine

(D) Radiation therapy

(E) Tumor necrosis factor-α

17 A 28-year-old radar technician aboard an aircraft carrier has been subjected to intense microwave radiation for 7 years. He has an elevated risk for developing which of the following?

(A) Aplastic anemia

(B) Hodgkin disease

(C) Lymphocytic leukemia

(D) Myelogenous leukemia

(E) None of the above

18 A 15-year-old African boy has a history of tooth loss, gingivitis, skin hemorrhages, multiple infections, and poor wound healing. Physical examination shows that the child is in the 20th percentile for height and 10th percentile for weight. This patient most likely has which of the following underlying conditions?

(A) Beri-beri

(B) Impetigo

(C) Kwashiorkor

(D) Pellagra

(E) Scurvy

19 A 24-year-old woman, who is a food faddist, eats only corn-based foods. She presents with dermatitis, diarrhea, and dementia. This patient most likely suffers from which of the following conditions?

(A) Beri-beri

(B) Impetigo

(C) Kwashiorkor

(D) Marasmus

(E) Pellagra

20 A 45-year-old woman with longstanding Crohn disease and severe fat malabsorption experiences a fracture of the femoral neck after a minor contusion. This woman most likely has a deficiency of which of the following vitamins?

(A) Vitamin B_1 (thiamine)

(B) Vitamin C

(C) Vitamin D

(D) Vitamin K

(E) Niacin

21 A homeless man, who is a chronic alcoholic, is brought to the hospital in a wasted state. He is noted to have a peripheral

neuropathy, difficulty balancing, and dementia. He dies suddenly of an arrhythmia, and at autopsy, lesions are found in the mamillary bodies and the vicinity of the third ventricle. The vitamin deficiency associated with these signs and symptoms is which of the following?

(A) Vitamin B_1 (thiamine)

(B) Vitamin B_{12}

(C) Vitamin D

(D) Niacin

(E) Pyridoxine

22 A 40-year-old, malnourished woman presents with a 6-month history of night blindness. Physical examination reveals keratomalacia and corneal ulceration. Which of the following vitamin deficiencies would be suspected in this patient?

(A) Vitamin A

(B) Vitamin B_2 (riboflavin)

(C) Vitamin C

(D) Vitamin E

(E) Folic acid

23 A 26-year-old woman presents to the emergency room with fever and shaking chills. Her temperature is 38.7°C (103°F), pulse 120 per minute, and blood pressure 140/80 mm Hg. Physical examination reveals a harsh systolic murmur. The patient develops a headache, slips into a coma and expires. The aortic valve is examined at autopsy (shown in the image). Which of the following is the most important risk factor for this pathologic finding?

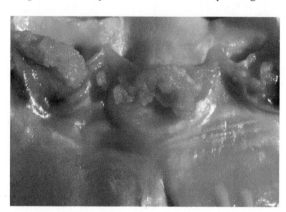

(A) Alcoholism

(B) Autoimmune disease

(C) Cigarette smoking

(D) Intravenous drug abuse

(E) Oral contraceptive use

24 A 50-year-old woman presents with easy fatigability, a smooth sore tongue, numbness and tingling of the feet, and weakness of the legs. A complete blood count shows a megaloblastic anemia that is not reversed by folate therapy. Hemoglobin is 5.6 g/dL, WBC count is 5,100/μL, and platelets are 240,000/μL. This patient most likely has a deficiency of which of the following vitamins?

(A) Vitamin B_1 (thiamine)

(B) Vitamin B_2 (riboflavin)

(C) Vitamin B_{12}

(D) Vitamin K

(E) Niacin

25 A starving, 4-year-old, African boy presents with apathy, generalized edema, and an enlarged fatty liver. The physician notes that, despite generalized growth failure, subcutaneous fat is preserved. What is the appropriate diagnosis?

(A) Beri-beri
(B) Kwashiorkor
(C) Marasmus
(D) Pellagra
(E) Scurvy

26 Petechial hemorrhages were noticed on the upper and lower extremities of a 5-day-old infant. Hemorrhagic disease of the neonate was most likely caused by a deficiency of which of the following vitamins?

(A) Vitamin B_2 (riboflavin)
(B) Vitamin D
(C) Folic acid
(D) Vitamin K
(E) Pyridoxine

27 A 6-year-old girl is examined at a clinic in central Africa. Physical examination reveals wasting of muscle and fat, and a protuberant abdomen. Her pulse, blood pressure, and temperature are low. The face appears wrinkled. There is no evidence of generalized edema. What is the appropriate diagnosis?

(A) Beri-beri
(B) Kwashiorkor
(C) Marasmus
(D) Pellagra
(E) Scurvy

28 A 40-year-old, chronically ill man from a Vietnamese village presents with painful sores around his mouth. Physical examination reveals prominent fissures at the angles of his mouth. Cheilosis in this patient is most likely caused by a deficiency of which of the following vitamins?

(A) Vitamin A
(B) Vitamin B_1 (thiamine)
(C) Vitamin B_2 (riboflavin)
(D) Vitamin B_{12}
(E) Vitamin C

29 A 32-year-old woman is a vegan (i.e., a strict vegetarian who eats no animal products of any kind). She is weak and pale, and laboratory studies show a macrocytic, normochromic anemia (hemoglobin = 6.2 g/dL). This patient most likely has which of the following vitamin deficiencies?

(A) Vitamin A
(B) Vitamin B_{12}
(C) Vitamin D
(D) Vitamin E
(E) Niacin

30 A 46-year-old man complains of weakness, dyspnea on exertion, and palpitations. His temperature is 37°C (98.6°F), pulse 95 per minute, respirations 24 per minute, and blood pressure 120/80 mm Hg. Physical examination reveals pulmonary rales and peripheral edema. Laboratory studies show normal serum cholesterol (180 mg/dL) and elevated fasting blood sugar (160 mg/dL). An echocardiogram discloses significant cardiomegaly but no valvular abnormalities or evidence of old myocardial infarcts. An angiogram shows normal coronary arteries. What is the most likely cause of his disease?

(A) Chronic alcoholism
(B) Cigarette smoking
(C) Diabetes mellitus
(D) Diffuse alveolar damage
(E) Rheumatic heart disease

31 A 28-year-old pregnant woman weighs 86.4 kg (190 lb) and gives birth after 39 weeks of gestation to a small baby weighing 2,300 g (5 lb, 1 oz). The baby has no congenital anomalies. Which of the following maternal factors in this case may be associated with the infant's low birth weight?

(A) Folic acid deficiency
(B) Obesity
(C) Premature delivery
(D) Previous oral contraceptive use
(E) Smoking

32 A 52-year-old man presents with sudden crushing chest pain and tachycardia. He admits to cigarette smoking, consumption of alcohol, and abuse of illicit drugs. An ECG is consistent with ischemic change in the anteroseptal region of the heart. Laboratory studies show elevated serum levels of CK-MB and troponin I. Serum cholesterol is 240 mg/dL. Which of the following most likely contributed to this patient's condition?

(A) Alcohol consumption
(B) Cigarette smoking
(C) Heroin addiction
(D) Inadequate calcium intake
(E) Marijuana use

33 A 52-year-old man presents with a chronic cough and shortness of breath. He admits to smoking two packs of cigarettes a day for 30 years. Pulmonary function tests reveal chronic obstructive pulmonary disease. In counseling this patient, you advise him to stop smoking immediately. You also mention that, in addition to emphysema, which of the following organs carries a significantly increased risk of smoking-related cancer?

(A) Brain
(B) Liver
(C) Pancreas
(D) Skin
(E) Small bowel

34 A homeless, poorly nourished man collapses on the street and cannot be revived by the emergency medical technicians. A social service agency notes that he had a long history of abusing many illicit drugs. An autopsy is performed and reveals a moderately enlarged heart, with patent coronary arteries and no valvular abnormalities. Microscopic examination shows patchy fibrosis of the myocardium. Which of the following substances most likely caused this cardiomyopathy?

(A) Cocaine
(B) Heroin
(C) Lysergic acid diethylamide (LSD)
(D) Marijuana
(E) Methamphetamine

35 A 52-year-old, obese man (BMI = 34 kg/m²) presents to his physician with complaints of hoarseness for 2 months. He has worked in a chemical factory for 25 years and gives a history of smoking, consumption of one or two beers a day, and occasional use of illicit drugs. Physical examination reveals enlarged and firm cervical lymph nodes. Direct laryngoscopy reveals a fixed and enlarged left vocal cord, which appears ulcerated. A biopsy of the lesion is interpreted by the pathologist as squamous cell carcinoma. What is the most likely cause of this man's disease?

(A) Alcohol
(B) Benzene inhalation
(C) Cigarette smoking
(D) Cocaine use
(E) High-fat diet

36 A 48-year-old man complains of weakness and easy fatigability for 6 weeks. He has worked for 20 years in a chemical factory that produces a variety of plastics and other synthetic compounds. A complete blood count shows a hemoglobin level of 8.2 g/dL, WBC count of 45,000/μL, and a platelet count of 40,000/μL. Examination of a bone marrow aspirate reveals numerous malignant myeloblasts, and a diagnosis of acute myeloid leukemia is made. Exposure to which of the following agents is the most likely cause of this patient's hematologic disease?

(A) Benzene
(B) Benzopyrene
(C) Carbon tetrachloride
(D) Glycerin
(E) Trichloroethylene

37 A 48-year-old woman complains she has had weakness, fatigue, and easy bruisability for 2 months. She had worked as a technician in a nuclear energy plant for 15 years and was involved in an accident during which she was exposed to considerable radiation. Physical examination reveals an enlarged liver and spleen. What disease should you suspect as a likely cause of her condition?

(A) Chronic myelogenous leukemia
(B) Hairy cell leukemia
(C) Metastatic carcinoma of the breast
(D) Metastatic carcinoma of the stomach
(E) Osteogenic sarcoma

38 A 16-year-old girl has suffered from severe celiac disease for years and reports continued steatorrhea. She suddenly develops abdominal pain in the right lower quadrant. A complete blood count shows a hemoglobin level of 14 g/dL, WBC of 18,000/μL, with 84% neutrophils, and a platelet count of 280,000/μL. A diagnosis of appendicitis is made, and tests before surgery reveal a prolonged prothrombin time of 17 seconds (control = 2). What is the most likely cause of her coagulation problem?

(A) Hemophilia A
(B) Hemophilia B
(C) Hypolipidemia
(D) Lymphoblastic leukemia
(E) Vitamin K deficiency

39 A 24-year-old beating victim is brought to the emergency room with a 4-cm linear tear of the skin caused by blunt trauma. Which of the following terms best describes this patient's skin lesion?

(A) Abrasion
(B) Avulsion
(C) Blast injury
(D) Contusion
(E) Laceration

ANSWERS

1 **The answer is B: Aromatic hydrocarbons.** These compounds (e.g., benzopyrene, methyl cholanthrene) are potent experimental carcinogens. Aflatoxins (choice A) produce experimental liver cancer. The tumor in this patient is a squamous cell carcinoma, which bears a strong resemblance to normal squamous cells and synthesizes keratin, as evidenced by epithelial pearls.
Diagnosis: Squamous cell carcinoma of the lung

2 **The answer is A: Asbestos.** Occupational exposure to asbestos poses a risk for the development of a pleural tumor termed malignant mesothelioma. Malignant disease may become evident 20 to 30 years following exposure. The inhalation of asbestos fibers also causes interstitial fibrosis of the lungs and pleural plaques consisting of dense connective tissue. Asbestos fibers coated with protein and iron are termed asbestos (ferruginous) bodies. The other choices do not produce ferruginous bodies or cause mesothelioma.
Diagnosis: Mesothelioma, asbestosis

3 **The answer is B: Iron.** Gastrointestinal hemorrhage leads to the loss of heme iron at a rate faster than it is replaced from dietary sources. The result is microcytic hypochromic anemia. The anemias associated with deficiencies of folic acid (choice A) and vitamin B_{12} (choice D) are macrocytic.
Diagnosis: Iron-deficiency anemia

4 **The answer is C: Kidney.** The major toxicity of ethylene glycol is acute tubular necrosis of the kidney, which results in renal failure. The compound has little effect on the other organs.
Diagnosis: Acute renal failure

5 **The answer is A: Alcohol.** Fetal alcohol syndrome is the most common acquired cause of mental retardation in the United States. The common features of the syndrome include intrauterine growth retardation, facial dysmorphology, neurologic impairment, and other congenital anomalies. In cases with lesser manifestations, termed fetal alcohol effect, children later suffer from mental retardation and minor dysmorphic features. Cocaine (choice B) may cause neonatal difficulties and heroin (choice D) intake may result in neonates that are addicted to that opiate, but they are not associated with characteristic facial dysmorphology.
Diagnosis: Fetal alcohol syndrome

6 **The answer is C: Lead.** Chronic lead poisoning inhibits delta-aminolevulinic acid dehydratase and ferrochelatase (enzymes essential for heme synthesis), thereby causing microcytic hypochromic anemia. The inhibition of heme synthesis leads to basophilic stippling of erythrocytes, which is due to residual ribosome clusters in the cytoplasm. Chronic exposure of children to lead also leads to cognitive loss. Mercury (choice D) poisoning has neurologic sequelae, but not these hematologic characteristics.

Diagnosis: Lead poisoning

7 **The answer is A: Angiosarcoma of the liver.** Occupational exposure to vinyl chloride (used in the production of plastics) is associated with the development of this malignant tumor of endothelial cells in the liver. Angiosarcoma is also associated with exposure to arsenic (a component of pesticides) and Thorotrast (a radioactive contrast medium used by radiologists prior to 1950). None of the other tumors have been associated with occupational exposure to vinyl chloride. Hepatic adenoma (choice C) is associated with the use of oral contraceptives.

Diagnosis: Angiosarcoma of the liver

8 **The answer is A: Displacement of oxygen on hemoglobin by CO.** CO combines with hemoglobin with an affinity 240 times greater than that of oxygen to form carboxyhemoglobin. At concentrations above 50% carboxyhemoglobin, cerebral anoxia, coma, convulsions, and death ensue. The other choices do not reflect the strong binding affinity of CO for hemoglobin.

Diagnosis: Carbon monoxide poisoning

9 **The answer is D: Mercury.** Mercury released into the environment may be bioconcentrated and enter the food chain, particularly predatory fish. Organic mercurials principally damage the brain, whereas inorganic mercury is toxic to the kidneys. Large outbreaks attributed to methyl mercury poisoning have been reported in Japan (fish) and Iraq (fungicides). Poisonings by the other choices do not elicit these neurologic symptoms.

Diagnosis: Mercury poisoning

10 **The answer is D: Membrane disruption by water crystals.** Exposure of the extremities to severe cold results in the crystallization of tissue water, which causes cellular disruption and vascular changes, resulting in frostbite. Localized thrombosis often leads to focal ischemia and gangrene of toes and fingers. Mechanical disruption of cellular membranes by ice crystals occurs during both freezing and thawing. The other choices are associated with cell death, but they are not early events in frostbite-induced necrosis.

Diagnosis: Frostbite

11 **The answer is E: Sepsis.** The most common cause of death in seriously burned patients is sepsis after infection of the burned skin. Gastric ulcers (stress or Curling ulcers, choice B) are occasionally encountered in burn patients, but they do not represent a common cause of death. Cushing ulcers of the stomach (choice C) are associated with trauma to the central nervous system.

Diagnosis: Sepsis, thermal injury

12 **The answer is B: Heat stroke.** Exertional heat stroke occurs in healthy men during unusually vigorous exercise, particularly when the ambient temperature is high. Lactic acidosis, hypocalcemia, and rhabdomyolysis may be severe problems. Myoglobinuric acute renal failure is not uncommon. Malignant

hyperthermia (choice C) occurs in surgical patients after anesthesia.

Diagnosis: Heat stroke

13 **The answer is A: Cardiac arrhythmia.** Electrical energy disrupts the electrical system within the heart and frequently causes death through ventricular fibrillation. The force produced by high-voltage currents vaporizes tissue water and produces extensive damage. The other choices are not consequences of powerful electrical currents. Although myocardial infarction (choice C) can cause an immediate arrhythmia, it reflects obstruction of the coronary circulation.

Diagnosis: Electrical injury, cardiac arrhythmia

14 **The answer is D: 300.** Acute total-body irradiation of about 300 rads causes depression of the bone marrow, and symptoms related to granulocytopenia and thrombocytopenia develop within 2 weeks. Anemia follows more slowly because red blood cells have a longer lifespan than leukocytes and platelets. Exposure to 3,000 rads (choice E) is rapidly fatal owing to central nervous system damage.

Diagnosis: Radiation sickness

15 **The answer is E: 1,000.** A radiation dose of 1,000 rads causes destruction of tissues composed of proliferating cells. Damage to the gastrointestinal tract is the most serious consequence and ensues within days of exposure. Death results from massive fluid loss from the denuded intestinal mucosa and superimposed passage of bacteria through the damaged intestine. The lower doses listed in the question do not destroy the gastrointestinal epithelium.

Diagnosis: Radiation sickness

16 **The answer is D: Radiation therapy.** Ionizing radiation administered for the treatment of cancer must first traverse the skin, leading to radiation dermatitis. Skin biopsy shows atrophy of the epidermis and dense fibrosis of the dermis, which displays dilated superficial blood vessels. In some cases, persistent ulcers require skin grafts. The other choices do not cause these dermal findings.

Diagnosis: Radiation injury

17 **The answer is E: None of the above.** The absorption of microwave energy produces only heat and is not associated with any known health risks.

Diagnosis: Radiation injury

18 **The answer is E: Scurvy.** Vitamin C is essential for collagen synthesis, and its deficiency results in poor wound healing. Perifollicular hemorrhages arise from capillaries that have weak walls and are easily damaged by minor trauma. Impaired collagen synthesis leads to gingivitis and alveolar bone resorption, resulting in loss of teeth. Wound healing requires collagen synthesis and is impaired in patients with vitamin C deficiency (scurvy).

Diagnosis: Scurvy, vitamin C deficiency

19 **The answer is E: Pellagra.** Niacin deficiency leads to the 3 "Ds": dermatitis, diarrhea, and dementia. A swollen, fissured tongue and chronic watery diarrhea are also characteristic. Dementia reflects degeneration of ganglion cells in the cerebral cortex.

Diagnosis: Pellagra, niacin deficiency

20 **The answer is C: Vitamin D.** Lipid malabsorption interferes with the absorption of vitamin D, thereby leading to a deficiency state. In adults, vitamin D deficiency results in osteomalacia, a disorder characterized by inadequate mineralization of newly formed bone matrix. The consequent weakness of bone is associated with a vulnerability to spontaneous fractures. Vitamin D deficiency in children is termed rickets. Deficiencies in the other choices are not associated with these bone abnormalities.

Diagnosis: Osteomalacia, vitamin D deficiency

21 **The answer is A: Vitamin B$_1$ (thiamine).** This man suffers from beri-beri (heart) and Wernicke-Korsakoff syndrome (brain). Thiamine deficiency in deteriorated alcoholics results in encephalopathy, peripheral neuropathy, and other disorders. Atrophy of the mammillary bodies, with loss of ganglion cells and rupture of small blood vessels, is characteristic. Deficiencies of the other vitamins are not related to these disorders.

Diagnosis: Beri-beri, Wernicke encephalopathy

22 **The answer is A: Vitamin A.** Vitamin A deficiency causes squamous metaplasia at a number of sites. In the cornea, it leads to xerophthalmia (dry eye), which may progress to softening of the tissue (keratomalacia) and corneal ulceration. Deficiencies of the other vitamins are not related to these clinical and pathologic findings.

Diagnosis: Vitamin A deficiency, keratomalacia

23 **The answer is D: Intravenous drug abuse.** The introduction of bacteria by intravenous drug abuse may lead to septic complications in many organs. Bacterial endocarditis, often involving *Staphylococcus aureus*, may occur on both sides of the heart. Infected emboli can occlude vessels leading to gangrene. Infected emboli in the brain can cause cerebral abscess. The photograph shows adherent vegetations on the aortic valve. These vegetations are composed of platelets, fibrin, cell debris, and masses of organisms. In addition to intravenous drug abuse, risk factors for bacterial endocarditis include congenital heart disease (children), rheumatic heart disease, prosthetic heart valves, transient bacteremia, and diabetes. Although certain autoimmune diseases (choice B) are associated endocarditis (e.g., Libman-Sacks), the verrucous vegetations are sterile (nonbacterial). The other choices are not associated with a significantly increased risk of bacterial endocarditis.

Diagnosis: Bacterial endocarditis

24 **The answer is C: Vitamin B$_{12}$.** Except for a few rare situations, vitamin B$_{12}$ (cyanocobalamin) deficiency is usually a result of pernicious anemia, an autoimmune disease of the stomach. Vitamin B$_{12}$ is required for DNA synthesis, and its deficiency results in large (megaloblastic) nuclei.

Diagnosis: Vitamin B$_{12}$ deficiency, pernicious anemia

25 **The answer is B: Kwashiorkor.** Kwashiorkor is a syndrome that results from a deficiency of protein in a diet relatively high in carbohydrates. It is one of the most common diseases of infancy and childhood in the nonindustrialized world. It usually occurs after an infant is weaned, when a protein-poor diet, consisting principally of staple carbohydrates, replaces mother's milk. Unlike marasmus (choice C), the disorder features edema, large fatty liver, and depigmentation of the skin. Extreme apathy is notable, diarrhea is common, and anemia

is the rule. These changes are reversible if and when sufficient protein is made available.

Diagnosis: Kwashiorkor

26 **The answer is D: Vitamin K.** Hemorrhagic disease of the newborn may be caused by a deficiency of vitamin K. Vitamin K is an important coagulation factor, which is necessary for the carboxylation and activation of prothrombin, as well as of clotting factors VII, IX, and X. Newborn infants frequently exhibit vitamin K deficiency because the vitamin is not transported well across the placenta, and the sterile gut of the newborn does not have bacteria to produce it. The other vitamin deficiencies do not impair coagulation.

Diagnosis: Vitamin K deficiency, hemolytic disease of the newborn

27 **The answer is C: Marasmus.** Deficiency of all elements of the diet leads to marasmus. The condition is common throughout the nonindustrialized world, particularly when breast feeding is stopped, and a child must subsist on a calorically inadequate diet. The pathological changes are similar to those in starving adults and consist of decreased body weight, diminished subcutaneous fat, a protuberant abdomen, muscle wasting, and a wrinkled face. In general, the child appears as a "shrunken old person." Wasting and increased lipofuscin pigment are seen in most visceral organs, especially the heart and the liver. No edema is present. The pulse, blood pressure, and temperature are low, and diarrhea is common. Because immune responses are impaired, the child suffers from numerous infections. An important consequence of marasmus is growth failure. If these children are not provided with an adequate diet during childhood, they will not reach their full potential stature as adults. Kwashiorkor (choice B) results from deficiency of protein in the diet. Choices A, D, and E result from deficiencies of vitamin B$_1$, nicacin, and vitamin C, respectively.

Diagnosis: Marasmus

28 **The answer is C: Vitamin B$_2$ (riboflavin).** Cheilosis refers to fissures at the angles of the mouth and is a common finding in patients with vitamin B$_2$ (riboflavin) deficiency. Riboflavin participates in the synthesis of flavin mononucleotides. Seborrheic keratosis and interstitial keratitis of the cornea also occur in patients with vitamin B$_2$ (riboflavin) deficiency. Except for vitamin A deficiency (which does not cause cheilosis), the other choices (B, D, and E) do not affect the skin.

Diagnosis: Cheilosis, vitamin B$_2$ (riboflavin) deficiency

29 **The answer is B: Vitamin B$_{12}$.** Vitamin B$_{12}$, which is necessary for DNA synthesis, is contained only in animal products, including eggs. Extreme vegetarians may suffer vitamin B$_{12}$ deficiency after many years of a restricted diet. The result is a macrocytic anemia similar to that seen in pernicious anemia. Macrocytic anemia is not a consequence of the other choices.

Diagnosis: Vitamin B$_{12}$ deficiency, megaloblastic anemia

30 **The answer is A: Chronic alcoholism.** Alcoholic cardiomyopathy correlates with the total lifetime dose of alcohol and leads to dilation and hypertrophy of the heart. As in this case, the disorder may cause congestive heart failure. Cigarette smoking (choice B) and diabetes mellitus (choice C) are associated with coronary artery disease, and rheumatic heart disease (choice E) features valvular abnormalities.

Diagnosis: Alcoholic cardiomyopathy

31 **The answer is E: Smoking.** Fetal tobacco syndrome refers to the deleterious effects of maternal cigarette smoking on the development of the fetus. Infants born to women who smoke during pregnancy are, on average, 200 g lighter than infants born to women who do not smoke. These infants are not born preterm, but rather, are small for gestational age. The noxious effect of smoking on the fetus is mirrored by its effect on the uteroplacental unit. The incidences of abruptio placentae, placenta previa, uterine bleeding, and premature rupture of the membranes are all increased in women who smoke. Evidence indicates that the injurious effects of maternal cigarette smoking are not limited to the fetus but extend to the physical, cognitive, and emotional development of children at older ages. Choices A, B, and D are not associated with low birth weight infants.
Diagnosis: Fetal tobacco syndrome

32 **The answer is B: Cigarette smoking.** Cigarette smoking is recognized as a major independent risk factor for myocardial infarction and acts synergistically with other risk factors such as high blood pressure and elevated blood cholesterol levels. It not only serves to precipitate initial myocardial infarction but also increases the risk for second heart attacks and diminishes survival after a heart attack among those who continue to smoke. Smoking also increases the incidence of sudden cardiac death, possibly by exacerbating regional ischemia. Atherosclerosis of the coronary arteries and the aorta is more severe and extensive among cigarette smokers than among nonsmokers, and the effect is dose related. Chronic alcohol consumption (choice A) actually protects against coronary artery disease, although dilated cardiomyopathy may develop. The other choices are not related to heart disease.
Diagnosis: Myocardial infarction

33 **The answer is C: Pancreas.** Cancer of the pancreas has shown a steady increase in incidence, which is partly related to cigarette smoking. The risk for adenocarcinoma of the pancreas in male smokers is elevated two- to threefold, and a clear dose-response relationship exists. In fact, men who smoke more than two packs a day have a five times greater risk of developing pancreatic cancer than nonsmokers. Smoking does not increase the risk of cancer for the other choices.
Diagnosis: Chronic obstructive pulmonary disease

34 **The answer is A: Cocaine.** Cocaine overdose leads to anxiety, delirium, and occasionally seizures. Cardiac arrhythmias and other effects on the heart may cause sudden death in otherwise healthy persons. Chronic abuse of cocaine is associated with the occasional development of a characteristic dilated cardiomyopathy, probably because of its effects in small, intramyocardial, coronary arteries. The other choices do not cause cardiomegaly.
Diagnosis: Cocaine cardiomyopathy

35 **The answer is C: Cigarette smoking.** Cancers of the lip, tongue, and buccal mucosa occur principally (>90%) in tobacco users. Cancer of the larynx and esophagus also result from smoking (>80% of cases). In some large studies, all deaths from cancer of the larynx occurred in smokers. There is no epidemiologic evidence that the other choices are risk factors for laryngeal cancer, although chronic alcoholism may be associated with a slightly increased risk.
Diagnosis: Laryngeal carcinoma

36 **The answer is A: Benzene.** Virtually all cases of acute and chronic benzene toxicity have occurred against the background of industrial exposure. Acute benzene poisoning primarily affects the central nervous system, and death results from respiratory failure. However, the long-term effects of benzene exposure have attracted the most attention. The bone marrow is the principal target in chronic benzene intoxication. Patients who develop hematologic abnormalities characteristically exhibit hypoplasia or aplasia of the bone marrow and pancytopenia. Aplastic anemia usually is seen while the workers are still exposed to high concentrations of benzene. In a substantial proportion of cases of benzene-induced anemias, acute myeloblastic leukemia develops. Overall, the risk of leukemia is increased 60-fold in workers exposed to the highest atmospheric concentrations of benzene. The other choices are not linked to the development of leukemia.
Diagnosis: Acute myelogenous leukemia

37 **The answer is A: Chronic myelogenous leukemia.** The evidence that whole-body radiation can lead to cancer is incontrovertible and comes from animal experiments and studies of the effects of occupational exposure, radiation therapy for nonneoplastic conditions, the diagnostic use of certain radioisotopes, and the atom bomb explosions. Some survivors of the atom bomb explosions and patients subjected to spinal radiation later developed chronic myelogenous leukemia. Although the other choices may lead to hepatosplenomegaly, they are not linked to acute radiation exposure.
Diagnosis: Chronic myelogenous leukemia

38 **The answer is E: Vitamin K deficiency.** Vitamin K deficiency is common in severe fat malabsorption, as seen in celiac sprue and biliary tract obstruction. The destruction of intestinal flora by antibiotics may also result in vitamin K deficiency. Vitamin K, which confers calcium-binding properties to certain proteins, is important for the activity of four clotting factors: prothrombin, factor VII, factor IX, and factor X. Deficiency of vitamin K can be serious because it can lead to catastrophic bleeding.
Diagnosis: Vitamin K deficiency

39 **The answer is E: Laceration.** A laceration is a linear tear of the skin produced by a force that causes unidirectional displacement. A surgical incision is a controlled laceration. Internal organs may also be lacerated by trauma or by the surgeon. An abrasion (choice A) is a skin defect caused by crushes or scrapes. Avulsion (choice B) is a tearing away or forcible separation. A contusion (choice D) is a localized mechanical injury with focal hemorrhage.
Diagnosis: Laceration

Chapter 9

Infectious and Parasitic Diseases

QUESTIONS

Select the single best answer.

1   A 23-year-old man presents with a 6-day history of fever, sore throat, swollen lymph nodes, weight loss, and fatigue. Physical examination shows generalized lymphadenopathy, most prominent in the cervical lymph nodes, and mild hepatosplenomegaly. The peripheral blood smear shows 65% atypical lymphocytes. A Paul-Bunnell antigen test (heterophile antibody test) is positive. The serum ALT, AST, and bilirubin are slightly elevated. The atypical lymphocytes in this patient's peripheral blood are described as which of the following?
(A) Activated T cells
(B) Immature B cells
(C) Mature B cells
(D) Natural killer cells
(E) Plasma cells

2   Which of the following is the most likely complication for the patient described in Question 1?
(A) Burkitt lymphoma
(B) Cirrhosis
(C) Encephalitis
(D) Laryngeal stricture
(E) Rupture of the spleen

3   A 19-year-old woman presents with vague lower abdominal pain and a swollen, painful right knee. She denies any trauma to the knee or history of arthritic disorders. Physical examination reveals an enlarged joint that is red, warm, and painful. Pelvic examination is exquisitely painful and reveals an ill-defined thickening in both adnexae. A green-yellow purulent vaginal discharge is noted. The patient is febrile and has an elevated WBC count of 15,000/μL. Which of the following etiologic agents is most likely responsible for this patient's condition?
(A) *Escherichia coli*
(B) *Neisseria gonorrhoeae*
(C) *Streptococcus pyogenes*
(D) *Treponema pallidum*
(E) *Yersinia pestis*

4   A 54-year-old man presents with a worsening skin rash of 10 days in duration. Physical examination shows an extensive, desquamative maculopapular rash of the palms and soles (shown in the image). The VDRL and FT-ABS tests are both positive. Which of the following lesions is also expected in this patient at this stage of his disease?

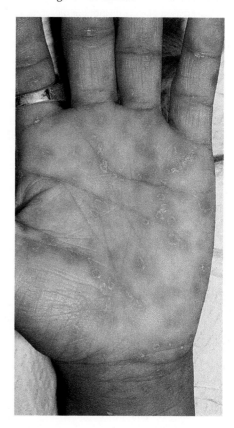

(A) Chancre
(B) Dementia
(C) Endarteritis obliterans
(D) Gummas
(E) Tabes dorsalis

81

5 A 35-year-old man presents with multiple skin lesions on his left forearm. He had worked in a garment factory, where he sorted wool imported from Iran. Physical examination shows an elevated cutaneous papule with bloody purulent exudate. An adjacent lesion displays a black scab. There is prominent axillary lymphadenopathy. This patient's necrotizing skin lesions are most likely caused by which of the following pathogens?

(A) *Bacillus anthracis*
(B) *Clostridium perfringens*
(C) *Escherichia coli*
(D) *Streptococcus pyogenes*
(E) *Treponema pallidum*

6 A 24-year-old man, who has just returned from a trip to India, complains of fatigue and severe, unremitting, watery diarrhea. Laboratory studies show severe hypernatremia and hypokalemia. Which of the following metabolic changes in enterocytes is chiefly responsible for the pathogenesis of this patient's acute gastrointestinal disorder?

(A) Decreased intracellular calcium
(B) Decreased plasma membrane biosynthesis
(C) Decreased water secretion
(D) Increased intracellular cAMP
(E) Increased intracellular water

7 A 12-year-old girl develops fever, abdominal pain, and bloody diarrhea 1 to 2 days after eating a hamburger at a fast food restaurant. Physical examination reveals an extensive purpuric skin rash. The patient develops oliguria, and laboratory studies show elevated serum levels of BUN and creatinine. Which of the following is the most likely etiologic agent responsible for this patient's condition?

(A) *Campylobacter jejuni*
(B) *Escherichia coli* 0157-H7
(C) *Salmonella typhi*
(D) *Shigella dysenteriae*
(E) *Yersinia pestis*

8 A 65-year-old man undergoes cardiac bypass surgery and is placed on postoperative, broad-spectrum, antibiotic prophylaxis. Several days later, he develops fever, abdominal pain, and bloody diarrhea. Colonoscopic biopsy demonstrates a thick mucopurulent exudate. Which of the following is the most likely etiology of this patient's gastrointestinal disorder?

(A) *Clostridium botulinum*
(B) *Clostridium difficile*
(C) *Clostridium perfringens*
(D) *Clostridium tetani*
(E) *Escherichia coli* 0157-H7

9 A 24-year-old woman develops an expanding erythematous skin lesion after hiking through the woods in Connecticut. The rash disappears, but 1 year later, the patient develops arthralgias and right facial nerve palsy. Which of the following is the most likely etiologic agent responsible for this patient's symptoms?

(A) Chlamydia
(B) Mycobacterium
(C) Protozoa
(D) Rickettsia
(E) Spirochete

10 A 3-year-old child attending a daycare center develops fever, chills, generalized rash, and a stiff neck. The child becomes hypotensive and expires the next day. Postmortem examination demonstrates bilateral adrenal hemorrhages (shown on right). Which of the following etiologic agents is the most likely cause of this child's disease?

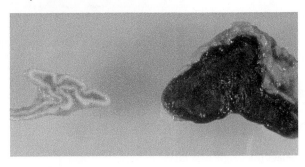

(A) *Haemophilus influenzae*
(B) *Klebsiella pneumoniae*
(C) *Neisseria meningitides*
(D) *Streptococcus pneumoniae*
(E) *Treponema pallidum*

11 A 45-year-old woman from India develops paroxysms of fever, chills, and severe headache while visiting her brother in the United States. Physical examination demonstrates hepatosplenomegaly and general pallor. Laboratory studies show anemia and hyperbilirubinemia. Her urine appears dark on visual inspection, and a urine dipstick is positive for hemoglobin. The patient develops tonic-clonic seizures and becomes comatose. Which of the following pathogens is most likely responsible for this patient's symptoms?

(A) *Naegleria fowleri*
(B) *Plasmodium falciparum*
(C) *Plasmodium vivax*
(D) *Schistosoma haematobium*
(E) *Trypanosoma bruceii*

12 A 56-year-old woman undergoes multidrug chemotherapy for breast cancer. After 10 days, she develops cough, fever, and respiratory distress. An X-ray film of the chest shows multiple areas of consolidation, with a large cavity in the right upper lobe. Despite vigorous therapy, the patient dies. Examination of the lungs at autopsy discloses multiple, sharply delineated, gray foci with hemorrhagic borders. A section of lung impregnated with silver is shown in the image. Which of the following mechanisms of disease best accounts for these pathologic findings?

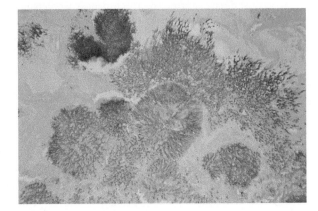

(A) Allergic inflammation

(B) Necrosis of type I pneumocytes and formation of hyaline membranes

(C) Perivascular plasma cell infiltrate with obliterative endarteritis

(D) Production of toxins that inhibit protein synthesis

(E) Thrombosis of blood vessels invaded by hyphae

13 A 30-year-old woman presents with persistent dry cough, fatigue, and low-grade fever. Physical examination shows marked pallor, respiratory distress, nasal flaring, and intercostal retractions. A chest X-ray reveals diffuse, bilateral interstitial infiltrates. A photomicrograph of bronchoalveolar lavage is shown. Which of the following etiologic agents is most likely responsible for this patient's pulmonary disease?

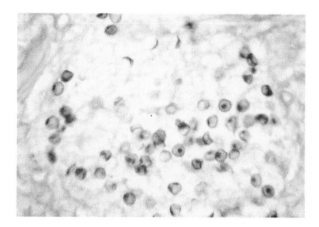

(A) *Aspergillus fumigatus*

(B) *Legionella pneumoniae*

(C) *Mycoplasma pneumoniae*

(D) *Pneumocystis jiroveci*

(E) Respiratory syncytial virus

14 A 28-year-old man presents with sudden onset of fever, chills, and a productive cough with blood-tinged sputum. His past medical history is significant for a splenectomy following a motor vehicle accident 3 years ago. An X-ray of the chest demonstrates consolidation of the right middle lobe. Sputum culture shows Gram-positive diplococci. Which of the following is the most likely cause of this patient's respiratory infection?

(A) *Klebsiella pneumoniae*

(B) *Legionella pneumophila*

(C) *Mycoplasma pneumoniae*

(D) *Staphylococcus aureus*

(E) *Streptococcus pneumoniae*

15 An 11-year-old boy presents with tea-colored urine and reduced urine output. He was seen for acute pharyngitis 3 weeks previously. Physical examination shows puffiness around the eyes and pitting edema of the lower extremities. Temperature and blood pressure are normal. Urinalysis reveals 2+ hematuria and 3+ proteinuria. Blood analysis discloses reduced serum levels of C3 and an elevated titer of antistreptolysin O antibodies. This patient's renal disease is most likely mediated by which of the following mechanisms?

(A) Antineutrophil cytoplasmic autoantibodies

(B) Deposition of circulating immune complexes

(C) Directly cytotoxic IgG and IgM antibodies

(D) IgE–mediated mast cell degranulation

(E) T cell–mediated delayed hypersensitivity reaction

16 A 59-year-old man with colon cancer is treated with chemotherapy. Two months later, he develops increasing cough and respiratory distress. A chest X-ray shows diffuse bilateral interstitial infiltrates. Sputum cultures are negative, and the patient does not respond to antibiotic therapy. A lung biopsy reveals acute and chronic interstitial pneumonitis. There are enlarged cells with prominent, dark-blue nuclear inclusions (shown in the image). Which of the following is most likely responsible for this patient's pulmonary condition?

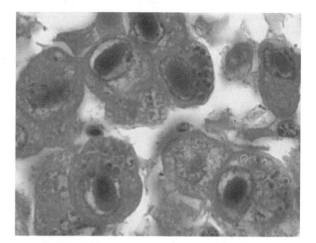

(A) Cytomegalovirus

(B) Epstein-Barr virus

(C) Herpes simplex virus

(D) Mycoplasma

(E) *Pneumocystis jiroveci*

17 A 6-month-old female infant is brought to the physician with a 2-day history of severe cough, wheezing, and respiratory distress. Physical examination shows rhinitis, mild cyanosis, and fever. Which of the following is the most likely etiology of this child's pulmonary infection?

(A) Adenovirus

(B) Cytomegalovirus

(C) Parainfluenza virus

(D) Respiratory syncytial virus

(E) Rhinovirus

18 A 75-year-old woman died in February of respiratory failure after a febrile disease of 1 week in duration. An autopsy shows necrotizing bronchitis and diffuse, hemorrhagic necrotizing pneumonia. Which of the following pathogens was most likely responsible for this patient's fatal pulmonary infection?

(A) Influenza virus

(B) Norwalk-like viruses

(C) Respiratory syncytial virus

(D) Rhinovirus

(E) Rotavirus

19 A 4-year-old girl, whose parents recently immigrated from Ecuador, presents with high fever, cough, and skin rash of 3 days in duration. Her parents report that her rash began in the form of pink papules behind the ears and spread around her body. Physical examination shows an extensive maculo-papular rash over the child's face, neck, trunk, and limbs. She displays small white spots on buccal surfaces. This patient's skin rash is most likely caused by infection with which of the following agents?

(A) *Candida albicans*
(B) Epstein-Barr virus
(C) Measles virus
(D) Mumps virus
(E) Rotavirus

20 A 50-year-old woman presents with increasing dry cough and shortness of breath that has lasted for 3 weeks. She is a bird fancier, and her house is filled with parrots. An X-ray film of the chest shows diffuse lung infiltrates. Sputum cultures are negative, and the patient does not respond to antibiotic therapy. A transbronchial aspirate reveals chronic interstitial pneumonia. The patient responds well to tetracycline. Which of the following is the most likely etiologic agent responsible for this patient's symptoms?

(A) Chlamydia
(B) Fungus
(C) Gram-positive bacterium
(D) Mycobacterium
(E) Rickettsia

21 A 5-year-old boy dies of respiratory insufficiency and complications of pneumonia. Histologic examination of the lungs at autopsy shows giant cells with up to 100 nuclei (shown in the image). Which of the following viruses most likely caused this child's fatal respiratory tract infection?

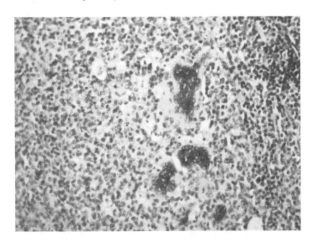

(A) Adenovirus
(B) Cytomegalovirus
(C) Measles virus
(D) Mumps virus
(E) Rubellavirus

22 A 45-year-old man who is a heavy smoker complains of sudden onset of high fever and chills, nonproductive cough, and chest pain. An X-ray film of the chest shows bilateral, diffuse, patchy infiltrates. The patient reports that a number of similar cases have occurred recently in the building where he works. He responds to antibiotics and recovers. Which of the following is the most likely a reservoir for the microorganism that is responsible for this patient's respiratory tract infection?

(A) Cooling towers
(B) Elevator shafts
(C) Floor cleaners
(D) Heat pumps
(E) Industrial solvents

23 A 37-year-old man is admitted to the hospital with a productive cough, fever, and night sweats. An X-ray film of the chest shows an ill-defined area of consolidation at the periphery of the right middle lobe and mediastinal lymphadenopathy. Sputum culture grows acid-fast bacilli. Lymph node biopsy in this patient would most likely show which of the following pathologic findings?

(A) Caseating granulomas
(B) Follicular hyperplasia
(C) Nodular amyloidosis
(D) Noncaseating granulomas
(E) Purulent abscess

24 A 24-year-old woman with insulin-dependent (type 1) diabetes mellitus presents to the emergency room with severe respiratory distress and pleuritic chest pain. The patient has a history of antibiotic-resistant sinusitis. Physical examination reveals periorbital edema and a mucopurulent postnasal discharge. Despite therapy, the patient dies of acute respiratory failure. Cross section of the lung at autopsy shows hemorrhagic infarction. The vessel in the center of the field is occluded by a septic thrombus (shown in the image). These clinicopathologic features are typical of which of the following pulmonary diseases?

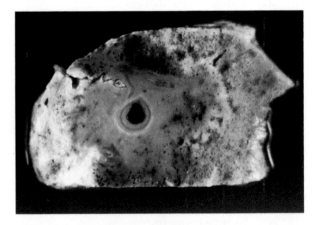

(A) *Haemophilus influenzae* pneumonia
(B) Mucormycosis
(C) Parainfluenza virus pneumonia
(D) *Pneumocystis jiroveci* pneumonia
(E) Psittacosis

25 A 3-year-old boy is brought to the emergency room by his parents with a high fever, sore throat, hoarse voice, and acute respiratory distress. On physical examination, the child is observed to be leaning forward with a hyperextended neck.

The epiglottis appears swollen and erythematous. Which of the following is the most likely cause of this child's upper respiratory tract infection?

(A) *Bordetella pertussis*
(B) *Haemophilus influenzae*
(C) *Klebsiella pneumoniae*
(D) Parainfluenza virus
(E) Respiratory syncytial virus

26 A 31-year-old man with AIDS complains of painful swallowing. Physical examination of his oral cavity demonstrates a whitish membrane covering much of his tongue and palate. Endoscopic examination reveals the same whitish membrane covering his esophageal mucosa. An endoscopic biopsy is shown in the image. Which of the following is the most likely etiologic agent responsible for this patient's symptoms?

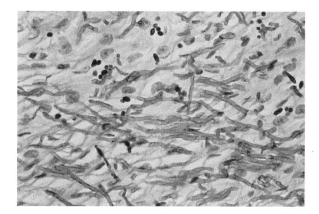

(A) Chlamydia
(B) Fungus
(C) Protozoon
(D) Rickettsia
(E) Spirochete

27 A 35-year-old man with AIDS presents to the emergency room with a 2-week history of progressive weight loss and productive cough with bloody sputum. An X-ray film of the chest shows a cavitary lesion in the right middle lobe. A smear of the sputum reveals many acid-fast rods. Which of the following is the most likely diagnosis?

(A) Ghon complex
(B) Miliary tuberculosis
(C) Primary tuberculosis
(D) Secondary tuberculosis
(E) Tuberculous pleuritis

28 A 1-year-old girl is brought to the clinic in January by her parents because of a fever, runny nose, congestion, "barking" cough, and difficulty breathing. Physical examination shows a red throat. Parainfluenza virus is isolated. Which of the following is chiefly responsible for the barking cough and inspiratory stridor seen in this patient?

(A) Laryngeal fibrosing strictures
(B) Laryngotracheal papillomatosis
(C) Laryngotracheitis
(D) Tonsillar hyperplasia
(E) Vocal cord paralysis

29 A 7-year-old black girl with sickle cell anemia presents with sudden onset of fatigue and joint pain. Physical examination shows marked pallor of the skin and mucous membranes and arthralgias of the lower limbs. The mother indicated that the child had recently recovered from a minor "flu." The CBC shows pancytopenia. Which of the following agents is responsible for this patient's symptoms?

(A) Adenovirus
(B) Norwalk virus
(C) Parainfluenza virus
(D) Parvovirus B19
(E) Rubellavirus

30 A 2-day-old premature infant develops tonic-clonic seizures in the nursery. A CT scan of the head shows microcalcifications. Three days later, the neonate dies. The brain at autopsy reveals large areas of subependymal necrosis with calcification (shown in the image, see arrows). Which of the following pathogens is the most likely cause of death in this neonate?

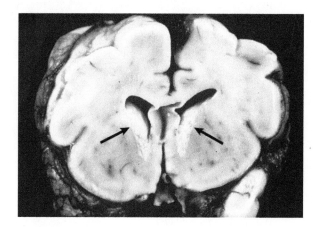

(A) Cytomegalovirus
(B) Herpes simplex type 1
(C) Human immunodeficiency virus
(D) *Toxoplasma gondii*
(E) *Treponema pallidum*

31 A 2-month-old infant presents with fever to 38.6°C (103°F) and neck rigidity. Cerebrospinal fluid shows numerous neutrophils, decreased glucose, and increased protein. Gram-positive cocci are present. Which of the following is the most likely cause of meningitis in this neonate?

(A) Group B streptococcus
(B) *Haemophilus influenzae*
(C) *Neisseria gonorrhoeae*
(D) *Neisseria meningitidis*
(E) *Staphylococcus aureus*

32 A 40-year-old man, who works in a grain silo in the American Southwest, presents with skin rash, headache, and fever. As part of his duties, he is required to trap rodents. Physical examination shows bilateral swelling of the parotid glands and a purpuric, maculopapular rash that spares the palms, face, and soles. Biopsy of lesional skin discloses intracellular microorganisms up to 1 μm in length within capillary endothelial cells. Which of the following pathogens is responsible for this patient's disease?

(A) *Borrelia burgdorferi*
(B) *Chlamydia psittaci*
(C) *Coxiella burnetii*
(D) *Rickettsia typhi*
(E) *Toxoplasma gondii*

33 A 40-year-old immigrant from Brazil presents with a 2-month history of fever, weight loss, and prominent muscle pain. She reports a "strange feeling around her heart." Physical examination shows tachycardia and an irregular heart beat. Laboratory studies reveal marked peripheral eosinophilia. The patient dies 2 days later of an arrhythmia. A photomicrograph of the heart at autopsy is shown. Which of the following pathogens is the most likely cause of cardiac arrest?

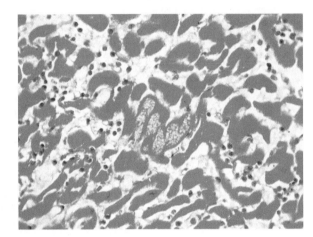

(A) *Pneumocystis jiroveci*
(B) *Schistosoma mansoni*
(C) *Treponema pallidum*
(D) *Trichuris trichiura*
(E) *Trypanosoma cruzi*

34 A 45-year-old man presents with chest pain, fever, productive cough, and rust-colored sputum. The patient was diagnosed with tuberculosis in his early 20s. A chest X-ray shows multiple, nodular infiltrates and cavitary lesions. A lung biopsy reveals necrotizing inflammation and vascular thrombi with branching fungal hyphae. Which of the following is the most likely diagnosis?
(A) Actinomycosis
(B) Aspergillosis
(C) Candidiasis
(D) Cryptococcosis
(E) Histoplasmosis

35 A 25-year-old man, who recently returned from a trip to Central America, presents with right upper quadrant pain and fever of 3 weeks in duration. A CT scan of the abdomen shows a large cystic cavity of the liver, after which a 12-cm abscess is excised (shown in the image). Histologic examination of the lesion reveals chocolate-colored, odorless debris, surrounded by a shaggy fibrin lining, scant inflammatory reaction, and organisms attached to adjacent cells. Which of the following pathogens is responsible for this patient's liver abscess?

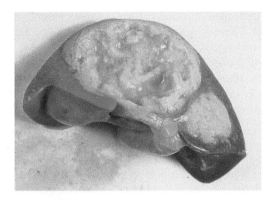

(A) *Clonorchis sinensis*
(B) *Entamoeba histolytica*
(C) *Giardia lamblia*
(D) *Schistosoma mansoni*
(E) *Streptococcus pyogenes*

36 A 24-year-old woman presents with severe vomiting, abdominal cramps, and diarrhea 2 hours after dining at a local restaurant. Many of the customers that night reported similar symptoms. Which of the following mechanisms of disease is chiefly responsible for the development of gastrointestinal symptoms in this patient?
(A) Activation of membrane-associated tyrosine kinase
(B) Exposure to preformed enterotoxin
(C) IgE-mediated mast cell degranulation
(D) Immune-complex deposition and complement activation
(E) Receptor-mediated stimulation of intracellular cAMP

37 A 48-year-old man with AIDS is admitted to the hospital with a fever of 38°C (103°F), night sweats, persistent cough, and prolonged diarrhea. His CD4 cell count is less than 300/μL. Stool culture reveals the presence of acid-fast bacilli. Which of the following pathogens is responsible for this patient's respiratory and gastrointestinal disease?
(A) *Campylobacter jejuni*
(B) *Cryptosporidium*
(C) *Clostridium perfringens*
(D) *Mycobacterium avium-intracellulare*
(E) *Streptococcus pyogenes*

38 A 14-year-old girl presents with yellow and red crusted lesions around her mouth and arms (shown in the image). She has a recent history of intermittent low-grade fever. This patient's skin lesions are most likely caused by which of the following microorganisms?

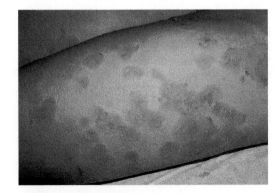

(A) *Staphylococcus epidermidis*

(B) *Streptococcus pneumoniae*

(C) *Streptococcus pyogenes*

(D) *Streptococcus viridans*

(E) *Treponema pallidum*

39 A 28-year-old drug abuser presents with high fever, chills, productive cough, hemoptysis, and right-sided chest pain. Physical examination shows the stigmata of intravenous drug abuse, as well as splenomegaly and pleuritis. Auscultation reveals a systolic ejection murmur over the tricuspid area. Which of the following is the most likely etiology of this patent's valvular heart disease?

(A) *Candida albicans*

(B) *Legionella pneumophila*

(C) *Mycobacterium tuberculosis*

(D) *Mycoplasma pneumoniae*

(E) *Staphylococcus aureus*

40 A 50-year-old woman presents with sudden-onset, crampy abdominal pain and watery diarrhea. She also complains of low-grade fever with chills, nausea, and vomiting. She ate partially cooked eggs 24 hours prior to the onset of these symptoms. Which of the following pathogens is most likely responsible for this patient's gastrointestinal disorder?

(A) *Clostridium perfringens*

(B) *Escherichia coli*

(C) Hepatitis A virus

(D) *Salmonella* sp.

(E) *Staphylococcus aureus*

41 A 30-year-old man presents with inguinal swelling and painless penile and perianal ulcers. He admits to having unprotected sexual intercourse with multiple partners. A silver stain of a biopsy from a skin lesion (shown in the image) reveals organisms clustered in large macrophages. Which of the following is the most likely diagnosis?

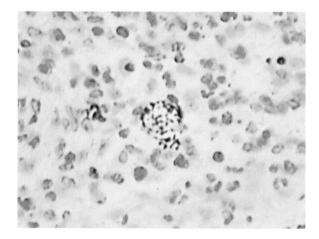

(A) Chancroid

(B) Genital herpes

(C) Gonorrhea

(D) Granuloma inguinale

(E) Syphilis

42 A 42-year-old man presents with a 1-week history of myalgia, low-grade fever, and swelling of the left calf. The patient reports recently attending a fireman's pig-roast. Laboratory data show elevated serum levels of creatine kinase. Examination of a muscle biopsy in this patient would most likely reveal an infiltrate of which of the following cell types?

(A) Eosinophils

(B) Mast cells

(C) Plasma cells

(D) Segmented neutrophils

(E) Smooth muscle cells

43 A 32-year-old immigrant from Vietnam presents with a 4-year history of progressive loss of eyebrows; patchy hypopigmentation of skin; coarse facial features; and multiple, firm subcutaneous nodules. Acid-fast organisms are seen on skin biopsy. Which of the following is the most likely etiology of this patient's condition?

(A) *Bacillus anthracis*

(B) *Mycobacterium leprae*

(C) *Mycobacterium tuberculosis*

(D) *Treponema pallidum*

(E) *Trypanosoma cruzi*

44 A 16-year-old girl presents with fever and swollen lymph nodes. Physical examination reveals painful lymphadenopathy in her left axilla. The girl remembers that she was scratched by her cat 3 weeks ago. A silver stain of a lymph node biopsy is shown in the image. Which of the following is the most likely cause of lymphadenopathy in this patient?

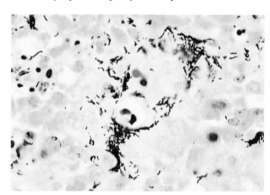

(A) *Bartonella henselae*

(B) *Eikenella corrodens*

(C) *Pasteurella multocida*

(D) *Staphylococcus aureus*

(E) *Streptococcus pyogenes*

45 A 12-year-old farm boy from Mexico complains of generalized weakness and abdominal pain. Physical examination shows pallor and pitting edema of the lower extremities. A CBC reveals severe microcytic, hypochromic anemia (hemoglobin = 8.2 g/dL). Which of the following pathogens is the most likely cause of anemia in this patient?

(A) *Ascaris lumbricoides*

(B) *Giardia lamblia*

(C) Hookworm (*Ancylostoma duodenale*)

(D) Pinworm (*Enterobius vermicularis*)

(E) Whipworm (*Trichuris trichiura*)

46 A 65-year-old man with a history of Hodgkin lymphoma develops a painful erythematous rash with a band-like distribution over the left side of his chest, which becomes vesicular over the next several days. Biopsy of lesional skin is shown in the image. Which of the following is the most likely etiology of this patient's rash?

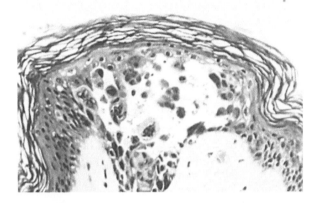

(A) Cytomegalovirus
(B) Epstein-Barr virus
(C) Human herpesvirus-6
(D) Human herpesvirus-8
(E) Varicella-zoster virus

47 A 23-year-old woman presents with low-grade fever and multiple, painful, vesicular lesions on the vulva. A Pap smear shows multinucleated giant cells with intranuclear inclusions. Which of the following pathogens is the most likely cause of this patient's genital lesions?
(A) *Calymmatobacterium granulomatis*
(B) Epstein-Barr virus
(C) Herpes simplex virus type 2
(D) Human papillomavirus
(E) *Treponema pallidum*

48 The patient described in Question 47 asks you about the possibility of future outbreaks and the risks of sexual transmission. In addressing her concerns, you might consider that the virus is harbored in a latent form in which of the following anatomic locations?
(A) Germ cells of the ovary
(B) Glandular epithelium of the endocervix
(C) Mucosa of the external genitalia
(D) Sensory neurons of sacral ganglia
(E) Squamous mucosa of the exocervix

49 A 6-year-old girl presents with intense perianal itching, especially at night. Physical examination reveals perianal excoriation. An adhesive tape test is positive for worms. Which of the following is the most likely parasite in this patient?
(A) *Ancylostoma duodenale*
(B) *Ascaris lumbricoides*
(C) *Enterobius vermicularis*
(D) *Necator americanus*
(E) *Toxocara canis*

50 An Egyptian fisherman develops lower abdominal pain and pain on urination, and reports seeing blood in his urine. Which of the following parasites is the most likely cause of urinary symptoms in this patient?
(A) *Clonorchis sinensis*
(B) *Diphyllobothrium latum*
(C) *Fasciola hepatica*
(D) *Schistosoma haematobium*
(E) *Schistosoma mansoni*

51 A 34-year-old man with history of diabetes mellitus presents with a fever of 3 days duration and a painful, swollen finger (shown in the image). Physical examination reveals erythema and edema affecting the fourth digit. Which of the following is the most likely etiology of this lesion?

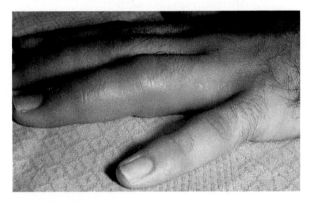

(A) *Pseudomonas aeruginosa*
(B) *Sporothrix schenckii*
(C) *Staphylococcus aureus*
(D) *Staphylococcus epidermidis*
(E) *Streptococcus pyogenes*

52 A 22-year-old student living in a college dormitory presents with a 4-week history of a nonproductive cough and previous low-grade fever. An X-ray film of the chest shows patchy consolidation of the right lower lobe, with evidence of interstitial involvement. Which of the following is the most likely etiology of this patient's pulmonary infection?
(A) *Klebsiella pneumoniae*
(B) *Mycobacterium tuberculosis*
(C) *Mycoplasma pneumoniae*
(D) *Staphylococcus aureus*
(E) *Streptococcus pneumoniae*

53 A 47-year-old woman receiving chemotherapy for leukemia complains of headache, cough, and dyspnea. An X-ray film of the chest shows nodular pulmonary infiltrates and thin-walled cavities. A mucicarmine stain of a lung biopsy discloses budding yeast surrounded by a mucin-rich capsule. Which of the following is the most likely pathogen?
(A) *Aspergillus flavus*
(B) *Candida albicans*
(C) *Coccidioides immitis*
(D) *Cryptococcus neoformans*
(E) *Histoplasma capsulatum*

54 A 30-year-old man presents with abrupt onset of fever, chills, myalgia, nausea, and vomiting. He had just returned from a month-long trip to the jungles of South America. If this patient has yellow fever, pathologic changes would most likely be observed in which of the following organs?

(A) Brain
(B) Kidney
(C) Liver
(D) Lung
(E) Stomach

55 A 50-year-old man, who recently returned from a trip to Africa, complains of darkening of his skin, weight loss, and an increased tendency to bleed. His temperature is 38°C (101°F), pulse rate 22 per minute, and blood pressure 90/80 mm Hg. Physical examination reveals a pale cachectic man with massive splenomegaly. CBC shows anemia, thrombocytopenia, and leukopenia. A bone marrow biopsy (silver stain) displays macrophages filled with proliferating organisms. Which of the following infectious diseases is most likely responsible for this patient's condition?

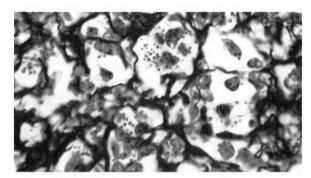

(A) Bilharziasis
(B) Chagas disease
(C) Cysticercosis
(D) Fascioliasis
(E) Leishmaniasis

56 A 6-year-old boy presents with a 10-month history of diarrhea, crampy abdominal pain, and progressive weight loss. He recently immigrated to the United States from Mexico. Physical examination shows mild abdominal distension and evidence of malabsorption. The stool guaiac test is negative. Which of the following is the most likely etiology of this child's gastrointestinal disease?

(A) *Campylobacter jejuni*
(B) *Escherichia coli*
(C) *Giardia lamblia*
(D) *Shigella dysenteriae*
(E) *Staphylococcus aureus*

57 A 52-year-old man presents with a 3-day history of sore throat, cough, fever, and runny nose. The symptoms of this patient's common upper respiratory tract infection are primarily caused by which of the following infectious agents?

(A) Adenovirus
(B) Epstein-Barr virus
(C) Herpes simplex virus
(D) Lentivirus
(E) Rhinovirus

58 A 29-year-old woman (gravida III, para II) delivers a premature infant at 28 weeks of gestation. At birth, the neonate shows signs of profound anemia and generalized edema (hydrops fetalis). The disease is most likely caused by an intrauterine infection with which of the following TORCH agents?

(A) Cytomegalovirus
(B) Herpes simplex virus
(C) Parvovirus B19
(D) Rubellavirus
(E) *Toxoplasma gondii*

59 A 36-year-old woman presents with a 2-day history of fever, myalgias, headache, and watery diarrhea (5 to 10 per day) that contains some blood. A stool smear shows leukocytes and Gram-negative curved bacilli. The patient reports drinking raw milk 7 days ago. Which of the following microorganisms is the most likely cause of this woman's gastrointestinal disorder?

(A) *Campylobacter jejuni*
(B) *Escherichia coli*
(C) *Salmonella typhi*
(D) *Shigella dysenteriae*
(E) *Staphylococcus aureus*

60 A 45-year-old construction worker suffers a penetrating wound of the left leg, which is cleaned and sutured. Three days later, the patient presents with sudden onset of severe pain at the site of injury. Physical examination shows darkening of the surrounding skin, hemorrhage, and cutaneous necrosis. The wound shows a thick serosanguinous discharge with gas bubbles and a fragrant odor. Which of the following is the most likely etiology of this patient's wound infection?

(A) *Clostridium botulinum*
(B) *Clostridium perfringens*
(C) *Staphylococcus aureus*
(D) *Staphylococcus epidermidis*
(E) *Streptococcus pyogenes*

61 A 32-year-old man presents with the sudden onset of tonic-clonic seizures and dies the next day. The brain at autopsy is shown in the image. This patient most likely contracted which of the following infectious diseases?

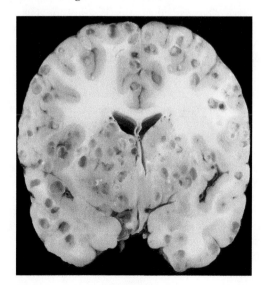

(A) Aspergillosis
(B) Clonorchiasis
(C) Cysticercosis
(D) Fascioliasis
(E) Paragonimiasis

62 A 5-year-old boy is brought to the emergency room with a fever of 103°F (38.7°C), chest pain, and productive cough. The patient has a history of recurrent pulmonary disease and respiratory distress. What microorganism recovered from the lungs of this child is virtually diagnostic of cystic fibrosis?

(A) *Klebsiella* sp.
(B) *Legionella* sp.
(C) *Pneumocystis* sp.
(D) *Pseudomonas* sp.
(E) *Streptococcus* sp.

ANSWERS

1 **The answer is A: Activated T cells.** Infectious mononucleosis is characterized by fever, pharyngitis, lymphadenopathy, and circulating atypical lymphocytes. This systemic viral infection is caused by Epstein-Barr virus (EBV), a herpesvirus that is transmitted through respiratory droplets and saliva and binds to nasopharyngeal cells and B lymphocytes. T cells proliferate in response to activated B lymphocytes and appear in the peripheral blood as atypical lymphocytes. Anemia and thrombocytopenia are common. In developed countries, infectious mononucleosis commonly affects teenagers and young adults and is often referred to as the "kissing disease." In underdeveloped countries, EBV infections are typically seen as subclinical infections in childhood and are associated with an increased risk of Burkitt lymphoma and nasopharyngeal carcinoma. Although EBV infects B cells, the circulating atypical lymphocytes seen in patients with infectious mononucleosis are not immature B cells (choice B), but rather indirectly activated T cells.
Diagnosis: Infectious mononucleosis

2 **The answer is E: Rupture of the spleen.** Splenomegaly often develops in patients with infectious mononucleosis due to lymphoid infiltration, hyperplasia, and edema. The enlarged spleen may rupture after minor trauma. Burkitt lymphoma (choice A) is associated with Epstein-Barr virus infection in certain parts of the world but is uncommon in North America.
Diagnosis: Infectious mononucleosis

3 **The answer is B: Neisseria gonorrhoeae.** *N. gonorrhoeae* causes an acute suppurative infection of the genital tract, which presents as urethritis in men and endocervicitis in women. It is one of the most common sexually transmitted diseases. Gonorrhea may involve the throat, anus, rectum, epididymis, cervix, fallopian tubes, prostate gland, or joints. Septic arthritis due to *N. gonorrhoeae*, a suppurative inflammation most commonly caused by hematogenous spread, is usually monoarticular, most commonly affecting hips and knees. The other choices do not typically exhibit arthritis and acute pelvic disease. Primary syphilis (choice D) presents with chancre.
Diagnosis: Gonorrhea

4 **The answer is C: Endarteritis obliterans.** Secondary syphilis represents systemic dissemination and proliferation of the spirochete, *Treponema pallidum*. This stage is characterized pathologically by lesions in skin, mucous membranes, lymph nodes, meninges, stomach, and liver. The lesions show a perivascular lymphocytic infiltration and endarteritis obliterans. In most cases, the rash appears 2 weeks to 3 months after the primary lesion (chancre) heals. Other lesions associated with secondary syphilis include condylomata lata, follicular syphilis, and nummular syphilis. Chancre (choice A) is a characteristic lesion of primary syphilis. Choices B, D, and E are encountered in patients with *tertiary* syphilis.
Diagnosis: Syphilis

5 **The answer is A: *Bacillus anthracis*.** Anthrax is a necrotizing disease caused by *B. anthracis*. The clinical presentation of anthrax depends on the site of inoculation and includes "malignant" pustule, pulmonary anthrax, septicemic anthrax, and gastrointestinal anthrax. *B. anthracis* typically produces extensive tissue necrosis at the site of infection, with a mild neutrophilic infiltration. Malignant pustule is seen in over 95% of all cases of anthrax and represents the cutaneous form of this infectious disease. The infected person presents with an elevated cutaneous papulae that enlarges and erodes into an ulcer. Local hemorrhagic pustules may progress to carbuncles. Cutaneous lesions contain numerous organisms that release a potent necrotizing toxin. The other choices do not typically present with these necrotizing cutaneous manifestations.
Diagnosis: Anthrax, malignant pustule

6 **The answer is D: Increased intracellular cAMP.** Cholera is a severe diarrheal illness caused by the enterotoxin of *Vibrio choleraE* an anaerobic Gram-negative rod. The organism proliferates in the lumen of the small intestine and causes profuse watery diarrhea and rapid dehydration. Shock and death can ensue within 24 hours from the onset of symptoms. The AB toxin secreted by the organism binds to ganglioside GM1 on intestinal epithelial cells and stimulates an increase in intracellular levels of cAMP, thereby leading to water secretion. The mucosa does not show significant pathologic changes. The other choices directly injure the intestinal mucosa and cause hemorrhage.
Diagnosis: Cholera, acute gastroenteritis

7 **The answer is B: *Escherichia coli* 0157-H7.** Enterohemorrhagic *E. coli* (serotype 0157-H7), which may contaminate meat or milk, causes bloody diarrhea, which can be followed by the hemolytic-uremic syndrome. The organism adheres to the colonic mucosa and releases an enterotoxin that destroys epithelial cells. Patients present with abdominal pain, low-grade fever, and bloody diarrhea. Stool examination shows leukocytes and erythrocytes. Hemolytic-uremic syndrome is manifested by microangiopathic hemolytic anemia, thrombocytopenia, and acute renal failure. Although they may be associated with bloody diarrhea, the other choices do not present with hemolytic-uremic syndrome.
Diagnosis: Hemolytic-uremic syndrome, enterohemorrhagic *E. coli*

8 **The answer is B: *Clostridium difficile.* *C. difficile*** is the most common cause of diarrhea in patients on antibiotic therapy (e.g., clindamycin or cephalosporins) who are hospitalized for more than 3 days. Necrotizing enterocolitis (pseudomembranous colitis) is a disease that may affect the colon in segments or in its entirety. The mucosa is covered by yellow-green, necrotic exudates (pseudomembranes). Food poisoning and necrotizing enterocolitis are caused by the enterotoxins of *C. perfringens* (choice C). About 48 hours after the ingestion of contaminated meal, patients present with abdominal pain and distention, vomiting, and passage of bloody stools. *C. perfringens* is also the most common cause of gas gangrene following wound infection or septic abortion. *C. tetani* (choice D) produces a potent neurotoxin that causes tetany and generalized muscle spasms. *Clostridium botulinum* (choice A) produces a neurotoxin that causes paralysis.

Diagnosis: Pseudomembranous colitis, *Clostridium difficile*

9 **The answer is E: Spirochete.** Lyme disease is a chronic infection that begins with a characteristic skin lesion and later variably manifests cardiac, neurologic, and joint disturbances. The causative agent is *Borrelia burgdorferi*, a large spirochete that is transmitted from its animal reservoir to humans by the bite of the deer tick (Ixodes). *B. burgdorferi* reproduces at the site of inoculation, spreads to regional lymph nodes, and is eventually disseminated throughout the body. Untreated Lyme disease is chronic, with periods of remission and exacerbation. Stage 1 is characterized by erythema chronicum migrans, a skin lesion that appears at the site of the tick bite. Stage 2 features migratory musculoskeletal pain and the development of cardiac or neurologic abnormalities (meningitis and facial nerve palsy). Stage 3 begins months to years after infection and involves joint, skin, and neurologic abnormalities. Over half of these patients develop a severe arthritis of the hips and knees, which is indistinguishable from the symptoms of rheumatoid arthritis.

Diagnosis: Lyme disease

10 **The answer is C: *Neisseria meningitides.*** Acute meningococcal meningitis may develop rapidly and is often fatal. Meningococcal sepsis is marked by profound endotoxemic shock and disseminated intravascular coagulation, known as Waterhouse-Friderichsen syndrome. Airborne transmission in crowded places (e.g., schools or barracks) can cause "epidemic meningitis." Fever, malaise, petechial rash, and adrenal hemorrhages are common. Although they may cause meningitis, choices A, B, and D are not typically associated with Waterhouse-Friderichsen syndrome.

Diagnosis: Meningococcal meningitis, Waterhouse-Friderichsen syndrome

11 **The answer is B: *Plasmodium falciparum.*** Malaria is a mosquito-borne illness that infects over 200 million persons per year worldwide. There are four species of *Plasmodium*: *P. falciparum*, *P. vivax*, *P. ovale*, and *P. malariae*. All of these organisms infect erythrocytes, but *P. falciparum* causes the most severe disease. In "malignant" malaria caused by *P. falciparum*, ischemic injury to the brain causes a range of symptoms, including somnolence, hallucinations, behavioral changes, seizures, and even coma. The liver, spleen, and lymph nodes are darkened by macrophages that are filled with hemosiderin and malaria pigments. *Naegleria fowleri* (choice A) is associated with a fatal type of meningitis. *Schistosoma haematobium* (choice D) is associated with bladder infections but does not cause the hematologic symptoms seen in this patient.

Diagnosis: Malaria

12 **The answer is E: Thrombosis of blood vessels invaded by hyphae.** The photomicrograph displays invasive aspergillosis. This is the most serious manifestation of *Aspergillus* infection, occurring almost exclusively as an opportunistic infection in persons with compromised immunity. *Aspergillus* readily invades blood vessels and causes thrombosis and local infarction. Branching hyphae (visualized by silver stain) are found in the walls and lumens of pulmonary vessels.

Diagnosis: Invasive aspergillosis

13 **The answer is D: *Pneumocystis jiroveci.*** *P. jiroveci* (formerly *P. carinii*) was identified in malnourished infants at the end of World War II. It causes progressive, often fatal pneumonia in persons with impaired cell-mediated immunity and is one of the most common opportunistic pathogens in persons with AIDS. The organism is now classified with the fungi. The infection begins with the attachment of trophozoites to the alveolar lining. Trophozoites feed, enlarge, and transform into cysts within the host cells. Eventually, the cysts burst, releasing new trophozoites. Progressive consolidation of the lung ensues. Although the other choices cause pneumonia, they do not exhibit these characteristic cysts.

Diagnosis: *Pneumocystis* pneumonia

14 **The answer is E: *Streptococcus pneumoniae.*** *S. pneumoniae* (pneumococcus) causes pyogenic infections involving the lungs (pneumonia), middle ear (otitis media), sinuses (sinusitis), and meninges (meningitis). It is one of the most common causes of community-acquired pneumonia. Consolidation of lung parenchyma typically produces lobar pneumonia, which passes through four stages: (1) congestion and edema, (2) red hepatization, (3) gray hepatization, and (4) resolution. During the acute phase, the alveoli are packed with neutrophils, fibrin, and debris. Pneumonia is caused by the other organisms with much lower frequency.

Diagnosis: Pneumococcal pneumonia

15 **The answer is B: Deposition of circulating immune complexes.** Infection with *Streptococcus pyogenes* causes two major nonsuppurative complications, namely rheumatic fever and acute poststreptococcal glomerulonephritis. Poststreptococcal glomerulonephritis is a classic immune complex–mediated disease that is associated with nephritic syndrome. Poststreptococcal illnesses are not mediated by any of the other choices.

Diagnosis: Poststreptococcal glomerulonephritis

16 **The answer is A: Cytomegalovirus (CMV).** CMV infection induces interstitial pneumonia in infants and immunocompromised persons. Infected alveolar cells show cytomegaly and display a single, dark basophilic nuclear inclusion surrounded by a halo. The virus may be transmitted from mother to child in utero or acquired during delivery. In adults, CMV is transmitted through sexual encounters, blood transfusions, transplantation, and even through the inhalation of infectious

viral particles. Central nervous symptoms predominate in symptomatic infants and children. In adults, the virus produces mostly respiratory and gastrointestinal symptoms but does not cause encephalitis. Herpes simplex virus (choice C) also features intranuclear inclusions (also surrounded by a clear halo) but does not cause chronic interstitial pneumonia.
Diagnosis: Interstitial pneumonitis, cytomegalovirus pneumonitis

17 **The answer is D: Respiratory syncytial virus (RSV).** RSV is an RNA virus, which is the major cause of bronchiolitis and pneumonia in infants. RSV bronchiolitis or pneumonitis presents with expiratory and inspiratory wheezing, cough, and hyperexpansion of both lung fields. Hyperinflation, interstitial infiltrates, and segmented atelectasis are expected findings on chest X-ray. The illness is usually self-limited and typically resolves within 1 to 2 weeks. Mortality is low in healthy babies. The other viruses cause pneumonia much less frequently.
Diagnosis: Respiratory syncytial virus, bronchiolitis

18 **The answer is A: Influenza virus.** Influenza A and B are RNA viruses. Influenza infections are common in the wintertime, with the severity of the illness depending on the immune status of the individual. Patients typically present with fever, tachypnea, conjunctivitis, and pharyngeal inflammation. In severe cases, they may develop extreme respiratory distress and prostration. Influenza affects all segments of the population, but severe cases are more commonly seen among the very young and the elderly. Rhinovirus (choice D) is the most frequent cause of the "common cold." Norwalk-like virus (choice B) and rotavirus (choice E) cause diarrhea in children. Infection with respiratory syncytial virus (choice C) is commonly seen in children under 2 years of age.
Diagnosis: Influenza virus, pneumonitis

19 **The answer is C: Measles virus.** Measles virus is an RNA virus that causes an acute, highly contagious, self-limited illness that is characterized by upper respiratory tract symptoms, fever, and rash. The measles virus, which is transmitted in respiratory droplets and secretions, is primarily a disease of children, but its effects may be particularly severe in adults. The skin rash results from the reaction of T cells with infected cells of the vascular endothelium. "Koplik spots" appear on the posterior buccal mucosa and consist of minute gray-white dots on an erythematous base. Although measles is usually a self-limited disease, measles pneumonia (particularly in adults) is a serious malady that may be fatal. Epstein-Barr virus infection and mumps (choices B and D) do not present with generalized rash. Rotavirus infection (choice E) is the most common cause of severe diarrhea worldwide. The yeast, *Candida albicans* (choice A), usually causes localized infection.
Diagnosis: Measles

20 **The answer is A: Chlamydia.** Psittacosis is a self-limited pneumonia transmitted to humans from birds. The etiologic agent, *Chlamydia psittaci*, is present in blood, feces, and feathers of infected birds. The organism first infects alveolar macrophages, which carry it to the liver and spleen, where it reproduces. The organism is then distributed hematogenously to produce a systemic infection. *C. psittaci* reproduces in alveolar lining cells, whose destruction elicits an inflammatory response

and interstitial pneumonia. Type II pneumocytes are hyperplastic and may show characteristic chlamydial cytoplasmic inclusions. Clinically, the disease presents with persistent dry cough, fever, headache, malaise, myalgias, and arthralgias. The other agents listed do not cause chronic interstitial pneumonia.
Diagnosis: Psittacosis

21 **The answer is C: Measles virus.** Measles virus can cause fusion of infected cells, producing multinucleated cells termed "Warthin-Finkeldey giant cells." These multinucleated giant cells are pathognomonic of measles infections. Cytomegalovirus-infected cells (choice B) are very large and contain nuclear and cytoplasmic viral inclusions, but they are not multinucleated. Adenovirus (choice A) also features intranuclear inclusions but not multinucleation. Mumps and rubella viruses (choices D and E) induce a mononuclear infiltrate composed of lymphocytes, macrophages, and plasma cells (no giant cells).
Diagnosis: Measles

22 **The answer is A: Cooling towers.** *Legionella pneumophila* causes a pneumonia that ranges from mild to a severe life-threatening, necrotizing pneumonia referred to as "Legionnaire disease." The bacterium is found in natural bodies of fresh water and survives chlorination, allowing it to proliferate in cooling towers, water heaters, humidifiers, and ventilation systems. Legionella pneumonia begins when microorganisms enter alveoli, where they are phagocytized by resident macrophages. Bacteria multiply within macrophages and are released to infect new macrophages. The disease presents as an acute bronchopneumonia, with a diffuse and patchy pattern of infiltration. None of the other situations creates suitable conditions for bacteria to multiply.
Diagnosis: Legionnaire disease

23 **The answer is A: Caseating granulomas.** Tuberculosis is a chronic, communicable disease in which the lungs are the prime target. The disease is caused principally by *Mycobacterium tuberculosis hominis* (Koch bacillus), but infection with other species occurs, notably *M. tuberculosis bovis* (bovine tuberculosis). Primary tuberculosis consists of lesions in the lower lobes and subpleural space, referred to as the Ghon focus. The infection then drains to hilar lymph nodes. The combination of Ghon focus and hilar lymphadenopathy is known as "Ghon complex." The typical lesion of tuberculosis is a caseous granuloma, with a soft core surrounded by epithelioid macrophages, Langhans giant cells, lymphocytes, and peripheral fibrosis. Noncaseating granulomas (choice D) are a feature of sarcoidosis, among other causes.
Diagnosis: Primary tuberculosis

24 **The answer is B: Mucormycosis.** Environmental fungi, such as *Rhizopus*, *Mucor*, *Rhizomucor*, and *Absidia* species, can produce necrotizing opportunistic infections that begin in the nasal sinuses or lungs. Mucor is ubiquitous in the nasal sinuses and invades surrounding tissues. The hard palate or nasal cavity is typically covered by a black crust, and the underlying tissues become friable and hemorrhagic. The fungal hyphae grow into arteries, causing devastating and rapidly progressive septic embolic infarctions. There are three principal forms of mucormycosis, namely rhinocerebral, pulmonary, and subcutaneous. Pulmonary mucormycosis is usually fatal. Microscopic examination shows a purulent arteritis with thrombi composed of hyphae. Mucormycosis should be suspected in patients who present with a paranasal sinusitis unresponsive to antibiotic treatment, particularly those who also have an underlying chronic disease (e.g., diabetes or leukemia). The other choices do not show rapidly progressive, septic, embolic infarctions of the lungs. Parainfluenza virus (choice C) does not cause thrombosis or infarction. *Pneumocystis jiroveci* pneumonia (choice D) is noninvasive and causes interstitial pneumonitis.

Diagnosis: Pulmonary mucormycosis

25 **The answer is B: *Haemophilus influenzae.*** *H. influenzae* is a Gram-negative coccobacillus that is the leading cause of meningitis and epiglottitis in children worldwide. Infections may also involve the middle ear, sinuses, facial skin, lungs, and joints. *H. influenzae* spreads from person to person in respiratory droplets and secretions. Inflammation of the epiglottis, aryepiglottis sinus, and pyriform recess produces significant airway obstruction, which can be fatal. Since the widespread use of the HiB vaccine in the United States, invasive disease due to *H. influenzae* type B in pediatric patients has been reduced by 80% to 90%. Other agents, such as *Streptococcus pyogenes*, *S. pneumoniae*, and *Staphylococcus aureus*, now represent a larger proportion of pediatric cases of epiglottitis in the United States.

Diagnosis: Acute epiglottitis, *Haemophilus influenzae*

26 **The answer is B: Fungus.** The genus *Candida* comprises over 20 species of fungi, which include the most common opportunistic pathogens. Many *Candida* species are endogenous human flora. When the normal bacterial flora that limit fungal growth are suppressed, the yeast converts to an invasive form, eliciting an inflammatory reaction. Thrush signifies candidal infection of the tongue and mucous membranes of the mouth. It consists of friable, white, curd-like membranes adherent to the affected area. Removal of this membrane leaves a painful bleeding surface. The other choices do not form thrush.

Diagnosis: Thrush, *Candida* esophagitis

27 **The answer is D: Secondary tuberculosis.** Secondary tuberculosis results from the proliferation of *M. tuberculosis* in a person who has been previously infected and has mounted an immunologic response. The source of infection is usually dormant bacteria from old granulomas but may also represent a newly acquired infection. Various conditions may predispose to the reemergence of endogenous microorganisms, including immunosuppressive states such as cancer, chemotherapy, immunosuppressive therapy, AIDS, and old age. The lungs are the most common sites of reinfection. The bacilli elicit an acute inflammatory response that leads to extensive tissue necrosis and the production of tuberculous cavities. Clinically, patients present with cough, low-grade fever, malaise, fatigue, anorexia, weight loss, and night sweats. The other conditions are not associated with pulmonary cavitation.

Diagnosis: Secondary tuberculosis

28 **The answer is C: Laryngotracheitis.** Parainfluenza viruses cause acute upper and lower respiratory tract infections particularly in young children. These RNA viruses are the most common cause of laryngotracheobronchitis, which is referred to as "croup." The infection is characterized by a subglottic swelling and airway obstruction, which lead to acute respiratory distress. The infection spreads from person to person through contaminated respiratory aerosols and secretions. The parainfluenza virus infects and kills ciliated respiratory epithelial cells and elicits an inflammatory response. When laryngotracheitis occurs, localized edema compresses the upper airway enough to obstruct breathing. Symptoms associated with croup include fever, hoarseness, barking cough, and inspiratory stridor. The other conditions are not features of parainfluenza infection.

Diagnosis: Croup, parainfluenza virus

29 **The answer is D: Parvovirus B19.** Human parvovirus B19 is a DNA virus that causes systemic infections characterized by rash, arthralgias, and a transient defect in erythropoiesis. The virus is spread from person to person through respiratory secretions. Infections are common in children. The virus is cytopathic for erythroid precursor cells in the bone marrow. The nuclei of infected cells are enlarged, and the chromatin is displaced to the periphery. Most patients suffer a mild exanthem known as erythema infectiosum. However, in patients with chronic hemolytic anemia (e.g., sickle cell disease), this transient interruption in erythropoiesis causes a potentially fatal condition known as "aplastic crisis." The other choices are not associated with anemia.

Diagnosis: Aplastic crisis

30 **The answer is D: *Toxoplasma gondii.*** Toxoplasmosis is a worldwide disease caused by the protozoan *T. gondii*. Most infections are asymptomatic, but a devastating necrotizing disease may occur when they involve the fetus or an immunocompromised adult. Infection of the central nervous system produces a necrotizing meningoencephalitis, which, in the most severe cases, results in destruction of brain parenchyma, cerebral calcification, and hydrocephalus. Ocular infections cause chorioretinitis. None of the other pathogens induce these characteristic pathologic findings.

Diagnosis: Congenital toxoplasmosis, TORCH syndrome

31 **The answer is A: Group B streptococcus.** Several thousand neonatal infections with group B streptococci occur in the United States every year. About 30% of infected infants die. The other choices are much less common causes of meningitis in this age group. Meningococci are Gram-negative organisms.

Diagnosis: Neonatal bacterial meningitis

32 **The answer is D: Rickettsia typhi.** Endemic typhus is a severe vasculitis transmitted by *R. typhi* through the bite of infected lice. The disease begins with localized infection of capillary endothelium, which progresses to systemic vasculitis. Mononuclear cell infiltrates are found in multiple organs and are typically arranged in typhus nodules. Louse-borne typhus is characterized clinically by fever, severe headache, and myalgias, followed by the appearance of a maculopapular rash on the upper trunk and axillary folds, spreading centrifugally to the extremities. The other choices do not infect endothelial cells or produce a vasculitis.

Diagnosis: Endemic typhus

33 The answer is E: *Trypanosoma cruzi.* Chagas disease is an insect-borne systemic infection in humans caused by the protozoan *T. cruzi*. Acute manifestations and long-term sequelae of infection occur primarily in the heart and gastrointestinal tract. The infections are endemic in Central and South America, where they are transmitted by the Reduviid ("kissing") bug, which hides within the cracks and straw roofs of older homes. The parasite reproduces within the myocardium and causes myocarditis. The other pathogens do not cause myocarditis.
Diagnosis: Chagas disease

34 The answer is B: Aspergillosis. Fungus balls (aspergillomas) consist of rounded, lobulated masses of hyphae and occur in patients with a previous history of cavitating pulmonary disease (e.g., pulmonary tuberculosis). *Aspergillus* is a common environmental fungus that causes opportunistic infections in the lungs. Inhaled spores germinate in the warm humid atmosphere provided by cavitary lung lesions, filling them with masses of hyphae. The organisms generally do not invade the lung parenchyma. There are three different types of pulmonary aspergillosis, namely allergic bronchopulmonary aspergillosis, aspergillomas, and invasive aspergillosis. Candidiasis (choice C) is incorrect because *Candida* infections are not typically angioinvasive. The other choices do not show characteristic branching fungal hyphae.
Diagnosis: Pulmonary aspergillosis, aspergilloma

35 The answer is B: *Entamoeba histolytica.* *E. histolytica* resides in the colon of infected persons and is transmitted by fecal-oral contact. The trophozoites invade submucosal veins of the colon, enter the portal circulation, and gain access to the liver. The amebae kill hepatocytes, producing a slowly expanding, necrotic cavity. The abscess is filled with a dark brown material that resembles anchovy paste. An amebic liver abscess can rupture and extend into the peritoneal cavity. Although the other choices may involve the liver, they do not cause hepatic abscess.
Diagnosis: Amebic liver abscess

36 The answer is B: Exposure to preformed enterotoxin. *Staphylococcus aureus* food poisoning is caused by the ingestion of food contaminated with preformed, heat-stable enterotoxin B. Outbreaks occur when food handlers inoculate foods such as meat or dairy products (salad dressings, cream sauces, and custard-filled pastries) with contaminated wounds or infected nasal droplets. Staphylococcal food poisoning typically begins less than 6 hours after a meal. Nausea and vomiting usually resolve within 12 hours. The other choices do not initiate rapid gastrointestinal symptoms.
Diagnosis: Staphylococcal food poisoning

37 The answer is D: *Mycobacterium avium-intracellulare.* *M. avium* and *M. intracellulare* are similar mycobacterial species that cause identical diseases and are, therefore, classified together as *M. avium-intracellulare* complex (MAC). MAC is a rare, granulomatous, pulmonary disease in immunocompetent persons, but it is a progressive systemic disorder in patients with AIDS. One third of all AIDS patients develop overt MAC infections. The proliferation of organisms and the recruitment of macrophages produce expanding lesions, ranging from epithelioid granulomas containing few organisms to loose aggregates with foamy macrophages. Symptoms associated with MAC resemble those of tuberculosis; however, progressive involvement of the small bowel produces malabsorption and diarrhea. *Camplyobacter jejuni* (choice A) produces a self-limited bacterial diarrhea. *Cryptosporidium* (choice B) is a protozoan that causes diarrhea in immunocompromised patients but is not associated with respiratory infections.
Diagnosis: Atypical mycobacterial infection in AIDS

38 The answer is C: *Streptococcus pyogenes.* Impetigo in this patient represents a localized, intraepidermal infection with *S. pyogenes*. It spreads by close contact and most commonly affects children. Minor trauma allows inoculation of the bacteria, forming an intraepithelial pustule that eventually ruptures and leaks a purulent exudate. *S. pneumoniae* (choice B) is a major cause of lobar pneumonia, otitis media, sinusitis and meningitis. *S. viridans* (choice D) is a major cause of bacterial endocarditis. *Treponema pallidum* (choice E) produces a maculopapular rash of the palms and soles in secondary syphilis.
Diagnosis: Impetigo

39 The answer is E: *Staphylococcus aureus.* *S. aureus* is a Gram-positive coccus that is the most common cause of suppurative infections involving the skin, joints, and bones. It is also one of the most common causes of acute bacterial endocarditis. This infection features colonization of heart valves or mural endocardium, leading to the formation of friable vegetations composed of thrombotic debris and microorganisms. Bacterial growth is often associated with destruction of the underlying valve tissue. Tricuspid insufficiency secondary to bacterial endocarditis is one of the most common complications of IV drug abuse. The most common source of bacteria in these patients is the skin. The tricuspid valve is infected in half of the cases. The other choices do not cause endocarditis.
Diagnosis: Bacterial endocarditis

40 The answer is D: *Salmonella.* Nontyphoidal species of *Salmonella* contaminate a variety of foods, including poultry, eggs, meat, and dairy products. *Salmonella* infections are characterized clinically by diarrhea, which begins 12 to 24 hours after ingestion of the contaminated food. Salmonella food poisoning is self-limited, lasting from 1 to 3 days. The bacteria proliferate in the small intestine and invade enterocytes, where they produce several toxins that contribute to the dysfunction of the intestinal epithelium. The mucosal surface of the ileum and colon become acutely inflamed and occasionally ulcerated. Pathogenic *Escherichia coli* (choice B) does not typically infect eggs. *Staphylococcus aureus* (choice E) characteristically causes diarrhea 1 to 6 hours after ingestion.
Diagnosis: *Salmonella* enterocolitis

41 The answer is D: Granuloma inguinale. Granuloma inguinale is a sexually transmitted, chronic, superficial ulceration of the genital, inguinal, and perianal region. It is caused by *Calymmatobacterium granulomatis*, a small Gram-negative bacillus. The characteristic lesion is a beefy-red superficial ulcer. Microscopically, the dermis and subcutis are infiltrated by macrophages and plasma cells. Skin lesions show microorganisms, termed "Donovan bodies," clustered within enlarged macrophages. The other choices do not display visible intracellular microorganisms.

Diagnosis: Granuloma inguinale

42 **The answer is A: Eosinophils.** Trichinosis is produced by the roundworm *Trichinella spiralis*. After mating, the females liberate larvae into the circulation. The larvae can invade almost any tissue but survive only in skeletal muscle in an encapsulated form. Elevated serum levels of creatine kinase indicate muscle cell necrosis. Early muscle involvement elicits an intense inflammatory infiltrate rich in eosinophils. The other cells do not typically respond to acute parasitic infestations.

Diagnosis: Trichinosis

43 **The answer is B: *Mycobacterium leprae*.** Leprosy (Hansen disease) is caused by *M. leprae* and appears in two forms, namely tuberculoid and lepromatous. The tuberculoid type occurs in patients who mount an immunologic response, whereas those with the lepromatous form are anergic. Lepromatous leprosy is a chronic, slowly progressive, destructive process involving peripheral nerves, skin, and mucous membranes. Patients exhibit multiple nodular lesions of the skin, eyes, testes, nerves, lymph nodes, and spleen. The skin infiltrates expand slowly to distort and disfigure the face, ears, and upper airways. There is also involvement of the eyes, eyebrows, eyelashes, nerves, and testes. *M. tuberculosis* (choice C) is acid-fast, but does not cause the symptoms listed for this case. Anthrax (choice A), syphilis (choice D), and trypanosomiasis (choice E) manifest differently.

Diagnosis: Leprosy

44 **The answer is A: *Bartonella henselae*.** Cat-scratch disease is a self-limited infection caused by *B. henselae* or (more rarely) *B. quintana*. These bacteria are small, Gram-negative rods that are difficult to culture but easily seen in a lymph node biopsy when stained with silver. *B. henselae* multiplies in the walls of small vessels and extracellular collagen fibers at the site of inoculation. The organisms are carried to the lymph nodes, where they produce suppurative lymphadenitis. The lymph nodes enlarge and drain through the skin. About half of infected patients present with systemic symptoms such as fever, malaise, rash, and erythema nodosum. *Pasteurella multocida* (choice C) is associated with wound infection after animal bites. *Eikenella corrodens* (choice B) produces wound infections after human bites.

Diagnosis: Cat-scratch disease

45 **The answer is C: Hookworm (*Ancylostoma duodenale*).** Hookworms are intestinal nematodes that infect the small bowel. *A. duodenale* molts within the duodenum and attaches to the mucosa. With extensive infections, particularly with *A. duodenale*, considerable blood loss results in iron-deficiency anemia. The other choices do not cause intestinal bleeding and iron-deficiency anemia.

Diagnosis: Hookworm, ancylostomiasis

46 **The answer is E: Varicella-zoster virus.** Varicella-zoster virus initially infects cells of the respiratory tract or conjunctival epithelium. It then reproduces and spreads via the bloodstream and lymphatic system. First exposure to the virus produces chickenpox, an acute systemic illness whose dominant feature is a generalized vesicular skin eruption. Reactivation of latent virus in adults causes herpes zoster. Microscopically, intraepithelial vesicles contain multinucleated giant cells and nuclear inclusions. Human herpesvirus-8 (choice D) is associated with Kaposi sarcoma in patients with AIDS. The other choices do not produce vesicular eruptions.

Diagnosis: Herpes zoster

47 **The answer is C: Herpes simplex virus type 2.** Herpes simplex viruses are common human pathogens, which most frequently produce recurrent painful vesicular eruptions of the skin and mucous membranes. The other choices do not show grouped vesicles. *Calymmatobacterium granulomatis* (choice A) is associated with a painful genital ulcer (chancroid). Human papillomavirus (choice D) relates to genital warts. *Treponema pallidum* (choice E) causes syphilis.

Diagnosis: Genital herpes

48 **The answer is D: Sensory neurons of sacral ganglia.** Herpesvirus ascends from genital lesions along sensory neurons and survives in a latent form in the sacral ganglia. Nonspecific stimuli (including sexual intercourse and menses) can reactivate the virus, which then descends along axons to the genital mucosa, causing recurrent blisters on the external and internal genitalia.

Diagnosis: Genital herpes

49 **The answer is C: *Enterobius vermicularis*.** *E. vermicularis* ("pinworm") is an intestinal nematode that is encountered worldwide but is more common in temperate zones. Individuals can be infected at any age, but parasitism is more common in children. Most people complain of pruritus caused by migrating worms. *Ancylostoma duodenale* and *Necator americanus* (choices A and D) are hookworms associated with intestinal bleeding and iron-deficiency anemia.

Diagnosis: Enterobiasis

50 **The answer is D: *Schistosoma haematobium*.** Schistosomiasis is the most important helminthic disease of humans. It is characterized by intense inflammatory and immunologic responses that damage the liver, intestine, and urinary bladder. In this case, the patient presents with urogenital schistosomiasis. *S. haematobium* causes urogenital infections and increases the risk for developing squamous cell carcinoma of the bladder. *S. mansoni* (choice E) affects the liver.

Diagnosis: Schistosomiasis

51 **The answer is E: *Streptococcus pyogenes*.** Erysipelas is an erythematous swelling of the skin caused chiefly by *S. pyogenes* infection. *S. pyogenes*, also known as group A streptococcus, is one of the most frequent bacterial pathogens of humans, producing various diseases ranging from acute self-limited pharyngitis to rheumatic fever. The rash usually begins on the face but can affect any part of the body. Cutaneous microabscesses and foci of necrosis are common. The other choices are not typically associated with erysipelas.

Diagnosis: Erysipelas

52   **The answer is C: *Mycoplasma pneumoniae.*** *M. pneumoniae* produces an acute self-limited lower respiratory tract infection, primarily in children and young adults. Most infections occur in groups of persons living in close contact. *M. pneumoniae* tends to be milder than other bacterial pneumonias and has, therefore, earned the appellation "walking pneumonia." Fever usually persists for no more than 2 weeks, although a cough may linger for 6 weeks or more. Chest X-ray commonly shows patchy consolidation of a single segment of a lower lung lobe. *M. pneumoniae* is responsible for about 20% of all pneumonias in developed countries. The other choices do not cause interstitial pneumonia.

Diagnosis: *Mycoplasma pneumoniae*

53   **The answer is D: Cryptococcus neoformans.** Cryptococcosis is a mycosis that primarily affects the meninges and lungs. *C. neoformans* is unique among pathogenic fungi because it has a proteoglycan capsule, which is essential for pathogenicity. The main reservoir for this fungus is pigeon droppings. The organisms appear as faintly stained, basophilic yeast with a clear, 3- to 5-μm thick mucinous capsule. Cryptococcus almost exclusively affects persons with impaired cell-mediated immunity. The other choices do not stain with mucicarmine.

Diagnosis: Cryptococcosis

54   **The answer is C: Liver.** Yellow fever is an acute hemorrhagic fever, which is associated with hepatic necrosis and jaundice. The illness is caused by a mosquito-borne flavivirus. Extensive injury to vascular endothelial cells may cause hemorrhage and shock. This virus has a tropism for liver cells, where it causes extensive hepatocellular injury. Councilman bodies (apoptotic bodies) and microvesicular fatty change are evident. In severe cases, the entire liver lobule may become necrotic. The other choices are incorrect, because the yellow fever virus is hepatotropic.

Diagnosis: Yellow fever

55   **The answer is E: Leishmaniasis.** Leishmaniae are protozoans that are transmitted to humans through insect bites. They cause a spectrum of clinical syndromes, ranging from indolent self-resolving cutaneous ulcers to fatal disseminated disease. Leishmaniasis is transmitted by the bite of phlebotomus sandflies, which acquire infections from feeding on infected animals. The infestation is primarily a disease of less developed countries, where over 20 million people are believed to be infected. Three distinct clinical entities are recognized: (1) localized cutaneous leishmaniasis, (2) mucocutaneous leishmaniasis, and (3) visceral leishmaniasis. Patients with visceral leishmaniasis suffer persistent fever, progressive weight loss, hepatosplenomegaly, anemia, thrombocytopenia, and leukopenia. Light-skinned persons develop darkening of the skin. If untreated, the disease is fatal. Aside from clinical differences, the other choices do not represent infection of macrophages and do not lead to massive splenomegaly.

Diagnosis: Leishmaniasis

56   **The answer is C: *Giardia lamblia.*** Giardiasis is an infestation of the small intestine by the flagellated protozoan *G. lamblia*. The organisms can be acquired from contaminated water or food, and the infection is characterized by abdominal cramping and nonbloody diarrhea. The gastrointestinal symptoms usually resolve in 1 to 4 weeks, but chronic giardiasis may lead to malabsorption, weight loss, and growth retardation. The organisms are recovered from stool specimens, duodenal aspirates, or intestinal biopsies. The other choices do not lead to chronic infection.

Diagnosis: Giardiasis, *Giardia lamblia*

57   **The answer is E: Rhinovirus.** The common cold is an acute, self-limited disorder of the upper respiratory tract caused by infection with a variety of RNA viruses, including over 100 distinct rhinoviruses and several coronaviruses. These viruses infect nasal respiratory epithelial cells, causing edema and increased mucus production. Clinically, the common cold is characterized by rhinorrhea, pharyngitis, cough, and low-grade fever. Symptoms last about a week. HIV is a lentivirus (choice D).

Diagnosis: Common cold

58   **The answer is C: Parvovirus B19.** Human parvovirus B19 is a DNA virus that causes systemic infections characterized by rash, arthralgias, and transient interruption in erythropoiesis. The virus produces characteristic cytopathic effects in erythroid precursor cells. The nucleus of an affected cell is enlarged, and the chromatin is displaced peripherally by central, glassy, eosinophilic material. When the fetus is infected with parvovirus B19, a transient cessation of erythrocyte production leads to severe anemia, hydrops fetalis, and often death in utero. The other choices do not interfere with erythropoiesis.

Diagnosis: Hydrops fetalis, TORCH syndrome

59   **The answer is A: *Campylobacter jejuni.*** *C. jejuni* causes an acute, self-limited, inflammatory diarrheal illness. The organism is distributed worldwide and is acquired through contaminated food or water. It is a major cause of childhood mortality in developing countries and is responsible for many cases of travelers' diarrhea. *C. jejuni* causes a superficial enterocolitis primarily involving the terminal ileum and colon. Focal necrosis of the intestinal epithelium is accompanied by an acute inflammatory infiltrate. In severe cases, focal disease progresses to small ulcers and patchy inflammatory exudates (pseudomembranes). The symptoms typically resolve in 5 to 7 days. A few patients develop a severe, protracted illness resembling acute ulcerative colitis. The other choices are characterized by a more rapid onset of symptoms after infection.

Diagnosis: *Campylobacter* enteritis

60   **The answer is B: *Clostridium perfringens.*** Gas gangrene (clostridial myonecrosis) is a necrotizing, gas-forming infection that begins in contaminated wounds and spreads rapidly to adjacent tissues. The disease can be fatal within hours of onset. Gas gangrene follows the deposition of *C. perfringens* into tissues under anaerobic conditions. Such conditions occur in areas of extensive necrosis (e.g., severe trauma, wartime injuries, and septic abortions). Clostridial myonecrosis is rare when the wound is subjected to prompt and thorough debridement of dead tissue. Damage to previously healthy muscle is mediated by a myotoxin. *C. botulinum* (choice A) secretes a preformed neurotoxin.

Diagnosis: Gas gangrene, clostridial myonecrosis

61 **The answer is C: Cysticercosis.** Pigs acquire cysticerci by ingesting eggs of *Taenia solium* shed in human feces. However, when humans accidentally ingest the eggs from human feces and become infected with cysticerci, the consequences may be catastrophic. The eggs release oncospheres, which penetrate the wall of the gut, enter the bloodstream, lodge in tissues, and differentiate to cysticerci. The cysticercus is a spherical milky white cyst of about 1 cm in diameter that contains fluid and an invaginated scolex (head of the worm). Viable cysts can be shelled out from the infected tissue. Multiple cysticerci in the brain may impart a "Swiss cheese" appearance and manifest clinically as headaches and seizures. The other worms (choices B, D, and E) do not infect the brain. Aspergillosis of the brain (choice A) is distinctly uncommon.

Diagnosis: Cysticercosis

62 **The answer is D: *Pseudomonas* sp.** Cystic fibrosis is the most common lethal autosomal recessive disorder in the white population. The disease is characterized by (1) chronic pulmonary disease, (2) deficient exocrine pancreatic function, and (3) other complications of inspissated mucus in a number of organs, including the small intestine, the liver, and the reproductive tract. It results from abnormal electrolyte transport caused by impaired function of the chloride channel of epithelial cells. The pulmonary symptoms of CF begin with cough, which eventually becomes productive of large amounts of tenacious and purulent sputum. Episodes of infectious bronchitis and bronchopneumonia become progressively more frequent, and eventually shortness of breath develops. Respiratory failure and the cardiac complications of pulmonary hypertension (cor pulmonale) are late sequelae. The most common organisms that infect the respiratory tract in CF are *Staphylococcus* and *Pseudomonas* species. As the disease advances, *Pseudomonas* may be the only organism cultured from the lung. In fact, the recovery of *Pseudomonas* sp., particularly the mucoid variety, from the lungs of a child with chronic pulmonary disease is virtually diagnostic of CF.

Diagnosis: Cystic fibrosis

Chapter 10

Blood Vessels

QUESTIONS

Select the single best answer.

1 An 80-year-old man with long-standing diabetes and systemic hypertension dies of congestive heart failure. The luminal surface of the abdominal aorta is shown in the image. Which of the following pathologic changes would you expect to see on microscopic examination?

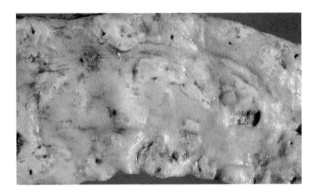

(A) Acute inflammation of the vessel wall
(B) Bacterial colonies in the vessel wall
(C) Cystic medial necrosis
(D) Lipid deposition and smooth muscle cell hyperplasia
(E) Obliterative endarteritis of the vasa vasorum

2 A 60-year-old mildly obese woman is admitted to the hospital with a chief complaint of recurrent chest pain on exertion. The patient reports several episodes of chest pain over the past several years and painful leg cramps when walking. Fasting blood glucose (160 mg/dL) and total serum cholesterol (370 mg/dL) are high. The ECG is normal and blood tests for cardiac-specific proteins are negative. Chest pain in this patient is most likely due to which of the following underlying conditions?
(A) Atherosclerosis of coronary artery
(B) Congenital anomalous origin of coronary artery
(C) Coronary arteritis
(D) Intramural course of the LAD coronary artery
(E) Thrombosis of coronary artery

3 A 69-year-old woman presents with crushing substernal chest pain and nausea. Laboratory studies show elevated serum levels of cardiac proteins (CK-MB = 8.5 ng/mL; troponin-I = 3.2 ng/mL). A diagnosis of myocardial infarction is confirmed by ECG. Despite treatment, the patient becomes hypotensive, and resuscitation attempts are unsuccessful. A cross section of the patient's right coronary artery at autopsy is shown in the image. Which of the following pathologic changes are evident in this autopsy specimen?

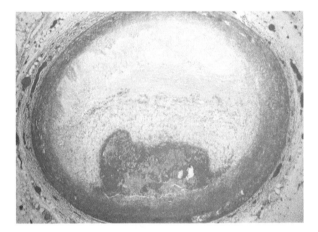

(A) Arteritis and atherosclerosis
(B) Atherosclerosis and thrombosis
(C) Microaneurysm and canalization
(D) Thrombosis and calcification
(E) Vasodilation and arteritis

4 Lipids sequestered by foam cells within the coronary arteries of the patient described in Question 3 were derived primarily from which of the following sources?
(A) Apoptotic bodies of smooth muscle cells
(B) Lipids found in platelet granules
(C) Membranes of dead cells at the site of vascular injury
(D) Secretory product of activated macrophages
(E) Serum lipoproteins

5 A 55-year-old man with a history of hypertension and type 2 diabetes is rushed to the emergency room after collapsing. He describes "tearing chest pain" radiating to the back. His blood pressure is 90/50 mm Hg, and pulse is diminished. Cardiac auscultation reveals a diastolic murmur, consistent with aortic regurgitation. The ECG is normal, and blood tests for cardiac-specific proteins and enzymes are negative. The patient dies within 24 hours of admission. The thoracic aorta at autopsy is shown in the image. The pathogenesis of this lesion is most closely related to which of the following underlying conditions?

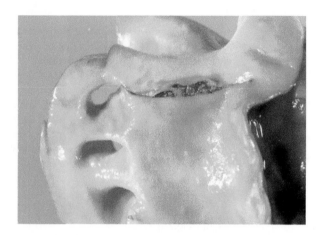

(A) Connective tissue weakness of the aortic wall
(B) Fibrinoid necrosis and smooth muscle hyperplasia
(C) Immune complex-mediated vasculitis
(D) Neovascularization of a complicated atheromatous plaque
(E) Subintimal lipid deposition and smooth muscle necrosis

6 A previously healthy 67-year-old man presents to the emergency room with numbness of his left leg. Temperature and blood pressure are normal. Physical examination shows pallor and a cool left leg with absence of distal pulse. An ECG reveals no abnormalities. An arteriogram demonstrates a markedly dilated abdominal aorta and occlusion of the left popliteal artery. The blockage is removed surgically, and the patient recovers. Which of the following is the most likely source of the arterial thromboembolus in this patient?

(A) Deep venous thrombosis
(B) Left ventricular mural thrombus
(C) Nonbacterial endocarditis
(D) Paradoxical emboli
(E) Thrombus from an atheromatous aorta

7 A 28-year-old man develops the "worst headache of his life" and then becomes comatose. A CT scan of the head reveals subarachnoid hemorrhage. The patient eventually dies, and autopsy reveals an aneurysm at the base of the brain (shown in the image; see arrow). The pathogenesis of this abnormality is most closely linked to which of the following conditions?

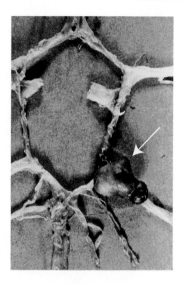

(A) Arterial wall defect due to diabetes
(B) Atherosclerotic plaque deposition
(C) Muscle weakness of the arterial wall
(D) Cystic medial necrosis
(E) Endarteritis of the vasa vasorum

8 A 45-year-old man presents with pain in the legs upon exercise and destruction of the tips of his fingers. He has an 80-pack-year history of smoking. Laboratory values include hemoglobin of 16 g/dL, WBC of 8,500/μL, serum cholesterol of 220 mg/dL, fasting blood sugar of 90 mg/dL, and negative tests for antinuclear antibodies. Biopsy of the affected area (shown in the image) reveals intraluminal thrombi in medium-sized arteries and inflammation extending from arteries to neighboring veins and nerves. What is the appropriate diagnosis?

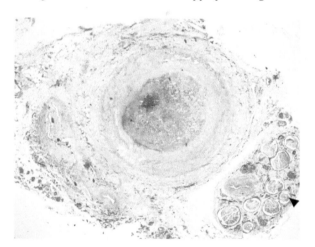

(A) Buerger disease
(B) Churg-Strauss disease
(C) Kawasaki disease
(D) Polyarteritis nodosa
(E) Takayasu arteritis

9 A 45-year-old man is brought to the emergency room with rapid pulse and cold and clammy skin. Blood pressure is 90/50 mm Hg. An X-ray film of the chest demonstrates dilation of the ascending aorta. Cardiac auscultation reveals a diastolic murmur in the aortic region. Laboratory studies show that serum cholesterol is 160 mg/dL, hematocrit is 35%, and hemoglobin is 13.6 g/dL. The fluorescent *Treponema* antibody test is positive. The patient suddenly becomes hypotensive and dies. The luminal surface of the ascending aorta at autopsy is shown in the image. Which of the following was most likely involved in the pathogenesis of this aortic lesion?

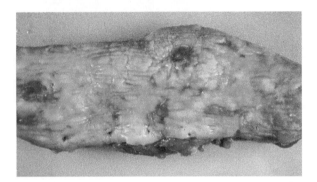

(A) Arterial wall defect due to diabetes
(B) Atherosclerosis
(C) Congenital defect of the arterial wall
(D) Cystic medial necrosis
(E) Endarteritis of the vasa vasorum

10 A 38-year-old woman with a history of ischemic heart disease presents with disfiguring skin lesions. Physical examination shows xanthomas on the dorsal surface of both hands (shown in the image) and xanthelasmas of the eyelids. Laboratory studies reveal serum cholesterol of 820 mg/dL and significantly elevated serum triglycerides and LDL. Which of the following histopathologic findings would be expected in a biopsy of this patient's skin lesions?

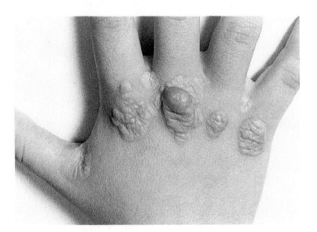

(A) Dermal calcium deposits
(B) Foamy macrophages
(C) Hypertrophic scar tissue
(D) Multinucleated giant cells
(E) Smooth muscle hyperplasia

11 A 55-year-old man suffers from an acute myocardial infarction after occlusion of the left anterior descending coronary artery. The patient undergoes coronary bypass surgery 3 days later. Which of the following is the most frequent cause of saphenous vein graft failure several years following coronary bypass surgery?

(A) Acute inflammation
(B) Atherosclerosis
(C) Graft-versus-host disease
(D) Metastatic calcification
(E) Microaneurysm

12 A 45-year-old black man undergoes renal biopsy for evaluation of chronic renal failure. The patient has a 60-pack-year history of smoking. Physical examination reveals a blood pressure of 190/120 mm Hg. A renal biopsy shows thickening of small arteries and arterioles, as well as edematous intimal expansion and fibrinoid necrosis. The Congo red stain is negative. Laboratory studies show hemoglobin is 10.2 g/dL and serum cholesterol is 250 mg/dL. BUN and serum creatinine are 42 and 5.5 mg/dL, respectively. Which of the following is the most likely cause of renal failure in this patient?

(A) Amyloid nephropathy
(B) Chronic pyelonephritis
(C) Malignant hypertension
(D) Polyarteritis nodosa
(E) Proliferative glomerulonephritis

13 A 32-year-old woman from Africa presents with a 4-month history of swelling of her right leg (patient shown in the image). Laboratory studies demonstrate a parasitic infestation. Soft tissue swelling of this patient's leg was most likely caused by which of the following conditions?

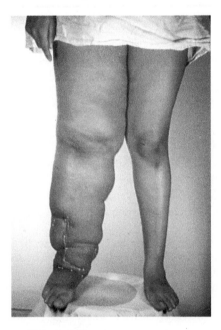

(A) Congestive heart failure
(B) Deep venous thrombosis
(C) Kidney disease
(D) Liver disease
(E) Lymphatic obstruction

14 A 60-year-old man presents with dizziness, nausea, and severe shortness of breath of several months' duration. Physical examination shows hepatomegaly, ascites, and anasarca. His blood pressure is 200/115 mm Hg. An X-ray film of the chest demonstrates cardiomegaly and mild pulmonary edema. Although different mechanisms may have contributed to the pathogenesis of hypertension in this patient, the common end result for all of them is which of the following?

(A) Arterial cystic medial necrosis
(B) Decreased plasma oncotic pressure
(C) Generalized vasodilation
(D) Increased peripheral vascular resistance
(E) Increased vascular permeability

15 A 40-year-old woman presents with an 8-month history of severe headaches, weakness, and dizziness. Blood pressure is 180/110 mm Hg. Physical examination shows diminished tendon reflexes. An abdominal CT scan reveals a 4-cm mass in the right adrenal gland. The results of laboratory studies include serum potassium of 2.3 mEq/L, serum sodium of 155 mEq/L, plasma cortisol of 25 µg/dL (8 AM) and 20 µg/dL (4 PM), and low plasma renin. These clinical and laboratory findings are consistent with an adrenal tumor that secretes which of the following hormones?

(A) Aldosterone
(B) Cortisol
(C) Epinephrine
(D) Renin
(E) Testosterone

16 A 25-year-old woman with a recent history of acute hepatitis B infection presents with reddish-blue lesions on her lower extremities, fever, muscle pain, and mild weight loss. Physical examination reveals numerous regions of red-purple discoloration affecting the skin of both legs. Laboratory tests demonstrate positive P-ANCA and an elevated erythrocyte sedimentation rate. Urinalysis shows 2+ proteinuria. Biopsy of lesional skin is shown in the image. Which of the following is the most likely diagnosis?

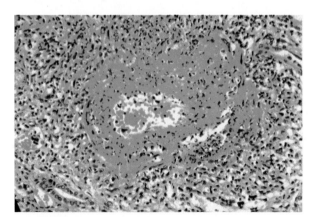

(A) Benign arteriosclerosis
(B) Fibromuscular dysplasia
(C) Henoch-Schönlein purpura
(D) Mönckeberg medial sclerosis
(E) Polyarteritis nodosa

17 A 33-year-old man with AIDS presents with multiple, purple-colored skin nodules on his hands and feet. The lesions vary in size from 1 mm to 1 cm in diameter. Biopsy of lesional skin is shown in the image. Which of the following viruses is implicated in the pathogenesis of this patient's skin neoplasm?

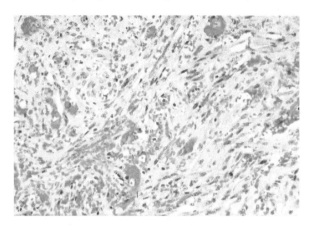

(A) Cytomegalovirus
(B) Human herpesvirus-6
(C) Human herpesvirus-8
(D) Human immunodeficiency virus
(E) Human papillomavirus

18 A 30-year-old woman presents with a widespread skin rash that she has had for 5 days. She is taking sulfa medication for recurrent cystitis. A skin biopsy shows leukocytoclastic vasculitis involving dermal venules. What is the appropriate diagnosis?

(A) Buerger disease
(B) Giant cell granulomatous arteritis
(C) Henoch-Schönlein purpura
(D) Hypersensitivity angiitis
(E) Polyarteritis nodosa

19 A 70-year-old woman complains of a throbbing unilateral headache and vision problems. She reports weight loss and mandibular pain while eating. The patient also has a history of recurrent bouts of fever accompanied by malaise and muscle aches. Physical examination reveals nodular enlargement of the temporal artery with pain on palpation. A biopsy is obtained (shown in the image). What is the appropriate diagnosis?

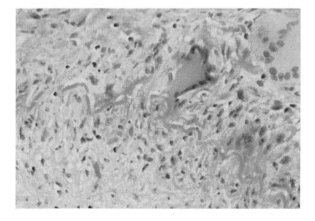

(A) Giant cell arteritis

(B) Hypersensitivity angiitis

(C) Kawasaki disease

(D) Polyarteritis nodosa

(E) Wegener granulomatosis

20 A 48-year-old man presents with an exquisitely painful, raised, red lesion on the dorsal surface of his left hand. Histologic examination of a skin biopsy reveals nests of round regular cells within connective tissue associated with branching vascular spaces. Which of the following is the most likely diagnosis?

(A) Angiosarcoma

(B) Dermatofibroma

(C) Glomus tumor

(D) Hemangioma

(E) Lipoma

21 A 60-year-old man has his left forearm amputated because he has invasive rhabdomyosarcoma. The pathologist notes calcification in the wall of the radial artery, which otherwise appears unremarkable. Which of the following is the appropriate diagnosis?

(A) Churg-Strauss disease

(B) Complicated atherosclerotic plaque

(C) Fibromuscular dysplasia

(D) Mönckeberg medial sclerosis

(E) Polyarteritis nodosa

22 A 20-year-old woman complains of double vision, fainting spells, tingling of the fingers of her left hand, and numbness of the fingers of her right hand. Physical examination reveals absence of pulse in her right arm. Laboratory tests show elevated erythrocyte sedimentation rate and thrombocytosis. An aortogram demonstrates narrowing and occlusion of branching arteries, including the right subclavian artery. The patient subsequently develops heart failure and dies of massive pulmonary edema. At autopsy, the aorta has a thickened wall and shows vasculitis and fragmentation of elastic fibers. Which of the following is the most likely diagnosis?

(A) Buerger disease

(B) Churg-Strauss disease

(C) Kawasaki disease

(D) Polyarteritis nodosa

(E) Takayasu arteritis

23 A 19-year-old man with a history of recent-onset asthma presents with chest pain, intermittent claudication, and respiratory distress that is unresponsive to bronchodilators and antibiotics. Physical examination reveals mild hypertension (blood pressure = 150/100 mm Hg), bilateral wheezing, and numerous purpuric skin lesions on the feet. Laboratory studies demonstrate that leukocytes are increased to 14,000/μL with increased eosinophils and platelets are increased to 450,000/μL. BUN is elevated to 30 mg/dL, and serum creatinine is elevated to 3.5 mg/dL. The serum antineutrophil cytoplasmic antibody test is positive. Urinalysis discloses 3+ proteinuria and RBCs. A renal biopsy demonstrates vasculitis of medium-sized arteries, accompanied by eosinophilia. Which of the following is the most likely diagnosis?

(A) Churg-Strauss disease

(B) Henoch-Schönlein purpura

(C) Loeffler syndrome

(D) Polyarteritis nodosa

(E) Wegener granulomatosis

24 A 40-year-old man presents with a 2-week history of recurrent oral ulcers, genital ulcers, intermittent arthritic pain of the knees, and abdominal pain. Physical examination reveals shallow ulcerations of the mucosa of the glans penis, as well as oral aphthous ulcers and conjunctivitis. Which of the following is the most likely diagnosis?

(A) Behçet disease

(B) Genital herpes

(C) Gonorrhea

(D) Polyarteritis nodosa

(E) Syphilis

25 A neonate has a well-demarcated lesion in the upper eyelid and forehead resembling a tumor (shown in the image). A biopsy shows large vascular channels interspersed with small, capillary type vessels. What is the appropriate diagnosis?

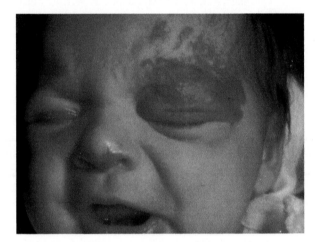

(A) Angiosarcoma

(B) Capillary lymphangioma

(C) Cavernous hemangioma

(D) Hemangioendothelioma

(E) Hemangiopericytoma

26 A 48-year-old man with diabetes presents with a history of progressive pain in both legs for several years. The pain is severe after walking two blocks or climbing one flight of stairs. Blood pressure is 145/90 mm Hg. Laboratory studies show a serum cholesterol of 320 mg/dL. He neither smokes nor drinks. Bruits are evident upon auscultation of both femoral arteries. The pathogenesis of intermittent claudication in this patient is most closely associated with which of the following risk factors?

(A) Hyperglycemia

(B) Hyperlipidemia

(C) Obesity

(D) Sedentary lifestyle

(E) Systemic hypertension

27 A 70-year-old, previously healthy man presents with right upper quadrant pain. Physical examination demonstrates hepatomegaly. A liver biopsy reveals a vascular lesion composed of pleomorphic endothelial cells with hyperchromatic nuclei and numerous mitoses. Laboratory tests for HIV infection are negative. Which of the following is the most likely diagnosis?

(A) Angiosarcoma
(B) Dermatofibroma
(C) Glomus tumor
(D) Hemangioma
(E) Kaposi sarcoma

28 A 60-year-old man with a history of recurrent headaches and blurred vision presents to the emergency room with excruciating pain radiating to his back, beginning 2 hours prior to admission. Blood pressure on admission is 110/70 mm Hg. He appears pale and sweaty. Echocardiogram shows an enlargement of the left ventricular wall. ECG is normal, and blood tests for cardiac proteins are negative. One hour after admission, the patient experiences pain radiating to his left flank and right side of his neck. The patient suddenly becomes hypotensive and expires. Microscopic examination of the thoracic aorta at autopsy is shown in the image (aldehyde fuchsin stain). Which of the following best characterizes these pathologic findings?

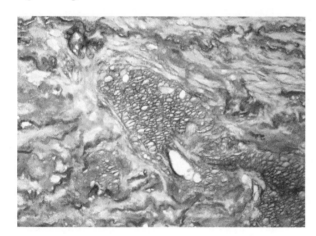

(A) Acute inflammation
(B) Atherosclerosis
(C) Chronic inflammation
(D) Cystic medial necrosis
(E) Fibrinoid necrosis

29 A 65-year-old man presents with a 2-week history of abdominal discomfort. Physical examination reveals a pulsatile, abdominal mass in the periumbilical region. A CT scan shows a segment of abdominal aorta proximal to the bifurcation that is dilated (5 cm) and calcified. The patient is scheduled for corrective surgery but suffers a massive stroke and expires. The abdominal aorta is examined at autopsy (shown in the image). Which of the following is the most likely underlying cause of this patient's abdominal mass?

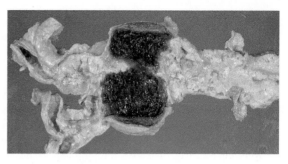

(A) Angiosarcoma
(B) Atherosclerosis
(C) Cystic medial necrosis
(D) Hypercalcemia
(E) Thromboembolism

30 A 48-year-old woman with familial hypercholesterolemia complains of severe, crushing, substernal chest pain. The pain is relieved by administration of sublingual nitroglycerin or bed rest. The patient subsequently goes into cardiorespiratory arrest and expires. The left coronary artery at autopsy is shown in the image. The material that has acutely occluded the lumen of this blood vessel is largely composed of which of the following cellular components?

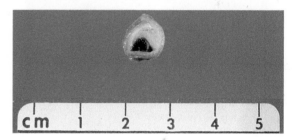

(A) Activated endothelial cells
(B) Lipid-laden (foamy) macrophages
(C) Multinucleated giant cells
(D) Platelets and red blood cells
(E) Segmented neutrophils

31 A 30-year-old woman with Sjögren syndrome presents with a 24-hour history of a purpuric skin rash. Which of the following is the most likely diagnosis?
(A) Buerger disease
(B) Giant cell granulomatous arteritis
(C) Hypersensitivity vasculitis
(D) Thrombotic thrombocytopenic purpura
(E) Wegener granulomatosis

32 A 62-year-old man is discovered to have hyperlipidemia on screening tests after a routine physical examination. Laboratory studies show total serum cholesterol of 285 mg/dL, LDL of 215 mg/dL, HDL of 38 mg/dL, and triglycerides of 300 mg/dL. This patient is most at risk of developing an aneurysm in which of the following anatomic locations?
(A) Abdominal aorta
(B) Ascending aorta
(C) Circle of Willis
(D) Coronary artery
(E) Renal artery

33 A 3-year-old girl presents with high fever, extensive skin rash, and conjunctival congestion. Physical examination reveals cervical lymphadenopathy, erythematous palms and soles, and a dry and red oral mucosa. A throat culture is negative. Routine CBC is normal, and the monospot test for infectious mononucleosis is negative. Additional laboratory tests rule out cytomegalovirus infection and toxoplasmosis. Two months later, the child develops signs and symptoms of heart failure and eventually goes into cardiac arrest. The heart at autopsy is shown in the image. What is the appropriate diagnosis?

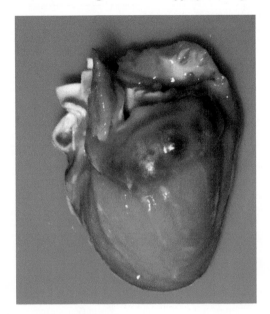

(A) Buerger disease
(B) Churg-Strauss disease
(C) Giant cell granulomatous arteritis
(D) Kawasaki disease
(E) Takayasu arteritis

34 A 45-year-old woman presents with a 4-month history of severe headaches and pain, and blanching of the hands upon exposure to cold. She is a nonsmoker. Over the past 6 months, she has noticed progressive difficulty in swallowing solid food. Physical examination reveals smooth and tight skin over the face and fingers. The serologic test for anti–Scl-70 (antitopoisomerase) is positive. Painful hands in this patient are best described using which of the following terms?

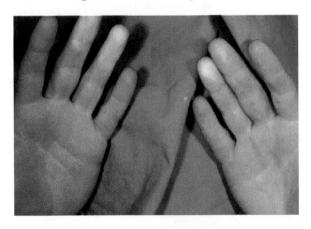

(A) Chilblains
(B) Homans' sign
(C) Intermittent claudication
(D) Raynaud phenomenon
(E) Trousseau phenomenon

35 A 6-year-old girl presents with a 2-week history of a skin rash over her buttocks and legs and joint pain. The parents report seeing blood in the urine. Physical examination reveals palpable purpuric skin lesions and markedly swollen knees. The results of laboratory studies reveal abnormally high erythrocyte sedimentation rate (30 mm/h), BUN of 25 mg/dL, and serum creatinine of 3 mg/dL. Urinalysis demonstrates RBCs and RBC casts. The stool guaiac test is positive. Biopsy of lesional skin reveals deposits of IgA in the walls of small blood vessels. Which of the following is the most likely diagnosis?

(A) Henoch-Schönlein purpura
(B) Hypersensitivity vasculitis
(C) Kawasaki disease
(D) Polyarteritis nodosa
(E) Poststreptococcal glomerulonephritis

36 A 50-year-old woman with type 2 diabetes and hypertension undergoes renal biopsy for evaluation of chronic renal disease. The biopsy is shown in the image. What is the appropriate diagnosis?

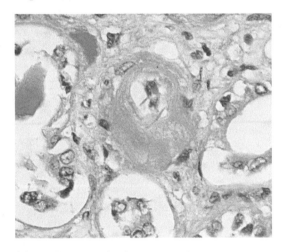

(A) Hyaline arteriolosclerosis
(B) Kimmelstiel-Wilson disease
(C) Mönckeberg medial sclerosis
(D) Papillary necrosis
(E) Polyarteritis nodosa

37 A 79-year-old man presents with a history of extensive ulcers on both legs for 4 years. A photograph of the patient's legs is shown in the image. What is the appropriate diagnosis?

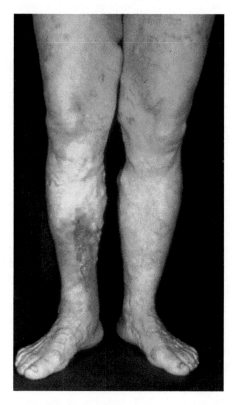

(A) Deep venous thrombosis
(B) Lymphangitis
(C) Milroy disease
(D) Severe arteriolosclerosis
(E) Varicose veins

38 A 76-year-old woman presents with a 1-hour history of substernal chest pain. Shortly after admission the patient expires. At autopsy, extensive calcium deposits are noted in the coronary and other arteries affected by severe atherosclerosis. Which of the following terms best describes these autopsy findings?

(A) Dystrophic calcification
(B) Hyperplastic calcification
(C) Hypertrophic calcification
(D) Metastatic calcification
(E) Physiologic calcification

39 A 48-year-old man with a longstanding history of chronic constipation complains of anal itching and discomfort toward the end of the day. He describes a perianal pain when sitting and finds himself sitting sideways to avoid discomfort. Physical examination reveals painful varicose dilations in the anal region, associated with edema. Which of the following is the most likely diagnosis?

(A) Anal cancer
(B) Anal fissure
(C) Hemorrhoids
(D) Ischiorectal abscess
(E) Rectal cancer

40 A 45-year-old woman complains that her fingers feel stiff. On physical examination the skin of the patient's face appears tense and radial furrows are evident around the mouth. Laboratory studies establish a diagnosis of scleroderma. Several years later, the patient subsequently develops renal insufficiency. A renal biopsy is shown in the image. Which of the following best describes the pathogenesis of renal vascular involvement in this patient with progressive systemic sclerosis?

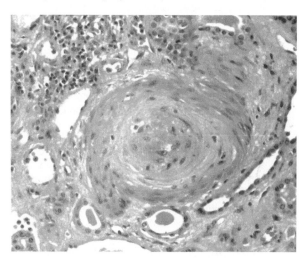

(A) Accelerated atherosclerosis
(B) Cystic medial necrosis
(C) Organization of microthrombi
(D) Perivascular arteritis
(E) Subintimal fibromuscular thickening

41 An 80-year-old woman with a history of smoking experiences acute chest pain and is rushed to the emergency room. Laboratory studies and ECG confirm a diagnosis of myocardial infarction; however, coronary artery angiography 2 hours later does not demonstrate evidence of vessel occlusion. Which of the following proteins mediated fibrinolysis at the site of temporary blockage in this patient's coronary artery?

(A) Bradykinin
(B) Collagenase
(C) Kallikrein
(D) Plasmin
(E) Thrombin

ANSWERS

1 **The answer is D: Lipid deposition and smooth muscle cell hyperplasia.** Atherosclerosis is a disease of large- and medium-sized elastic and muscular arteries that results in the progressive accumulation within the intima of inflammatory cells, hyperplastic smooth muscle cells, lipids, and connective tissue. The resulting characteristic lesion, the lipid plaque (atheroma), contains pools of extracellular lipid and numerous lipid-laden macrophages (foam cells). It is not an acute inflammatory or infectious process (choices A and B). Obliterative endarteritis (choice E) is a syphilitic lesion.
Diagnosis: Atherosclerosis

2 **The answer is A: Atherosclerosis of coronary artery.** Patients with severe atherosclerosis present with organ-specific vascular disorders, including intermittent claudication, abdominal aortic aneurysms, coronary artery disease (chest pain), cerebrovascular disease, and peripheral vascular disease. Angina pectoris is the pain of myocardial ischemia. It typically occurs in the substernal portion of the chest and may radiate to the left arm, jaw, and epigastrium. It is the most common symptom of ischemic heart disease. Laboratory findings in this patient show evidence of diabetes mellitus and hyperlipidemia, which are risk factors for atherosclerosis. Thrombosis of a ruptured atheromatous plaque (choice E) usually precipitates acute myocardial infarction. The other conditions (choices C, D, and E) may limit coronary blood flow and present with chest pain on exertion, but they are less common than coronary atherosclerosis.
Diagnosis: Ischemic heart disease, atherosclerosis

3 **The answer is B: Atherosclerosis and thrombosis.** The photomicrograph shows severe atherosclerosis and a recent thrombus in the narrowed lumen. The mature atheroma is highly thrombogenic, and thrombosis of an atherosclerotic plaque can abruptly occlude the lumen of medium-sized muscular arteries causing ischemic necrosis of dependent tissues. Thrombotic occlusion may manifest as myocardial infarction, stroke, or gangrene of intestinal loops or lower extremities. Arteritis (choice A) would exhibit inflammatory cells. Calcification (choice D) would appear as irregular blue material with H&E stain.
Diagnosis: Myocardial infarction

4 **The answer is E: Serum lipoproteins.** Hyperlipidemia is correlated with the early onset of atherosclerosis and cardiovascular disease. Cholesterol carried by serum lipoproteins is deposited in the atheroma, where it is endocytosed by macrophages (lipid-laden foam cells).
Diagnosis: Myocardial infarction, atherosclerosis

5 **The answer is A: Connective tissue weakness of the aortic wall.** Dissecting aneurysm refers to the entry of blood into the arterial wall and its extension along the length of the vessel, which is associated with a degeneration and weakening of the aortic media. Some cases are seen in patients with Marfan syndrome, a systemic connective tissue disorder associated with mutations in the gene encoding the extraceullar matrix glycoprotein, fibrillin. Although the other choices may lead to saccular or fusiform aneurysms in other locations, they do not cause an aortic dissection.
Diagnosis: Dissecting aortic aneurysm

6 **The answer is E: Thrombus from an atheromatous aorta.** This patient has an abdominal aortic aneurysm. A thrombus that forms over the aneurysm may embolize and lodge in a distal vessel. In this case, a thromboembolus occluded the popliteal artery, causing ischemia of the patient's left leg. Although a mural thrombus of the left ventricle (choice B) can embolize, there is no evidence of underlying myocardial infarction in this case. Choices B, C, and D are much rarer causes of thromboembolism.
Diagnosis: Arterial thromboembolism

7 **The answer is C: Muscle weakness of the arterial wall.** The most common type of cerebral aneurysm is a saccular aneurysm, also referred to as a berry aneurysm. The lesion results from a congenital defect in smooth muscle distribution at a branch point of the arterial wall. The most common site of berry aneurysm formation is between the anterior communicating and the anterior cerebral arteries in the circle of Willis. In this case, the berry aneurysm arose from the posterior cerebral artery (see photograph). Diabetes (choice A) and atherosclerosis (choice B) do not cause berry aneurysms. Cystic medial necrosis (choice D) is associated with dissecting aortic aneurysm. Endarteritis of the vasa vasorum (choice E) is associated with syphilitic aneurysm of the ascending aorta.
Diagnosis: Berry aneurysm, subarachnoid hemorrhage

8 **The answer is A: Buerger disease.** Buerger disease (thromboangiitis obliterans) is an occlusive inflammatory disease of medium and small arteries of the distal arms and legs. The etiologic role of smoking has been emphasized by the observation that cessation of smoking can be followed by remission. Microscopic examination of affected vessels shows polymorphonuclear infiltrates extending to neighboring veins and nerves. Inflammation of the endothelium is associated with thrombosis and obliteration of the affected vessels. The other choices are not associated with smoking and do not exhibit these characteristic histologic findings.
Diagnosis: Buerger disease

9 **The answer is E: Endarteritis of the vasa vasorum.** The results of laboratory tests indicate that the patient has syphilis. Syphilitic aneurysm typically affects the ascending aorta. Microscopic examination shows obliterative endarteritis and periarteritis of the vasa vasorum. The vasa vasorum ramify in the adventitia and penetrate the outer and middle third of the aorta. In syphilitic disease, they become encircled by lymphocytes, plasma cells, and macrophages. Obliteration of the vasa vasorum causes focal necrosis and scarring of the media, with disruption and disorganization of the elastic lamellae. The inner surface of the affected aorta shows a typical "tree bark" appearance. The other choices are not involved in the pathogenesis of syphilitic aneurysm.
Diagnosis: Syphilitic aneurysm

10 **The answer is B: Foamy macrophages.** This patient has familial hypercholesterolemia and has inherited mutations in the LDL receptor gene. The LDL receptor is a cell surface glycoprotein that regulates plasma cholesterol by mediating endocytosis and recycling of apolipoprotein (apo)E. Lacking LDL receptor function, high levels of LDL circulate, are taken up by tissue macrophages, and accumulate to form occlusive arterial plaques (atheromas) and papules or nodules of lipid-laden, foamy macrophages (xanthomas). The other choices are not expected findings in xanthomas.
Diagnosis: Familial hypercholesterolemia, xanthoma

11 **The answer is B: Atherosclerosis.** Saphenous veins are used as autografts in coronary artery bypass surgery. These grafts usually undergo a series of adaptive and reparative changes. Venous grafts in place for 5 to 10 years typically show atherosclerotic plaques that are indistinguishable from those found in native coronary arteries, a process referred to as atherosclerotic "restenosis."

Diagnosis: Atherosclerosis

12 **The answer is C: Malignant hypertension.** Malignant hypertension refers to an elevated blood pressure that may result in rapidly progressive vascular disease affecting the brain, heart, and kidney. The disease injures endothelial cells, causing increased vascular permeability, which leads to the insudation of plasma proteins into the vessel wall and morphologic evidence of fibrinoid necrosis. Polyarteritis nodosa (choice D) is an inflammatory process. In this patient, acute vascular injury is followed by smooth muscle proliferation with an increase in concentric layers of smooth muscle cells that yield the so-called "onion skin" appearance. Poor perfusion of the kidneys stimulates the release of renin, which serves to elevate systemic blood pressure even further (renovascular hypertension).

Diagnosis: Hypertensive nephrosclerosis

13 **The answer is E: Lymphatic obstruction.** The patient has filarial worm infestation of an inguinal lymph node which has caused elephantiasis. Under normal circumstances, more fluid is filtered into the interstitial spaces than is reabsorbed into the vascular bed. This excess interstitial fluid is removed by the lymphatics. Thus, obstruction to the lymphatic flow leads to localized edema formation. Lymphatic channels can be obstructed by (1) malignant neoplasms, (2) fibrosis resulting from inflammation or irradiation, and (3) surgical ablation. The inflammatory response to filarial worms (Bancroftian and Malayan filariasis) can result in lymphatic obstruction that produces massive lymphedema of the scrotum or extremity (elephantiasis). Lymphatic edema differs from other forms of edema in its high protein content, since lymph is the vehicle by which proteins and interstitial cells are returned to the circulation. This increased protein concentration may be a fibrogenic stimulus in the formation of dermal fibrosis in chronic edema (indurated edema). Congestive heart failure (choice A), kidney disease (choice C), and liver disease (choice D) can cause generalized noninflammatory edema, but the swelling is bilateral. Although deep venous thrombosis can cause tenderness and swelling, it does not cause elephantiasis.

Diagnosis: Elephantiasis, lymphedema

14 **The answer is D: Increased peripheral vascular resistance.** In patients with systemic hypertension, the end result of autoregulation is always increased peripheral resistance. Most cases of hypertension represent an imbalance between renal function and sodium homeostasis. In this context, the renin-angiotensin system increases blood pressure, whereas this axis is antagonized by atrial natriuretic factor. Cystic medial necrosis (choice A) is a factor in aortic dissecting aneurysm. Vasodilation (choice C) decreases blood pressure. Choices B and E may be a consequence of uncontrolled hypertension, but do not cause it.

Diagnosis: Hypertensive heart disease

15 **The answer is A: Aldosterone.** This patient has Conn syndrome, an endocrine disorder most commonly caused by an adrenal cortical adenoma. Aldosterone secreted by the adrenal cortical tumor causes hypertension, hypernatremia, and

hypokalemia. Epinephrine, renin, and testosterone (choices C, D, and E) are not produced by adrenal cortical tumors. Cortisol (choice B) may be produced by adrenal cortical tumors but does not significantly alter electrolyte homeostasis.

Diagnosis: Conn syndrome, hyperaldosteronism

16 **The answer is E: Polyarteritis nodosa (PAN).** PAN is an acute necrotizing vasculitis that affects medium-sized and smaller muscular arteries. On occasion, PAN extends into larger arteries, such as the renal, splenic, or coronary arteries. The most common morphologic feature of affected arteries is fibrinoid necrosis, in which the medial muscle and adjacent tissue are fused into an eosinophilic mass that stains for fibrin. PAN affecting small vessels is frequently associated with the presence of P-ANCA. Approximately 15% of patients with PAN demonstrate either HBsAg or anti-HCV antibodies. Choices A, B, and D are not characterized by necrosis of the arterial wall. The immune complexes seen in Henoch-Schönlein purpura (choice C) are unrelated to hepatitis B.

Diagnosis: Polyarteritis nodosa

17 **The answer is C: Human herpesvirus-8 (HHV-8).** Patients with AIDS may develop Kaposi sarcoma. Microscopic examination of a skin lesion shows numerous poorly differentiated spindle-shaped neoplastic cells and vascular lesions filled with red blood cells, characteristic of Kaposi sarcoma. HHV-8 is implicated in the pathogenesis of this tumor in HIV-infected patients. HIV (choice D) by itself is not a cause of Kaposi sarcoma.

Diagnosis: Kaposi sarcoma, AIDS

18 **The answer is D: Hypersensitivity angiitis.** Hypersensitivity angiitis refers to a broad spectrum of inflammatory lesions that represent a reaction to foreign materials (e.g., bacterial products or more commonly drugs). When the vascular lesions are confined to the skin, the terms leukocytoclastic vasculitis, cutaneous vasculitis, or cutaneous necrotizing venulitis are applied. The other choices are not caused by sulfa drugs.

Diagnosis: Hypersensitivity angiitis

19 **The answer is A: Giant cell arteritis.** Giant cell (temporal) arteritis is the most common vasculitis. The disease is a local, chronic granulomatous inflammation of the temporal arteries. The average age at onset is 70 years. Histologic examination shows giant cell granulomatous inflammation, which destroys the media of the temporal artery and predisposes to thrombosis (see photomicrograph). Headaches, typically in the form of throbbing temporal pain and visual problems, may appear. A palpable, tortuous, and swollen temporal artery may be the only finding on physical examination. Wegener granulomatosis (choice E) causes granulomatous inflammation, but not in the temporal artery. The other choices are not associated with multinucleated giant cells.

Diagnosis: Giant cell granulomatous arteritis, temporal arteritis

20 **The answer is C: Glomus tumor.** A glomus tumor is a benign tumor of the glomus body, which is often extremely painful. Glomus bodies are normal neuromyoarterial receptors that are sensitive to temperature and regulate arteriolar blood flow. The lesions are small, usually smaller than 1 cm in diameter. The two main histologic components are branching vascular channels in connective tissue stroma and aggregates of specialized glomus cells. The other choices tend not to be painful.

Diagnosis: Glomus tumor

21   The answer is D: Mönckeberg medial sclerosis. Mönckeberg medial sclerosis is characterized by calcification of the media of large- and medium-sized arteries of older persons who are not otherwise affected by atherosclerosis (choice B). On gross examination, the involved arteries are hard and dilated. These arterial changes are usually asymptomatic. None of the other choices display calcification.

Diagnosis: Mönckeberg medial sclerosis

22   The answer is E: Takayasu arteritis. Takayasu arteritis is an inflammatory disorder of large arteries, classically the aortic arch and its major branches. On gross examination, the aorta is thickened, and the intima exhibits focal, raised plaques. The branches of the aorta often display localized stenosis or occlusion, which interferes with blood flow and accounts for the symptoms of "pulseless" disease. Ischemic cerebrovascular episodes in a young woman and a differential between the blood pressure in the left and the right arm suggest the diagnosis of Takayasu disease. More than 90% of patients are women under 30 years of age. The other choices are diseases of arteries that have different clinical and pathologic manifestations.

Diagnosis: Takayasu arteritis

23   The answer is A: Churg-Strauss disease. Churg-Strauss disease is an idiopathic, systemic, granulomatous disease of small- and medium-size arteries characterized by vasculitis of many organs, fluctuating eosinophilia, and late-onset asthma. The majority of patients display antineutrophil cytoplasmic antibodies. The disease is also known as allergic granulomatosis and angiitis. Transbronchial lung biopsy shows granulomatous lesions in vascular and extravascular sites, accompanied by intense eosinophilia. The vasculitis histologically resembles the lesions of polyarteritis nodosa (choice D) and Wegener granulomatosis (choice E), but these diseases do not typically present with an asthmatic syndrome.

Diagnosis: Churg-Strauss disease

24   The answer is A: Behçet disease. Behçet disease is a systemic vasculitis characterized by oral aphthous ulcers, genital ulceration, and ocular inflammation, with occasional involvement of the nervous, gastrointestinal, and cardiovascular systems. The mucocutaneous lesions show a nonspecific vasculitis of arterioles, capillaries, and venules. The cause of the necrotizing inflammation of small blood vessels is not known, but an association with specific HLA subtypes suggests an immune basis. Herpes (choice B) does not present with arthritis.

Diagnosis: Behçet disease

25   The answer is C: Cavernous hemangioma. Congenital cavernous hemangioma is a benign lesion consisting of large vascular channels, frequently interspersed with small capillary-type vessels. These lesions occur primarily in the skin, where they are termed port-wine stains. Cavernous hemangiomas may also be found in the brain, where, after a long quiescent period, they may slowly enlarge and cause neurologic symptoms. Cavernous hemangiomas can undergo a variety of changes, including thrombosis and fibrosis, cystic cavitations, and intracystic hemorrhage. Capillary lymphangioma (choice B) is a tumor of the lymphatic system and is not discolored. The other choices are not characteristically encountered as congenital lesions of the face.

Diagnosis: Congenital cavernous hemangioma

26   The answer is B: Hyperlipidemia. The pathogenesis of atherosclerosis is believed to involve injury to the intima, insudation of cholesterol, activation of platelets, and growth factor–mediated recruitment of fibroblasts, macrophages, and smooth muscle cells. The principal risk factors for atherosclerosis are age, male sex, heredity, lipid metabolism (hypercholesterolemia), obesity, hypertension, diabetes mellitus, smoking, and sedentary lifestyle. Although several of these risk factors apply to this patient (choices A, D, and E), hyperlipidemia is considered to be the major factor in the pathogenesis of atherosclerosis. Chronic ischemia of the lower limbs due to atherosclerosis causes hypoperfusion of the leg muscles. When the blood supply becomes inadequate, usually upon exertion, the muscles develop cramps (intermittent claudication).

Diagnosis: Atherosclerosis

27   The answer is A: Angiosarcoma. Angiosarcoma is a highly malignant tumor composed of masses of malignant endothelial cells. The most common locations are the skin, breast, bone, liver, and spleen. Angiosarcoma exhibits varying degrees of differentiation, ranging from tumors composed of distinct vascular elements to undifferentiated tumors with nuclear pleomorphism, and frequent mitosis. Kaposi sarcoma (choice E) is most commonly associated with AIDS patients who are infected by HHV-8.

Diagnosis: Angiosarcoma

28   The answer is D: Cystic medial necrosis. Dissecting aneurysms typically affect the thoracic aorta, but may extend to other vessels. The morphologic findings are characteristic of a degenerative process known as cystic medial necrosis (of Erdheim). Focal loss of elastic and muscle fibers in the aortic media leads to "cystic" spaces filled with pools of metachromatic myxoid material (see photomicrograph). Neither inflammation (choices A and C), atherosclerosis (choice B), nor fibrinoid necrosis (choice E) are present.

Diagnosis: Dissecting aortic aneurysm, cystic medial necrosis

29   The answer is B: Atherosclerosis. Aneurysms are localized dilations of blood vessels caused by either congenital or acquired weakness. An aneurysm is defined as an increase in the vessel's diameter by at least 50%. Forms of aneurysm include saccular, fusiform, and dissecting (tear in the media). The large majority of aneurysms of the abdominal aorta in elderly patients are related to atherosclerosis. The aneurysm in this patient was opened longitudinally to reveal a large mural thrombus within the lumen (see photograph). The risk of rupture of an abdominal aortic aneurysm is a function of its size. Aneurysms under 4 cm in diameter rarely rupture, whereas up to 40% of those larger than 5 cm rupture within 5 years. Cystic medial necrosis (choice C) is associated with dissecting aortic aneurysm. The other choices do not cause abdominal aneurysm.

Diagnosis: Aneurysm, atherosclerotic

30 The answer is D: Platelets and red blood cells. Patients with familial hyperlipidemia develop complications of atherosclerosis at an early age, including coronary artery thrombosis. A thrombus is a collection of fibrin and retained blood elements (e.g., platelets and RBCs) that adhere to the vascular wall. Thrombi may result in complete arterial occlusion, followed by ischemia and infarction. The other choices do not represent cellular components of a thrombus.

Diagnosis: Myocardial infarction

31 The answer is C: Hypersensitivity vasculitis. Purpura or skin rash in a patient with a known autoimmune disease, such as Sjögren syndrome or systemic lupus erythematosus, is usually attributed to hypersensitivity vasculitis. This vasculitis is caused by the deposition of immune complexes in dermal venules. The other choices are not primarily immune complex diseases.

Diagnosis: Hypersensitivity vasculitis

32 The answer is A: Abdominal aorta. Abdominal aortic aneurysms, which are defined as an increase in aortic diameter of 50% or more, are the most frequent aneurysms, usually developing after the age of 50 years. The most common cause of these abdominal aortic aneurysms is atherosclerosis. Aneurysms secondary to atherosclerosis are less common in the other anatomic locations listed.

Diagnosis: Atherosclerosis

33 The answer is D: Kawasaki disease. Kawasaki disease, or mucocutaneous lymph node syndrome, is a vasculitis of unknown etiology that presents with fever, skin rash, mucosal inflammation, and lymph node enlargement. The disease usually has a self-limited course but may involve the coronary arteries and lead to aneurysm formation. Heart failure occurs in 1% to 2% of cases. The other choices are not associated with aneurysms of coronary arteries.

Diagnosis: Kawasaki disease

34 The answer is D: Raynaud phenomenon. This patient suffers from scleroderma complicated by Raynaud phenomenon. The latter refers to intermittent, bilateral attacks of vasospasm of the fingers or toes (sometimes affecting the ears or nose), resulting in pallor, paresthesias, and pain from ischemia. The symptoms are precipitated by cold or emotional stimuli and relieved by heat. Raynaud phenomenon may occur as an isolated disorder or as a feature of a number of systemic diseases, including systemic lupus erythematosus and scleroderma. Intermittent claudication (choice C) is associated with peripheral vascular disease (atherosclerosis). Chilblains (choice A) represent itchy or tender red or purple bumps that occur as a reaction to cold.

Diagnosis: Scleroderma

35 The answer is A: Henoch-Schönlein purpura. Henoch-Schönlein purpura is the most common type of childhood vasculitis and is caused by vascular localization of immune complexes, containing predominantly IgA. Purpuric skin lesions and glomerulonephritis in a child suggest the diagnosis of Henoch-Schönlein purpura. The other choices do not include deposits of IgA in the blood vessels.

Diagnosis: Henoch-Schönlein purpura

36 The answer is A: Hyaline arteriolosclerosis. Hyaline arteriolosclerosis is demonstrated by vessels (smallest arteries and arterioles) that are markedly thickened by the deposition of basement membrane material and accumulation of plasma proteins. Hyaline arteriolosclerosis is often seen in the elderly, but more advanced lesions are observed in persons with diabetes or long-standing hypertension. The other choices are incorrect because they are not diseases of arterioles. Kimmelstiel-Wilson disease (choice B) affects glomeruli in patients with diabetes mellitus.

Diagnosis: Hyaline arteriolosclerosis

37 The answer is E: Varicose veins. The principle diseases affecting the veins are thrombophlebitis (thrombosis-induced local inflammation) and varicosities. A varicose vein is an enlarged and tortuous blood vessel. Superficial varicosities of the leg veins, usually in the saphenous system, are among the most common ailments of humans due to our upright posture. Blood flow becomes turbulent and slow, and leaks from the engorged capillaries into the surrounding tissue cause stasis dermatitis (as shown here). Varicose veins predispose to deep venous thrombosis (choice A), but there is no specific evidence for this condition in the patient's clinical history. Lymphangitis and Milroy disease (choices B and C) represent diseases of the lymphatic system.

Diagnosis: Varicose veins

38 The answer is A: Dystrophic calcification. Dystrophic calcification is a response to cell injury. Serum levels of calcium are normal, and the calcium deposits are located in previously damaged tissue. This patient suffered from coronary artery atherosclerosis. The pathogenesis of the atherosclerotic plaque is a dynamic process that usually occurs over decades, leading to erosion, ulceration or fissuring of the surface of the plaque; plaque hemorrhage; mural thrombosis; and calcification. Calcification is thought to depend on a balance of mineral deposition and resorption in areas of vascular necrosis. These apposing metabolic processes are regulated by osteoblast-like and osteoclast-like cells in the vessel wall. Metastatic calcification (choice D) is associated with hypercalcemia. Physiologic calcification (choice E) occurs in normal bone.

Diagnosis: Atherosclerosis, dystrophic calcification

39 The answer is C: Hemorrhoids. Hemorrhoids are dilations of veins of the rectum and anal canal, which may occur inside or outside the anal sphincter. This condition may be aggravated by constipation and pregnancy and can also result from venous obstruction by rectal tumors. Thrombosis of hemorrhoids is exquisitely painful. Of interest, internal hemorrhoids typically bleed without pain, whereas external hemorrhoids typically hurt but do not bleed. The other choices do not feature dilated veins.

Diagnosis: Hemorrhoids, varicose veins

40   **The answer is E: Subintimal fibromuscular thickening.** Scleroderma is characterized by vasculopathy and excessive collagen deposition in the skin and a variety of internal organs. The disease occurs four times as often in women as in men, mostly in persons between 25 and 50 years of age. Lesions in the arteries, arterioles, and capillaries are typical, and in some cases may be the first demonstrable pathological finding in the disease. The kidneys are involved in more than half of patients with scleroderma. They show marked vascular changes, often with focal hemorrhage and cortical infarcts. Among the most severely affected vessels are the interlobular arteries and afferent arterioles. Early fibromuscular thickening of the subintima causes luminal narrowing, followed by fibrosis. The other pathologic lesions may occur, but they are not the principal cause of vasculopathy in patients with scleroderma.

Diagnosis: Scleroderma

41   **The answer is D: Plasmin.** A thrombus may undergo several fates including (1) lysis, (2) growth and propagation, (3) detachment and embolization, or (4) organization and canalization. The combination of aggregated platelets and clotted blood is made unstable by the activation of plasmin. Plasmin is a fibrinolytic enzyme that is formed from plasminogen by tissue plasminogen activator (tPA). tPA is a serine protease that catalyzes the conversion of plasminogen to plasmin. Once formed, plasmin lyses fibrin and dissolves the thrombus. Occlusive thrombi can also be dissolved by enzymes, such as streptokinase, that activate plasma fibrinolytic activity. The conversion of plasminogen to plasmin, and the activity of plasmin, are regulated by specific inhibitors. None of the other choices are involved in fibrinolysis.

Diagnosis: Myocardial infarction, thrombolysis

Chapter 11

The Heart

QUESTIONS

Select the single best answer.

1 A heart murmur is noted during the preschool physical examination of a 4-year-old girl. An echocardiogram reveals a defect between the right and left atrium involving the limbus of the foramen ovale. What is the most likely diagnosis?
(A) Atrial septal defect (ASD), ostium primum
(B) ASD, ostium secundum
(C) Tetralogy of Fallot
(D) Truncus arteriosus
(E) Ventricular septal defect

2 A 15-year-old girl is brought to the emergency room with heart palpitations and dyspnea. Her past medical history is significant for an unrepaired atrial septal defect (ASD). Physical examination reveals cyanosis, distended jugular veins, hepatosplenomegaly, and a systolic ejection murmur. This patient has most likely developed which of the following complications of congenital heart disease?
(A) Aortic aneurysm
(B) Myocardial infarction
(C) Paradoxical embolism
(D) Pneumonia
(E) Pulmonary hypertension

3 A 5-year-old boy is found to have a harsh holosystolic murmur heard at the left 4th intercostal space. The child has a history of recurrent pneumonias and respiratory tract infections. An echocardiogram reveals a heart defect and biventricular cardiac hypertrophy. Cardiac catheterization discloses pulmonary hypertension. This patient likely has which of the following congenital heart diseases?
(A) Coarctation of aorta
(B) Hypoplastic left ventricle
(C) Patent ductus arteriosus
(D) Pulmonic stenosis
(E) Ventricular septal defect

4 An 8-month-old girl with Turner syndrome is brought to the emergency room by her parents, who complain that their daughter is breathing rapidly and not eating. Physical examination reveals tachypnea, pallor, absent femoral pulses, and a murmur heard at the left axilla. There is hypertension in the upper extremities and low blood pressure in both legs. A chest X-ray shows notching or scalloping of the ribs. What is the appropriate diagnosis?
(A) Aortic valve stenosis
(B) Atrial septal defect
(C) Coarctation of aorta
(D) Patent ductus arteriosus
(E) Tetralogy of Fallot

5 A 2-week-old boy is irritable and feeding poorly. On physical examination, the infant is irritable, diaphoretic, tachypneic, and tachycardic. There is circumoral cyanosis, which is not alleviated by nasal oxygen. A systolic thrill and holosystolic murmur are heard along the left sternal border. An echocardiogram reveals a heart defect in which the aorta and pulmonary artery form a single vessel that overrides a ventricular septal defect. What is the appropriate diagnosis?
(A) Atrial septal defect
(B) Coarctation of aorta, preductal
(C) Patent ductus arteriosus
(D) Tetralogy of Fallot
(E) Truncus arteriosus

6 A 2-week-old girl is found to have a harsh murmur along the left sternal border. The parents report that the baby gets "bluish" when she cries or drinks from her bottle. Echocardiogram reveals a congenital heart defect associated with pulmonary stenosis, ventricular septal defect, dextroposition of the aorta, and right ventricular hypertrophy. What is the appropriate diagnosis?
(A) Atrial septal defect
(B) Coarctation of aorta, postductal
(C) Coarctation of aorta, preductal
(D) Tetralogy of Fallot
(E) Truncus arteriosus

7 A 2-month-old boy is admitted to the pediatric ward in acute respiratory distress. Physical examination shows pallor, peripheral cyanosis, tachypnea, intercostal retractions, and nasal flaring with grunting. Cardiac auscultation reveals third heart sounds. An X-ray film of the chest shows severe cardiomegaly and bilateral pleural effusion. The patient expires 2 days after admission. The heart at autopsy is shown in the image. Which of the following is the most likely diagnosis?

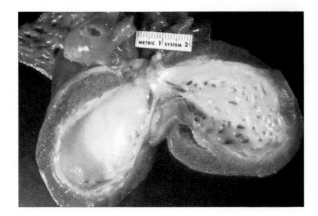

(A) Cardiac amyloidosis
(B) Endocardial fibroelastosis
(C) Hypoplastic left heart syndrome
(D) Patent ductus arteriosus
(E) Tetralogy of Fallot

8 A 29-year-old woman complains of a 3-month history of nervousness and weakness. She feels hot and sweaty and has experienced a 9-kg (20-lb) weight loss over the past 2 months, despite increased caloric intake. She frequently finds her heart racing and can feel it pounding in her chest. Physical examination reveals an enlarged thyroid, warm hands, and bulging eyes. This patient is at risk of developing which of the following cardiovascular complications?

(A) Cardiac tamponade
(B) Cor pulmonale
(C) High-output heart failure
(D) Pericardial effusion
(E) Ventricular aneurysm

9 A 56-year-old man presents to the emergency room with 1 hour of chest pain. Laboratory studies show an increased leukocyte count and increased serum levels of cardiac enzymes. ECG confirms a massive transmural myocardial infarction of the left ventricle. The patient dies 2 days later. Histologic examination of the left main coronary artery at autopsy is shown in the image. Examination of injured heart muscle would be expected to show which of the following pathologic changes by light microscopy?

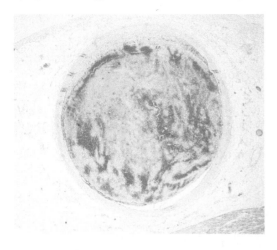

(A) Collagen-rich scar tissue
(B) Extensive infiltration of myocardium with mononuclear cells
(C) Necrosis of cardiac myocytes and infiltrates of neutrophils
(D) No obvious changes evident by light microscopy
(E) Proliferation of fibroblasts and capillary endothelial cells

10 A 44-year-old man presents to the emergency room with acute chest pain. The ECG is normal. Analysis of which pair of serum markers given below would be most helpful in excluding a diagnosis of acute myocardial infarction in this patient?

(A) Cardiac troponin-I and myoglobin
(B) CK-BB and myoglobin
(C) CK-MB and cardiac troponin-I
(D) CK-MM and lactate dehydrogenase (LDH)-1
(E) Myoglobin and CK-BB

11 A 35-year-old man presents with acute chest pain and nausea. ECG and laboratory studies confirm the diagnosis of myocardial infarction. The patient expires 2 days later. A photomicrograph of his left main coronary artery is shown in the image. This patient most likely suffered from which of the following hereditary diseases?

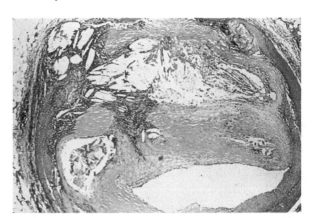

(A) Ehlers-Danlos syndrome
(B) Familial hypercholesterolemia
(C) Kawasaki disease
(D) Marfan syndrome
(E) Systemic hypertension

12 A 60-year-old man with a history of emphysema returns home from the hospital after suffering a myocardial infarction involving the apex of the left ventricle. Six months later, an echocardiogram reveals the development of a ventricular bulge that does not contract during systole. The patient subsequently suffers a massive stroke and suddenly expires. Which of the following is an expected pathologic finding at autopsy?

(A) Calcific aortic stenosis
(B) Dilated cardiomyopathy
(C) Mitral valve prolapse
(D) Mural thrombus
(E) Ventricular rupture

13 A 50-year-old man with familial hyperlipidemia undergoes resection of an abdominal aneurysm. Signs of congestive heart failure develop shortly after surgery. Despite treatment, the patient becomes hypotensive and expires 2 days later. Autopsy reveals marked narrowing of coronary arteries, without thrombosis. Multiple foci of necrosis are found circumferentially around the inner walls of both ventricles. Which of the following is the most likely cause of congestive heart failure in this patient?

(A) Calcific aortic stenosis

(B) Dilated cardiomyopathy

(C) Rupture of papillary muscle

(D) Subendocardial myocardial infarction

(E) Transmural myocardial infarction

14 A 68-year-old obese woman (BMI = 32 kg/m²) presents with substernal chest pain and a history of recurrent angina pectoris and intermittent claudication. The following day, she develops a fever of 38°C (101°F). Results of laboratory studies include an elevated WBC count (13,000/μL), CK-MB of 6.6 ng/mL, and troponin-I of 2.5 ng/mL. ECG confirms a myocardial infarction of the left ventricular wall. Which of the following mechanisms is most likely responsible for the myocardial infarction in this patient?

(A) Coronary artery thrombosis

(B) Coronary artery vasospasm

(C) Decreased collateral blood flow

(D) Deep venous thrombosis

(E) Paradoxical embolism

15 Two months later, the patient described in Question 14 experiences several days of severe, sharp, retrosternal chest pain radiating to the neck and shoulders. The pain is worse when she is in the supine position and less intense when she is sitting upright and leaning forward. Which of the following is the most likely cause of the patient's symptoms?

(A) Congestive heart failure

(B) Dressler syndrome

(C) Left ventricular aneurysm

(D) Mural thrombi

(E) Ruptured papillary muscle

16 A 65-year-old man with a 2-year history of angina pectoris is admitted to the hospital with excruciating substernal chest pain that is not relieved by rest or medication. Physical examination shows diaphoresis and dyspnea. Results of laboratory studies include WBC of 13,000/μL, CK-MB of 6.8 ng/mL, and troponin-I of 3.0 ng/mL. An ECG shows ST segment elevation. The patient expires 1 hour after admission. At autopsy, the heart is found to be enlarged but otherwise anatomically normal. Which of the following is the most likely cause of death?

(A) Cardiac tamponade

(B) Postmyocardial infarction syndrome

(C) Ruptured myocardial infarct

(D) Septal perforation

(E) Ventricular fibrillation

17 After suffering an acute myocardial infarction, a 54-year-old man presents to the emergency room 3 weeks later, complaining of sharp pain on the left side of his chest. On physical examination, the patient is apprehensive and sweating. His blood

pressure is 80/40 mm Hg and the pulse rate is 100 per minute. The patient dies within minutes. The ventricular wall at autopsy is shown in the image. What is the most likely cause of death?

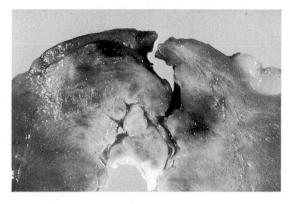

(A) Cardiac tamponade

(B) Dissecting aortic aneurysm

(C) Pulmonary edema

(D) Pulmonary thromboembolism

(E) Septic shock

18 A 48-year-old man complains of chest pain upon exertion. He had been well until 4 months previously, when he first developed a chest discomfort while jogging. His symptoms have progressed to the point that he now develops chest pain after climbing a single flight of stairs. He has a history of diabetes controlled by diet and of 25 pack-years of cigarette smoking. His father and maternal grandfather both died of heart disease before the age of 60. On the 5th hospital day, the patient develops chest pain during periods of mild activity, which is minimally responsive to sublingual nitroglycerin. Results of laboratory studies include WBC of 8,100/μL, CK-MB of 4.5 ng/mL, and troponin-I of 0.5 ng/mL. Which of the following is the most likely diagnosis?

(A) Acute myocardial infarction

(B) Cardiac arrhythmia

(C) Dressler syndrome

(D) Pulmonary thromboembolism

(E) Unstable angina

19 On the morning of the sixth day, the patient described in Question 18 experiences acute, substernal chest pain and nausea. He is treated with plasminogen activator and oxygen but expires several hours later. A cross section of the heart at autopsy is shown in the image. This infarct was most likely caused by thrombotic occlusion of which of the following coronary arteries?

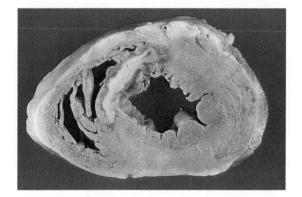

(A) Left anterior descending
(B) Left circumflex
(C) Main right
(D) Posterior descending
(E) Sinoatrial nodal

20   A 69-year-old woman presents with crushing substernal chest pain and nausea. She is treated with plasminogen activator, oxygen, and morphine sulfate. Laboratory studies show a WBC count of 13,000/μL, CK-MB of 6.6 ng/mL, and troponin-I of 2.5 ng/mL. An ECG shows ST segment elevation. Cardiac catheterization reveals diffuse atherosclerosis of all major coronary arteries. The patient subsequently becomes acutely hypotensive and undergoes cardiac arrest. The surface of the heart at autopsy is shown in the image. At what point in time following acute myocardial infarction did this pathologic condition most likely occur?

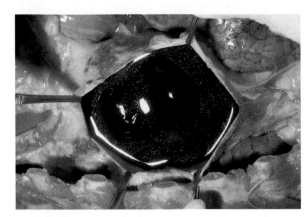

(A) 0 to 6 hours
(B) 6 to 12 hours
(C) 12 to 24 hours
(D) 1 to 4 days
(E) 6 months to 1 year

21   A 66-year-old woman collapses while shopping and expires suddenly of cardiac arrest. Her past medical history is significant for long-standing type 2 diabetes mellitus. Her relatives note that she had complained of chest heaviness and shortness of breath for the past 2 weeks. Sterile fibrinous pericarditis and pericardial effusion are observed at autopsy. What additional finding would be expected during autopsy of this patient?
(A) Endocardial fibroelastosis
(B) Marantic endocarditis
(C) Mitral valve prolapse
(D) Myocardial infarct
(E) Right ventricular hypertrophy

22   A 68-year-old woman with a history of diabetes mellitus expires suddenly of cardiac arrest. The patient suffered a massive anterior myocardial infarction 1 year earlier. The heart at autopsy is shown in the image. Which of the following is the most likely complication of this condition?

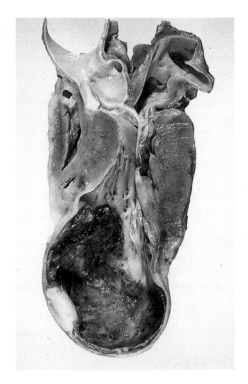

(A) Aortic stenosis
(B) Coronary artery aneurysm
(C) Hypertrophic cardiomyopathy
(D) Pulmonary embolism
(E) Stroke

23   A 60-year-old woman with a 30-pack-year history of smoking and a 10-year history of emphysema expires of congestive heart failure. There is no evidence of coronary artery disease or valvular heart disease. The heart at autopsy is shown in the image. Which of the following is the most likely cause of right ventricular hypertrophy?

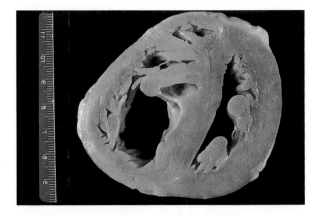

(A) Endocardial fibroelastosis
(B) Essential hypertension
(C) Pulmonary hypertension
(D) Pulmonary stenosis
(E) Systemic hypertension

24 A 72-year-old man presents with difficulty breathing. He says that he becomes short of breath at night unless he uses three pillows to prop himself up. Measurements of vital signs reveal normal temperature, mild tachypnea, and a blood pressure of 180/100 mm Hg. Physical examination discloses obesity, bilateral 2+ pitting leg edema, hepatosplenomegaly, and rales at the bases of both lungs. An X-ray film of the chest shows mild enlargement of the heart and a mild pleural effusion. Echocardiography reveals left ventricular hypertrophy without valvular heart defects. Which of the following is the most likely diagnosis?

(A) Acute cor pulmonale
(B) Constrictive pericarditis
(C) Dilated cardiomyopathy
(D) Hypertensive heart disease
(E) Renal failure

25 A 62-year-old man with a history of hypertension is brought to the emergency room with severe left chest and back pain. His blood pressure is 80/50 mm Hg. Physical examination shows pallor, diaphoresis, and a murmur of aortic regurgitation. An ECG does not show myocardial infarction. An X-ray film of the chest reveals mediastinal widening. Which of the following is the most likely diagnosis?

(A) Bacterial endocarditis
(B) Dissecting aneurysm
(C) Pericarditis
(D) Pulmonary thromboembolism
(E) Ruptured myocardial wall

26 A 30-year-old woman presents with a heart murmur. There is a history of recurrent episodes of arthritis, skin rash, and glomerulonephritis. Blood cultures are negative. Laboratory tests for antinuclear antibodies (ANA) and anti–double-stranded DNA are positive. Which of the following is the most likely cause of heart murmur in this patient?

(A) Libman-Sacks endocarditis
(B) Mitral valve prolapse
(C) Myocardial infarct
(D) Mitral valve prolapse
(E) Rheumatic fever

27 A 50-year-old man with adenocarcinoma of the pancreas is brought to the emergency room in a comatose state. A CT scan of the brain is consistent with a recent infarct in the left temporal lobe. Blood cultures are negative. The patient never regains consciousness and expires 2 days later. The heart at autopsy is shown in the image. Which of the following is the most likely underlying cause of stroke in this patient?

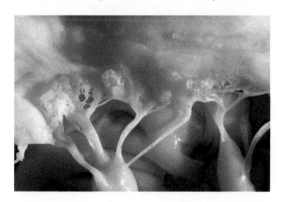

(A) Calcific aortic stenosis
(B) Carcinoid heart disease
(C) Cardiac metastases
(D) Nonbacterial thrombotic endocarditis
(E) Subacute bacterial endocarditis

28 A 78-year-old man with a history of recurrent syncope undergoes surgery for aortic valve disease. A hard, markedly deformed valve is observed, but the patient expires during surgery. The aortic valve at autopsy is shown in the image. What is the appropriate diagnosis?

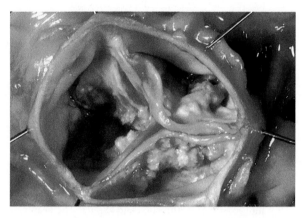

(A) Bacterial endocarditis
(B) Bicuspid aortic valve
(C) Calcific aortic stenosis
(D) Hypertrophic subaortic stenosis
(E) Marantic endocarditis

29 A 16-year-old girl, who arrived in the United States from Africa, comes to the hospital with chest pain and respiratory distress. On physical examination, the patient is short of breath, wheezing, and gasping for air. A prominent pansystolic heart murmur and a prominent third heart sound are heard on cardiac auscultation. An X-ray study of the chest shows marked enlargement of the heart. The patient expires despite intense supportive measures. At autopsy, microscopic examination of the myocardium discloses aggregates of mononuclear cells arranged around centrally located deposits of eosinophilic collagen. What is the appropriate diagnosis?

(A) Acute bacterial endocarditis
(B) Rheumatic heart disease
(C) Subacute bacterial endocarditis
(D) Systemic lupus erythematosus
(E) Viral myocarditis

30 A 10-year-old boy with a 2-week history of an upper respiratory infection was admitted to the hospital with malaise, fever, joint swelling, and diffuse rash. The patient is treated and discharged. However, the patient suffers from recurrent pharyngitis and, a few years later, develops a heart murmur. This patient's heart murmur is most likely caused by exposure to which of the following pathogens?

(A) Beta-hemolytic streptococcus
(B) *Candida albicans*
(C) Epstein-Barr virus
(D) *Staphylococcus aureus*
(E) *Streptococcus viridans*

31 For the patient described in Question 30, which of the following is the most common life-threatening complication of his valvular heart disease?
(A) Congestive heart failure
(B) Dissecting aneurysm
(C) Hemolytic anemia
(D) Myocardial infarction
(E) Pulmonary thromboembolism

32 A 34-year-old intravenous drug abuser presents to the emergency room with a 24-hour history of fever and shaking chills. His temperature is 38.7°C (103°F), pulse rate 110 per minute, and blood pressure 140/80 mm Hg. Physical examination reveals a harsh systolic murmur. The patient rapidly develops a headache and right-arm paralysis. A CT scan of the brain demonstrates an infarct of the right frontal lobe. Which of the following is the most likely cause of stroke in this patient?
(A) Atrial myxoma
(B) Bacterial endocarditis
(C) Dissecting aortic aneurysm
(D) Myocardial infarction
(E) Paradoxical embolus

33 A 68-year-old woman with metastatic breast cancer develops multiple organ dysfunction and expires. The heart at autopsy weighs 380 g (normal = 230 to 280 g in women). The patient's myocardium (right) is compared to normal myocardium (left). These pathologic findings are mostly likely due to which of the following conditions?

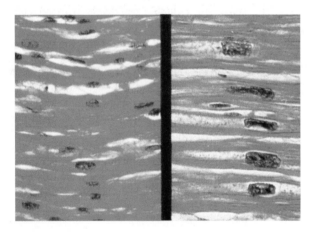

(A) Amyloidosis
(B) Chemotherapy
(C) Hypertension
(D) Inflammation
(E) Ischemia

34 A 45-year-old woman presents with sudden attacks of wheezing, shortness of breath, episodic hot flashes, abdominal cramps, and diarrhea. Physical examination shows facial redness, as well as hepatomegaly and pitting edema of the lower legs. A 24-hour urine specimen reveals elevated levels of 5-hydroxyindoleacetic acid (5-HIAA). A CT scan of the abdomen demonstrates multiple 2- to 3-cm nodules throughout the liver and a 2-cm nodule in the jejunum. An echocardiogram would be most expected to demonstrate which of the following?

(A) Aortic stenosis
(B) Bacterial endocarditis
(C) Mitral valve prolapse
(D) Nonbacterial thrombotic endocarditis
(E) Pulmonic stenosis

35 A 40-year-old woman with a history of rheumatic fever presents with shortness of breath, weight loss, fatigue, and abdominal distension. Physical examination shows rales in the lungs, hepatosplenomegaly, and 2+ pitting edema of the legs. A chest X-ray reveals only left atrial enlargement and pulmonary edema. What is the most likely cause of pulmonary edema in this patient?
(A) Aortic insufficiency
(B) Aortic stenosis
(C) Mitral stenosis
(D) Pulmonic stenosis
(E) Tricuspid insufficiency

36 A 55-year-old man with idiopathic dilated cardiomyopathy receives a heart transplant. Which of the following is the most likely cause of death in this patient 2 years after transplantation?
(A) Acute cellular graft rejection
(B) Aortic valve stenosis
(C) Chronic vascular rejection
(D) Hyperacute graft rejection
(E) Pulmonary fibrosis

37 A 19-year-old college basketball player suddenly collapses on the court. A cardiac monitor shows ventricular tachycardia and then ventricular fibrillation. He is successfully resuscitated and hospitalized. The patient's history indicates that his father died suddenly at 38 years of age. The boy's echocardiogram reveals a thickened left ventricular wall, with a small slit-like chamber. The interventricular septum is also markedly thickened. Five years later the patient expires suddenly. Histologic examination of the heart muscle at autopsy is shown in the image. Which of the following is the most likely diagnosis?

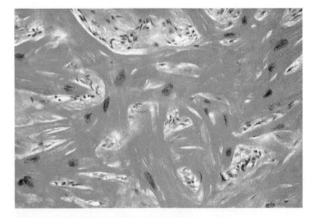

(A) Amyloidosis
(B) Cardiac myxoma
(C) Dilated cardiomyopathy
(D) Hypertrophic cardiomyopathy
(E) Toxic cardiomyopathy

38 A 58-year-old man presents with dyspnea on exertion and fatigue. Physical examination shows evidence of congestive heart failure and echocardiography discloses a dilated left ventricle and a left ventricular ejection fraction of 20%. The liver appears fatty by MRI. Cardiac catheterization demonstrates minimal coronary artery atherosclerosis. Which of the following is the most likely cause of these signs and symptoms?

(A) Alcoholic cardiomyopathy
(B) Aortic stenosis
(C) Amyloidosis of the heart
(D) Hypertrophic cardiomyopathy
(E) Viral myocarditis

39 A 60-year-old man presents with increasing girth and fatigue. Physical examination reveals peripheral edema, ascites, and hepatomegaly. Liver function tests are normal. An echocardiogram shows a remarkably enlarged right heart and no signs of valvular heart disease. Endomyocardial biopsy discloses interstitial, pink amorphous deposits between cardiac myocytes. Which of the following is the appropriate diagnosis?

(A) Carcinoid heart disease
(B) Cardiac amyloidosis
(C) Dilated cardiomyopathy
(D) Hypertrophic cardiomyopathy
(E) Rheumatic heart disease

40 A 50-year-old man underwent heart transplantation for low-output heart failure that was unresponsive to medical treatment. The affected heart at autopsy is shown in the image. It weighs 950 g (normal up to 350 g) and shows no evidence of coronary artery atherosclerosis. Histologically, the myocardium demonstrates hypertrophic myocytes and foci of myocardial fibrosis but no evidence of inflammation or myofiber disarray. Which of the following is the most likely diagnosis?

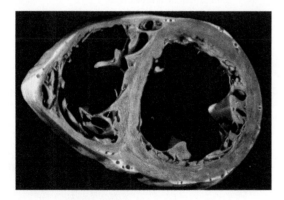

(A) Cardiac amyloidosis
(B) Dilated cardiomyopathy
(C) Hypertrophic cardiomyopathy
(D) Restrictive cardiomyopathy
(E) Ventricular aneurysm

41 A 40-year-old woman presents with dyspnea, heart palpitations, and pitting edema. She was seen for flu-like symptoms and prominent muscle pain 3 weeks ago. Physical examination shows tachycardia and irregular heart beats. A chest X-ray reveals cardiomegaly and pulmonary edema. The patient subsequently dies of cardiorespiratory failure. Histopathology of the heart muscle at autopsy is shown in the image. What is the appropriate diagnosis?

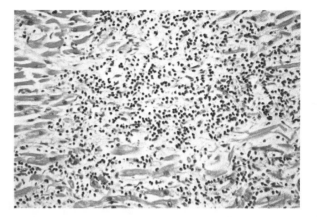

(A) Acute bacterial endocarditis
(B) Acute myocardial infarction
(C) Endocardial fibroelastosis
(D) Rheumatic heart disease
(E) Viral myocarditis

42 A 50-year-old woman presents with fatigue and shortness of breath. Physical examination shows clinical evidence of pulmonary edema, enlargement of the left atrium, and calcification of the mitral valve. A CT scan demonstrates a large mass in the left atrium. Before open heart surgery can be performed, the patient expires of an ischemic stroke. The heart at autopsy is shown in the image. Which of the following is the most likely diagnosis?

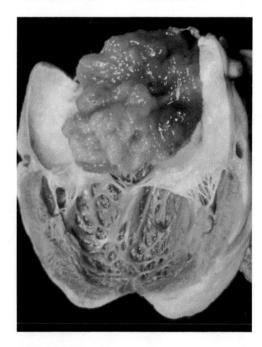

(A) Calcific aortic stenosis
(B) Cardiac myxoma
(C) Fibroelastoma
(D) Metastatic melanoma
(E) Mural thrombus

43 A 45-year-old male immigrant from Haiti presents with a 3-week history of difficulty breathing, chest pain, and abdominal discomfort. Physical examination shows hepatomegaly, ascites, and 2+ pitting edema of the legs. The patient was diagnosed with active pulmonary tuberculosis 2 years before. Cardiac auscultation reveals a pericardial friction rub and respiratory crackles in at the bases of both lungs. An X-ray film of the chest shows an enlarged cardiac silhouette without visible borders. The patient eventually dies and the heart at autopsy is shown in the image. What is the most likely underlying cause of death in this patient?

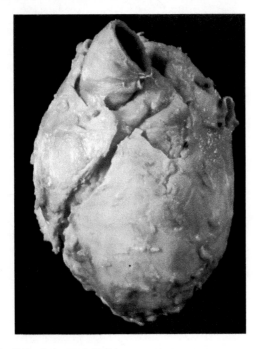

(A) Constrictive pericarditis
(B) Infective endocarditis
(C) Restrictive cardiomyopathy
(D) Rheumatic heart disease
(E) Viral myocarditis

44 A 43-year-old woman with Marfan syndrome suffers a dissecting aneurysm of the aortic arch and expires. An abnormal mitral valve is noted at autopsy (shown in the image). Patients with this valve disorder are at greater risk for developing which of the following conditions?

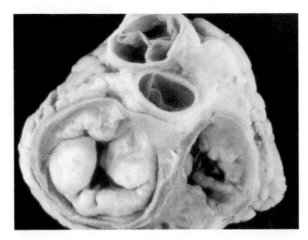

(A) Cardiac tamponade
(B) Cerebral embolism
(C) Dressler syndrome
(D) Libman-Sacks endocarditis
(E) Ventricular aneurysm

45 A 40-year-old man with a history of intravenous drug abuse develops rapidly progressive right-sided heart failure. These symptoms are most likely due to which of the following conditions?
(A) Aortic insufficiency
(B) Mitral regurgitation
(C) Ruptured chordae tendineae
(D) Tricuspid insufficiency
(E) Tricuspid stenosis

46 A 53-year-old woman presents with a 6-week history of fever, fatigue, and weight loss. Her temperature is 38.7°C (103°F), pulse rate 110 per minute, and blood pressure 140/80 mm Hg. Physical examination reveals petechiae and clubbing of the fingers. The patient develops mental status changes, suffers a massive stroke, and expires. The mitral valve is examined at autopsy (shown in the image). Which of the following is the appropriate pathologic diagnosis?

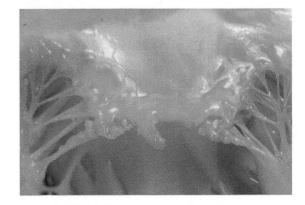

(A) Bacterial endocarditis
(B) Carcinoid heart disease
(C) Libman-Sacks endocarditis
(D) Marantic endocarditis
(E) Mitral valve prolapse

47 A 72-year-old woman dies of congestive heart failure. The aortic valve is examined at autopsy (shown in the image). Which of the following is the most likely cause of aortic stenosis in this patient?

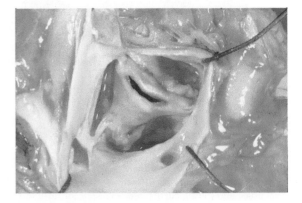

(A) Acute bacterial endocarditis
(B) Aging-related degeneration
(C) Chronic rheumatic valvulitis
(D) Congenital bicuspid valve
(E) Hypertrophic cardiomyopathy

ANSWERS

1 **The answer is B: ASD, ostium secundum.** Ostium secundum–type ASD accounts for 90% of all ASDs. It reflects a true deficiency of the atrial septum and should not be confused with patent foramen ovale. Ostium secundum defects commonly occur in the middle portion of the septum and vary in size from a trivial opening to a large defect of the entire fossa ovalis. A small ASD is unlikely to be functional, but left-to-right shunting may occur in large defects, causing dilation and hypertrophy of the right atrium and ventricle. The ostium primum anomaly occurs adjacent to the AV valves and is usually associated with a cleft anterior mitral leaflet. Ventricular septal defect (choice E) occurs in the interventricular septum. The diagnoses in choices C and D are characterized by multiple congenital abnormalities and early cyanosis.

Diagnosis: Atrial septal defect

2 **The answer is E: Pulmonary hypertension.** Patients with uncorrected ASDs may develop narrowing of the pulmonary vasculature, in which case the flow of blood through the defect may be reversed, thereby creating a right-to-left shunt. The increase in pulmonary capillary pressure is transmitted to the pulmonary arteries, a condition termed pulmonary hypertension, ultimately resulting in right-sided heart failure. Complications of ASDs include cyanosis, atrial arrhythmias, right ventricular hypertrophy, right heart failure, bacterial endocarditis, and paradoxical emboli. None of the other choices are associated with a right-to-left shunt.

Diagnosis: Eisenmenger syndrome, atrial septal defect

3 **The answer is E: Ventricular septal defect (VSD).** VSD is the most common congenital heart lesion. Such anomalies occur as isolated lesions or in combination with other malformations. VSDs vary in size, occurring as a small hole in the membranous septum, a large defect involving more than the membranous portion, defects in the muscular portion, or a complete absence of septum. Small VSDs may have little functional significance and often close spontaneously. Large VSDs are initially characterized by a left-to-right shunt, with left ventricular dilation and congestive heart failure. If the patient survives long enough, pulmonary hypertension may cause reversal of the direction of the shunt and lead to cyanosis. Coarctation of aorta (choice A) presents only with left ventricular hypertrophy and does not typically cause pulmonary hypertension. Pulmonic stenosis (choice D) presents with right ventricular hypertrophy.

Diagnosis: Ventricular septal defect

4 **The answer is C: Coarctation of aorta.** Aortic coarctation is common, accounting for 6% of all cases of congenital heart disease. Coarctation usually occurs in the thoracic portion of the descending aorta, distal to the takeoff of the left subclavian artery at the site of the ductus arteriosus. The incidence of a bicuspid aortic valve in association with coarctation is 80% to -85%. The cardinal physical finding is diminution or absence of femoral pulses and hypertension in the upper extremities. Notching or scalloping of the ribs caused by marked enlargement of the intercostal collaterals can be seen on X-ray. None of the other choices exhibit these characteristics. Aortic valve stenosis (choice A) does not present with hypertension in the upper extremities.

Diagnosis: Coarctation of aorta

5 **The answer is E: Truncus arteriosus.** Truncus arteriosus refers to a common trunk for the origin of the aorta, pulmonary arteries, and coronary arteries. It results from absent or incomplete partitioning of the truncus arteriosus by the spiral septum during development. Most infants with persistent truncus arteriosus have torrential pulmonary blood flow, which leads to heart failure. None of the other choices are distinguished by a single vessel that carries blood from the heart.

Diagnosis: Truncus arteriosus

6 **The answer is D: Tetralogy of Fallot.** Tetralogy of Fallot is defined by four anatomic changes: pulmonary stenosis, ventricular septal defect, dextroposition of the aorta, and right ventricular hypertrophy. It is the most common cyanotic congenital heart disease, accounting for 10% of all congenital heart defects. Cyanosis appears shortly after birth or in early infancy due to right-to-left shunting of venous blood from the right ventricle into the dextroposed aorta. The aorta overrides the ventricular septal defect and receives blood from both ventricles. Narrowing of the pulmonary artery impedes the entry of blood into the lung, thereby increasing the pressure in the right ventricle. None of the other choices exhibit this particular constellation of congenital heart defects.

Diagnosis: Tetralogy of Fallot

7 **The answer is B: Endocardial fibroelastosis (EF).** EF is characterized by fibroelastotic thickening of the endocardium of the left ventricle, which may also affect the valves. The endocardium and valves of the left ventricle show irregular gray-white patches of fibroelastotic thickening usually accompanied by degeneration of subendocardial myocytes. EF occurs in association with underlying cardiovascular anomalies that lead to left ventricular hypertrophy in the face of an inability to meet the increased oxygen demands of the myocardium (e.g., aortic stenosis and coarctation of the aorta). Endocardial thickening observed in the photograph is not a feature of the other choices.

Diagnosis: Endocardial fibroelastosis

8 **The answer is C: High-output heart failure.** The patient suffers from hyperthyroidism (Graves disease). This autoimmune condition causes decreased peripheral resistance, which in time requires increased cardiac output. Hyperthyroidism may lead to high-output heart failure. None of the other choices are characterized by increased cardiac output.

Diagnosis: Graves disease, hyperthyroidism

9 **The answer is C: Necrosis of cardiac myocytes and infiltrates of neutrophils.** Two days after myocardial infarction, the affected heart muscle will show myofiber necrosis, edema, and focal hemorrhage. Polymorphonuclear leukocytes accumulate at the border of the zone of infarction and infiltrate the necrotic tissue. Lack of changes evident by light microscopy (choice D) is expected during the first 24 hours but not at 2 days. The other changes (choices A, B, and E) occur after longer periods of time.

Diagnosis: Acute myocardial infarction

10 **The answer is C: CK-MB and cardiac troponin-I.** Laboratory evaluation of myocardial infarction is based on measuring blood levels of intracellular macromolecules that leak out of necrotic myocardial cells. These proteins include myoglobin, cardiac troponin-T and -I, creatine kinase (CK), and LDH. The preferred biomarkers for myocardial damage are cardiac-specific proteins, particularly troponin-I and troponin-T. The MB isoform of creatine kinase (CK-MB; choice C) is also cardiac specific. CK-BB (choice B) is elevated primarily in patients with infarction of brain tissue. CK-MM (choice D) and myoglobin are usually elevated following necrosis of skeletal muscle.

Diagnosis: Ischemic heart disease

11 **The answer is B: Familial hypercholesterolemia.** Patients with familial hypercholesterolemia have a defective LDL receptor, which inhibits cholesterol uptake by the liver. They develop complications of atherosclerosis at an early age. Cholesterol and serum lipoproteins are deposited in the atheroma, where they are continuously endocytosed by macrophages (lipid-laden foam cells). The mature atheroma is highly thrombogenic. Although systemic hypertension (choice E) may accelerate atherosclerosis, it is not a common cause of early myocardial infarction. The other choices (choices A, C, and D) do not accelerate the development of atherosclerosis.

Diagnosis: Myocardial infarction, familial hypercholesterolemia

12 **The answer is D: Mural thrombus.** Mural thrombi form on the endocardium, over the affected myocardium, early after infarction and are found in half of all patients who die after myocardial infarction. Mural thrombi also form over ventricular aneurysms, as in this case, which are found at the site of a healed, transmural myocardial infarct. Such thrombi are a source of systemic emboli. Mural thrombi may form in cases of dilated cardiomyopathy (choice B), but there is no clinical evidence for that disease in this vignette.

Diagnosis: Mural thrombus, ventricular aneurysm

13 **The answer is D: Subendocardial myocardial infarction.** Subendocardial circumferential infarcts generally occur as a consequence of hypoperfusion of the heart secondary to poor coronary blood flow, often in the setting of hypotension. Coronary artery narrowing is common, but total occlusion is usually not seen. Subendocardial myocardial infarcts affect the inner one third to one half of the ventricle. They may arise within the territory of one of the major coronary arteries or may involve the subendocardial distribution of all coronary arteries. Transmural myocardial infarction (choice E) generally follows occlusion of a major coronary artery.

Diagnosis: Subendocardial myocardial infarction

14 **The answer is A: Coronary artery thrombosis.** Coronary artery thrombosis is the most common cause of acute myocardial infarction and is often secondary to rupture of an atherosclerotic plaque. Coronary artery vasospasm (choice B) would be unlikely in this clinical setting.

Diagnosis: Myocardial infarction

15 **The answer is B: Dressler syndrome.** Postmyocardial infarction syndrome (Dressler syndrome) refers to a delayed form of pericarditis that develops 2 to 10 weeks after myocardial infarction. The pain associated with pericarditis may be confused with that resulting from postinfarction angina or recurrent infarction. The other choices would not present with a prolonged history of chest pain or the clinical features seen in this case.

Diagnosis: Dressler syndrome

16 **The answer is E: Ventricular fibrillation.** Arrhythmias account for half of all deaths within the first 24 hours after an acute myocardial infarction. Acute infarction is often associated with premature ventricular beats, ventricular tachycardia, complete heart block, and ventricular fibrillation. The cause of arrhythmias is multifactorial but acute ischemia may promote conduction disturbances and myocardial irritability. The other choices occur after longer time periods.

Diagnosis: Myocardial infarction

17 **The answer is A: Cardiac tamponade.** The gross specimen shows a ruptured myocardial wall, which causes cardiac tamponade. This catastrophe reflects the accumulation of pericardial fluid (blood in this case), which restricts the motion of the heart. Pulsus paradoxus (>10 mm Hg fall in arterial blood pressure with inspiration) is commonly observed in such cases. Although aortic dissection (choice B) can break through to the pericardium, it does not cause rupture of the myocardium. The other choices do not cause cardiac tamponade.

Diagnosis: Hemopericardium

18 **The answer is E: Unstable angina.** Unstable angina refers to a pattern of pain that occurs progressively and with increasing frequency. It often occurs at rest and tends to be of more prolonged duration. Unstable angina is often a prodrome of myocardial infarction. Acute myocardial infarction (choice A) is ruled out in this case because blood analysis does not show evidence of infarction.

Diagnosis: Ischemic heart disease

19 **The answer is A: Left anterior descending.** The left anterior descending coronary artery supplies the anterior and part of the lateral portions of the left ventricle. Acute blockage of this artery produces an infarct of the apical, anterior, and anteroseptal walls of the left ventricle. Sinoatrial (SA) nodal artery (choice E) primarily supplies the right atrium and the SA node. The distribution of choices C and D largely encompass the posterior wall of the heart.

Diagnosis: Myocardial infarction

20 **The answer is D: 1 to 4 days.** The autopsy reveals hemopericardium (see photograph). Myocardial rupture and hemorrhage into the pericardial sac may occur at almost any time during the first 3 weeks following infarction, but is most commonly seen between the 1st and 4th days. During this critical interval, the infarcted wall is weak, being composed of soft necrotic tissue. The extracellular matrix within the infarct is degraded by proteases released by inflammatory cells. Choices A, B, and C are incorrect because the strength of the ventricular wall is maintained during the first 24 hours. Choice E is incorrect because the scar tissue that has formed by this time provides mechanical stability to the site of injury.

Diagnosis: Hemopericardium, cardiac tamponade

21 The answer is D: Myocardial infarct. Fibrinous pericarditis may develop 2 to 10 weeks after a transmural myocardial infarction. Patients with long-standing diabetes mellitus are particularly susceptible to coronary atherosclerosis and myocardial infarction. One fourth to one half of all nonfatal myocardial infarctions are asymptomatic. In such patients, sudden death usually reflects a cardiac arrhythmia. Right ventricular hypertrophy (choice E) may be encountered but is not related to the development of pericarditis.
Diagnosis: Myocardial infarction

22 The answer is E: Stroke. As myocardial infarcts heal, newly deposited collagenous matrix is susceptible to stretching and may become dilated. Mural thrombosis in the aneurysm is common and may lead to the release of emboli to the brain (stroke). Pulmonary embolism (choice D) involves the venous system and the right-sided circulation of the heart.
Diagnosis: Ventricular aneurysm, mural thrombus

23 The answer is C: Pulmonary hypertension. Cor pulmonale is defined as right ventricular hypertrophy and dilation secondary to pulmonary hypertension. The most common cause of cor pulmonale is chronic obstructive pulmonary disease usually as a result of smoking. Pulmonary stenosis (choice D) is a rare cause of cor pulmonale.
Diagnosis: Cor pulmonale, pulmonary hypertension

24 The answer is D: Hypertensive heart disease. Systemic hypertension is one of the most prevalent and serious causes of coronary artery and myocardial disease in the United States. It is defined as a persistent increase in systemic blood pressure to levels above 140 mm Hg systolic or 90 mm Hg diastolic, or both. Chronic hypertension causes compensatory hypertrophy of the left ventricle as a result of the increased workload imposed on the heart muscle. The left ventricular wall and interventricular septum become uniformly thickened. Congestive heart failure is the most common cause of death in untreated hypertensive patients. Intracerebral hemorrhage is also a frequent fatal complication. In addition, death may result from coronary atherosclerosis and myocardial infarction, dissecting aneurysm of the aorta, or ruptured berry aneurysm of the cerebral circulation. Renal failure may supervene when nephrosclerosis induced by hypertension becomes severe. Although dilated cardiomyopathy (choice C) may present with similar clinical findings, it does not feature hypertension. The other choices do not exhibit left ventricular hypertrophy.
Diagnosis: Hypertensive heart disease

25 The answer is B: Dissecting aneurysm. Aortic dissection reflects hemorrhage between and along the laminar planes of the media, with the formation of a blood-filled channel within the aortic wall. If it begins in the ascending aorta, it may extend backward toward the aortic valve or distally to involve the thoracic and abdominal aorta. More than 90% of dissections occur in men between the ages of 40 and 60 with antecedent hypertension. The second major group of patients, usually younger, has a systemic or localized abnormality of connective tissue that affects the aorta (e.g., Marfan syndrome). Although bacterial endocarditis (choice A) can result in aortic regurgitation, it does not lead to acute chest pain. The other choices are not associated with aortic regurgitation.
Diagnosis: Aortic dissection

26 The answer is A: Libman-Sacks endocarditis. In patients with systemic lupus erythematosus, endocarditis is the most striking cardiac lesion, termed Libman-Sacks endocarditis. Nonbacterial vegetations are seen on the undersurface of the mitral valve close to the origin of the leaflets from the valve ring (Libman-Sacks endocarditis). There is fibrinoid necrosis of small vessels with focal degeneration of interstitial tissue. Rheumatic fever (choice E) is not commonly associated with ANAs seen in this case.
Diagnosis: Systemic lupus erythematosis

27 The answer is D: Nonbacterial thrombotic endocarditis. Nonbacterial thrombotic endocarditis, also known as marantic endocarditis, refers to the presence of sterile vegetations on apparently normal cardiac valves, almost always in association with cancer or some other wasting disease. The cause of marantic endocarditis is poorly understood, but it has been attributed to increased blood coagulability and immune-complex deposition. The principal danger is embolization to distant organs. Subacute bacterial endocarditis (choice E) features positive blood cultures and is not particularly associated with cancer.
Diagnosis: Marantic endocarditis

28 The answer is C: Calcific aortic stenosis. The aortic valve shows calcific aortic stenosis in a three-cuspid valve in an elderly person. There is no commissural fusion. Calcific aortic stenosis refers to a narrowing of the aortic valve orifice as a result of the deposition of calcium in the valve cusps and ring. There are three main causes of calcific aortic stenosis: rheumatic disease, senile calcific stenosis, and congenital bicuspid aortic stenosis. Calcific aortic stenosis is related to the cumulative effect of years of trauma due to turbulent blood flow around the valve. Bicuspid aortic valve (choice B) is incorrect because three valve cusps are shown. Vegetations of marantic endocarditis (choice E) are absent. Patients with hypertrophic cardiomyopathy may develop subvalvular obstruction of the aortic outflow tract (choice D), but the autopsy specimen does not show this pathology.
Diagnosis: Calcific aortic stenosis

29 The answer is B: Rheumatic heart disease. Focal inflammatory lesions are found in various tissues in patients with acute rheumatic fever. These inflammatory lesions are most distinctive within the heart, where they are termed "Aschoff bodies." They consist of foci of eosinophilic material surrounded by T lymphocytes, occasional plasma cells, and plump macrophages called "Anitschkow cells." These distinctive cells have abundant cytoplasm and central round-to-ovoid nuclei, in which the chromatin is disposed in a central, slender, wavy ribbon (caterpillar cells). These lesions are pathognomonic for rheumatic fever and are not encountered in the other choices.
Diagnosis: Rheumatic heart disease

30 The answer is A: Beta-hemolytic streptococcus. Rheumatic fever develops after antibodies to surface antigens of group A (beta-hemolytic) streptococci cross react with similar antigens found in the heart, joints, and connective tissue of the skin. Cardiac lesions caused by acute rheumatic fever include endocarditis, myocarditis, and pericarditis, or all three combined. Chronic rheumatic endocarditis causes fibrous scarring and deformity of cardiac valves, leading to heart murmurs and functional defects. None of the other pathogens cause rheumatic heart disease.

Diagnosis: Rheumatic heart disease

31 The answer is A: Congestive heart failure. Chronic rheumatic disease was a frequent cause of heart failure, secondary to valvular stenosis or insufficiency. Although the disease is uncommon in the industrialized world today, it remains a problem in underdeveloped countries. None of the other choices are related to left-sided rheumatic valvulitis.

Diagnosis: Rheumatic heart disease

32 The answer is B: Bacterial endocarditis. Septicemia and cardiac murmurs in an intravenous drug abuser suggest bacterial endocarditis. Infected thromboemboli from the heart valves cause infarcts and abscesses in various organs, including the brain, kidneys, spleen, intestines, and upper and lower extremities. One third of the victims of bacterial endocarditis manifest some evidence of neurological dysfunction, owing to the frequency of embolization to the brain. Mycotic aneurysms of cerebral vessels, brain abscesses, and intracerebral bleeding are observed. The prognosis depends, to some extent, on the offending organism and the stage at which the infection is treated. The most common source of bacteria in intravenous drugs users is the skin (*Staphylococcus aureus*). Although atrial myxoma (choice A) is theoretically correct, the condition is rare and not associated with either increased temperature or tachycardia. The other choices are not associated with septicemia.

Diagnosis: Bacterial endocarditis

33 The answer is C: Hypertension. Chronic hypertension causes compensatory left ventricular hypertrophy. The overall weight of the heart increases, exceeding 375 g in men and 350 g in women. Microscopically, hypertrophic myocardial cells exhibit an increased diameter with enlarged, hyperchromatic, rectangular ("boxcar") nuclei (see photomicrograph). Myocardial hypertrophy adds to the ability of the heart to handle an increased workload. However, there is a limit beyond which additional hypertrophy is no longer compensatory. This upper limit to useful hypertrophy may reflect the increasing diffusion distance between the interstitium and the center of each myofiber; if the distance becomes too great, the supply of oxygen to the myofiber will be deficient. Interstitial fibrosis typically develops as part of the hypertrophic response, causing left ventricular stiffness. Hypertension also increases the severity of atherosclerosis. The combination of increased cardiac workload (systolic dysfunction), diastolic dysfunction, and narrowed coronary arteries leads to a greater risk of myocardial ischemia, infarction, and heart failure. None of the other choices feature boxcar nuclei.

Diagnosis: Hypertensive heart disease, boxcar nuclei

34 The answer is E: Pulmonic stenosis. Carcinoid syndrome reflects the release of active tumor products and features diarrhea, flushing, bronchospasm, and skin lesions. Carcinoid heart disease typically affects the right heart, causing changes in the pulmonary and tricuspid valves. It is associated with intestinal carcinoids that have metastasized to the liver. The cardiac lesions consist of plaque-like deposits of dense fibrous tissue on the tricuspid and pulmonary valves, producing tricuspid insufficiency and pulmonic stenosis. Elevated levels of HIAAA, a metabolite of serotonin, are diagnostic of carcinoid syndrome. The other choices are not complications of carcinoid syndrome.

Diagnosis: Carcinoid heart disease

35 The answer is C: Mitral stenosis. The mitral valve is the most commonly and severely affected valve in chronic rheumatic disease. The mitral valve snaps shut under systolic pressure and thus bears the greatest mechanical burden of all cardiac valves. Chronic rheumatic valvulitis is characterized by irregular thickening and calcification of the leaflets, with fusion of the commissures and chordae tendineae. Eventually, the valve orifice becomes reduced to a "fish mouth" appearance with a narrow orifice. The pressure in the left atrium rises and is transmitted via the pulmonary veins to the pulmonary vasculature. In cases of aortic insufficiency (choice A) or stenosis (choice B), the left atrium is initially protected by closure of the mitral valve. The other choices are not associated with atrial enlargement or pulmonary edema.

Diagnosis: Mitral stenosis, rheumatic heart disease

36 The answer is C: Chronic vascular rejection. Chronic vascular rejection, also referred to as accelerated coronary artery disease, is the most common cause of death in heart transplant patients after the first year of transplantation. It usually affects the proximal and distal coronary arteries and their penetrating branches. Microscopically, the disorder is characterized by concentric intimal proliferation, leading to occlusion and myocardial infarction. This complication is painless because the transplanted heart is denervated. Acute cellular graft rejection (choice A) occurs during the first few months after transplantation, and hyperacute graft rejection (choice D) occurs quickly after transplantation.

Diagnosis: Coronary artery disease

37 The answer is D: Hypertrophic cardiomyopathy. Hypertrophic cardiomyopathy (HCM) refers to a condition in which cardiac hypertrophy is out of proportion to the hemodynamic load placed on the heart. This disorder is an autosomal dominant trait in about half of the patients, usually involving mutations of contractile proteins. The wall of the left ventricle is thickened (hypertrophic), and its cavity is small. The most notable histologic characteristic of this disorder is myofiber disarray, which is most extensive in the interventricular septum. Despite an absence of symptoms, persons with HCM are at risk of sudden death, particularly during vigorous exercise. The other choices do not demonstrate this distinctive histopathology.

Diagnosis: Cardiomyopathy, hypertrophic

38 The answer is A: Alcoholic cardiomyopathy. Alcoholic cardiomyopathy is the most common identifiable cause of dilated cardiomyopathy in the United States and Europe. The mechanism by which alcohol injures the heart remains unclear, but the degree of myocardial damage has been correlated with the total lifetime dose of ethanol. Abstinence ameliorates or even reverses the early stages of alcoholic cardiomyopathy, but this is not true in late-stage disease. Viral myocarditis (choice E) might also present in this manner, but it is much less common than alcoholic cardiomyopathy.

Diagnosis: Cardiomyopathy, alcoholic

39 **The answer is B: Cardiac amyloidosis.** Cardiac amyloidosis causes restrictive cardiomyopathy, which is characterized by reduced diastolic filling and right-sided heart failure. Infiltration of the conduction system can result in arrhythmias or sudden cardiac death. Amyloid appears amorphous, glassy, and eosinophilic. It is readily documented using a Congo red stain, which demonstrates red-green birefringence when viewed under polarized light. None of the other choices exhibit such amorphous, eosinophilic extracellular deposits.
Diagnosis: Cardiac amyloidosis

40 **The answer is B: Dilated cardiomyopathy.** Dilated cardiomyopathy (DCM) is the most common type of cardiomyopathy and is characterized by biventricular dilation, impaired contractility, and eventually congestive heart failure. In the majority of cases, the cause is unknown (idiopathic DCM), although genetic factors often play a role. The disorder can also develop in response to a large number of insults that may directly affect the myocardium (secondary DCM), including alcohol, cytotoxic drugs, and viral infections. The heart is typically enlarged, often to remarkable proportions ("cor bovinum"). Hypertrophic cardiomyopathy (choice C) displays myofiber disarray. The other choices do not lead to biventricular dilation and hypertrophy.
Diagnosis: Cardiomyopathy, dilated

41 **The answer is E: Viral myocarditis.** The pathogenesis of viral myocarditis is believed to involve direct viral cytotoxicity, as well as cell-mediated immune reactions directed against virally infected myocytes. The hearts of patients with myocarditis who develop congestive heart failure typically show biventricular dilation and hypokinesis. Histologic changes in myocarditis are nonspecific, but most cases show a patchy or diffuse interstitial mononuclear inflammatory infiltrate, composed primarily of T lymphocytes and macrophages (as seen in this case). Coxsackievirus type B is one of the most common pathogens associated with myocarditis.
Diagnosis: Viral myocarditis

42 **The answer is B: Cardiac myxoma.** Cardiac myxoma is the most common primary tumor of the heart. Most myxomas arise in the left atrium, but they can occur in any chamber or valve. Unlike a mural thrombus (choice E), these tumors appear as a glistening, gelatinous polypoid mass, usually 5 to 6 cm in diameter. Microscopically, cardiac myxoma has a loose myxoid stroma, containing abundant proteoglycans. More than half the patients have clinical evidence of mitral valve dysfunction. Although the tumor does not metastasize, it may embolize.
Diagnosis: Cardiac myxoma

43 **The answer is A: Constrictive pericarditis.** Constrictive pericarditis is a chronic fibrosing disease of the pericardium that compresses the heart and restricts inflow. It results from an exuberant healing response following acute pericardial injury in which the pericardial space becomes obliterated and the visceral and parietal layers are fused in a dense mass of fibrous tissue. Pericarditis may be caused by bacteria, viruses, or fungi. Active tuberculosis (as in this case) is a major cause of this condition in underdeveloped countries. Previous radiation therapy to the mediastinum and cardiac surgery account for one third of the cases, whereas, in the other cases, constrictive pericarditis evolves from chronic infection. The other choices are not pericardial diseases, as illustrated in the photograph shown.
Diagnosis: Constrictive pericarditis

44 **The correct answer is B: Cerebral embolism.** The heart displays mitral valve prolapse (MVP), a condition in which the mitral valve leaflets become enlarged and redundant. The chordae tendineae are thinned and elongated, and the billowed leaflets prolapse into the left atrium during systole. Valves from patients with MVP exhibit a striking accumulation of myxomatous connective tissue. Many cases are transmitted as an autosomal dominant trait, related to an unidentified defect in extracellular matrix metabolism. Most (>90%) of patients with Marfan syndrome have clinical evidence of MVP. Although most patients with MVP are asymptomatic, they are at higher risk for developing complications, including bacterial endocarditis, a condition in which vegetations on the valve can break off and embolize to the brain. Libman-Sacks endocarditis (choice D) occurs in patients with systemic lupus erythematosus.
Diagnosis: Mitral valve prolapse

45 **The answer is D: Tricuspid insufficiency.** Tricuspid insufficiency secondary to bacterial endocarditis is one of the most common complications of intravenous drug abuse. Intravenous drug abusers inject pathogenic organisms along with their illicit drugs. In such patients, 80% have no underlying cardiac lesion, and the tricuspid valve is infected in half of cases. Septic pulmonary emboli characterize tricuspid valve endocarditis in drug addicts. Despite antibiotic therapy, a third of cases of endocarditis caused by *S. aureus* are fatal. Other risk factors for bacterial endocarditis include aging, diabetes, pregnancy, transient bacteremia, and prosthetic valves. The most common predisposing condition for bacterial endocarditis in children is congenital heart disease. Choices A, B, and C primarily affect the left ventricle. Tricuspid stenosis (choice E) is distinctly uncommon and does not occur rapidly.
Diagnosis: Bacterial endocarditis

46 **The answer is A: Bacterial endocarditis.** The mitral valve in this case shows destructive vegetations that have eroded through the free margins of the valve leaflets. Vegetations in bacterial endocarditis form on the atrial side of the atrioventricular valves and the ventricular side of the semilunar valves, often at points of closure of the leaflets or cusps. They are composed of platelets, fibrin, cell debris, and masses of organisms. The underlying valve tissue may become so damaged that the leaflet perforates, causing regurgitation. The disease begins with nonspecific symptoms of low-grade fever, fatigue, anorexia, and weight loss. Heart murmurs develop almost invariably. In cases of more than 6 weeks duration, splenomegaly, petechiae, and clubbing of the fingers are frequent. In a third of patients, systemic emboli (e.g., petechiae) are recognized at some time during the illness. More than half of adults with bacterial endocarditis have no predisposing cardiac lesion. Mitral valve prolapse and congenital heart disease are today the most frequent bases for bacterial endocarditis in adults. Carcinoid heart disease affects the right side of the heart and produces tricuspid regurgitation and pulmonary stenosis. The other choices do not cause destructive aortic valve lesions.

Diagnosis: Bacterial endocarditis

47 **The answer is C: Chronic rheumatic valvulitis.** Recurrent episodes of rheurmatic fever result in progressive damage to the mitral and aortic valves. In this case, the aortic valve shows severe aortic stenosis. Three sinuses of Valsalva are recognizable, but the valve cusps are rigidly fibrotic and calcified, and there is extensive fusion of the commissures. Chronic rheumatic valvulitis has narrowed the orifice into a fixed slitlike configuration that does not change during the cardiac cycle. None of the other choices display such fusion of the commissures.

Diagnosis: Rheumatic heart disease, aortic stenosis

Chapter 12

The Respiratory System

QUESTIONS

Select the single best answer.

1 A 63-year-old man with small cell carcinoma of the left mainstem bronchus begins chemotherapy. During the treatment period, he becomes febrile and develops a productive cough. The temperature is 38.7°C (103°F), respirations are 32 per minute, and blood pressure is 125/85 mm Hg. A CBC shows leukocytosis (WBC = 18,500/μL). The patient's cough worsens, and he begins expectorating large amounts of foul-smelling sputum. A chest X-ray shows a distinct cavity with an air/fluid level distal to the tumor area. Which of the following is the most likely diagnosis?

(A) Atelectasis

(B) Bronchiectasis

(C) Ghon complex

(D) Lobar pneumonia

(E) Pulmonary abscess

2 A 64-year-old man presents with fever, chills, and increasing shortness of breath. The patient appears in acute respiratory distress and complains of pleuritic chest pain. Physical examination shows crackles and decreased breath sounds over both lung fields. The patient exhibits tachypnea, with flaring of the nares. The sputum is rusty-yellow and displays numerous neutrophils and erythrocytes. Which of the following pathogens is the most common cause of this patient's pulmonary infection?

(A) *Legionella pneumophila*

(B) *Mycoplasma pneumoniae*

(C) *Pseudomonas aeruginosa*

(D) *Staphylococcus aureus*

(E) *Streptococcus pneumoniae*

3 If the patient described in Question 2 is appropriately treated with antibiotics, which of the following is the most likely outcome?

(A) Abscess formation

(B) Bronchopleural fistula

(C) Bullous emphysema

(D) Resolution

(E) Scar formation

4 A 40-year-old alcoholic man is admitted to the hospital in severe respiratory distress. The temperature is 38.7°C (103°F), respirations are 32 per minute, and blood pressure is 130/90 mm Hg. He coughs constantly and expectorates "currant-jelly" sputum. A chest X-ray reveals bilateral diffuse pulmonary consolidation. Physical examination shows bilateral crackles, dullness to percussion over both pulmonary fields, and use of accessory muscles. The patient subsequently dies from complications of bacterial sepsis. The left lung at autopsy (shown in the image) shows a red, engorged lower lobe. What is the appropriate diagnosis?

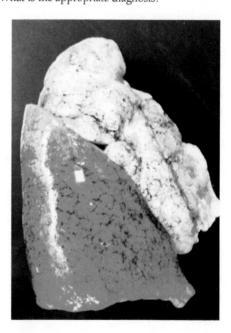

(A) Atypical pneumonia

(B) Bronchopneumonia

(C) Interstitial pneumonia

(D) Lobar pneumonia

(E) Pulmonary abscess

5 A 28-year-old woman with cystic fibrosis presents with increasing shortness of breath and production of abundant foul-smelling sputum. The sputum in this patient is most likely associated with which of the following pulmonary conditions?

(A) Atelectasis
(B) Bronchiectasis
(C) Empyema
(D) Pneumothorax
(E) Pyothorax

6 A 60-year-old alcoholic woman presents to the emergency room with fever, chills, and shortness of breath. The sputum is rusty-yellow and contains numerous neutrophils, red blood cells, and Gram-positive cocci. A chest X-ray shows diffuse haziness over both lungs. One week following admission, the patient develops empyema. This pulmonary condition is associated with the spread of bacterial infection to which of the following anatomic locations?
(A) Blood
(B) Bronchi
(C) Interstitial space
(D) Pericardium
(E) Pleural space

7 A 10-year-old boy suffers head trauma and lies unconscious for 2 weeks. He is now intubated. His temperature rises to 38.7°C (103°F), and oxygenation becomes more difficult. A chest X-ray reveals a pleural effusion and multiple abscesses in the lung parenchyma. Which of the following microorganisms is the most likely cause of this pulmonary infection?
(A) *Legionella pneumophila*
(B) *Mycoplasma pneumoniae*
(C) *Pneumocystis carinii*
(D) *Staphylococcus aureus*
(E) *Streptococcus pneumoniae*

8 A 22-year-old man with AIDS complains of persistent cough, night sweats, low-grade fever, and general malaise. A chest X-ray reveals an area of consolidation in the periphery of the left upper lobe, as well as hilar lymphadenopathy. Sputum cultures show acid-fast bacilli. Which of the following is the most likely diagnosis?
(A) Bronchopneumonia
(B) Pulmonary abscess
(C) Sarcoidosis
(D) Tuberculosis
(E) Wegener granulomatosis

9 A 53-year-old man develops weakness, malaise, cough with bloody sputum, and night sweats. A chest X-ray reveals numerous apical densities bilaterally, some of which are cavitary. Exposure to *Mycobacterium tuberculosis* was documented 20 years ago, and *M. tuberculosis* is identified in his sputum. Which of the following describes the expected lung pathology in this patient?
(A) Dense fibrosis
(B) Eosinophilic infiltration
(C) Granulomas
(D) Interstitial pneumonia
(E) Plasma cell infiltration

10 A 3-day-old girl shows signs of cyanosis and respiratory distress. Her temperature is 38.7°C (103°F), pulse rate is 140 per minute, respirations are 60 per minute, and blood pressure is 90/58 mm Hg. Laboratory studies indicate that the baby is positive for HIV. The infant does not respond to conventional antibiotic therapy and expires. Histologic examination of the lungs at autopsy is shown in the image. The alveolar cells are very large and display single basophilic nuclear inclusions, with a peripheral halo and multiple cytoplasmic basophilic inclusions. Which of the following is the most likely etiologic agent in this child's pulmonary infection?

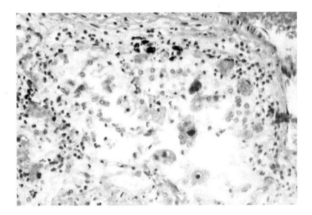

(A) Adenovirus
(B) Cytomegalovirus (CMV)
(C) Herpesvirus
(D) *Pneumocystis carinii*
(E) Rubellavirus

11 A 56-year-old woman with disseminated breast cancer undergoes multidrug chemotherapy. Ten days later, she develops cough and a fever of 38.7°C (103°F). A chest X-ray shows multiple areas of consolidation and a large cavity in the right upper lobe. Multiple pulmonary infarcts are also identified. The patient subsequently dies of multisystem organ failure. Histologic examination of the lungs at autopsy is shown in the image. Which of the following is the most likely diagnosis?

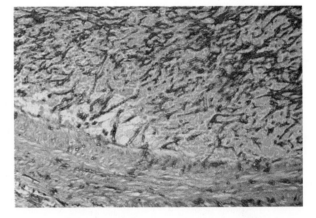

(A) Actinomycosis
(B) Blastomycosis
(C) Coccidioidomycosis
(D) Cryptococcosis
(E) Invasive aspergillosis

12 A 40-year-old woman with leukemia is treated with chemotherapy. During treatment she develops increasing cough and shortness of breath. A chest X-ray shows diffuse lung infiltrates. Sputum cultures are negative, and the patient does not respond to routine antibiotic therapy. An open lung biopsy is diagnosed by the pathologist as viral pneumonia. Which of the following histopathologic findings would be expected in the lungs of this patient?
(A) Clusters of epithelioid macrophages
(B) Confluent areas of caseous necrosis
(C) Fibrous scarring of lung parenchyma
(D) Hyaline membranes and interstitial inflammation
(E) Sheets of bacilli-filled macrophages

13 A 38-year-old woman, who is being treated with corticosteroids for systemic lupus erythematosus, presents with chronic nonproductive cough. She breeds pigeons for avian hobbyists. A chest X-ray reveals a 2-cm nodule in the upper lobe of the right lung. The lung nodule is resected. Histologic examination reveals granulomas and budding yeast forms, which stain positively for polysaccharides (mucicarmine stain, shown in the image). What is the appropriate diagnosis?

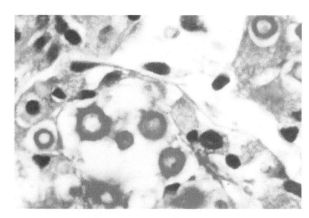

(A) Actinomycosis
(B) Coccidioidomycosis
(C) Cryptococcosis
(D) Histoplasmosis
(E) Mycoplasma pneumonia

14 A 36-year-old man with AIDS presents with fever, dry cough, and dyspnea. A chest X-ray shows bilateral and diffuse infiltrates. Laboratory studies reveal a CD4$^+$ cell count of less than 50/μL. A lung biopsy discloses a chronic interstitial pneumonitis and an intra-alveolar foamy exudate. A silver stain of a bronchoalveolar lavage is shown in the image. Which of the following organisms is the most likely pathogen responsible for these pulmonary findings?

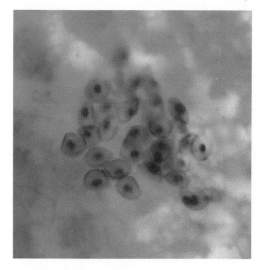

(A) *Cryptococcus neoformans*
(B) Cytomegalovirus
(C) *Histoplasma capsulatum*
(D) *Mycoplasma pneumoniae*
(E) *Pneumocystis jiroveci*

15 A 48-year-old man with AIDS is admitted to the hospital with a fever of 38.7°C (103°F). The patient has a 2-week history of persistent cough and diarrhea. Laboratory studies show that the CD4$^+$ cell count is less than 500/μL. A sputum culture reveals acid-fast organisms, which are further identified as *Mycobacterium avium-intracellulare*. This patient's pneumonia is characterized by extensive pulmonary infiltrates of which of the following cell types?
(A) CD4$^+$ helper T cells
(B) Eosinophils
(C) Macrophages
(D) Mast cells
(E) Neutrophils

16 A 65-year-old man who is a heavy smoker complains of sudden onset of malaise, fever, productive cough, abdominal pain, and muscle aches. A chest X-ray shows bilateral, diffuse, patchy, alveolar infiltrates. Laboratory studies reveal that the patient is infected with *Legionella pneumophila*. This patient's pneumonia is characterized by extensive pulmonary infiltrates of which of the following cell types?
(A) CD4$^+$ helper T cells
(B) CD8$^+$ killer T cells
(C) Eosinophils
(D) Macrophages
(E) Mast cells

17 A 16-year-old boy is rushed to the emergency room after sustaining a stab wound to the chest during a fight. Physical examination reveals a 1-cm entry wound at the right 5th intercostal space in the midclavicular line. His temperature is 37°C (98.6°F), respirations are 35 per minute, and blood pressure is 90/50 mm Hg. A chest X-ray shows air in the right pleural space. Which of the following pulmonary conditions is the expected complication of pneumothorax arising in this patient?

(A) Atelectasis
(B) Chylothorax
(C) Diffuse alveolar damage
(D) Empyema
(E) Pyothorax

18 A 62-year-old woman is rushed to the emergency room following an automobile accident. She has suffered internal injuries and massive bleeding and appears to be in a state of profound shock. Her temperature is 37°C (98.6°F), respirations are 42 per minute, and blood pressure is 80/40 mm Hg. Physical examination shows cyanosis and the use of accessory respiratory muscles. A CT scan of the chest is normal on arrival. Her condition is complicated by fever, leukocytosis, and a positive blood culture for staphylococci (sepsis). Two days later, the patient develops rapidly progressive respiratory distress, and a pattern of "interstitial pneumonia" can be seen on a chest X-ray. Which of the following is the most likely diagnosis?

(A) Acute bronchiolitis
(B) Alveolar proteinosis
(C) Atelectasis
(D) Desquamative interstitial pneumonitis
(E) Diffuse alveolar damage

19 A 64-year-old woman who has suffered shock and sepsis experiences declining respiratory function and is placed on a ventilator. Despite intensive therapy, the patient dies 3 weeks later in respiratory failure. Histologic examination of the lungs at autopsy is shown in the image. Which of the following best describes the pathologic findings in this autopsy specimen?

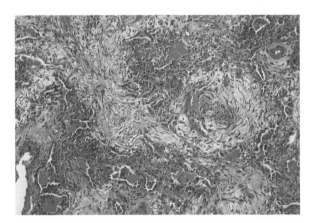

(A) Atelectasis
(B) Bronchiectasis
(C) Bronchopneumonia
(D) Lobar pneumonia
(E) Pulmonary fibrosis

20 A 22-year-old man who is being treated for leukemia complains of shortness of breath on exertion, pleuritic chest pain, and a low-grade fever. Physical examination reveals crackles in both lung bases and clubbing of the fingers. Bronchoalveolar lavage demonstrates PAS-positive material and elevated levels of surfactant proteins. An open-lung biopsy is shown in the image. Which of the following is the most likely diagnosis?

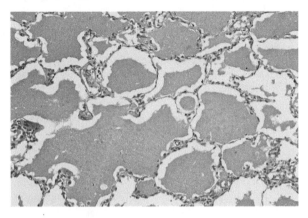

(A) Alveolar proteinosis
(B) Eosinophilic pneumonia
(C) Goodpasture syndrome
(D) Hyaline membrane disease
(E) Radiation pneumonitis

21 A 50-year-old woman presents with a 4-week history of fever, shortness of breath, and dry cough. She reports that her chest feels "tight." The patient is a pigeon fancier. Blood tests show leukocytosis and neutrophilia, an elevated erythrocyte sedimentation rate, and increased levels of immunoglobulins and C-reactive protein. A lung biopsy reveals poorly formed granulomas composed of epithelioid macrophages and multinucleated giant cells. Which of the following is the appropriate diagnosis?

(A) Actinomycosis
(B) Goodpasture syndrome
(C) Hypersensitivity pneumonitis
(D) Nocardiosis
(E) Wegener granulomatosis

22 A 55-year-old man is admitted to the hospital with increasing shortness of breath and dry cough for the past few years. He smokes 1.5 packs of cigarettes and drinks about four bottles of beer a day. He is constantly "gasping for air" and now walks with difficulty because he becomes breathless after only a few steps. Prolonged expiration with wheezing is noted. Physical examination shows a barrel chest, hyperresonance on percussion, and clubbing of the digits. The patient's face is puffy and red, and he has pitting edema of the legs. A chest X-ray discloses hyperinflation, flattening of the diaphragm, and increased retrosternal air space. Which of the following is the appropriate diagnosis?

(A) Asthma
(B) Chronic bronchitis
(C) Emphysema
(D) Hypersensitivity pneumonitis
(E) Usual interstitial pneumonia

23 Which of the following best describes the expected histopathology of the lungs in the patient described in Question 22?

(A) Destruction of the walls of airspaces without fibrosis
(B) Interstitial fibrosis of the lung parenchyma
(C) Lymphocytes restricted to the interstitium
(D) Prominent bronchial smooth muscle cell hyperplasia
(E) Thickening of the epithelial basement membrane

24 A 35-year-old woman with a long history of dyspnea, chronic cough, sputum production, and wheezing dies of respiratory failure following a bout of lobar pneumonia. She was a non-smoker and did not drink alcoholic beverages. The lung at autopsy is shown in the image. Which of the following underlying conditions was most likely associated with the pathologic changes shown here?

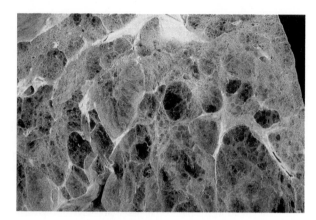

(A) α_1-Antitrypsin deficiency
(B) Cystic fibrosis
(C) Goodpasture syndrome
(D) Hypersensitivity pneumonitis
(E) Kartagener syndrome

25 A 55-year-old man was admitted to the hospital with a chief complaint of increasing shortness of breath over the past several years. The patient was a heavy smoker over the past 40 years. Physical examination reveals cyanosis, elevated jugular venous pressure, and peripheral edema. A high-resolution CT scan shows bullae over both lungs. Chronic intra-alveolar exposure to which of the following proteins is most likely associated with the pathogenesis of chronic obstructive pulmonary disease in this patient?

(A) Alkaline phosphatase
(B) α_1-Antitrypsin
(C) Collagenase
(D) Elastase
(E) α_2-Macroglobulin

26 A 48-year-old man with a history of heavy smoking presents with a 3-year history of persistent cough and frequent upper respiratory infections, associated with sputum production. Physical examination reveals prominent expiratory wheezes and peripheral edema. Analysis of arterial blood gases reveals hypoxia and CO_2 retention. Which of the following is the appropriate diagnosis?

(A) Atelectasis
(B) Chronic obstructive pulmonary disease
(C) Goodpasture syndrome
(D) Hypersensitivity pneumonitis
(E) Usual interstitial pneumonia

27 An 8-year-old girl is brought into the physician's office in mild respiratory distress. She has a history of allergies to cats and wool, and her parents state that she has recurrent episodes of upper respiratory tract infections. Physical examination shows expiratory wheezes, use of accessory respiratory muscles, and a hyperresonant chest to percussion. Analysis of arterial blood gases discloses respiratory alkalosis, and the peripheral eosinophil count is increased. What is the appropriate diagnosis?

(A) Acute bronchiolitis
(B) Asthma
(C) Cystic fibrosis
(D) Kartagener syndrome
(E) Usual interstitial pneumonia

28 A 10-year-old boy dies following a severe episode of status asthmaticus. Histologic examination of the lung at autopsy is shown in the image. Which of the following best describes the pathologic features evident in this autopsy specimen?

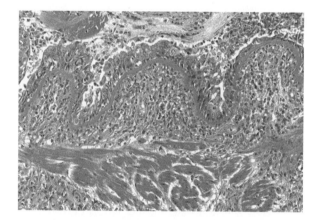

(A) Destruction of the walls of airspaces without fibrosis
(B) Hyaline membranes and interstitial edema
(C) Interstitial fibrosis of the lung parenchyma
(D) Intra-alveolar hemorrhage and exudates containing neutrophils
(E) Smooth muscle hyperplasia and basement membrane thickening

29 A 60-year-old mason complains of shortness of breath, which has become progressively worse during the past year. A chest X-ray shows small nodular shadows in both lungs. Pulmonary function studies reveal a pattern consistent with restrictive lung disease. The patient subsequently develops congestive heart failure and expires. Autopsy discloses numerous small, fibrotic nodules in both lungs. Histologic examination of these nodules is shown in the image. Which of the following is the most likely diagnosis?

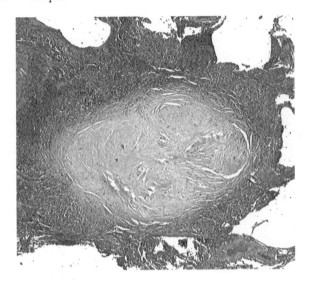

(A) Anthracosis
(B) Asbestosis
(C) Sarcoidosis
(D) Silicosis
(E) Wegener granulomatosis

30 A 65-year-old coal miner is admitted for evaluation of chronic lung disease. The patient admits to smoking one pack of cigarettes a day for 40 years. On physical examination, he is noticed to have a barrel chest and use accessory muscles for inspiration. His face is puffy and red. He has 2+ pitting edema of the lower extremities. A chest X-ray is compatible with diffuse fibrosis, with some nodularity in central areas. Which of the following is the most likely diagnosis?
(A) Anthracosilicosis
(B) Asbestosis
(C) Diffuse alveolar damage
(D) Psittacosis
(E) Sarcoidosis

31 A 75-year-old man who had worked in a shipyard dies of a chronic lung disease. Autopsy reveals extensive pulmonary fibrosis, and iron stains of lung tissue show numerous ferruginous bodies. The dome of the diaphragm is shown in the image. What is the appropriate diagnosis?

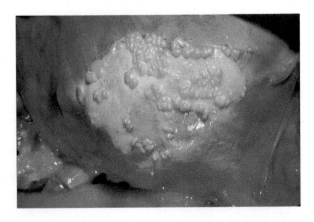

(A) Anthracosis
(B) Asbestosis
(C) Berylliosis
(D) Sarcoidosis
(E) Silicosis

32 A 69-year-old retired man is brought to the emergency department because he experienced sudden onset of left-sided chest pain, which is exacerbated upon inspiration. He is taking no medications and has been in good health. Physical examination reveals dyspnea and hemoptysis. Temperature is 38°C (101°F), pulse rate is 98 per minute, respirations are 35 per minute, and blood pressure is 158/100 mm Hg. A pleural friction rub is present on auscultation. The left leg is markedly edematous, with a positive Homans' sign. An ECG shows a normal sinus rhythm. A chest X-ray reveals a left pleural effusion. What is the most likely cause of this patient's pulmonary condition?
(A) Congestive heart failure
(B) Cor pulmonale
(C) Mitral stenosis
(D) Subacute endocarditis
(E) Thromboembolism

33 A 25-year-old black woman presents with a 3-month history of cough and shortness of breath on exertion. A chest X-ray reveals enlargement of hilar and mediastinal lymph nodes. Laboratory studies show elevated serum levels of angiotensin-converting enzyme and an increase in 24-hour urine calcium excretion. An open-lung biopsy is shown in the image. Stains for microorganisms in the tissue are negative. Which of the following is the most likely diagnosis?

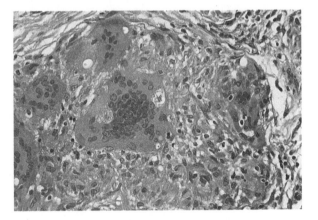

(A) Goodpasture syndrome
(B) Sarcoidosis
(C) Silicosis
(D) Tuberculosis
(E) Wegener granulomatosis

34 A 43-year-old woman with Sjögren syndrome and a 5-year history of cough and shortness of breath develops end-stage lung disease and dies of respiratory failure. Histologic examination of the lung at autopsy is shown in the image. Which of the following is the most likely diagnosis?

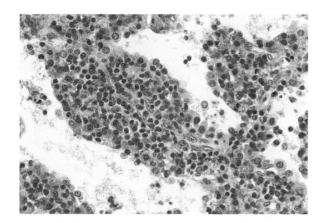

(A) Alveolar proteinosis
(B) Churg-Strauss syndrome
(C) Langerhans cell histiocytosis
(D) Lymphangioleiomyomatosis
(E) Lymphocytic interstitial pneumonia

35 A 23-year-old man complains of nasal obstruction, serosanguinous discharge, cough, and bloody sputum. A chest X-ray shows cavitated lesions and multiple nodules over both lung fields. A CT scan discloses obliteration of several maxillary sinuses. Urinalysis reveals hematuria and RBC casts. Laboratory studies demonstrate anemia and elevated serum levels of C-ANCA. An open-lung biopsy is shown in the image. Which of the following is the most likely diagnosis?

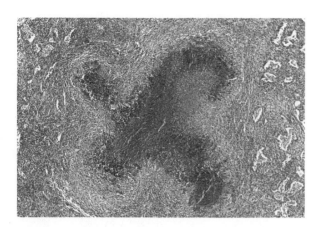

(A) Adenocarcinoma of lung
(B) Churg-Strauss syndrome
(C) Necrotizing sarcoid granulomatosis
(D) Tuberculosis
(E) Wegener granulomatosis

36 A 31-year-old woman smoker complains of nonproductive cough, chest pain, shortness of breath on exertion, and fatigue. A CBC is normal. A chest X-ray shows ill-defined nodules, reticulonodular infiltrates, a small cavitary lesion in the right middle lobe, and mediastinal adenopathy. A transbronchial biopsy is shown in the image. Which of the following is the most likely diagnosis?

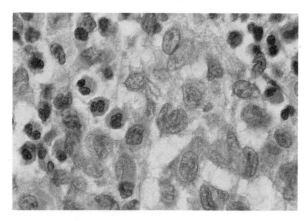

(A) Goodpasture syndrome
(B) Langerhans cell histiocytosis
(C) Lymphangioleiomyomatosis
(D) Pulmonary interstitial fibrosis
(E) Wegener granulomatosis

37 A 30-year-old woman presents with shortness of breath and bloody sputum. Physical examination reveals pulmonary crackles and abdominal ascites. A chest X-ray shows bilateral pleural effusions and marked hyperinflation of the lungs. A CT scan of the chest discloses thin-walled, air-containing cysts in a diffuse symmetric pattern. A lung biopsy is shown in the image. The patient responds favorably to antiestrogen and antiprogesterone therapy. Which of the following is the most likely diagnosis?

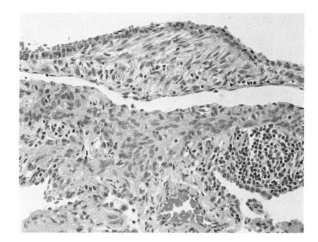

(A) Bronchiectasis
(B) Histiocytosis X
(C) Lymphangioleiomyomatosis
(D) Tuberculosis
(E) Wegener granulomatosis

38 A 22-year-old man presents with a 6-month history of increasing shortness of breath and persistent cough with rusty sputum. A chest X-ray shows diffuse bilateral alveolar infiltrates. Urine dipstick analysis reveals 2+ hematuria. A transbronchial lung biopsy is shown in the image. Linear deposits of IgG and complement C3 are detected in the alveolar basement membrane by immunofluorescence. Which of the following is the most likely diagnosis?

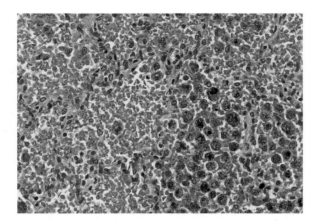

(A) Churg-Strauss syndrome
(B) Goodpasture syndrome
(C) Hypersensitivity pneumonitis
(D) Loeffler syndrome
(E) Wegener granulomatosis

39 A 28-year-old man presents with 6 days of fever and shortness of breath. His temperature is 38.7°C (103°F), respirations are 30 per minute, and blood pressure is 120/80 mm Hg. A chest X-ray reveals diffuse interstitial and alveolar infiltrates. Sputum cultures are negative, and the patient does not respond to standard antibiotic therapy. A transbronchial lung biopsy is shown in the image. Which of the following is the appropriate diagnosis?

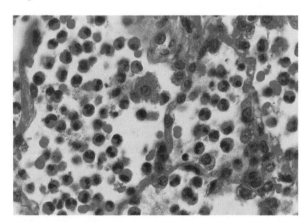

(A) Eosinophilic pneumonia
(B) Lipid pneumonia
(C) Pneumococcal pneumonia
(D) Pneumocystis pneumonia
(E) Usual interstitial pneumonia

40 A 53-year-old man presents with increasing shortness of breath on exertion and dry cough that has developed over a period of a few years. Physical examination shows clubbing of the fingers. A chest X-ray discloses diffuse bilateral infiltrates, predominantly in the lower lobes, in a reticular pattern. Two years later, the patient suffers a massive stroke and expires. Histologic examination of the lung at autopsy is shown in the image. Patchy scarring with extensive areas of honeycomb cystic change predominantly affects the lower lobes. Which of the following is the most likely diagnosis?

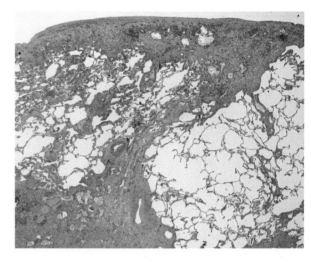

(A) Churg-Strauss syndrome
(B) Desquamative interstitial pneumonia
(C) Goodpasture syndrome
(D) Usual interstitial pneumonia
(E) Wegener granulomatosis

41 A 55-year-old woman complains of sudden onset of fever, dry cough, and shortness of breath. She was seen for flu-like symptoms 6 weeks ago. A chest X-ray shows bilateral patchy alveolar consolidations. An open-lung biopsy reveals narrow inflamed airways containing plugs of fibrous tissue (shown in the image). Which of the following is the most likely diagnosis?

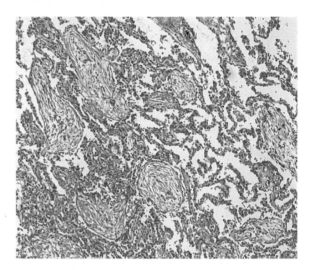

(A) AIDS-related pneumonia
(B) Alveolar proteinosis
(C) Cryptogenic organizing pneumonia
(D) Diffuse alveolar damage
(E) Wegener granulomatosis

42 A 45-year-old woman with severe kyphoscoliosis presents with fatigue, shortness of breath on exertion, fainting spells, and bloody sputum. A CBC is normal. Physical examination shows splitting of the second heart sound with accentuation of the pulmonic component, distended neck veins with a prominent V wave, a right ventricular third heart sound, and peripheral edema. A chest X-ray film shows enlargement of the central pulmonary arteries. A transbronchial lung biopsy is shown in the image. Which of the following is the most likely diagnosis?

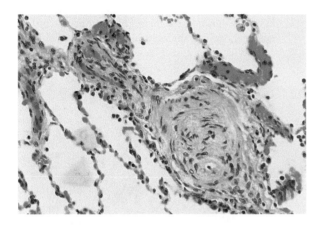

(A) Churg-Strauss syndrome
(B) Diffuse alveolar damage
(C) Eosinophilic granuloma
(D) Pulmonary hypertension
(E) Wegener granulomatosis

43 A 56-year-old man with a history of cigarette smoking presents with difficulty swallowing and a muffled voice. Laryngoscopy reveals a 2-cm laryngeal mass. If this mass is a malignant neoplasm, which of the following is the most likely histologic diagnosis?
(A) Adenocarcinoma
(B) Leiomyosarcoma
(C) Small cell carcinoma
(D) Squamous cell carcinoma
(E) Transitional cell carcinoma

44 A 56-year-old man undergoes a routine chest radiograph as part of a comprehensive physical examination. The X-ray film of the chest shows a solitary, centrally located coin lesion, with a "popcorn" pattern of calcification. A lung biopsy is performed and reveals nodules of benign mature cartilage and respiratory epithelium (shown in the image). What is the most likely diagnosis?

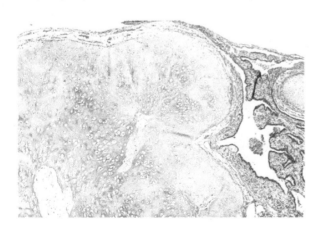

(A) Carcinoid tumor
(B) Extralobar sequestration
(C) Leiomyoma
(D) Pulmonary fibroma
(E) Pulmonary hamartoma

45 A 68-year-old man complains of shortness of breath, hoarseness, productive cough, and bloody sputum of 2 weeks in duration. He admits to smoking two packs a day for 45 years and drinks occasionally. Recently, he has experienced a significant loss of appetite and weight loss. Physical examination shows pallor, cachexia, clubbing of the fingers, and barrel-shaped chest. A chest X-ray reveals a mass at the right lung apex. Histologic examination of a transbronchial biopsy is shown in the image. What is the appropriate histologic diagnosis?

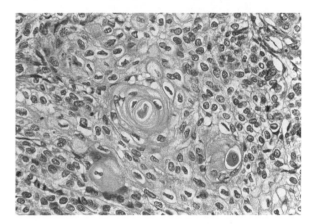

(A) Adenocarcinoma
(B) Mesothelioma
(C) Metastatic adenocarcinoma
(D) Small cell carcinoma
(E) Squamous cell carcinoma

46 A 53-year-old woman with a history of cigarette smoking presents with a 3-month history of chest pain, cough, and mild fever. A chest X-ray reveals a peripheral mass in the left upper lobe. The surgical specimen is shown in the image. What is the most likely diagnosis?

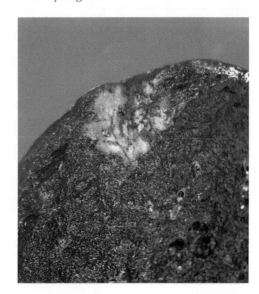

(A) Adenocarcinoma
(B) Large cell carcinoma
(C) Mesothelioma
(D) Small cell carcinoma
(E) Squamous cell carcinoma

47 A 67-year-old woman with a history of smoking presents with a 3-week history of chest pain and bloody sputum. A chest X-ray reveals a bulky mass within the pulmonary parenchyma. An open-lung biopsy is shown in the image. Immunohistochemical stains for keratin and chromogranin are negative. What is the appropriate diagnosis?

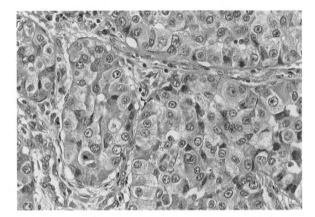

(A) Adenocarcinoma
(B) Carcinoid tumor
(C) Large cell carcinoma
(D) Metastatic adenocarcinoma
(E) Small cell carcinoma

48 A 58-year-old man presents with a long history of persistent cough, chest pain, and recurrent pneumonia. He denies smoking or consuming alcohol. The patient subsequently dies of sepsis. Autopsy reveals malignant cells that diffusely infiltrate the lung parenchyma. Histopathologic examination of the lung shows well-differentiated, mucus-producing, columnar neoplastic cells lining the alveolar spaces (shown in the image). Neoplastic cells are not found in any other organ. What is the most likely diagnosis?

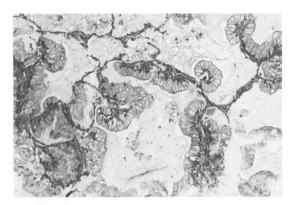

(A) Bronchioloalveolar carcinoma
(B) Carcinoid tumor
(C) Large cell carcinoma
(D) Mesothelioma
(E) Small cell carcinoma

49 A 52-year-old woman presents with a 1-year history of upper truncal obesity and moderate depression. Physical examination shows hirsutism and moon facies. Endocrinologic studies reveal hypokalemia, high plasma corticotropin levels, and increased concentrations of serum and urine cortisol. CT scan of the thorax demonstrates a hilar mass. A transbronchial lung biopsy is shown in the image. Electron microscopy discloses neuroendocrine granules within the cytoplasm of some tumor cells. What is the appropriate diagnosis?

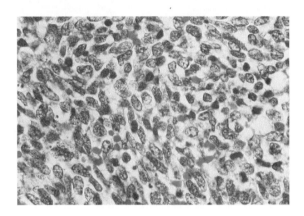

(A) Adenocarcinoma
(B) Bronchioloalveolar carcinoma
(C) Carcinoid tumor
(D) Metastatic carcinoma
(E) Small cell carcinoma

50 A 55-year-old man presents with increasing chest pain, bloody sputum, and weight loss over the past 3 months. A high-resolution CT scan reveals a mass circumscribing the right main bronchus, extending into its lumen. Histologic examination of an open-lung biopsy is shown in the image. Electron microscopy shows numerous neuroendocrine granules within tumor cells. What is the appropriate diagnosis?

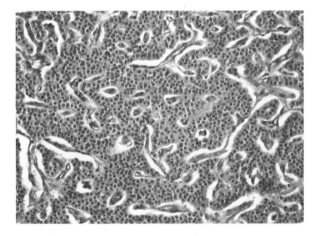

(A) Adenocarcinoma
(B) Bronchioloalveolar carcinoma
(C) Carcinoid tumor
(D) Large cell carcinoma
(E) Squamous cell carcinoma

51 A 64-year-old man who has worked in a manufacturing plant all his life complains of an 8-month history of chest discomfort, malaise, fever, night sweats, and weight loss. A chest X-ray reveals a pleural effusion and pleural mass encasing the lung. The patient subsequently dies of cardiorespiratory failure. Histologic examination of the pleural mass at autopsy shows a biphasic pattern of epithelial and sarcomatous elements. What is the most likely diagnosis?

(A) Carcinoid tumor
(B) Large cell carcinoma
(C) Malignant melanoma
(D) Malignant mesothelioma
(E) Metastatic carcinoma

52 A 48-year-old woman with a long-standing history of ulcerative colitis presents with anemia and shortness of breath. Laboratory studies show increased serum levels of carcinoembryonic antigen. A chest X-ray reveals multiple, round masses in both lungs. Histologic examination of an open-lung biopsy discloses nodules that are composed of gland-like structures. What is the most likely diagnosis?

(A) Adenocarcinoma
(B) Bronchioloalveolar carcinoma
(C) Eosinophilic granuloma
(D) Large cell undifferentiated carcinoma
(E) Metastatic carcinoma

53 A 72-year-old woman complains of shortness of breath upon exertion. She states that she also becomes short of breath at night unless she uses three pillows. Physical examination reveals mild obesity, bilateral pitting leg edema, an enlarged liver and spleen, and fine crackling sounds on inspiration. A chest X-ray is consistent with pulmonary edema and cardiomegaly. Which of the following is the most likely pulmonary complication in this patient?

(A) Chylothorax
(B) Hemothorax
(C) Hydrothorax
(D) Pneumothorax
(E) Pyothorax

54 A 27-year-old man with history of alcoholism and repeated bouts of aspiration pneumonia comes to the emergency room with a high fever and pleuritic chest pain. Physical examination reveals dullness on percussion and absence of breath sounds in the right lower lung field. A chest X-ray demonstrates pleural fluid on the right side. Thoracentesis returns a thick, foul-smelling fluid. Which of the following is the most likely diagnosis?

(A) Chylothorax
(B) Empyema
(C) Hemothorax
(D) Hydrothorax
(E) Pneumothorax

55 A 22-year-old man has been treated for lymphoma and comes to the emergency room complaining of severe shortness of breath. Physical examination reveals decreased breath sounds and shifting dullness. Cervical adenopathy is prominent.

Thoracocentesis yields a milky-white fluid with a high lipid content. Which of the following is the most likely diagnosis?

(A) Chylothorax
(B) Empyema
(C) Hemothorax
(D) Hydrothorax
(E) Pyothorax

ANSWERS

1 **The answer is E: Pulmonary abscess.** Lung abscess is a localized accumulation of pus accompanied by the destruction of pulmonary parenchyma, including alveoli, airways, and blood vessels. The most common cause of pulmonary abscess is aspiration, often in the setting of depressed consciousness. Pulmonary abscess is also a common complication of lung cancer. A cystic abscess contains purulent exudates and is contained by a fibrous wall. Abscess cavities are often partially filled with pus and air, which accounts for the X-ray finding of an "air/fluid level." Inflammation is usually present in the surrounding pulmonary parenchyma. Foul-smelling sputum may be expectorated if an abscess is connected to a bronchus. None of the other choices present as cavitary lesions.
Diagnosis: Pulmonary abscess, small cell carcinoma of lung

2 **The answer is E: *Streptococcus pneumoniae*.** All of the choices cause pneumonia. However, despite the impact of antibiotic therapy, pneumonia caused by *Streptococcus pneumoniae* (pneumococcus) remains the most significant problem. The onset of pneumococcal pneumonia is acute with fever and chills.
Diagnosis: Pneumonia, *Streptococcus pneumoniae*

3 **The answer is D: Resolution.** Although abscesses and fistulas may occur (choices A and B), the most common outcome of acute bacterial pneumonia is resolution, particularly with appropriate antibiotic treatment.
Diagnosis: Pneumonia, *Streptococcus pneumoniae*

4 **The answer is D: Lobar pneumonia.** The term lobar pneumonia refers to consolidation of an entire lobe; bronchopneumonia (choice B) signifies scattered solid foci in the same or several lobes. Lobar pneumonia presents with a diffuse consolidation of one or more pulmonary lobes. In contrast to lobar pneumonia, interstitial pneumonia (choice C) primarily involves the alveolar septa. Atypical pneumonia (choice A) is most often encountered in mycoplasma pneumonia. Pulmonary abscess (choice E) may be a complication of lobar pneumonia or bronchopneumonia.
Diagnosis: Lobar pneumonia

5 **The answer is B: Bronchiectasis.** Bronchiectasis refers to the irreversible dilation of bronchi, which is caused by the destruction of the muscular and elastic elements of bronchial walls. Bronchiectasis is often localized to a segment of the lung distal to mechanical obstruction of a bronchus by a variety of lesions, including tumors, inhaled foreign bodies, mucous plugs (e.g., cystic fibrosis and asthma), and compressive lymphadenopathy. Nonobstructive bronchiectasis is usually a complication of chronic pulmonary infections. Patients with bronchiectasis present with chronic productive cough, often with copious mucopurulent sputum. Pyothorax (choice E) is infection of pleural effusion.

Diagnosis: Bronchiectasis, cystic fibrosis

6 The answer is E: Pleural space. Complications of bacterial pneumonia include pleuritis (extension of inflammation to the pleural surface), pleural effusion, pyothorax (infection of pleural effusion), pulmonary abscess, and pulmonary fibrosis. Empyema is a loculated collection of pus with fibrous walls that follows the spread of bacterial infection to the pleural space. All of the other choices are possible routes of spread, but do not describe empyema.

Diagnosis: Bacterial pneumonia, empyema

7 The answer is D: *Staphylococcus aureus*. Staphylococcal pneumonia is an uncommon community-acquired disease, accounting for only 1% of bacterial pneumonias. However, pulmonary infection with *Staphylococcus aureus* is common as a superinfection after influenza and other viral respiratory tract infections. Nosocomial (hospital acquired) staphylococcal pneumonia typically occurs in chronically ill patients who are prone to aspiration or who are intubated. Although lung abscess can conceivably follow any respiratory infection, the other choices do not usually do so.

Diagnosis: Bacterial pneumonia

8 The answer is D: Tuberculosis. Tuberculosis represents infection with *Mycobacterium tuberculosis*, although atypical mycobacterial infections may mimic it. The Ghon complex includes parenchymal consolidation and enlargement of ipsilateral hilar lymph nodes and is often accompanied by a pleural effusion. The sputum contains *M. tuberculosis*, which is acid-fast in smears stained by the Ziehl-Neelsen technique. After resolution of primary tuberculosis, reemergence may occur (secondary tuberculosis). None of the other choices feature acid-fast organisms.

Diagnosis: Tuberculosis, *Mycobacterium tuberculosis*

9 The answer is C: Granulomas. Secondary (reactivation) tuberculosis is characterized by the formation of granulomas and extensive tissue destruction (caseous necrosis). Mycobacteria typically spread to the apices of the lungs and produce large cavities, which are associated with hemoptysis. Miliary tuberculosis refers to widespread seeding of bacteria in the lungs and distant organs. Granulomatous inflammation may induce fibrosis (choice A) as a secondary feature.

Diagnosis: Tuberculosis, *Mycobacterium tuberculosis*

10 The answer is B: Cytomegalovirus (CMV). CMV produces a characteristic interstitial pneumonia. Initially described in infants, it is now well recognized in immunocompromised persons. The virus may be transmitted from mother to child transplacentally (a feature of TORCH syndrome). Although infected children are usually asymptomatic, in symptomatic infants and children, central nervous symptoms predominate. As implied by its name, CMV causes marked enlargement of infected cells, which contain typical intranuclear and often cytoplasmic inclusions. The other TORCH agents may

cause pneumonia, but only CMV exhibits this cellular morphology.

Diagnosis: Cytomegalovirus, viral pneumonia

11 The answer is E: Invasive aspergillosis. Invasive aspergillosis is the most serious manifestation of *Aspergillus* infection, occurring almost exclusively as an opportunistic infection in immunocompromised persons (e.g., undergoing cytotoxic therapy or diagnosed with AIDS). Invasion of blood vessels and tissue infarcts are common. *Aspergillus* species may also grow in preexisting cavities caused by tuberculosis or bronchiectasis. They proliferate to form fungus balls, which are also referred to as aspergillomas or mycetomas. Vascular invasion is not a feature of the other choices.

Diagnosis: Pulmonary aspergillosis

12 The answer is D: Hyaline membranes and interstitial inflammation. Viral infections of the pulmonary parenchyma produce diffuse alveolar damage (DAD) and interstitial pneumonia. Necrosis of type I pneumocytes and the formation of hyaline membranes result in an appearance that is indistinguishable from DAD in other settings. Choices A, B, and D are not characteristic of interstitial pneumonia. Choice C (fibrous scarring) may be a late complication of some forms of this disorder.

Diagnosis: Diffuse alveolar damage, viral pneumonia

13 The answer is C: Cryptococcosis. Cryptococcosis results from the inhalation of spores of *Cryptococcus neoformans*, an organism frequently encountered in pigeon droppings. Most serious cases occur in immunocompromised persons. Other examples of fungal infections of the lungs are histoplasmosis (choice D), coccidioidomycosis (choice B), and aspergillosis. However, cryptococcus stains positively with a mucicarmine stain for capsular polysaccharides. These diseases are also acquired by inhaling spores.

Diagnosis: Cryptococcal pneumonia, pigeon breeder lung disease

14 The answer is E: *Pneumocystis jiroveci*. *P. jiroveci* (formerly *P. carinii*) is the most frequent cause of infectious pneumonia in patients with AIDS. Once considered a protozoan, the organism has been reclassified as a fungus. The classic lesion of *Pneumocystis* pneumonia comprises an interstitial infiltrate of plasma cells and lymphocytes, diffuse alveolar damage, and hyperplasia of type II pneumocytes. The alveoli are filled with a characteristic foamy exudate. The organisms appear as small bubbles in a background of proteinaceous exudates. In this case, a centrifuged bronchoalveolar lavage specimen impregnated with silver shows a cluster of cysts. The cysts appear as round or indented ("crescent moon") bodies, which are approximately 5 μm in diameter. *Cryptococcus neoformans* (choice A) and *Histoplasma capsulatum* (choice C) do not typically cause interstitial pneumonia.

Diagnosis: *Pneumocystis* pneumonia, AIDS

15 The answer is C: Macrophages. *Mycobacterium avium-intracellulare* (MAI) complex is a progressive systemic disorder, often occurring in patients who have AIDS. One third of all patients with AIDS develop overt MAI infections because depletion of CD4⁺ helper T cells cripples the immune response. This pneumonia is characterized by an extensive infiltrate of macrophages. The proliferation of MAI and the recruitment of macrophages produce expanding lesions, ranging from epithelioid granulomas containing few organisms to loose aggregates of foamy macrophages. Symptoms associated with MAI resemble those of tuberculosis. The other inflammatory cells listed are not characteristic of infection with MAI.

Diagnosis: *Mycobacterium avium-intracellulare,* AIDS

16   The answer is D: Macrophages. *Legionella* pneumonia begins when microorganisms enter the alveoli, where they are phagocytozed by macrophages. Bacteria multiply within macrophages and are released to infect new macrophages. Smoking, alcoholism, and chronic pulmonary diseases interfere with normal host defenses thereby increasing the risk of developing *Legionella* pneumonia. Patients typically present with an acute bronchopneumonia. One third of cases of *Legionella* pneumonia are complicated by subsequent emphysema. The other inflammatory cells listed are scarce or absent in the alveolar exudate.

Diagnosis: Legionnaire disease

17   The answer is A: Atelectasis. Pneumothorax, which is defined as the presence of air in the pleural cavity, may be due to traumatic perforation of the pleura or may be spontaneous. Traumatic causes include penetrating wounds of the chest wall (e.g., stab wound or a rib fracture). Traumatic pneumothorax is most commonly iatrogenic and is seen after aspiration of fluid from the pleura (thoracentesis), pleural or lung biopsies, transbronchial biopsies, and positive pressure-assisted ventilation. Pneumothorax causes collapse of a previously expanded lung, a condition that is termed atelectasis. Additional causes of atelectasis include deficiency of surfactant, compression of the lungs, and bronchial obstruction. Chylothorax (choice B) is the accumulation of lymphatic fluid within the pleural space and is a rare complication of trauma.

Diagnosis: Atelectasis

18   The answer is E: Diffuse alveolar damage (DAD). DAD refers to a nonspecific pattern of reaction to injury of alveolar epithelial and endothelial cells from a variety of acute insults. The clinical counterpart of severe DAD is acute respiratory distress syndrome. In this disorder, a patient with apparently normal lungs sustains pulmonary damage and then develops rapid progressive respiratory failure. DAD is a final common pathway of pathologic changes caused by a variety of insults, including respiratory infections, sepsis, shock, aspiration of gastric contents, inhalation of toxic gases, near-drowning, radiation pneumonitis, and a large assortment of drugs and other chemicals. Desquamative interstitial pneumonia (choice D) is a chronic, fibrosing, interstitial pneumonitis of unknown etiology.

Diagnosis: Diffuse alveolar damage

19   The answer is E: Pulmonary fibrosis. The photomicrograph shows hyaline membranes, thickening of the alveolar walls, and loose connective tissue. This organizing phase of diffuse alveolar damage begins about 1 week after the initial injury. This phase is marked by the proliferation of fibroblasts within the alveolar walls. Alveolar macrophages digest the remnants

of hyaline membranes and other cellular debris. Loose fibrosis then thickens the alveolar septa. This fibrosis resolves in mild cases, but in severe cases, it may progress to restructuring of the pulmonary parenchyma and cyst formation. The photograph does not display features of the other choices.

Diagnosis: Diffuse alveolar damage

20   The answer is A: Alveolar proteinosis. Alveolar proteinosis (also termed lipoproteinosis) is a rare condition in which the alveoli are filled with a granular, proteinaceous, eosinophilic material, which is PAS-positive, diastase resistant, and rich in lipids. The disease was initially described as idiopathic, but recent studies have associated alveolar proteinosis with compromised immunity, leukemia and lymphoma, respiratory infections, and exposure to environmental inorganic dusts. Repeated bronchoalveolar lavage is used to remove the alveolar material, and repeated lavage may halt progression of the disease. None of the other choices exhibit an acellular eosinophilic material that fills the alveoli.

Diagnosis: Alveolar proteinosis

21   The answer is C: Hypersensitivity pneumonitis. Hypersensitivity pneumonitis (extrinsic allergic alveolitis) is a response to inhaled antigens. The inhalation of a variety of antigens leads to acute or chronic interstitial inflammation in the lung. Hypersensitivity pneumonitis may develop in response to repeated exposure to a variety of organic materials (e.g., bird droppings, feathers, mushrooms, and tree bark). Histologically, the lung contains poorly formed granulomas, which differ from the compact (solid) noncaseating granulomas of sarcoidosis and the caseating granulomas of tuberculosis or histoplasmosis. Actinomycosis and nocardiosis (choices A and D) do not induce granulomas. Wegener granulomatosis (choice E) is not known to be associated with environmental exposure.

Diagnosis: Hypersensitivity pneumonitis, pigeon breeder lung disease

22   The answer is C: Emphysema. Chronic obstructive pulmonary disease is a nonspecific term that describes patients with chronic bronchitis or emphysema who evidence a decrease in forced expiratory volume. Emphysema is characterized principally by hyperinflated lungs. Chronic bronchitis (choice B) occurs after recurrent infections and, like asthma (choice A), is not generally associated with hyperinflated lungs. The major cause of emphysema is cigarette smoking, and moderate-to-severe emphysema is rare in nonsmokers.

Diagnosis: Emphysema

23   The answer is A: Destruction of the walls of airspaces without fibrosis. Emphysema is a chronic lung disease characterized by enlargement of the airspaces distal to the terminal bronchioles, with destruction of their walls, but without fibrosis or inflammation.

Diagnosis: Emphysema

24   The answer is A: α₁-Antitrypsin deficiency. Hereditary deficiency of α₁-antitrypsin accounts for about 1% of all patients with a clinical diagnosis of chronic obstructive pulmonary disease and is considerably more common in young persons with severe emphysema. Emphysema in patients with this genetic disease is diffuse and is classified as panacinar. In the lung, the most important action of α_1-antitrypsin is its inhibition of neutrophil elastase, an enzyme that digests elastin and other structural components of the alveolar septa. Most patients with clinically-diagnosed emphysema who are younger than 40 years of age have α_1-antitrypsin (PiZZ phenotype) deficiency. Emphysema is not a feature of the other choices.

Diagnosis: α_1-Antitrypsin deficiency, emphysema

25 The answer is D: Elastase. The dominant hypothesis concerning the pathogenesis of emphysema is the proteolysis-antiproteolysis theory. In most patients with emphysema, it is thought that tobacco smoke induces an inflammatory reaction. Serine elastase in neutrophils is a particularly potent elastolytic agent, which injures the elastic tissue of the lung. Over time, an imbalance in elastin generation and catabolism in the lung leads to emphysema (i.e., emphysema results when elastolytic activity is increased or antielastolytic activity is reduced). α_1-Antitrypsin (choice B), a circulating glycoprotein produced in the liver, is a major inhibitor of a variety of proteases, including elastase, and accounts for 90% of antiproteinase activity in the blood.

Diagnosis: Emphysema

26 The answer is B: Chronic obstructive pulmonary disease. Chronic obstructive pulmonary disease is a nonspecific term that describes patients with chronic bronchitis, emphysema, or both who evidence obstruction to air flow in the lungs. It is often difficult to separate the relative contribution of each disease to the clinical presentation. Chronic bronchitis is defined clinically as the presence of a chronic productive cough without a discernible cause for more than half the time over a period of 2 years. It is primarily a disease of cigarette smoking, with 90% of all cases occurring in smokers. The frequency and severity of acute respiratory tract infections is increased in patients with chronic bronchitis. Exertional dyspnea and cyanosis supervene, and cor pulmonale may ensue. The combination of cyanosis and edema secondary to cor pulmonale has led to the label "blue bloater" for such patients. In contrast to patients with predominantly chronic bronchitis, those with emphysema are at lower risk of recurrent pulmonary infections and are not so prone to the development of cor pulmonale. The clinical course of emphysema is marked by an inexorable decline in respiratory function and progressive dyspnea, for which no treatment is adequate.

Diagnosis: Chronic obstructive pulmonary disease, chronic bronchitis, emphysema

27 The answer is B: Asthma. Asthma is a chronic lung disease caused by increased responsiveness of the airways to a variety of stimuli. Patients typically have paroxysms of wheezing, dyspnea, and cough. Acute episodes of asthma may alternate with asymptomatic periods or they may be superimposed on a background of chronic airway obstruction. The consensus hypothesis attributes bronchial hyperresponsiveness in asthma to an inflammatory reaction to diverse stimuli, either extrinsic (e.g., pollen) or intrinsic (e.g., exercise). Extrinsic asthma is typically a childhood disease, whereas intrinsic asthma usually begins in adults. The other choices do not lead to wheezing and eosinophilia.

Diagnosis: Asthma

28 The answer is E: Smooth muscle hyperplasia and basement membrane thickening. When severe acute asthma is unresponsive to therapy, it is referred to as status asthmaticus. Histological examination of lung from a patient who died in status asthmaticus often shows a bronchus containing a luminal mucous plug, submucosal gland hyperplasia, smooth muscle hyperplasia, basement membrane thickening, and increased numbers of eosinophils. All of the other choices concern alveolar damage, whereas the photograph demonstrates a section of bronchus.

Diagnosis: Asthma

29 The answer is D: Silicosis. Silicosis is caused by inhalation of small crystals of quartz (silicon dioxide), which are generated by stone cutting, sandblasting, and mining. The condition is marked by the insidious development of fibrotic pulmonary nodules containing quartz crystals. The disease may be asymptomatic for prolonged periods of time or may cause only mild to moderate dyspnea. Continued exposure may lead to progressive fibrosis and severe respiratory embarrassment. Anthracosis (choice A) by itself does not cause restrictive lung disease, whereas asbestosis (choice B) is characterized by interstitial fibrosis. The nodules of sarcoidosis (choice C) and Wegener granulomatosis (choice E) are not fibrotic.

Diagnosis: Silicosis

30 The answer is A: Anthracosilicosis. Coal dust is composed of amorphous carbon and other constituents of the earth's surface, including variable amounts of silica. Amorphous carbon by itself is not fibrogenic owing to its inability to kill alveolar macrophages. It is simply a nuisance dust that causes an innocuous anthracosis. By contrast, silica is highly fibrogenic, and the inhalation of rock particles may therefore lead to the lesions of anthracosilicosis. Coal workers' pneumoconiosis is also known as "black lung disease" due to massive deposits of carbon particles. The characteristic pulmonary lesions of complicated coal workers' pneumoconiosis include palpable coal-dust nodules scattered throughout the lung as 1- to 4-mm black foci. Nodules consist of dust-laden macrophages associated with a fibrotic stroma. Coal miners are not predisposed to the other choices.

Diagnosis: Coal workers' pneumoconiosis, anthracosilicosis

31 The answer is B: Asbestosis. Asbestosis refers to the diffuse interstitial fibrosis that results from the inhalation of asbestos fibers. The disease occurs as a result of the processing and handling of asbestos, rather than mining, which is a surface operation. Asbestosis is characterized by bilateral, diffuse interstitial fibrosis and asbestos bodies in the lung. These ferruginous bodies are golden brown and beaded, with a central colorless core fiber. Asbestos bodies are encrusted with protein and iron. In this patient, the dome of the diaphragm is covered by a smooth, pearly white, nodular fibrotic lesion (pleural plaque), a common feature of asbestos exposure. A clear-cut relationship between occupational asbestos exposure and malignant mesothelioma is established. None of the other choices display pleural plaques or ferruginous bodies.

Diagnosis: Asbestosis

32 The answer is E: Thromboembolism. Pulmonary arterial embolism is potentially fatal. Most pulmonary emboli arise from the deep veins of the lower extremities. This patient had signs of deep venous thrombosis of the leg. However, only half of patients with pulmonary thromboembolism have deep vein thrombosis. In this patient, pulmonary embolism was associated with pulmonary infarction, pleuritic chest pain, hemoptysis, and pleural effusion. None of the other choices feature pleuritic signs and symptoms.

Diagnosis: Pulmonary thromboembolism

33 The answer is B: Sarcoidosis. Sarcoidosis is a granulomatous disease of unknown etiology. In sarcoidosis, the lung is the most frequently involved organ, but the lymph nodes, skin, and eyes are also common targets. Angiotensin-converting enzyme (ACE) is produced by epithelioid macrophages and is elevated in the blood. Spontaneous regression of lesions is common, but in some cases, the disease causes pulmonary fibrosis and respiratory failure. Symptoms of pulmonary disease include dyspnea, cough, and wheezing. None of the other choices are associated with increased serum levels of ACE.

Diagnosis: Sarcoidosis

34 The answer is E: Lymphocytic interstitial pneumonia. Lymphocytic interstitial pneumonia (LIP) is a rare pneumonitis in which lymphoid infiltrates are distributed diffusely in the interstitial spaces of the lung. In this case, the walls of the alveolar septa are diffusely infiltrated with chronic inflammatory cells. LIP often occurs in a variety of clinical settings, including Sjögren syndrome and HIV infection. The course of the disease varies from an indolent condition to one that progresses to end-stage lung disease and respiratory failure. Langerhans cell histiocytosis (choice C) features nodular infiltrates. Interstitial lymphocytic infiltrates are not characteristic of the other choices.

Diagnosis: Lymphocytic interstitial pneumonia

35 The answer is E: Wegener granulomatosis (WG). WG is a disease of unknown cause that is characterized by aseptic, necrotizing, granulomatous inflammation and vasculitis. This disease affects the upper and lower respiratory tract and kidneys. Pulmonary features of WG include necrotizing granulomatous inflammation, parenchymal necrosis, and vasculitis. In most cases, multiple nodules averaging 2 to 3 cm in diameter are seen in the lungs. WG most commonly affects the head and neck, followed by the lung, kidney, and eye. Respiratory manifestations include sinusitis, cough, hemoptysis, and pleuritis. Sinus involvement is not common in the incorrect choices. Churg-Strauss syndrome (choice B) shares some features with WG, but is characterized by asthma, peripheral eosinophilia and P-ANCA.

Diagnosis: Wegener granulomatosis

36 The answer is B: Langerhans cell histiocytosis. Different presentations of Langerhans cell histiocytosis have been called eosinophilic granuloma, Hand-Schuller-Christian disease, and Letterer-Siwe disease. In adults, the disorder occurs most often as an isolated form known as pulmonary eosinophilic granuloma. Virtually all of these patients are cigarette smokers. The pulmonary lesions consist of varying proportions of Langerhans cells admixed with lymphocytes, eosinophils, and macrophages. Eosinophils are not typical of the other choices.

Diagnosis: Langerhans histiocytosis

37 The answer is C: Lymphangioleiomyomatosis. Lymphangioleiomyomatosis is a rare interstitial lung disease that occurs in women of childbearing age. It is characterized by the widespread abnormal proliferation of smooth muscle in the lung (see photomicrograph), mediastinal and retroperitoneal lymph nodes, and the major lymphatic ducts. On gross examination, the lungs show bilateral, diffuse enlargement, with extensive cystic changes resembling those of emphysema. Hormonal ablation through oophorectomy and antiestrogen and progesterone therapy has shown some promise. None of the other choices exhibit this morphologic pattern.

Diagnosis: Lymphangioleiomyomatosis

38 The answer is B: Goodpasture syndrome. Goodpasture syndrome is an autoimmune disease in which autoantibodies bind to the noncollagenous domain of type IV collagen. This connective tissue protein is a major structural component of both pulmonary and glomerular basement membranes. Local complement activation results in the recruitment of neutrophils, tissue injury, pulmonary hemorrhage, and glomerulonephritis. Anti–type IV collagen antibodies are not encountered in the other choices.

Diagnosis: Goodpasture syndrome

39 The answer is A: Eosinophilic pneumonia. Eosinophilic pneumonia is principally an allergic disorder. It refers to the accumulation of eosinophils in alveolar spaces and is classified as either idiopathic or secondary to an underlying illness. In acute eosinophilic pneumonia, the alveolar spaces are filled with an inflammatory exudate composed of eosinophils and macrophages. The alveolar septa are thickened by the presence of numerous eosinophils and hyaline membranes are present. Patients respond dramatically to corticosteroids, and, in contrast to chronic eosinophilic pneumonia, acute eosinophilic pneumonia does not recur. Excess eosinophils are not encountered in the other choices.

Diagnosis: Eosinophilic pneumonia

40 The answer is D: Usual interstitial pneumonia (UIP). UIP is one of the most common types of interstitial pneumonia and demonstrates a histologic pattern that occurs in a variety of clinical settings, including collagen vascular disease, chronic hypersensitivity pneumonitis, and drug toxicity. Most commonly, it has no known cause, although viral, genetic, and immunologic factors may be implicated. A microscopic view of the lung in this case shows patchy, subpleural fibrosis with microscopic "honeycomb" cystic change. Diffuse fibrosis is not characteristic of the other choices.

Diagnosis: Usual interstitial pneumonia

41 The answer is C: Cryptogenic organizing pneumonia. Organizing pneumonia was previously referred to as bronchiolitis obliterans-organizing pneumonia. The histologic pattern is not specific for any particular etiologic agent and may be observed in many settings, including respiratory tract infections, inhalation of toxic materials, and collagen vascular diseases. In the absence of a specific etiology, the term cryptogenic organizing pneumonia is applied. Loose fibrous tissue in the alveoli and bronchioles is a typical finding in patients with cryptogenic organizing pneumonia. Diffuse alveolar damage (choice D) features intra-alveolar fibrin (hyaline membranes).

Diagnosis: Cryptogenic organizing pneumonia

42 The answer is D: Pulmonary hypertension. Pulmonary hypertension is characterized by thickening of the media of pulmonary muscular arteries. As pulmonary hypertension becomes more severe, there is extensive intimal fibrosis and muscle thickening within arteries and arterioles, which may be occlusive. Churg-Strauss syndrome (choice A) exhibits vasculitis and eosinophilia but is excluded in this case on the basis of a normal CBC. The other choices do not principally affect arteries.

Diagnosis: Pulmonary hypertension

43 The answer is D: Squamous cell carcinoma. The vast majority of laryngeal cancers are squamous cell carcinomas and occur principally in smokers. Adenocarcinoma (choice A), leiomyosarcoma (choice B), and small cell carcinoma (choice C) are rarely encountered in the larynx.

Diagnosis: Laryngeal cancer

44 The answer is E: Pulmonary hamartoma. Although the term hamartoma implies a malformation, hamartomas are true tumors. They are composed of cartilage, fibromyxoid connective tissue, fat, bone, and occasional smooth muscle. They typically occur in adults, with a peak in the sixth decade of life. Hamartomas are the cause of approximately 10% of "coin" lesions discovered incidentally on chest radiographs. A characteristic "popcorn" pattern of calcification is often seen by X-ray. Cartilage is not encountered in the other choices.

Diagnosis: Pulmonary hamartoma

45 The answer is E: Squamous cell carcinoma. Squamous cell carcinoma accounts for 30% of all invasive lung cancers in the United States. Well-differentiated squamous cell carcinoma displays keratin "pearls," which appear as a small round nest of brightly eosinophilic aggregates of keratin surrounded by concentric ("onion skin") layers of squamous cells. Gland formation is exhibited in adenocarcinoma (choices A and C).

Diagnosis: Squamous cell carcinoma of lung

46 The answer is A: Adenocarcinoma. Adenocarcinoma usually presents as a peripheral subpleural mass composed of neoplastic gland-like structures. Central (hilar) cancers of the lung can be of any of the histologic types (e.g., choices B, D, and E), whereas peripheral lung cancers are most commonly diagnosed as adenocarcinomas. They are often associated with pleural fibrosis and subpleural scars. At initial presentation, adenocarcinomas usually appear as irregular masses, although they may be so large that they completely replace the entire lobe of the lung. Mesothelioma (choice C) is pleural based.

Diagnosis: Adenocarcinoma of lung

47 The answer is C: Large cell carcinoma. Large cell undifferentiated carcinoma is composed of atypical neoplastic cells that do not resemble any normal cells in the lung. These cells do not form glands (like adenocarcinoma) and do not express cytokeratin (choices A and D). Chromogranin is expressed in carcinoid tumors (choice B) and often in small cell carcinomas (choice E).

Diagnosis: Large cell carcinoma of lung

48 The answer is A: Bronchioloalveolar carcinoma. Bronchioloalveolar carcinoma is a primary pulmonary adenocarcinoma originating from stem cells in the terminal bronchioles. The cells may be columnar and mucus producing or cuboidal and similar to type II pneumocytes. They tend to grow along the alveolar septa, as depicted in the photomicrograph. A similar growth pattern may be seen in metastatic adenocarcinomas. None of the other tumors produce alveolar mucus or display alveolar spaces lined by a columnar epithelium.

Diagnosis: Bronchioloalveolar carcinoma

49 The answer is E: Small cell carcinoma. Small cell carcinoma (previously referred to as "oat-cell" carcinoma) is a highly malignant epithelial tumor of the lung that exhibits neuroendocrine features. It accounts for 20% of all lung cancers and is strongly associated with cigarette smoking. Metastases occur early and are widespread. Carcinoid tumors (choice C) also contain neuroendocrine granules, but the tumor cells are arranged in a distinctive pattern. Moreover, Cushing syndrome is often encountered in patients with small cell carcinoma, but not carcinoid tumor (choice C).

Diagnosis: Small cell carcinoma of lung

50 The answer is C: Carcinoid tumor. Carcinoid tumors account for 2% of all primary lung cancers. They comprise a group of neuroendocrine neoplasms derived from the pluripotential basal layer of the respiratory epithelium. Carcinoid tumors occur most often in the wall of the major bronchus and may protrude into its lumen. The tumors are characterized by an organoid growth pattern and uniform cytologic features. Carcinoid tumors exhibit a neuroendocrine differentiation similar to that of resident Kulchitsky cells. The indolent nature of carcinoid tumors is reflected in the finding that half of the patients are asymptomatic at the time of presentation, but regional lymph node metastases occur in 20% of patients. Atypical carcinoids exhibit a more aggressive behavior. Neuroendocrine features are absent in the other tumors.

Diagnosis: Carcinoid tumor of lung

51 The answer is D: Malignant mesothelioma. Mesothelioma is a malignant neoplasm of mesothelial cells that is most common in the pleura, but also occurs in the peritoneum, pericardium, and the tunica vaginalis of the testis. The tumor is strongly linked to occupational inhalation of asbestos. Patients are often first seen with a pleural effusion or a pleural mass, chest pain, and nonspecific symptoms, such as weight loss and malaise. Pleural mesotheliomas tend to spread locally and extensively within the chest cavity, but do not typically invade the pulmonary parenchyma. Widespread metastases can occur. Mesothelioma is typically composed of both epithelial and sarcomatous elements (i.e., biphasic pattern). The other choices do not ordinarily encase the lung.

Diagnosis: Malignant mesothelioma

52 The answer is E: Metastatic carcinoma. Pulmonary metastases represent the most common neoplasm of the lung. In one third of all fatal cancers, pulmonary metastases are evident at autopsy. Metastatic carcinomas typically present as multiple, round masses scattered at random throughout the parenchyma of lungs and liver. Although pulmonary adenocarcinoma (choice A) and bronchoalveolar carcinoma (choice B) cannot be excluded on histologic grounds, this patient with ulcerative colitis is predisposed to develop adenocarcinoma of the colon, which most likely accounts for the anemia and lung metastases.

Diagnosis: Metastatic carcinoma of lung

53 **The answer is C: Hydrothorax.** The elevation of hydrostatic pressure in patients with congestive heart failure causes transudation of edema fluid into the pleural cavity (i.e., hydrothorax). Chylothorax (choice A) and hemothorax (choice B) refer to lymph and blood in the pleural space, respectively. Pneumothorax (choice D) and pyothorax (choice E) refer to air and acute inflammatory cells in the pleural space, respectively.

Diagnosis: Congestive heart failure, hydrothorax

54 **The answer is B: Empyema.** Pleuritis (inflammation of the pleura) may result from the extension of any pulmonary infection to the visceral pleura. Causes of pleuritis include bacterial infections, viral infections, and pulmonary infarction involving the surface of the lung. Pyothorax refers to a turbid effusion containing many neutrophils. Empyema is a variant of pyothorax in which thick pus accumulates within the pleural cavity, often with loculation and fibrosis. Hydrothorax (choice D) refers to transudation of edema fluid into the pleural cavity.

Diagnosis: Empyema

55 **The answer is A: Chylothorax.** Chylothorax is defined as the accumulation in the pleural cavity of a milky, lipid-rich fluid as a result of lymphatic obstruction. It has an ominous portent because obstruction of the lymphatics suggests disease of the lymph nodes in the posterior mediastinum. Chylothorax is thus found as a rare complication of malignant tumors in the mediastinum, such as lymphoma. Empyema (choice B) is a loculated collection of pus with fibrous walls that follows the spread of bacterial infection to the pleural space.

Diagnosis: Chylothorax

Chapter 13

The Gastrointestinal Tract

QUESTIONS

Select the single best answer.

1 A 35-year-old man complains of difficulty swallowing and a tendency to regurgitate his food. Endoscopy does not reveal any esophageal or gastric abnormalities. Manometric studies of the esophagus show a complete absence of peristalsis, failure of the lower esophageal sphincter to relax upon swallowing, and increased intraesophageal pressure. Which of the following is the most likely diagnosis?

(A) Achalasia
(B) Barrett esophagus
(C) Esophageal stricture
(D) Mallory-Weiss syndrome
(E) Schatzki ring

2 A 20-year-old woman presents with a 2-year history of difficulty swallowing and increasing fatigue. A CBC shows iron-deficiency anemia. Upper endoscopy reveals an annular narrowing in the upper third of the esophagus. A mucosal biopsy shows no evidence of inflammation or neoplasia. Which of the following is the most likely diagnosis?

(A) Achalasia
(B) Barrett esophagus
(C) Diverticulum
(D) Esophageal web
(E) Schatzki ring

3 A 45-year-old woman presents with general discomfort and increasing tightness in the skin of her face. She reports intermittent pain in the tips of her fingers when exposed to the cold. Physical examination shows "stone facies" and edema of the fingers and hands. Serologic tests for antinuclear and anti–Scl-70 antibodies are both positive. Which of the following gastrointestinal manifestations is expected in this patient?

(A) Adenocarcinoma of the esophagus
(B) Dysphagia
(C) Esophageal rupture
(D) Esophageal varices
(E) Squamous cell carcinoma of the esophagus

4 A 54-year-old man with a long history of indigestion after meals and "heartburn" presents with upper abdominal pain. He was treated with proton-pump inhibitors for gastroesophageal reflux 3 years previously. An endoscopic biopsy of the lower esophagus is shown in the image. Which of the following best describes these pathologic findings?

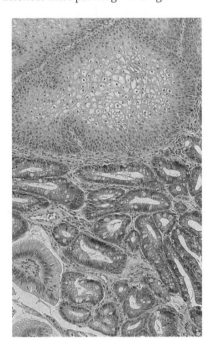

(A) *Candida* esophagitis
(B) Esophageal diverticulum
(C) Esophageal varices
(D) Glandular metaplasia
(E) Schatzki ring

5 The patient described in Question 4 is at increased risk of developing which of the following diseases of the esophagus?

(A) Achalasia
(B) Adenocarcinoma
(C) Candidiasis
(D) Plummer-Vinson syndrome
(E) Varices

6 A 65-year-old woman complains of a 4-month history of bad breath, regurgitation of undigested food, occasional aspiration of food, and change in the sound of her voice. A barium swallow examination shows a posterior, midline pouch greater than 2 cm in diameter arising just above the cricopharyngeal muscle. Which of the following is the most likely diagnosis?

(A) Epiphrenic diverticulum
(B) Intramural pseudodiverticulum
(C) Meckel diverticulum
(D) Traction diverticulum
(E) Zenker diverticulum

7 A 45-year-old man presents with long-standing heartburn and dyspepsia. An X-ray film of the chest shows a retrocardiac, gas-filled structure. This patient most likely has which of the following conditions?

(A) Boerhaave syndrome
(B) Esophageal varices
(C) Esophageal webs
(D) Hiatal hernia
(E) Mallory-Weiss syndrome

8 A 3-year-old boy is rushed to the emergency room in acute distress. The child has vague chest pain and difficulty swallowing. He refuses to drink water. Physical examination shows drooling and salivation. Vital signs are normal. The mother states that she saw the boy ingesting a liquid used to clear drains. If this chemical was a strong acid, which of the following histopathologic findings would be expected in the esophagus of this child?

(A) Apoptosis
(B) Coagulative necrosis
(C) Fat necrosis
(D) Hyaline sclerosis
(E) Liquefactive necrosis

9 A 70-year-old woman presents with difficulty swallowing and a 9-kg (20-lb) weight loss over the past several months. Endoscopy reveals irregular narrowing of the lower third of the esophagus. A biopsy shows markedly atypical cuboidal cells lining irregular gland-like structures. Which of the following is the most likely diagnosis?

(A) Adenocarcinoma
(B) Esophageal stricture
(C) Leiomyosarcoma
(D) Scleroderma
(E) Squamous cell carcinoma

10 A 60-year-old man presents with a 5-week history of difficulty swallowing. Physical examination is unremarkable. Upper endoscopy shows a large mass in the upper third of the esophagus. A biopsy is shown in the image. What is the appropriate histologic diagnosis for this esophageal mass?

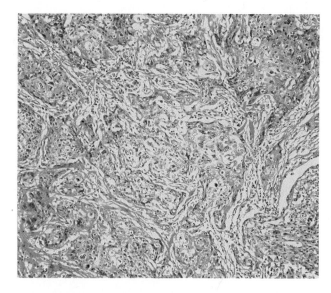

(A) Adenocarcinoma
(B) Glandular metaplasia
(C) Malignant melanoma
(D) Squamous cell carcinoma
(E) Transitional cell carcinoma

11 Which of the following is the most important risk factor for development of the esophageal mass identified in the patient described in Question 10?

(A) Cigarette smoking
(B) Exposure to aflatoxin
(C) Herpetic esophagitis
(D) Hot and spicy food
(E) Reflux esophagitis

12 A 50-year-old obese man (BMI = 32 kg/m²) comes to the physician complaining of indigestion after meals, bloating, and heartburn. Vital signs are normal. A CT scan of the abdomen reveals a hiatal hernia of the esophagus. Endoscopic biopsy shows thickening of the basal layer of the squamous epithelium, upward extension of the papillae of the lamina propria, and an increased number of neutrophils and lymphocytes. Which of the following is the most likely diagnosis?

(A) Esophageal varices
(B) Mallory-Weiss syndrome
(C) Reflux esophagitis
(D) Schatzki mucosal ring
(E) Squamous cell carcinoma

13 A 30-year-old man with AIDS complains of severe pain on swallowing. Upper GI endoscopy shows elevated, white plaques on a hyperemic and edematous esophageal mucosa. Which of the following is the most likely diagnosis?

(A) Barrett esophagus
(B) *Candida* esophagitis
(C) Herpetic esophagitis
(D) Reflux esophagitis
(E) Squamous cell carcinoma in situ

14 A 58-year-old woman is brought to the emergency department 4 hours after vomiting blood and experiencing bloody stools. The patient was diagnosed with alcoholic cirrhosis 2 years ago. The patient subsequently goes into shock and expires. The histologic appearance of the esophagus at autopsy is shown in the image. Which of the following is the most likely underlying cause of hematemesis and hematochezia in this patient?

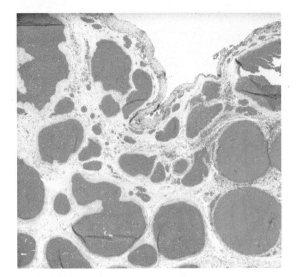

(A) Alcoholic hepatitis
(B) Ischemia of the gastric mucosa
(C) Mallory-Weiss syndrome
(D) Peptic ulcer disease
(E) Portal hypertension

15 A 3-week-old boy is brought to the physician by his parents, who report that he vomits forcefully immediately after nursing. Physical examination reveals an "olive-like" palpable mass and visible peristaltic movements within the infant's abdomen. What is the most likely cause of projectile vomiting in this infant?

(A) Appendicitis
(B) Congenital pyloric stenosis
(C) Hirschsprung disease
(D) Meconium ileus
(E) Tracheoesophageal fistula

16 A 50-year-old woman with long-standing rheumatoid arthritis complains of weakness and fatigue. She states that her stools have recently become black after taking a new nonsteroidal anti-inflammatory drug (NSAID). Gastroscopy shows numerous superficial, bleeding mucosal defects. Which of the following is the most likely diagnosis?

(A) Acute erosive gastritis
(B) Early gastric cancer
(C) *Helicobacter pylori* gastritis
(D) Ménétrier disease
(E) Peptic ulcer disease

17 A 34-year-old man presents with a 5-month history of weakness and fatigue. There is no history of drug or alcohol abuse. A CBC shows megaloblastic anemia and a normal reticulocyte count.

Further laboratory studies reveal vitamin B$_{12}$ deficiency. Anemia in this patient is most likely caused by which of the following?

(A) Acute erosive gastritis
(B) Autoimmune gastritis
(C) *Helicobacter pylori* gastritis
(D) Ménétrier disease
(E) Peptic ulcer disease

18 A 40-year-old woman presents with a 2-month history of burning epigastric pain that usually occurs between meals. The pain can be relieved with antacids or food. The patient also reports a recent history of tarry stools. She denies taking aspirin or NSAIDs. Laboratory studies show a microcytic, hypochromic anemia (serum hemoglobin = 8.5 g/dL). Gastroscopy reveals a bleeding mucosal defect in the antrum measuring 1.5 cm in diameter. An endoscopic biopsy shows that the lesion lacks mucosal lining cells and is composed of amorphous, cellular debris and numerous neutrophils. Which of the following is the most important factor in the pathogenesis of this patient's disease?

(A) Achlorohydria
(B) Acute ischemia
(C) Autoimmunity
(D) Gastrinoma
(E) *Helicobacter pylori* infection

19 A 58-year-old woman suffers a massive stroke and expires. The stomach at autopsy is shown in the image. Prior to her death, this patient would most likely have exhibited which of the following?

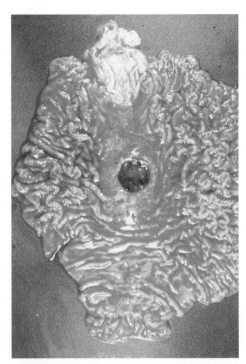

(A) Dysphagia
(B) Hypersecretion of gastric acid
(C) Melena
(D) Steatorrhea
(E) Variceal bleeding

20 A 45-year-old woman presents with a 6-month history of fatigue and swelling in her neck. Physical examination shows a goiter. A CBC discloses megaloblastic anemia and a normal reticulocyte count. Additionally, there is an elevated serum level of TSH and antithyroid antibodies. Needle aspiration of the left lobe of the thyroid reveals benign follicular cells and numerous lymphocytes. Anemia in this patient is most likely caused by antibodies directed to which of the following targets?

(A) Chief cells
(B) Intrinsic factor
(C) Paneth cells
(D) TSH receptor
(E) Vitamin D

21 A 45-year-old man describes burning epigastric pain 2 to 3 hours after eating. Foods, antacids, and over-the-counter medications provide no relief, and prescribed inhibitors of acid secretion are only moderately effective. Recently, the patient noticed that his stools were black. Physical examination reveals abdominal tenderness. The blood pressure is 120/80 mm Hg in the supine position and 90/50 mm Hg sitting up. The patient complains of lightheadedness upon returning to a standing position. CBC shows a hemoglobin of 6.3 g/dL. Endoscopy reveals multiple gastric and duodenal ulcers. Epigastric pain and anemia are most likely related to a neoplasm arising in which of the following anatomic locations?

(A) Adrenal medulla
(B) Ampulla of Vater
(C) Duodenum
(D) Esophagus
(E) Pancreas

22 A 60-year-old man presents with an 8-week history of progressive weight loss, nausea, and upper abdominal pain that does not respond to antacids or H2-receptor antagonists. Laboratory studies show iron-deficiency anemia. Gastroscopy reveals a crater-like, ulcerated lesion in the antrum, with raised, irregular, and indurated margins. The patient undergoes partial gastrectomy and the surgical specimen is shown in the image. Which of the following is the most likely diagnosis?

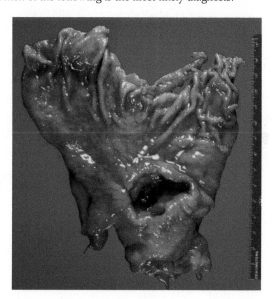

(A) Acute erosive gastritis
(B) Adenocarcinoma
(C) Curling ulcer
(D) Linitis plastica
(E) Peptic ulcer disease

23 A 58-year-old woman presents with a 2-month history of abdominal discomfort and dark stools. Physical examination shows pallor but no evidence of jaundice. Laboratory studies disclose a microcytic, hypochromic anemia, with a hemoglobin level of 6.7 g/dL. A barium swallow radiograph reveals a "leather bottle" appearance of the stomach. Microscopic examination shows diffusely infiltrating malignant cells, many of which are "signet ring" cells, in the stomach wall. Which of the following is the most likely diagnosis?

(A) Fungating adenocarcinoma
(B) Gastric leiomyosarcoma
(C) Gastric lymphoma
(D) Linitis plastica
(E) Ménétrier disease

24 A 42-year-old man presents with long-standing abdominal pain after meals, which is relieved by over-the-counter antacids. The patient has lost 9 kg (20 lb) in the past year. Physical examination reveals peripheral edema and ascites. Laboratory studies show decreased serum albumin but normal serum levels of transaminases and gastrin. Gross and microscopic examination of this patient's stomach would most likely show which of the following pathologic changes?

(A) Atrophic gastritis
(B) Enlarged rugal folds
(C) Intestinal metaplasia
(D) Multiple hemorrhagic ulcers
(E) Proliferation of neuroendocrine cells

25 A 55-year-old woman complains of upper gastrointestinal pain and tarry stools. Upper endoscopy shows a firm, smooth, yellowish submucosal ulcerated mass in the stomach. Gastroscopic biopsy reveals spindle cells with vacuolated cytoplasm. The mass is removed, and the surgical specimen is shown in the image. Which of the following is the most likely diagnosis?

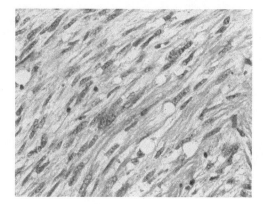

(A) Gastric adenocarcinoma
(B) Gastric lymphoma
(C) Gastrointestinal stromal tumor
(D) Peptic ulcer
(E) Tubular adenoma

26 A 56-year-old woman comes to the physician after noticing multiple lumps in her neck. Physical examination shows enlarged and nontender supraclavicular lymph nodes. Upper endoscopy discloses thickening of the gastric mucosa, without an obvious tumor. The results of gastric biopsy are shown in the image. Which of the following is the most likely diagnosis?

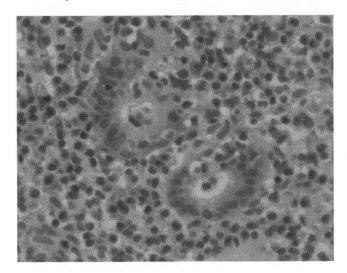

(A) Adenocarcinoma
(B) Gastric lymphoma
(C) Leiomyosarcoma
(D) Linitis plastica
(E) Ménétrier disease

27 A 23-year-old woman with a history of an eating disorder complains of vomiting, nausea, and severe abdominal pain. Physical examination shows abdominal distension and constipation. An X-ray film of the abdomen reveals air-fluid levels and a hyperlucent shadow at the epigastric area. The material obstructing the gastrointestinal tract is removed surgically and shown. Which of the following is the most likely diagnosis?

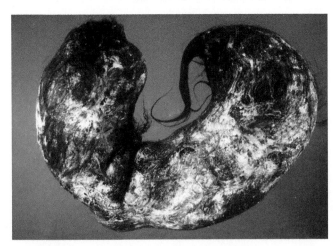

(A) Diverticulum of the stomach
(B) Gastric lymphoma
(C) Phytobezoar
(D) Trichobezoar
(E) Volvulus of the stomach

28 A 60-year-old man presents with epigastric pain after meals, with some nausea and vomiting. A burning sensation in the midepigastrium is relieved by antacids and H2 antagonists. Upper endoscopy demonstrates paired ulcers on both walls of the proximal duodenum. Which of the following represents the most common complication of this patient's duodenal disease?

(A) Bleeding
(B) Malignant transformation
(C) Obstruction
(D) Perforation
(E) Peritonitis

29 A 45-year-old woman presents with sudden attacks of wheezing, shortness of breath, and episodic hot flashes. She also reports abdominal cramps and diarrhea. Physical examination shows facial redness, pitting edema of the lower legs, and a murmur of tricuspid regurgitation. A 24-hour urine specimen contains elevated levels of 5-hydroxyindoleacetic acid (5-HIAA). A CT scan of the abdomen demonstrates multiple 1- to 2-cm nodules in distal ileum. A small bowel resection is performed (shown in the image). The arrows point to submucosal tumors. Microscopic examination shows nests of cells with round and uniform nuclei. Which of the following is the most likely diagnosis?

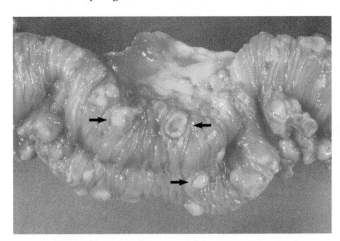

(A) Carcinoid tumor
(B) Mediterranean intestinal lymphoma
(C) Mucosa-associated lymphoid tissue (MALT) lymphoma
(D) Peutz-Jeghers syndrome
(E) Whipple disease

30 A 5-year-old girl is brought to the physician after her parents noticed red blood in her stool. Physical examination reveals mucocutaneous pigmentation. Small bowel radiography discloses multiple, small- to medium-sized polyps that are diagnosed pathologically as hamartomas. Which of the following is the most likely diagnosis?

(A) Congenital teratoma
(B) Hyperplastic polyp
(C) Peutz-Jeghers polyp
(D) Tubular adenoma
(E) Villous adenoma

31 A 55-year-old man undergoes routine colonoscopy. A small, raised, mucosal nodule measuring 0.4 cm in diameter is identified in the rectum and resected. The surgical specimen is shown in the image. Microscopic examination reveals goblet cells and absorptive cells with exaggerated crypt architecture, but no signs of nuclear atypia. Which of the following is the most likely diagnosis?

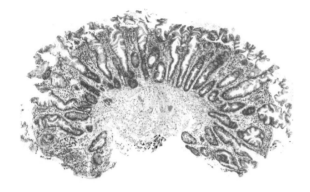

(A) Adenocarcinoma
(B) Hyperplastic polyp
(C) Inflammatory polyp
(D) Peutz-Jeghers polyp
(E) Villous adenoma

32 A 65-year-old woman undergoes routine colonoscopy. During the procedure, a 2-cm mass is identified in the rectosigmoid region and resected. The surgical specimen is shown in the image. Microscopic examination shows irregular crypts lined by pseudostratified epithelium with hyperchromatic nuclei, without dysplastic features. Which of the following is the most likely diagnosis for this patient's colonic lesion?

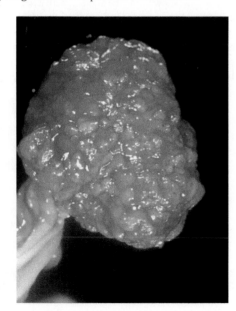

(A) Adenocarcinoma
(B) Carcinoid tumor
(C) Hyperplastic polyp
(D) Tubular adenoma
(E) Villous adenoma

33 A 63-year-old woman complains of rectal bleeding of 1 week in duration. Laboratory studies show hypochromic, microcytic anemia (hemoglobin = 7.6 g/dL and MCV = 70 μm³). Colonoscopy reveals a large polypoid mass, which is removed (surgical specimen shown in the image). The arrow points to a malignant tumor. The patient asks about the relative risk of cancer arising in various types of gastrointestinal polyps. Which of the following types of colonic polyps is most likely to undergo malignant transformation?

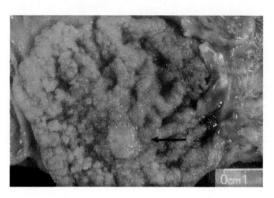

(A) Hyperplastic polyp
(B) Lymphoid polyp
(C) Peutz-Jeghers polyp
(D) Tubular adenoma
(E) Villous adenoma

34 A 59-year-old man complains of progressive weakness. His friends have noticed that he has become pale, and he reports that his stools are tinged with blood. On abdominal palpation, there is fullness in the right lower quadrant. Laboratory studies show iron-deficiency anemia, with a hemoglobin level of 7.4 g/dL. Stool specimens are positive for occult blood. Colonoscopy reveals an elevated and centrally ulcerated lesion of the sigmoid colon. The biopsy is shown in the image. Which of the following is the most likely diagnosis?

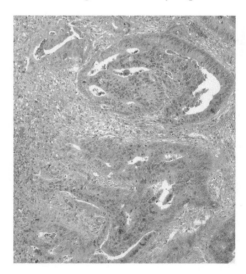

(A) Adenocarcinoma
(B) Carcinoid tumor
(C) Gastrointestinal stromal tumor
(D) Lymphoma
(E) Mucinous cystadenoma

35 A portion of the large bowel was removed from a 34-year-old man with a familial disease that affects his gastrointestinal tract. The surgical specimen is shown in the image. This patient most likely carries a germline mutation in which of the following genes?

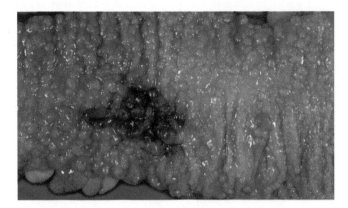

(A) *APC*
(B) *C-myc*
(C) *DCC*
(D) *p53*
(E) *Ras*

36 A 65-year-old woman presents with a 3-month history of diarrhea and abdominal pain. She has lost 9 kg (20 lb) in the past 6 months. The patient had two benign colonic polyps removed 3 years ago. Laboratory studies reveal mild iron-deficiency anemia, and stool specimens are positive for occult blood. Sigmoidoscopy demonstrates an ulcerated mass, and a biopsy shows malignant glands. A segment of the colon is resected, and the surgical specimen is shown in the image. Based on current models of colonic carcinogenesis, which of the following genes was most likely mutated in the transition from benign adenoma to carcinoma in this patient?

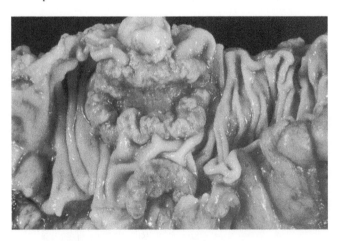

(A) *BRCA1*
(B) *C-myc*
(C) *p53*
(D) *Ras*
(E) *VHL*

37 A 60-year-old woman complains of increasing abdominal girth of 4 weeks in duration. Physical examination discloses ascites, and cytologic examination of the fluid reveals malignant cells. Exploratory laparotomy shows multiple tumor nodules on the serosal surface of the intestines. Which of the following is the most likely diagnosis?
(A) Carcinoid tumor
(B) Gastrointestinal stromal tumor
(C) Liposarcoma
(D) MALToma
(E) Metastatic carcinoma

38 A 34-year-old man with AIDS presents with a 3-month history of constipation and lower abdominal pain. The patient has a history of chronic diarrhea and persistent cough. Recently, he noticed blood in his stool. Laboratory studies reveal mild iron-deficiency anemia. Stool specimens are positive for occult blood. A CBC shows a CD4 count of less than 50/μL. Sigmoidoscopy discloses a mass in the rectosigmoid region. In addition to B-cell lymphoma, this patient is at increased risk of developing which of the following tumors of the gastrointestinal (GI) tract?
(A) Carcinoid tumor
(B) Colonic adenocarcinoma
(C) Kaposi sarcoma
(D) Leiomyosarcoma
(E) Melanoma

39 A 27-year-old woman presents with a 9-month history of bloody diarrhea and crampy abdominal pain. Three weeks ago, she noticed that her left knee was swollen, red, and painful. Her temperature is 38°C (101°F), respirations are 32 per minute, and blood pressure is 130/90 mm Hg. Abdominal palpation reveals tenderness over the left lower quadrant. Laboratory studies show moderate anemia, with a hemoglobin level of 9.3 g/dL. Microscopic examination of the stool reveals numerous red and white blood cells. A diffusely red, bleeding, friable colonic mucosa is visualized by colonoscopy. The colon is subsequently removed and the surgical specimen is shown in the image. Which of the following is the most likely diagnosis?

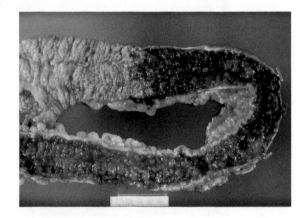

(A) Adenocarcinoma
(B) Carcinoid tumor
(C) Crohn disease
(D) Pseudomembranous colitis
(E) Ulcerative colitis

40 The patient described in Question 39 is at increased risk of developing which of the following complications?

(A) Adenocarcinoma
(B) Fistula
(C) Granulomatous lymphadenitis
(D) Transmural inflammation
(E) Volvulus

41 A 44-year-old woman complains of having yellow eyes, dark urine, and recurrent fever for about 3 months. She has a long history of chronic diarrhea. On physical examination, the patient is thin and jaundiced. The liver edge descends 1 cm below the right costal margin and is nontender. Laboratory studies show elevated serum bilirubin of 3.8 mg/dL, normal levels of AST and ALT, and an elevated level of alkaline phosphatase (440 U/dL). Endoscopic retrograde cholangiopancreatography demonstrates a beaded appearance of the extrahepatic biliary tree. Which of the following is the most likely underlying cause of diarrhea in this patient?

(A) Amebiasis
(B) Amyloidosis
(C) Carcinoma of the ampulla of Vater
(D) Celiac sprue
(E) Ulcerative colitis

42 A 25-year-old woman is brought to the emergency room with symptoms of acute intestinal obstruction. The patient has an 8-month history of blood-tinged diarrhea and cramping abdominal pain. Her temperature is 38°C (101°F), and respirations are 32 per minute. There is abdominal tenderness to palpation. Laboratory studies show moderate anemia, with serum hemoglobin of 9.3 g/dL. Microscopic examination of the stool reveals numerous RBCs and WBCs. A CT scan of the abdomen shows massive distention of the transverse colon. Which of the following is the most likely underlying cause of this patient's colonic disorder?

(A) Adenocarcinoma
(B) Carcinoid tumor
(C) Crohn disease
(D) Pseudomembranous colitis
(E) Ulcerative colitis

43 A 21-year-old man is brought to the emergency room with symptoms of acute intestinal obstruction. His temperature is 38°C (101°F), respirations are 25 per minute, and blood pressure is 120/80 mm Hg. Physical examination reveals a mass in the right lower abdominal quadrant. The patient subsequently undergoes surgery, and a segmental lesion involving the terminal ileum is resected (shown in the image). Which of the following is the most likely diagnosis?

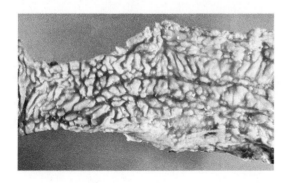

(A) Adenocarcinoma
(B) Carcinoid tumor
(C) Crohn disease
(D) Pseudomembranous colitis
(E) Ulcerative colitis

44 A 24-year-old man is brought to the emergency room with symptoms of acute intestinal obstruction. His temperature is 38°C (101°F), respirations are 25 per minute, and blood pressure is 120/80 mm Hg. Physical examination reveals a mass in the right lower abdominal quadrant. At laparoscopy, there are numerous small bowel strictures and a fistula extending into a loop of small bowel. Which of the following is the most likely diagnosis?

(A) Adenocarcinoma
(B) Carcinoid tumor
(C) Crohn disease
(D) Pseudomembranous colitis
(E) Ulcerative colitis

45 A 30-year-old woman presents with 2 days of abdominal cramping and diarrhea. Her temperature is 38°C (101°F), respirations are 32 per minute, and blood pressure is 100/65 mm Hg. Stool culture shows a toxigenic *Escherichia coli* infection. Which of the following best explains the pathogenicity of this organism in this patient?

(A) Destruction of Peyer patches
(B) Invasion of the mucosa of the colon
(C) Invasion of the mucosa of the ileum
(D) Stimulation of acute inflammation in the superficial bowel mucosa
(E) Stimulation of fluid transport into the lumen of the intestine

46 A 1-year-old girl is brought to the emergency room by her parents who report that she had a fever and diarrhea for 3 days. The child's temperature is 38°C (101°F). The CBC shows a normal WBC count and increased hematocrit. Which of the following microorganisms is the most likely cause of diarrhea in this young child?

(A) Cytomegalovirus
(B) Rotavirus
(C) *Salmonella typhi*
(D) *Shigella dysenteriae*
(E) *Yersinia jejuni*

47 A 70-year-old man is rushed to the emergency room complaining of severe abdominal pain and rectal bleeding of 2 hours in duration. He has a history of coronary artery disease. Bowel sounds are absent on physical examination. A CT scan of the abdomen shows distention of the stomach and air-fluid levels in the small bowel. Abdominal pain and bleeding in this patient most likely involved acute occlusion of which of the following arteries?

(A) Celiac trunk
(B) Gastroduodenal artery
(C) Inferior mesenteric artery
(D) Inferior rectal artery
(E) Superior mesenteric artery

48   A 16-year-old girl complains of chronic abdominal distention, flatulence, and diarrhea after drinking milk. Elimination of milk and other dairy products from the patient's diet relieves these symptoms. This example of malabsorption is caused by a functional deficiency of which of the following enzymes associated with the intestinal brush border membrane?

(A) Disaccharidase
(B) Glycogen phosphorylase
(C) Hyaluronidase
(D) Mannosidase
(E) Sphingomyelinase

49   A 2-year-old girl with a history of chronic constipation since birth is brought to the emergency room because of nausea and vomiting. Physical examination shows marked abdominal distension. Abdominal radiography reveals distended bowel loops with a paucity of air in the rectum. A rectal biopsy shows an absence of ganglion cells. Which of the following is the most likely diagnosis?

(A) Acquired megacolon
(B) Anorectal stenosis
(C) Hirschsprung disease
(D) Imperforate anus
(E) Rectal atresia

50   A 25-year-old woman presents with persistent bloody diarrhea of 4 weeks' duration. She has experienced severe abdominal cramping for the past 3 days. Her temperature is 38°C (101°F), respirations are 22 per minute, and blood pressure is 120/70 mm Hg. Physical examination reveals abdominal tenderness and mild abdominal distension. Bowel sounds are diminished. Laboratory studies show mild hypochromic, normocytic anemia. Stool cultures are negative for pathogens, and no ova or parasites are detected. A blood test for *Clostridium difficile* toxin is negative. Rectosigmoidoscopy shows hemorrhagic mucosal lesions in the distal colorectal region. A biopsy of the colon reveals crypt abscesses, basal lymphoplasmacytosis and crypt distortion. Which of the following represents the most common extraintestinal manifestation of the colonic disorder in this patient?

(A) Arthritis
(B) Cystitis
(C) Gastritis
(D) Pancreatitis
(E) Sepsis

51   A 10-year-old boy is brought to the emergency room after 48 hours of fever and severe abdominal pain. He had developed edema of the legs several weeks previously. The temperature on admission is 38.7°C (103°F). Physical examination shows rebound tenderness, guarding, and ascites. An abdominal tap returns numerous segmented neutrophils. This child's spontaneous bacterial peritonitis is most often associated with which of the following underlying conditions?

(A) Celiac sprue
(B) Diverticulosis
(C) Hirschsprung disease
(D) Meconium ileus
(E) Nephrotic syndrome

52   A 74-year-old woman presents with 3 weeks of left lower quadrant abdominal pain, changes in bowel habits, and intermittent fever. Her temperature is 38°C (101°F), respirations are 19 per minute, and blood pressure is 130/80 mm Hg. Physical examination shows left lower quadrant tenderness. A CBC reveals neutrophilia. An abdominal-pelvic ultrasound examination is normal. Which of the following is the most likely diagnosis?

(A) Appendicitis
(B) Diverticulitis
(C) Ovarian carcinoma
(D) Renal colic
(E) Uterine leiomyoma

53   A 9-year-old boy undergoes emergency surgery for presumptive acute appendicitis. During the operation, the surgeon notices that the boy's ileocecal lymph nodes are enlarged and matted together. One of the nodes is sent for a frozen section. The pathologist finds granulomatous inflammation with central necrosis. The specimen is cultured. Which of the following pathogens is the most likely cause of lymphadenopathy in this patient?

(A) *Campylobacter jejuni*
(B) *Shigella dysenteriae*
(C) Toxigenic *E. coli*
(D) *Vibrio cholerae*
(E) *Yersinia enterocolitica*

54   A 36-year-old man presents with fever and painful joints for 2 weeks. Physical examination shows skin pigmentation, glossitis, angular cheilitis, and generalized lymphadenopathy. The patient has lost 9 kg (20 lb) over the past 6 months. He reports that his stools are pale and foul smelling. Blood cultures are negative. The patient is started on antibiotic therapy and exhibits remarkable clinical improvement. Biopsy of the small intestine shows marked distortion of the intestinal villi, and a periodic acid-Schiff stain reveals large, foamy macrophages filled with glycoprotein-rich granules (shown in the image). Which of the following is the most likely diagnosis?

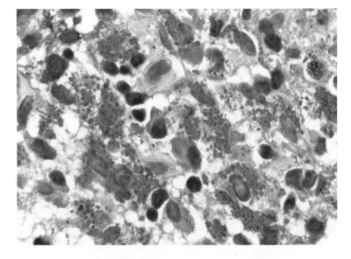

(A) Angiodysplasia of ileum

(B) Crohn disease

(C) Ménétrier disease

(D) Peutz-Jeghers syndrome

(E) Whipple disease

55 Which of the following cellular/biochemical mechanisms best explains the pathogenesis of malabsorption in the patient described in Question 54?

(A) Bile salt inactivation

(B) Blind loop syndrome

(C) Extrahepatic cholestasis

(D) Impaired mucosal function

(E) Obstruction of the common bile duct

56 A 4-year-old girl is brought to the physician because her parents noticed that she has been having pale, fatty, foul-smelling stools. The patient is at the 50th percentile for height and 10th percentile for weight. Her symptoms respond dramatically to a gluten-free diet. Which of the following is the most likely diagnosis?

(A) Celiac sprue

(B) Cystic fibrosis of the pancreas

(C) Ménétrier disease

(D) Tropical sprue

(E) Whipple disease

57 A 53-year-old woman complains of acute diarrhea and severe abdominal pain. She was recently treated with broad-spectrum antibiotics for community-acquired pneumonia. A CBC shows a WBC count of 24,000/μL. The patient subsequently develops septic shock and dies. A portion of her colon is shown at autopsy. These findings are typical of which of the following gastrointestinal diseases?

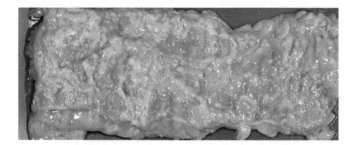

(A) Crohn disease

(B) Diverticulitis

(C) Ischemic colitis

(D) Pseudomembranous colitis

(E) Ulcerative colitis

58 Physical examination of a newborn female after delivery reveals an imperforate anus. Meconium is visible behind the thin, cutaneous membrane. The classification of this anorectal malformation is based on the relationship of the terminal bowel to which of the following anatomic structures?

(A) Ganglia in the wall of the rectum

(B) Inferior mesenteric artery

(C) Levator ani muscle

(D) Muscularis mucosae of rectum

(E) Urachus

59 In addition to anorectal malformation, the infant described in Question 58 is most likely to have which of the following birth defects?

(A) Cleft lip/cleft palate

(B) Congenital pyloric stenosis

(C) Esophageal atresia

(D) Gastrointestinal fistula

(E) Persistent urachus

60 A 2-year-old boy is brought to the emergency room with a 48-hour history of nausea, vomiting, and abdominal discomfort. Physical examination reveals right lower quadrant guarding. Ultrasound examination of the abdomen reveals a 2-cm mass in the right iliac fossa. A segment of the small intestine is removed (shown in the image). Which of the following best describes this pathologic finding?

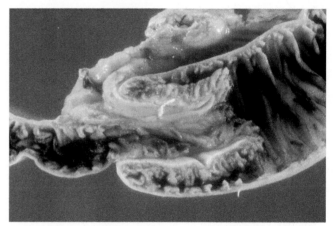

(A) Intestinal infarct

(B) Intussusception

(C) Meckel diverticulum

(D) Peutz-Jeghers polyps

(E) Volvulus

61 An 85-year-old man complains of abdominal pain and bright red blood in his stool. An X-ray film of the abdomen shows fecal impaction in the rectosigmoid region. Which of the following pathologic lesions is most likely to be found in this patient?

(A) Curling ulcer

(B) Cushing ulcer

(C) Melanosis coli

(D) Peptic ulcer

(E) Stercoral ulcer

62 A 45-year-old woman complains of chronic, right lower quadrant pain. An abdominal CT scan reveals a globular, smooth-walled mass protruding into the cecum. The patient subsequently has the mass removed and the surgical specimen is shown in the image. Which of the following is the most likely diagnosis?

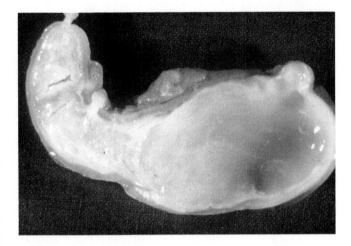

(A) Acute appendicitis
(B) Adenocarcinoma
(C) Carcinoid tumor
(D) Foreign body
(E) Mucocele of the appendix

63 A 70-year-old woman with a history of ovarian cancer presents with diarrhea. She completed radiation therapy for her cancer 3 months ago. Physical examination shows cachexia, hyperactive bowel sounds, and generalized pallor. The stools are found to contain blood. A CBC shows decreased hemoglobin (7.8 g/dL) and decreased mean corpuscular volume (70 μm³). Which of the following is the most likely cause of GI bleeding in this patient?
(A) Angiodysplasia
(B) Hemorrhoids
(C) Ischemic colitis
(D) Radiation enterocolitis
(E) Solitary rectal ulcer

ANSWERS

1 **The answer is A: Achalasia.** Achalasia is characterized by failure of the lower esophageal sphincter to relax in response to swallowing and the absence of peristalsis in the body of the esophagus. As a result of these defects in both the outflow tract and the pumping mechanisms of the esophagus, food is retained within the esophagus, and the organ hypertrophies and dilates. Achalasia is associated with a depletion or absence of ganglion cells in the myenteric plexuses, which regulate contraction of the esophagus. In Latin America, achalasia can be a manifestation of Chagas disease, in which the ganglion cells are destroyed by *Trypanosoma cruzi*. The other choices are usually associated with visible mucosal abnormalities and do not primarily affect peristalsis.
Diagnosis: Achalasia

2 **The answer is D: Esophageal web.** Esophageal rings and webs cause dysphagia. Webs are thin mucosal membranes that project into the lumen of the esophagus. Rings are thicker than webs and contain smooth muscle. The clinical symptoms of esophageal webs and rings include dysphagia, esophageal substernal pain, and aspiration or regurgitation of foods and liquids. Plummer-Vinson syndrome is characterized by a cervical esophageal web, mucosal lesions of the mouth and pharynx, and iron-deficiency anemia. Carcinoma of the oropharynx and upper esophagus are complications of Plummer-Vinson syndrome. The other choices are not associated with anemia. Schatzki ring (choice E) occurs near the gastroesophageal junction.
Diagnosis: Esophageal web

3 **The answer is B: Dysphagia.** This patient exhibits signs of scleroderma (progressive systemic sclerosis), which is characterized by vasculopathy and excessive collage deposition in the skin and internal organs. Patients often suffer from intermittent episodes of ischemia of the fingers, marked by pallor, paresthesias, and pain (Raynaud phenomenon). Anti–Scl-70 antibodies to nuclear topoisomerase are virtually specific for this autoimmune disease. Scleroderma can involve any portion of the gastrointestinal tract, although esophageal dysfunction is the most common and troublesome complication. The disease affects principally the lower esophageal sphincter, which may become so impaired that the lower esophagus and upper stomach are no longer distinct functional entities. In some affected patients, there may be a lack of peristalsis in the entire esophagus. The other choices are not associated with scleroderma.
Diagnosis: Scleroderma

4 **The answer is D: Glandular metaplasia** The biopsy shows Barrett esophagus, which is defined as a replacement of the esophageal squamous epithelium by columnar epithelium as a result of chronic gastroesophageal reflux. This disorder occurs typically in the lower third of the esophagus. The lesion is characterized histologically by distinctive intestine-like epithelium composed of goblet cells and surface cells similar to those of incompletely intestinalized gastric mucosa. Complete intestinal metaplasia, with Paneth cells and absorptive cells, may occur. Barrett esophagus is more resistant to peptic juices than normal squamous epithelium and appears to be an adaptive mechanism that serves to limit the harmful effects of gastroesophageal reflux. None of the other choices lead to metaplastic changes.
Diagnosis: Barrett esophagus, reflux esophagitis

5 **The answer is B: Adenocarcinoma.** Barrett esophagus carries a serious risk of malignant transformation to adenocarcinoma, and the risk correlates with the length of the involved esophagus and the degree of dysplasia. Virtually all esophageal adenocarcinomas arise in the background of the metaplastic epithelium of Barrett esophagus. The symptoms and clinical course of adenocarcinoma of the esophagus are similar to those of squamous cell carcinoma and include dysphagia, pain, and, occasionally, bleeding. None of the other choices reflect a complication of Barrett esophagus.
Diagnosis: Barrett esophagus

6 The answer is E: Zenker diverticulum. Zenker diverticulum is an uncommon lesion that appears high in the esophagus and affects men more than women. It was once believed to result from luminal pressure exerted in a structurally weak area and was, therefore, classed as a pulsion diverticulum. The cause is probably more complicated, but disordered function of the cricopharyngeal musculature is still thought to be involved in the pathogenesis of this false diverticulum. Most affected persons who come to medical attention are older than 60 years, an observation that supports the belief that Zenker diverticulum is an acquired lesion. Epiphrenic diverticuli (choice A) are located immediately above the diaphragm. Intramural pseudodiverticulum (choice B) is characterized by numerous small diverticula in the wall of the esophagus. Traction diverticuli (choice D) are outpouchings that occur principally in the midportion of the esophagus.

Diagnosis: Zenker diverticulum

7 The answer is D: Hiatal hernia. Hiatal hernia is a protrusion of the stomach through an enlarged esophageal hiatus in the diaphragm. Two basic types of hiatal hernia are observed. In sliding hiatal hernias, an enlargement of the hiatus and laxity of the circumferential connective tissue allows a cap of gastric mucosa to move upward above the diaphragm. Paraesophageal hiatal hernias are characterized by herniation of a portion of the gastric fundus alongside the esophagus through a defect in the diaphragmatic connective tissue membrane that defines the esophageal hiatus. Symptoms of hiatal hernia, particularly heartburn and regurgitation, are attributed to the reflux of gastric contents, which is primarily related to incompetence of the lower esophageal sphincter. Classically, the symptoms are exacerbated when the affected person is recumbent. Large herniations carry a risk of gastric volvulus or intrathoracic gastric dilation. Boerhaave syndrome (choice A) represents rupture of the esophagus as a result of vomiting. Mallory-Weiss syndrome (choice E) refers to mucosal laceration of the upper stomach and lower esophagus in the setting of severe retching.

Diagnosis: Paraesophagic hiatal hernia

8 The answer is B: Coagulative necrosis. Chemical injury to the esophagus usually reflects accidental poisoning in children, attempted suicide in adults, or contact with medication. Ingestion of strong acids produces an immediate coagulative necrosis in the esophagus, which results in a protective eschar that limits injury and further chemical penetration. By contrast, ingestion of strong alkaline solutions is accompanied by liquefactive necrosis (choice E), with inflammation and saponification of membrane lipids. Alkaline solutions are particularly insidious because they are generally odorless and tasteless and, therefore, easily swallowed before protective reflexes come into play.

Diagnosis: Chemical esophagitis

9 The answer is A: Adenocarcinoma. Adenocarcinoma of the esophagus is now more common (60%) in the United States than squamous carcinoma. Adenocarcinoma originates in the glandular metaplasia of Barrett esophagus. Endoscopic surveillance for adenocarcinoma is now commonly done in patients with Barrett esophagus, particularly those with dysplasia. Tumors tend to grow into the lumen of the esophagus.

The affected region of the esophagus is typically indurated and ulcerated, causing pain and bleeding. The other choices do not exhibit the histologic features described.

Diagnosis: Adenocarcinoma of the esophagus

10 The answer is D: Squamous cell carcinoma. Most cancers of the esophagus worldwide are squamous cell carcinomas, although adenocarcinoma is now more common in the United States. Squamous cell tumors range from well-differentiated cancers with "epithelial pearls" to poorly differentiated neoplasms that lack evidence of squamous differentiation. The most common presenting complaint of patients with esophageal cancer is dysphagia, but by this time, most tumors are unresectable. Adenocarcinoma (choice A) and Barrett esophagus (choice B) are incorrect because the biopsy does not show glandular features. Primary malignant melanoma (choice C) of the esophagus is extremely rare, although melanoma metastases to the esophagus may occur.

Diagnosis: Squamous cell carcinoma of the esophagus

11 The answer is A: Cigarette smoking. Risk factors for squamous cell carcinoma of the esophagus include chronic alcoholism, tobacco use, diets lacking in fresh fruits, exposure to aniline dyes, chronic esophagitis, and congenital disorders of the esophagus (e.g., Plummer-Vinson syndrome). Cigarette smoking is associated with a 5- to 10-fold increased risk of esophageal cancer, and the number of cigarettes smoked correlates with the presence of dysplasia in the esophageal epithelium. Epidemiologic data suggest that there are additional, as yet unidentified risk factors prevalent in certain geographical regions of the world (China, Iran, and South Africa). Reflux esophagitis (choice E) leads to Barrett esophagus and adenocarcinoma. Aflatoxin (choice B) is a well-known hepatotoxin linked to the development of hepatocellular carcinoma. Herpetic esophagitis (choice C) frequently occurs in immunocompromised persons but is not associated with the development of carcinoma.

Diagnosis: Esophageal cancer

12 The answer is C: Reflux esophagitis. Esophagitis may be caused by infections, reflux of gastric juice, or exogenous irritants. Of these, the most common type is reflux esophagitis, which is often found in conjunction with a sliding hiatal hernia but may also arise through an incompetent lower esophageal sphincter without any demonstrable anatomical lesion. Chronic exposure to stomach juice causes reactive thickening of the squamous epithelium (leukoplakia) and the underlying stroma. Areas affected by gastric reflux are susceptible to mucosal erosions and ulcers which appear as linear vertical streaks. Neutrophils and lymphocytes accumulate in the mucosa. The other choices are not typical complications of hiatal hernia.

Diagnosis: Reflux esophagitis, hiatal hernia

13 The answer is B: *Candida* esophagitis. *Candida* esophagitis has become commonplace because of an increasing number of immunocompromised persons. Esophageal candidiasis also occurs in patients with diabetes and in those receiving antibiotic therapy. The pseudomembranes are composed of fungal mycelia, fibrin, and necrotic debris. Involvement of deeper layers of the esophageal wall can lead to disseminated candidiasis, as well as fibrosis, which is sometimes severe enough to create esophageal stricture. Symptoms include dysphagia and odynophagia (pain on swallowing). Herpetic esophagitis (choice C) features mucosal vesicles. The other choices are not characterized by the formation of elevated white plaques on the esophageal mucosa.

Diagnosis: Infective esophagitis

14 The answer is E: Portal hypertension. Esophageal varices are dilated (varicose) veins immediately beneath the mucosa, which are prone to rupture and hemorrhage. They arise in the lower third of the esophagus, most often in the setting of portal hypertension, secondary to cirrhosis. The lower esophageal veins are linked to the portal system through gastroesophageal anastomoses. If the portal blood pressure exceeds a critical level, these anastomoses become prominent. When varices become greater than 5 mm in diameter, they are likely to rupture, in which case life-threatening hemorrhage may ensue. The other choices are not associated with bleeding esophageal varices. Alcoholic hepatitis (choice A) by itself does not cause varices, but long-term alcohol abuse often leads to cirrhosis and esophageal varices.

Diagnosis: Esophageal varices, cirrhosis

15 The answer is B: Congenital pyloric stenosis. Congenital pyloric stenosis is a concentric enlargement of the pyloric canal that obstructs the outlet of the stomach. The disorder is the most common indication for abdominal surgery in the first 6 months of life. Congenital pyloric stenosis has a familial tendency, and the condition is more common in identical twins than in fraternal ones. The only consistent microscopic abnormality is hypertrophy of the circular muscle coat. Projectile vomiting is not characteristic of the other choices, particularly in neonates.

Diagnosis: Congenital pyloric stenosis

16 The answer is A: Acute erosive gastritis. Acute hemorrhagic gastritis is characterized by necrosis of the mucosa and is commonly associated with the intake of aspirin, other NSAIDs, alcohol, or ischemic injury. The factor common to all forms of acute hemorrhagic gastritis is thought to be the breakdown of the mucosal barrier, which permits acid-induced injury. Mucosal injury causes bleeding from superficial erosions. Defects in the mucosa may extend into the deeper tissues to form an ulcer. The necrosis is accompanied by an acute inflammatory response and hemorrhage, which may be severe enough to result in exsanguination and hypovolemic shock. The other choices are not associated with the use of NSAIDs.

Diagnosis: Acute erosive gastritis

17 The answer is B: Autoimmune gastritis. Autoimmune gastritis refers to chronic, diffuse inflammatory disease of the stomach that is restricted to the body and fundus and is associated with other autoimmune phenomena. This disorder typically features diffuse atrophic gastritis, antibodies to parietal cells and the intrinsic factor, and increased serum gastrin due to G-cell hyperplasia. Immunologic destruction of parietal cells and antibody targeting of intrinsic factor interfere with intestinal absorption of vitamin B_{12}. As a result, all lineages of bone marrow precursors show asynchronous maturation between the nucleus and cytoplasm (megaloblastic cells), and the peripheral blood displays megaloblastic anemia. Megaloblastic

anemia that is caused by malabsorption of vitamin B_{12}, occasioned by a deficiency of the intrinsic factor, is referred to as "pernicious anemia." The other choices are not causes of pernicious anemia.

Diagnosis: Autoimmune atrophic gastritis, pernicious anemia

18 The answer is E: *Helicobacter pylori* infection. Peptic ulcer disease refers to breaks in the mucosa of the stomach and small intestine, principally the proximal duodenum, which are produced by the action of gastric secretions. The pathogenesis of peptic ulcer disease is believed to involve an underlying chronic gastritis caused by *H. pylori*. This pathogen has been isolated from the gastric antrum of virtually all patients with duodenal ulcers and from about 75% of those with gastric ulcers. *H. pylori* gastritis is the most common type of gastritis in the United States and is characterized by prominent chronic inflammation of the antrum and body of the stomach. In addition to peptic ulcer disease, *H. pylori* gastritis is a risk factor for development of gastric adenocarcinoma and lymphoma. Eradication of *H. pylori* infection is curative of peptic ulcer disease in most patients. Gastrinoma (choice D) is a rare cause of peptic ulcers. Achlorhydria (choice A) is incorrect because the formation of peptic ulcers requires at least some gastric acid secretion.

Diagnosis: Chronic infectious gastritis, peptic ulcer disease, gastric ulcer

19 The answer is C: Melena. Peptic ulcers of the stomach and duodenum are estimated to afflict 10% of the population of Western industrialized countries at some time during their lives. Peptic ulcers appear as punched out, rounded ulcers. Erosion through arteries causes bleeding and iron-deficiency anemia. Melena refers to black, tarry stools composed largely of blood from the upper digestive tract that has been processed by the action of gastric juices. Melena is commonly seen in patients who suffer from chronic peptic ulcer disease. Unlike duodenal ulcers, most patients with gastric ulcers secrete normal or decreased amounts of gastric acid (see choice B).

Diagnosis: Peptic ulcer disease, gastric ulcer

20 The answer is B: Intrinsic factor. This patient has chronic lymphocytic thyroiditis (Hashimoto thyroiditis) and pernicious anemia. Pernicious anemia is a megaloblastic anemia that is caused by malabsorption of vitamin B_{12} due to a deficiency of the intrinsic factor. In many cases, pernicious anemia is associated with other autoimmune diseases (e.g., Hashimoto thyroiditis, Graves disease, Addison disease, or diabetes mellitus type 1). Circulating antibodies to parietal cells, some of which are cytotoxic in the presence of complement, occur in 90% of patients with pernicious anemia. Two thirds of patients display an antibody to the intrinsic factor that prevents its combination with vitamin B_{12}, thereby preventing formation of the complex that is later absorbed in the ileum. Half of all patients with pernicious anemia have circulating antibodies to thyroid tissue.

Diagnosis: Pernicious anemia, Hashimoto thyroiditis

21 The answer is E: Pancreas. Zollinger-Ellison syndrome is characterized by unrelenting peptic ulceration in the stomach or duodenum (or even proximal jejunum) by the action of tumor-derived gastrin. Gastrin-producing neuroendocrine tumors (gastrinomas) usually arise in the pancreatic islets. Among islet cell tumors, pancreatic gastrinomas are second in frequency only to insulinomas. Duodenum (choice C) is incorrect because only 15% of cases of Zollinger-Ellison syndrome are due to gastrinomas outside the pancreas (e.g., duodenum). Most gastrinomas are malignant.

Diagnosis: Zollinger-Ellison syndrome, peptic ulcer disease, gastric ulcer

22 The answer is B: Adenocarcinoma. Adenocarcinoma of the stomach accounts for more than 95% of all malignant gastric tumors. Most patients have metastases by the time they are seen for examination. The most frequent initial symptom of gastric cancer is weight loss, usually associated with anorexia and nausea. Most patients complain of epigastric pain—a symptom that mimics benign gastric ulcer disease, and is often relieved by antacids or H2-receptor antagonists. On gross inspection, gastric cancer appears as a polypoid, fungating, or ulcerated mass, or diffuse infiltration of the stomach wall. This patient has an ulcerating carcinoma. Acute erosive gastritis (choice A) and peptic ulcer disease (choice E) do not typically present with rapid weight loss, and these benign ulcers usually do not have heaped-up (raised), ragged margins. Curling ulcers (choice C) occur in severely burned patients.

Diagnosis: Gastric adenocarcinoma

23 The answer is D: Linitis plastica. Diffuse adenocarcinoma constitutes10% of all stomach cancers. No true tumor mass is seen macroscopically. Instead, the wall of the stomach is conspicuously thickened and firm, accounting for the radiologic "leather bottle" appearance. When the entire stomach is involved, the term linitis plastica is applied. The invading tumor cells induce extensive fibrosis in the submucosa and muscularis of the stomach wall. Gastric carcinomas typically metastasize to regional lymph nodes and the liver. Signet ring cells are so named because intracellular mucin displaces the nuclei to the periphery of the tumor cells. Gastric carcinomas and linitis plastica, in particular, have a poor prognosis. The other choices do not show the characteristic morphologic appearance of linitis plastica and generally do not exhibit signet ring cells.

Diagnosis: Gastric adenocarcinoma

24 The answer is B: Enlarged rugal folds. Ménétrier disease (hyperplastic hypersecretory gastropathy) is an uncommon disorder of the stomach characterized by enlarged rugae. It is often accompanied by a severe loss of plasma proteins (including albumin) from the altered gastric mucosa. The disease occurs in two forms: a childhood form due to cytomegalovirus infection and an adult form attributed to overexpression of TGF-α. The folds of the greater curvature in the fundus and body of the stomach (occasionally in the antrum) are increased in height and thickness, forming a convoluted brain-like surface. The other choices do not feature protein-losing enteropathy.

Diagnosis: Ménétrier disease

25 The answer is C: Gastrointestinal stromal tumor (GIST). GISTs are derived from the pacemaker cells of Cajal. They include the vast majority of mesenchyme-derived stromal tumors of the entire gastrointestinal tract. Gastric GISTs are usually submucosal and covered by intact mucosa. Microscopically, the tumors show spindle cells with vacuolated cytoplasms. GISTs are considered to be of low malignant potential and are removed surgically. Gastric adenocarcinoma (choice A) does not often dedifferentiate to a spindle cell morphology.

Diagnosis: Gastrointestinal stromal tumor

26 The answer is B: Gastric lymphoma. Gastric lymphoma is the most common form of extranodal lymphoma, accounting for 20% of all such tumors. Gastric lymphoma has a considerably better prognosis than gastric carcinoma (45% 5-year survival). The clinical symptoms of gastric lymphoma are nonspecific and indistinguishable from those of gastric carcinoma (e.g., weight loss, dyspepsia, and abdominal pain). Most gastric lymphomas are low-grade B-cell neoplasms of the MALToma (mucosa-associated lymphoid tissue) type, which arise in the setting of chronic *Helicobacter pylori* gastritis with lymphoid hyperplasia. Some of these lymphomas regress after eradication of the infection. The other choices do not demonstrate the lymphoid lesion depicted here.

Diagnosis: Gastric lymphoma, MALToma

27 The answer is D: Trichobezoar. Bezoars are foreign bodies in the stomach that are composed of food or hair that have been altered by the digestive process. The mass removed from the stomach in this patient is a hairball (trichobezoar) within a gelatinous matrix. Trichobezoar is usually seen in long-haired girls or young women who eat their own hair as a nervous habit (trichotillomania; also called "Rapunzel" syndrome). Such a trichobezoar may grow by accretion to form a complete cast of the stomach. Strands of hair may extend into the bowel as far as the transverse colon (Rapunzel syndrome). Phytobezoars (choice C) are concretions of plant material, which usually occur in persons with conditions that interfere with gastric emptying.

Diagnosis: Trichobezoar, bezoar, Rapunzel syndrome

28 The answer is A: Bleeding. Bleeding is the most common complication of peptic ulcer disease, occurring in about 20% of patients. Chronic blood loss due to occult bleeding is often a feature of peptic ulcers, whereas massive bleeding occurs less often. Perforation (choice D) is a serious complication that occurs in 5% of patients. Perforating ulcers are commonly encountered in the duodenum. Duodenal peptic ulcers do not undergo malignant transformation (choice B). The other choices are uncommon. Diseases associated with peptic ulcers include cirrhosis, chronic renal failure, hereditary endocrine syndromes (MEN-1), α₁–antitrypsin deficiency, and chronic pulmonary disease.

Diagnosis: Duodenal ulcer, peptic ulcer disease

29 The answer is A: Carcinoid tumor. Carcinoid tumors are low-grade malignant neoplasms composed of neuroendocrine cells, which usually show considerable nuclear uniformity. They are most commonly located in the submucosa of the intestines (appendix, terminal ileum, and rectum). Carcinoids are distinguished from intestinal carcinomas based on their location, histologic features, malignant potential, endocrine activity, and clinical features. Carcinoid syndrome is a systemic paraneoplastic disease caused by the release of hormones from carcinoid tumors into venous blood. Clinical features of carcinoid tumors (e.g., flushing, bronchial wheezing, watery diarrhea, and abdominal colic) are presumably caused by the release of serotonin, bradykinin, and histamine. Release of tumor secretions from hepatic metastases leads to the formation of fibrous plaques in the tricuspid and pulmonic valves and may result in tricuspid insufficiency or pulmonic stenosis. The other choices are not associated with secretion of 5-HIAA acid or other neuroendocrine peptides.

Diagnosis: Carcinoid syndrome

30   The answer is C: Peutz-Jeghers polyp.   Peutz-Jeghers syndrome is an autosomal dominant, hereditary disorder characterized by intestinal hamartomatous polyps and mucocutaneous melanin pigmentation, which is particularly evident on the face, buccal mucosa, hands, feet, and perianal and genital regions. The polyps seen in Peutz-Jeghers syndrome are hamartomatous, characterized by a branching network of smooth muscle fibers continuous with the muscularis mucosa that support the glandular epithelium of the polyp. Congenital teratoma (choice A) does not involve the intestine. The other choices are principally colonic polyps that derive from the luminal epithelium.

Diagnosis: Gastrointestinal polyp, Peutz-Jeghers polyp

31   The answer is B: Hyperplastic polyp.   Hyperplastic polyps are small, sessile mucosal excrescences that display exaggerated crypt architecture. They are the most common polypoid lesions of the colon and are particularly frequent in the rectum. The crypts of hyperplastic polyps are elongated and may exhibit cystic dilations. The epithelium is composed of goblet cells and absorptive cells, without any dysplasia. There are no dysplastic features indicative of adenocarcinoma (choice A). Villous adenomas (choice E) are considerably larger and exhibit prominent thin, tall, fingerlike processes. Peutz-Jeghers polyps (choice D) are hamartomatous.

Diagnosis: Gastrointestinal polyp, hyperplastic polyp

32   The answer is D: Tubular adenoma.   Tubular adenomas constitute two thirds of benign colonic adenomas. They are typically smooth-surface lesions, usually less than 2 cm in diameter, and often have a stalk. Microscopically, tubular adenomas exhibit closely packed epithelial tubules, which may be uniform or irregular with excessive branching. Dysplasia and carcinoma often develop in tubular adenomas. As long as dysplastic foci remain confined to the polyp mucosa, the lesion is almost always cured by resection. Adenocarcinoma (choice A) is incorrect because the lesion does not have dysplastic features. Pseudostratified epithelium is not a feature of carcinoid tumor (choice B) or hyperplastic polyp (choice C). The incorrect choices do not typically exhibit a stalk.

Diagnosis: Gastrointestinal polyp, tubular adenoma

33   The answer is E: Villous adenoma.   These polyps comprise one third of colonic adenomas and are found predominantly in the rectosigmoid region. They are typically large, broad-based, elevated lesions that display a shaggy, cauliflower-like surface. Microscopically, villous adenomas are composed of thin, tall, fingerlike processes, which superficially resemble the villi of small intestine. Compared to tubular adenomas (choice D), villous adenomas more frequently contain foci of carcinoma. Hyperplastic polyps (choice A) have a much lower risk for malignant transformation.

Diagnosis: Gastrointestinal polyp, villous adenoma

34   The answer is A: Adenocarcinoma.   Adenocarcinoma of the rectum or sigmoid colon often presents as a circumferential mass narrowing the intestinal lumen. The gross appearance of the colorectal cancer is similar to that seen elsewhere in the gastrointestinal tract. The most important risk factors associated with the development of colonic adenocarcinoma are age, prior colorectal cancer, ulcerative colitis, genetic factors, and perhaps diet. Colorectal cancer invades lymphatic channels and initially involves the lymph nodes immediately underlying the tumor. As the tumor grows, the most common sign is occult blood in feces. Bright red blood more often occurs in distal lesions. In either case, bleeding typically causes iron-deficiency anemia. Choices B, C, and D are principally lesions of the intestinal wall. Choice E (mucinous cystadenoma) is an ovarian tumor.

Diagnosis: Colorectal cancer, adenocarcinoma of colon

35   The answer is A: _APC_.   The photograph shows numerous adenomas of the colon, consistent with familial adenomatous polyposis (FAP), also termed adenomatous polyposis coli (APC). This autosomal dominant inherited disease accounts for about 1% of colorectal cancers. It is characterized by the progressive development of innumerable adenomatous polyps of the colorectum, particularly in the rectosigmoid region. Germline mutations in the _APC_ gene, a putative tumor suppressor gene, are responsible for FAP. Carcinoma of the colon and rectum is inevitable in these patients, and the mean age of onset is 40 years. The _DCC_ gene ("deleted in colon cancer"— choice C) is a putative tumor suppressor gene that is often missing in colorectal cancers. Activating mutations of the _ras_ protooncogene (choice E) occur early in tubular adenomas of the colon.

Diagnosis: Adenomatous polyposis coli

36   The answer is C: _p53_.   In most cases of colorectal carcinoma, it has been estimated that a minimum of eight to ten mutational events must accumulate before the development of invasive cancer. This process is initiated in morphologically normal mucosa, proceeds through an adenomatous precursor, and terminates as invasive adenocarcinoma. The _APC_ gene is considered to play an important role in the early development of most colorectal neoplasms, whereas mutations in the _p53_ tumor suppressor gene are thought to participate in the late transition from adenoma to carcinoma. _BRCA1_ (choice A) has been implicated in the pathogenesis of breast and ovarian cancers. _VHL_ (choice E) has been incriminated in the pathogenesis of clear cell renal cell carcinoma.

Diagnosis: Adenocarcinoma of colon

37   The answer is E: Metastatic carcinoma.   Metastatic carcinoma is by far the most common malignant disorder affecting the peritoneum. Ovarian, gastric, and pancreatic carcinomas are particularly likely to seed the peritoneum, but any intra-abdominal carcinoma can spread to the peritoneum. Metastatic carcinoma to the abdomen presents in the form of multiple serosal nodules and ascites fluid that contains malignant cells.

Diagnosis: Metastatic carcinoma

38   The answer is C: Kaposi sarcoma.   Kaposi sarcoma of the GI tract is found almost exclusively in patients with AIDS. One third to one half of AIDS patients, with cutaneous Kaposi sarcoma, exhibit involvement of the GI tract. In most patients, intestinal Kaposi sarcoma does not lead to symptoms, although GI bleeding, obstruction, and malabsorption have been reported. The other choices are not specifically associated with AIDS.

Diagnosis: AIDS, Kaposi sarcoma

39 The answer is E: Ulcerative colitis. Ulcerative colitis is an inflammatory disease of the large intestine characterized by chronic diarrhea and rectal bleeding. It is associated with a pattern of remission and exacerbations and the possibility of serious local and systemic complications. The disorder occurs principally, but not exclusively, in young adults. Ulcerative colitis is essentially a disease of the mucosa. The process extends from the rectum for a variable distance proximally and is limited to the colon and rectum. Pseudomembranous colitis (choice D) is usually a complication of antibiotic therapy, and the mucosal surface of the colon is covered by raised, irregular plaques composed of necrotic debris and an acute inflammatory exudate. Crohn disease (choice C) typically affects the colon in a patchy distribution with transmural inflammation.

Diagnosis: Ulcerative colitis

40 The answer is A: Adenocarcinoma. Patients with long-standing ulcerative colitis have a higher risk of developing colorectal cancer (adenocarcinoma) than does the general population. This risk is related to the extent of colorectal involvement and the duration of the inflammatory process. Thus, people with involvement of the entire colon are at the greatest risk of developing colorectal cancer. Intestinal fistula (choice B) is a complication of Crohn disease. Ulcerations in ulcerative colitis are largely confined to the mucosa (not transmural, choice D).

Diagnosis: Ulcerative colitis

41 The correct answer is E: Ulcerative colitis. Primary sclerosing cholangitis (PSC) is characterized by inflammation and obliterative fibrosis of intrahepatic and extrahepatic bile ducts. Approximately 70% of patients with PSC have long-standing ulcerative colitis, although the prevalence of PSC in such patients is only 4%. The clinicopathologic findings are complemented by a characteristic radiographic appearance of a beaded biliary tree, representing sporadic strictures. The other choices are not associated with PSC.

Diagnosis: Primary sclerosing cholangitis, ulcerative colitis

42 The answer is E: Ulcerative colitis. Local complications of ulcerative colitis include toxic megacolon, perforation, inflammatory pseudopolyps, hemorrhage, and adenocarcinoma. The other choices are not associated with the development of toxic megacolon.

Diagnosis: Toxic megacolon, ulcerative colitis

43 The answer is C: Crohn disease. Crohn disease is a transmural, chronic inflammatory disease that may affect any part of the digestive tract but occurs principally in the distal small intestine and occasionally the right colon. It has variously been referred to as terminal ileitis and regional ileitis when it involves the ileum and granulomatous colitis when

it principally affects the colon. Skip lesions are common. The affected mucosa has a characteristic "cobblestone" appearance (shown in the image) due to the presence of linear ulcerations and edema, and inflammation of the intervening tissue. The other choices do not show the characteristic cobblestone morphology that is seen in this case.

Diagnosis: Crohn disease

44 The answer is C: Crohn disease. Crohn disease is a transmural, chronic inflammatory disease that may affect any part of the digestive tract. Intestinal obstruction and fistulas are the most common intestinal complications of Crohn disease. Occasionally, free perforation of the bowel occurs. The risk of small bowel cancer is increased at least threefold in patients with Crohn disease. Pseudomembranous colitis (choice D) and ulcerative colitis (choice E) are not associated with fistula formation. Adenocarcinoma (choice A) rarely, if ever, arises in the terminal ileum.

Diagnosis: Crohn disease

45 The answer is E: Stimulation of fluid transport into the lumen of the intestine. The most significant factor in infectious diarrhea is increased intestinal secretion, stimulated by bacterial toxins and enteric hormones. Organisms that produce diarrhea by secreting specific toxins include *Vibrio cholera* and toxigenic strains of *E. coli*. There is minimal or absent damage to the intestinal mucosa (choices A to D) in cases of toxigenic diarrhea. The organisms remain attached to the intestinal mucosa and elaborate toxins, which stimulate the transmucosal transport of fluid into the lumen, resulting in diarrhea. Patients may become severely dehydrated, particularly in the case of cholera.

Diagnosis: Bacterial diarrhea

46 The answer is B: Rotavirus. Rotavirus is the most common cause of infantile diarrhea and can be demonstrated in duodenal biopsy specimens in half the cases of acute diarrhea in hospitalized children under the age of 2 years. Choices C, D, and E can cause diarrhea, but are uncommon in developed countries.

Diagnosis: Viral diarrhea

47 The answer is E: Superior mesenteric artery. Sudden occlusion of a large artery by thrombosis or embolization leads to small bowel infarction before collateral circulation comes into play. Depending on the size of the artery, infarction may be segmental or may lead to gangrene of virtually the entire small bowel. The small intestine, which is supplied by the superior mesenteric artery, is more likely to suffer transmural hemorrhagic infarction than the large intestine. The inferior mesenteric artery (choice C), which supplies blood to the colon, is a less common site for atherosclerotic embolization than the superior mesenteric artery because of the smaller size of the latter and its oblique origin from the aorta. Pathologically, ischemic bowel disease is classified as occlusive or nonocclusive. Occlusive disease is caused by thrombi or emboli, whereas nonocclusive disease is secondary to arterial narrowing by atherosclerosis. The other choices are not specifically associated with small bowel ischemia.

Diagnosis: Ischemic colitis

48 The answer is A: Disaccharidase. Acquired lactase deficiency is a widespread disorder of carbohydrate absorption. The symptoms of this disease typically begin in adolescence, when patients complain of flatulence and diarrhea after the ingestion of dairy products. Lactose is one of the most common disaccharides in dairy products. The intestinal brush border contains disaccharidases that are important for cleavage of lactose to free glucose and galactose for absorption. Congenital lactase deficiency is rare but may be lethal if not recognized. The other choices do not hydrolyze lactose.

Diagnosis: Lactose intolerance

49 **The answer is C: Hirschsprung disease.** Hirschsprung disease, also referred to as congenital megacolon, results from a congenital defect in the innervation of the large intestine, usually in the rectum. Severe chronic constipation is typical. Marked dilation of the colon occurs proximal to the stenotic rectum, with clinical signs of intestinal obstruction. The other choices are not associated with loss of ganglion cells.

Diagnosis: Hirschsprung disease

50 **The answer is A: Arthritis.** The case history is indicative of ulcerative colitis. Arthritis is seen in 25% of patients with ulcerative colitis. Uveitis and skin lesions develop in approximately 10% of patients. The most common cutaneous lesions are erythema nodosum and pyoderma gangrenosum. Liver disease occurs in about 4% of patients, the most common pathologic findings being pericholangitis and fatty liver. The other choices do not represent extraintestinal manifestations of ulcerative colitis.

Diagnosis: Ulcerative colitis, arthritis

51 **The answer is E: Nephrotic syndrome.** Most cases of peritonitis are caused by bacteria that enter the abdominal cavity from a perforated viscus or through an abdominal wound. However, spontaneous bacterial peritonitis occurs in children without an obvious perforation. Most of these patients have a nephrotic syndrome and a systemic infection that seeds the ascitic fluid with bacteria. In adults, spontaneous bacterial peritonitis is a feared complication of cirrhosis. The other choices are not associated with the development of spontaneous bacterial peritonitis.

Diagnosis: Spontaneous bacterial peritonitis, nephrotic syndrome

52 **The answer is B: Diverticulitis.** Diverticular disease refers to two entities: a condition termed diverticulosis and an inflammatory complication called diverticulitis. Diverticulosis is generally asymptomatic. Diverticulitis results from the irritation caused by retained fecal material that obstructs the lumen of a diverticulum. Clinically, the most common symptoms of diverticulitis usually follow microscopic or gross perforation of the diverticulum. Diverticula are most common in the sigmoid colon, which is affected in 95% of cases. Peritonitis and sepsis are serious complications. Appendicitis (choice A) usually presents with right lower quadrant pain. None of the other choices presents with gastrointestinal symptoms and fever.

Diagnosis: Diverticulitis

53 **The answer is E: _Yersinia enterocolitica._** _Yersinia_ can cause mesenteric adenitis and pain in the right lower quadrant (pseudoappendicitis). Infected children not infrequently have undergone laparotomy because of a mistaken diagnosis of appendicitis. The lymph nodes show a granulomatous inflammation. Other symptoms are diarrhea, reactive arthritis, erythema nodosum, and septicemia. The other choices are not associated with the development of mesenteric adenitis and do not present with symptoms that mimic acute appendicitis.

Diagnosis: _Yersinia_ lymphadenitis

54 **The answer is E: Whipple disease.** Whipple disease is a rare infectious disorder of the small intestine in which malabsorption is the most prominent feature. The disorder typically features infiltration of the small bowel mucosa by macrophages that are packed with small, rod-shaped bacilli (_Tropheryma whippelii_). Infiltrates of macrophages containing bacilli may be found in other organs, including regional lymph nodes and the heart. The other choices do not feature these distinctive aggregates of foamy macrophages.

Diagnosis: Whipple disease

55 **The answer is D: Impaired mucosal function.** Normal intestinal absorption is characterized by a luminal phase and an intestinal phase. The intestinal phase includes those processes that occur in epithelial cells and transport channels. Injury to the mucosa in patients with Whipple disease (secondary to inflammation) results in impaired transport of nutrients through the intestinal wall. Histologic examination of the small intestine reveals flat, thickened villi and extensive infiltration of the lamina propria with foamy macrophages. The other choices pertain to luminal phase processes that are unaffected in patients with Whipple disease.

Diagnosis: Whipple disease

56 **The answer is A: Celiac sprue.** Celiac sprue, which is also referred to as gluten-sensitive enteropathy, is characterized by (1) generalized malabsorption, (2) small intestinal mucosal lesions, and (3) prompt clinical and histopathologic response to the withdrawal of gluten-containing food. Critical factors in the development of celiac sprue include genetic predisposition and gliadin exposure. The hallmark of celiac disease is a flat mucosa, with blunting of villi, damaged epithelial cells, intraepithelial T cells, and increased plasma cells in the lamina propria. The other choices do not respond to a gluten-free diet.

Diagnosis: Celiac sprue

57 **The answer is D: Pseudomembranous colitis.** Pseudomembranous colitis is a generic term for an inflammatory disease of the colon that is characterized by exudative plaques on the mucosa. Antibiotic therapy eliminates the normal mixed flora of the colon and facilitates the overgrowth of _Clostridium difficile_, leading to an acute infection of the colon. The exotoxins produced by _C. difficile_ cause intestinal necrosis, with superficial ulcers covered by a thick fibropurulent exudate. The other choices are not related to antibiotic therapy and are not associated with the development of these exudative plaques.

Diagnosis: Pseudomembranous colitis

58 **The answer is C: Levator ani muscle.** Anorectal malformations are among the most common anomalies and vary from minor narrowing to serious and complex effects. The classification of these anomalies is based on the relation of the terminal bowel to the levator ani muscle. The other choices are not associated with anorectal malformations.

Diagnosis: Anorectal malformation

59 **The answer is D: Gastrointestinal fistula.** Anorectal malformations result from arrested development of the caudal region of the gut in the first 6 months of fetal life. The cause is unknown. Fistulas between the malformation and the bladder, urethra, vagina, or skin may occur in all types of anorectal anomalies. The other choices are not associated with anorectal malformations.

Diagnosis: Anorectal malformation

60 **The answer is B: Intusssesception.** Mechanical obstruction to the passage of intestinal contents can be caused by (1) a luminal mass, (2) an intrinsic lesion of the bowel wall, or (3) extrinsic compression. Obstruction in this case was caused by intussusception, in which a segment of bowel (intussusceptum) protruded distally into a surrounding outer portion (intussuscipiens). This condition is usually a disorder of infants or young children, in whom it occurs without a known cause. In adults, the leading point of an intussusception is usually a lesion in the bowel wall, such as Meckel diverticulum or a tumor. Once the leading point is entrapped in the intussuscipiens, peristalsis drives the intussusceptum forward. In addition to acute intestinal obstruction, intussusception compresses the blood supply to the intussusceptum, which may become infarcted. If the obstruction is not relieved spontaneously, treatment requires surgery. None of the other choices display "telescoping" of the small intestine. Meckle diverticulum (choice C) is an outpouching of the gut caused by persistence of the embryonic vitelline duct. It is the most common congenital anomaly of the small intestine and is usually asymptomatic. Peutz-Jeghers polyps (choice D) are hamartomas of the small intestine. Volvulus (choice E) is an example of intestinal obstruction and acute abdomen, in which a segment of the gut twists on its mesentery, kinking the bowel and usually interrupting its blood supply.

Diagnosis: Intussusception

61 **The answer is E: Stercoral ulcer.** Incomplete evacuation of the feces, usually in association with debilitating disease or old age, may lead to the formation of a large mass of stool that cannot be passed, termed fecal impaction. Stercoral ulcers result from pressure necrosis of the mucosa caused by the fecal mass. Complications include rectal bleeding and perforation. The other ulcers do not occur in the rectum.

Diagnosis: Stercoral ulcer

62 **The answer is E: Mucocele of the appendix.** Mucocele refers to a dilated mucous-filled appendix. The pathogenesis may be neoplastic or nonneoplastic. In the nonneoplastic variety, chronic obstruction leads to the retention of mucus in the appendiceal lumen. In the presence of a mucinous cystadenoma (in this case) or mucinous cystadenocarcinoma, the dilated appendix is lined by a villous adenomatous mucosa. A mucocele may become secondarily infected and rupture. Rupture of a neoplastic mucocele may seed the peritoneal cavity with mucus-secreting tumor cells, a condition referred to as "pseudomyxoma peritonei."

Diagnosis: Mucocele

63 **The answer is D: Radiation enterocolitis.** Radiation therapy for malignant disease of the pelvis or abdomen may be complicated by injury to the small intestine and colon. Clinically significant radiation enterocolitis is most common in the rectum. The lesions produced by radiation therapy range from a reversible injury of the intestinal mucosa to chronic inflammation, ulceration, and fibrosis of the intestine.

Diagnosis: Radiation enterocolitis, ovarian cancer

Chapter 14

The Liver and Biliary System

QUESTIONS

Select the single best answer.

1 A 62-year-old man is brought to the emergency room in a disoriented state. Physical examination reveals signs of poor hygiene and an odor of alcohol, as well as jaundice, splenomegaly, and ascites. The patient has a coarse flapping tremor of the hands, palmar erythema, and diffuse spider angiomata. The abdomen displays dilated paraumbilical veins. Serum levels of ALT, AST, alkaline phosphatase, and bilirubin are all mildly elevated. Soon after admission, the patient vomits a large amount of blood. Which of the following is the most likely underlying cause of hematemesis in this patient?

(A) Acute alcoholic hepatitis
(B) Acute gastritis
(C) Cirrhosis
(D) Hepatic steatosis
(E) Mallory-Weiss tear

2 For the patient described in Question 1, which of the following pathophysiologic mechanisms is most directly associated with the development of ascites?

(A) Decreased aldosterone secretion
(B) Decreased intravascular volume
(C) Hyperalbuminemia
(D) Increased intravascular oncotic pressure
(E) Increased portal hydrostatic pressure

3 An 18-year-old man presents with a 2-week history of yellow skin and sclerae but is otherwise asymptomatic. He recalls a similar episode 2 years previously. His brother also has recurrent jaundice. The serum bilirubin is 5.2 mg/dL, mostly in the unconjugated form. Serum AST and ALT levels are normal, as is the urinalysis. Two weeks later, the jaundice resolves spontaneously. What is the most likely diagnosis?

(A) α_1-Antitrypsin deficiency
(B) Dubin-Johnson syndrome
(C) Gilbert syndrome
(D) Hereditary hemochromatosis
(E) Wilson disease

4 A 48-year-old woman has a 3-week history of fatigue as well as yellow skin and sclerae. Physical examination is unremarkable except for mild jaundice. The serum bilirubin level is 3.7 mg/dL, mostly in the unconjugated form. Liver function tests including serum AST, ALT, and alkaline phosphatase are normal. The hemoglobin level is 6.0 g/dL. After corticosteroids are administered, the jaundice resolves. Which of the following diseases is the most likely cause of hyperbilirubinemia in this patient?

(A) Acute hepatitis B infection
(B) Autoimmune hemolytic anemia
(C) Gallstone in the common bile duct
(D) Primary biliary cirrhosis
(E) Primary sclerosing cholangitis

5 A 20-year-old woman presents with a 2-week history of fever, malaise, and brown-colored urine. She recently visited Mexico. Physical examination reveals jaundice, mild hepatomegaly, and tenderness in the right upper quadrant. The serum bilirubin is 7.8 mg/dL, with 60% in the conjugated form. Serum levels of AST and ALT are markedly elevated (400 and 392 U/L, respectively). Serum albumin and immunoglobulin levels are normal. Serum IgM anti–hepatitis A virus (anti-HAV) is positive. IgG anti–hepatitis B surface antigen (anti-HBsAg) antibodies are positive. Anti–hepatitis C virus antibodies are negative. What is the most likely diagnosis?

(A) Acute viral hepatitis A
(B) Acute viral hepatitis B
(C) Acute viral hepatitis C
(D) Autoimmune hepatitis
(E) Chronic viral hepatitis B

6 A 3-day-old neonate born after a 32-week gestation develops yellow skin. Physical examination of the infant is unremarkable. Which of the following is most likely to be increased in this neonate's serum?

(A) Alanine aminotransferase
(B) Carotene
(C) Conjugated bilirubin
(D) Galactosyltransferase
(E) Unconjugated bilirubin

7 A previously healthy 38-year-old man complains of yellow discoloration of his eyes, abdominal pain, and low-grade fever of 1-month duration. Physical examination demonstrates a distended abdomen, right upper quadrant tenderness, and a palpable liver edge 2 cm below the right costal margin. Total serum bilirubin is 7.4 mg/dL. Serum levels of AST and ALT are elevated (229 and 495 U/L, respectively). The prothrombin time is prolonged (18 seconds). A liver biopsy is shown in the image. The arrows point to Councilman bodies. The pathologic findings are indicative of which of the following liver diseases?

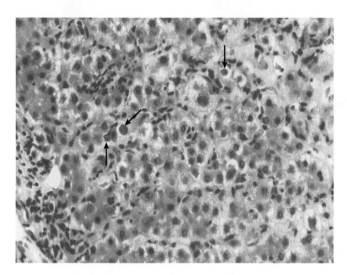

(A) Acute viral hepatitis
(B) Alcoholic cirrhosis
(C) Cardiac cirrhosis
(D) Hemochromatosis
(E) Primary biliary cirrhosis

8 A 30-year-old man presents with a 9-month history of fatigue and recurrent fever. He also complains of yellow skin and sclerae, abdominal tenderness, and dark urine. Physical examination reveals jaundice and mild hepatomegaly. Laboratory studies demonstrate elevated serum bilirubin (3.1 mg/ dL), decreased serum albumin (2.5 g/dL), and prolonged prothrombin time (17 seconds). Serologic tests reveal antibodies to hepatitis B core antigen (IgG anti-HBcAg). The serum is positive for HBsAg and HbeAg. A liver biopsy is shown in the image. What is the most likely diagnosis?

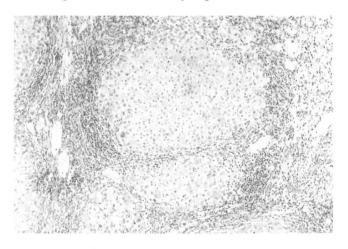

(A) Acute hepatitis B
(B) Alcoholic hepatitis
(C) Chronic hepatitis B
(D) Delta virus infection
(E) Subacute hepatic necrosis secondary to hepatitis B infection

9 The patient described in Question 8 is most likely to develop which of the following vascular inflammatory diseases?
(A) Allergic angiitis
(B) Buerger disease
(C) Giant cell arteritis
(D) Polyarteritis nodosa
(E) Wegener granulomatosis

10 A 40-year-old woman presents with a long history of vague upper abdominal pain and frequent indigestion. Physical examination reveals an obese woman with jaundice and abdominal tenderness. Serum bilirubin is elevated (4.2 mg/dL). There is a mild increase in serum AST and ALT (62 and 57 U/L, respectively) and a moderate increase in alkaline phosphatase (325 U/L). Markers for viral hepatitis are negative. Abdominal ultrasound examination shows echogenic stone-like material within the gallbladder and thickening of the gallbladder wall. An intrahepatic mass is also visualized adjacent to the gallbladder. A cholecystectomy is performed. Histologic examination shows dense fibrosis and glandular structures in the wall of the gallbladder. What is the most likely diagnosis?
(A) Carcinoma of the gallbladder
(B) Hemangiosarcoma
(C) Hepatic adenoma
(D) Hepatocellular carcinoma
(E) Metastatic carcinoma of the stomach

11 A 60-year-old man is found in a state of disorientation and is brought to the emergency room in a comatose state. He lived alone, ate poorly, and drank large amounts of hard liquor. Physical examination reveals an emaciated man with a distended abdomen, jaundice, ascites, and a slightly enlarged liver and spleen. A liver biopsy is shown in the image. What blood test would confirm a diagnosis of hepatic coma?

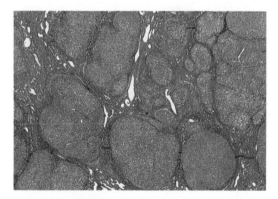

(A) Alanine aminotransferase
(B) Alkaline phosphatase
(C) Ammonia
(D) Bilirubin
(E) Urea nitrogen

12 A 20-year-old woman presents with a 4-week history of dry mouth, fatigue, fever, and yellow sclerae. Physical examination shows mild jaundice and hepatomegaly. Serum total bilirubin is 3.3 mg/dL. Serologic markers for viral hepatitis are negative. The anti–mitochondrial antibody test is negative. A liver biopsy discloses parenchymal and periportal inflammatory cell infiltrates composed primarily of lymphocytes and plasma cells. The patient's signs and symptoms abate following 2 months of treatment with steroids. Which of the following is the most likely diagnosis?

(A) Autoimmune hepatitis
(B) Extrahepatic jaundice
(C) Primary biliary cirrhosis
(D) Primary sclerosing cholangitis
(E) Wilson disease

13 A 52-year-old recent immigrant from Vietnam complains of abdominal swelling, weight loss, and upper abdominal pain of 3 weeks in duration. His past medical history includes malaria and infection with the liver fluke *Clonorchis sinensis*. The liver is hard to palpation. An abdominal CT scan shows a hypoattenuated mass with lobulated margins in the liver. A biopsy discloses well-differentiated neoplastic glands embedded in a dense fibrous stroma. Which of the following is the most likely diagnosis?

(A) Carcinoma of the gallbladder
(B) Cholangiocarcinoma
(C) Hemangiosarcoma
(D) Hepatocellular carcinoma
(E) Metastatic colon adenocarcinoma

14 A 58-year-old man with longstanding alcoholic cirrhosis presents with abdominal pain, fever, and an episode of hematemesis. Physical examination reveals jaundice and a markedly distended abdomen. The patient is disoriented and has a coarse flapping tremor of the hands. Laboratory studies reveal modestly elevated serum levels of AST and ALT (96 and 92 U/L, respectively) and a high serum level of alkaline phosphatase (320 U/L). Prothrombin time is prolonged (20 seconds). The WBC count is 18,000/μL. Shortly after admission, the patient develops coma, adult respiratory distress syndrome, and renal failure (oliguria and elevated serum levels of BUN and creatinine), leading to death within 3 days. Histologic examination of the patient's kidney at autopsy would most likely show which of the following?

(A) Interstitial nephritis
(B) Membranous nephropathy
(C) No histologic changes
(D) Proliferative glomerulonephritis
(E) Pyelonephritis

15 A liver biopsy in the patient described in Question 14 would definitely show which of the following pathologic changes?

(A) Dilated bile ducts and portal inflammation
(B) Fatty liver
(C) Nodular regeneration and scarring
(D) Periportal necrosis and peripheral cholestasis
(E) Scattered single cell necrosis and acidophilic bodies

16 A 40-year-old black woman has frequent indigestion after meals and abdominal pain. Physical examination demonstrates a moderately obese woman in no acute distress. An ultrasound examination demonstrates numerous echogenic objects within the gallbladder. A cholecystectomy is performed, and the surgical specimen is shown in the image. The gallstones seen in this patient are typically associated with which of the following diseases?

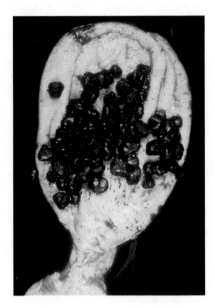

(A) Chronic pancreatitis
(B) Diabetes mellitus
(C) Familial hypercholesterolemia
(D) Hyperparathyroidism
(E) Sickle cell disease

17 A 25-year-old heroin addict presents in a disoriented state with a 5-day history of fatigue, malaise, and dark-colored urine. Physical examination reveals jaundice and multiple petechial hemorrhages on the upper extremities. Laboratory studies show serum bilirubin of 15.6 mg/dL, mostly in the conjugated form, 10-fold elevations of serum AST and ALT, high levels of blood ammonia, and increased prothrombin time (15 seconds). The patient's condition deteriorates and he develops stage 4 hepatic encephalopathy. A liver biopsy is shown in the image. Which of the following viruses is most likely responsible for the clinical and pathologic findings in this patient?

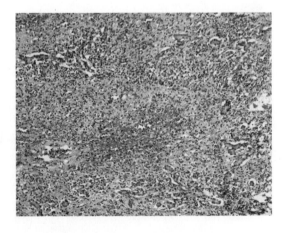

(A) Cytomegalovirus
(B) Hepatitis A virus
(C) Hepatitis B virus
(D) Hepatitis C virus
(E) Hepatitis E virus

18 A 25-year-old woman complains of sudden onset of acute abdominal pain. Physical examination shows abdominal distention. Her temperature is 37°C (98.6°F), respirations 22 per minute, heart rate 110 per minute, and blood pressure 70/50 mm Hg. A tap of the abdomen returns blood. A CT scan reveals a solitary 20-cm mass of the liver. A surgically resected portion of the liver is shown in the image. This patient's tumor was most likely associated with chronic exposure to which of the following?

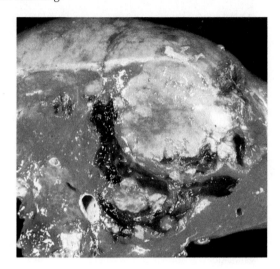

(A) Carbon tetrachloride
(B) Halothane
(C) L-thyroxine
(D) Oral contraceptives
(E) Vinyl chloride

19 A 15-year-old boy complains of a 2-month history of fatigue, abdominal pain, and yellow eyes and skin. Physical examination shows tremor of his hands, lack of coordination, and mild jaundice. The results of an ophthalmic examination are shown in the image. This patient most likely has an inborn error of metabolism associated with tissue overload of which of the following elements?

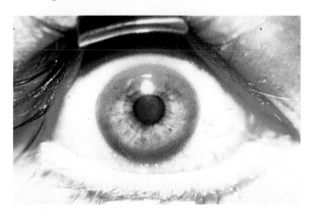

(A) Copper
(B) Iron
(C) Lead
(D) Magnesium
(E) Mercury

20 A 49-year-old woman presents with a 1-month history of yellow discoloration of her eyes, abdominal pain, malaise, weight loss, and low-grade fever (38.4°C, 101°F). Physical examination shows a distended abdomen with right upper quadrant tenderness and a palpable liver 2 cm below the right costal margin. Laboratory studies reveal decreased serum albumin (2.6 g/dL), elevated serum AST (225 U/L) and ALT (150 U/L), and increased alkaline phosphatase (210 U/L). The prothrombin time is prolonged (15 seconds). A moderate leukocytosis (13,500/μL, 80% neutrophils) is observed. A liver biopsy is shown in the image. These pathologic findings are most commonly associated with which of the following liver diseases?

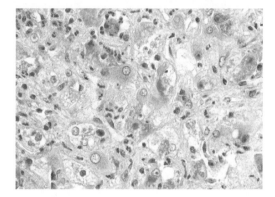

(A) Alcoholic hepatitis
(B) Chronic hepatitis B
(C) Chronic hepatitis C
(D) Hemochromatosis
(E) Primary biliary cirrhosis

21 A 36-year-old woman presents with a 6-month history of progressive generalized itching, weight loss, fatigue, and yellow sclerae. She denies use of oral contraceptives or any other medication. Physical examination reveals mild jaundice and steatorrhea. Blood studies show a high cholesterol level of 350 mg/dL, elevated serum alkaline phosphatase (240 U/L), and normal levels of AST and ALT. An intravenous cholangiogram shows no evidence of obstruction. An antimitochondrial antibody test is positive; antinuclear antibodies are not present. Which of the following skin manifestations is expected in this patient?

(A) Acanthosis nigricans
(B) Hyperpigmentation
(C) Keratoacanthoma
(D) Seborrheic keratosis
(E) Xanthoma

22 For the patient described in Question 21, a liver biopsy would most likely show which of the following pathologic findings?

(A) Central hyaline sclerosis
(B) Cholangiocarcinoma
(C) Hemosiderosis
(D) Intrahepatic bile duct damage
(E) Macrovesicular steatosis

23 A 60-year-old man has a 6-month history of abdominal swelling. On a daily basis, he smokes two packs of cigarettes, drinks five cups of coffee, and reports that he consumes 2 six-packs of beer. Physical examination shows a distended abdomen with a palpable liver 2 cm below the costal margin. A liver biopsy is shown in the image. If this patient becomes abstinent, his liver will most likely do which of the following?

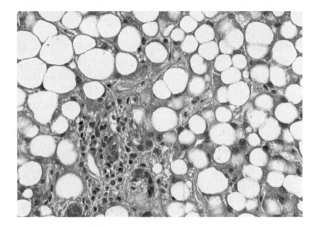

(A) Develop hepatocellular carcinoma
(B) Progress to cirrhosis
(C) Progress to inflammatory hepatitis
(D) Remain unchanged
(E) Revert to normal

24 A 54-year-old man presents with a 9-month history of progressive skin pigmentation. He passes large amounts of urine and is always thirsty. His father died of liver cancer. Physical examination reveals a dark skin color and an enlarged liver. Laboratory studies show normal serum levels of corticotropin. A glucose tolerance test indicates chemical diabetes. A liver biopsy stained with Prussian blue is shown in the image. If untreated, which of the following conditions is most likely to develop in this patient?

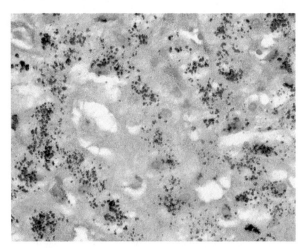

(A) Acute hepatitis
(B) Addison disease
(C) Cholangiocarcinoma
(D) Cholelithiasis
(E) Hepatocellular carcinoma

25 A 28-year-old woman presents with a 4-day history of abdominal pain and increasing abdominal girth. She does not drink alcoholic beverages, but smokes a pack of cigarettes a day. Except for oral contraceptives, she takes no medications. Physical examination shows hepatomegaly, ascites, and mild jaundice. A liver biopsy is obtained (shown in the image). Which of the following is the most likely diagnosis?

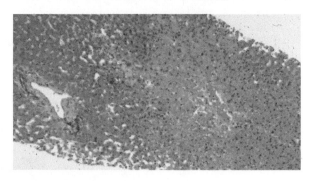

(A) Budd-Chiari syndrome
(B) Chronic hepatitis B
(C) Extrahepatic cholestasis
(D) Primary biliary cirrhosis
(E) Secondary biliary cirrhosis

26 A 47-year-old woman presents with a 3-month history of vague upper abdominal pain after fatty meals, some abdominal distension, and frequent indigestion. Physical examination shows an obese woman (BMI = 30 kg/m²) with right upper quadrant tenderness. An ultrasound examination discloses multiple echogenic objects in the gallbladder. The opened gallbladder is shown in the image. Which of the following metabolic changes is most likely associated with the formation of gallstones in this patient?

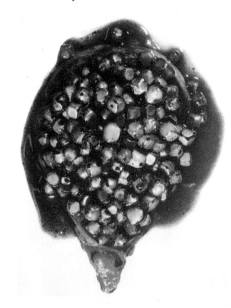

(A) Decreased hepatic bilirubin conjugation
(B) Decreased serum albumin
(C) Increased bilirubin uptake by the liver
(D) Increased hepatic calcium secretion
(E) Increased hepatic cholesterol secretion

27 For the patient described in Question 26, which of the following is a common complication?
(A) Bile peritonitis
(B) Chronic passive congestion of the liver
(C) Confluent hepatic necrosis
(D) Extrahepatic biliary obstruction
(E) Primary hepatocellular carcinoma

28 A 68-year-old man complains of vague abdominal pain, intermittent fever, and a 20-lb (9-kg) weight loss over the past 6 months. For the past 12 years, he has suffered from chronic hepatitis B. On physical examination, the patient shows diffuse abdominal tenderness, hepatomegaly, and mild jaundice. A CT scan of the abdomen reveals a diffusely nodular liver, with a dominant mass measuring 3 cm in diameter. A needle biopsy is shown in the image. Which of the following serum markers is useful for monitoring the progression of disease in this patient?

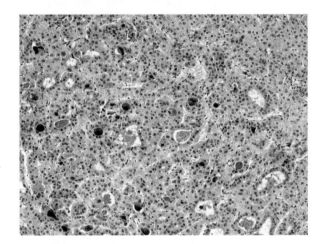

(A) Alkaline phosphatase
(B) Alpha-fetoprotein
(C) Anti-HBc antibody
(D) Carcinoembryonic antigen
(E) Human chorionic gonadotropin

29 A 30-year-old man presents with a 3-week history of fatigue, occasional fever, yellow skin and sclerae, tenderness below the right costal margin, and dark urine. Physical examination reveals jaundice and mild hepatomegaly. Laboratory studies show elevated serum levels of bilirubin, decreased albumin, and prolonged prothrombin time. Serologic tests disclose antibodies to hepatitis C virus. Which of the following tests is the most accurate method for assessing the extent of liver disease in this patient?
(A) Liver biopsy
(B) Serum alkaline phosphatase
(C) Serum ammonia
(D) Serum immunoglobulins
(E) Serum transaminases

30 A 38-year-old man is brought to the emergency room with clouded sensorium and lethargy. He had been degreasing the engine parts of an old car the previous day, using industrial solvents. Later that evening he felt ill, and by morning, he was difficult to rouse. Serum ALT is extremely high (2,400 U/L).

He dies 2 days later in hepatic coma. Which of the following liver injuries is the most likely diagnosis?
(A) Alcoholic hepatitis
(B) Allergic reaction
(C) Budd-Chiari syndrome
(D) Idiosyncratic reaction
(E) Predictable toxic liver injury

31 A 66-year-old man presents with a 2-week history of abdominal bloating, weight loss, and pain in the right upper quadrant. The patient had a serious motor vehicle accident 16 years ago, in which he required transfusion of 10 U of whole blood. On physical examination, he exhibits massive distension of the abdomen. The liver is hard on palpation and occupies the entire right side of the abdomen. Laboratory studies show a low serum albumin (2.2 g/dL) and a markedly elevated serum alpha-fetoprotein. An abdominal ultrasound examination reveals ascites. The patient expires 6 months later. The liver at autopsy is shown in the image. Which of the following is the most common cause of this disease worldwide?

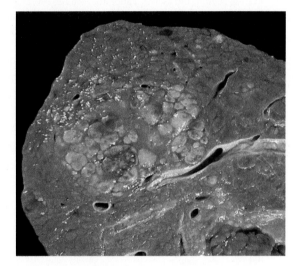

(A) Alcoholic hepatitis
(B) Autoimmune hepatitis
(C) Chronic hepatitis B
(D) Chronic hepatitis C
(E) Hepatitis E

32 A 60-year-old woman presents with several years of abdominal pain radiating to her back and a 5-day history of yellow skin and sclerae. She has lost 15 lb during the past several months, and her stools have become lighter in color. On physical examination, the patient is cachectic and jaundiced. The liver edge descends 1 cm below the right costal margin and is nontender. Her right calf is tender and erythematous. Serum AST and ALT are at the upper limits of normal, but alkaline phosphatase is increased to 430 U/L. A CT scan shows a mass in the head of the pancreas. What is the most likely cause of jaundice in this patient?
(A) Acute viral hepatitis
(B) Alcoholic hepatitis
(C) α_1-Antitrypsin deficiency
(D) Drug-induced hepatitis
(E) Extrahepatic biliary obstruction

33 A 40-year-old woman complains of having severe back pain for about 3 months and recurrent fever. Her past medical history is significant for ulcerative colitis. On physical examination, the patient is thin and jaundiced. The liver edge descends 1 cm below the right costal margin and is nontender. Laboratory studies show normal serum levels of AST and ALT but elevated serum levels of alkaline phosphatase (420 U/L). Endoscopic retrograde cholangiopancreatography demonstrates a beaded appearance of the extrahepatic biliary tree. Which of the following diseases is a late complication of this patient's condition?

(A) Adenocarcinoma of the gallbladder
(B) Cholangiocarcinoma
(C) Hepatic adenoma
(D) Hepatic angiosarcoma
(E) Hepatocellular carcinoma

34 A 32-year-old man presents with a 6-month history of yellow skin and sclerae. Physical examination shows mild jaundice, pitting edema, and ascites. Laboratory studies reveal decreased serum albumin (2.6 g/dL) and increased serum AST and ALT (120 and 140 U/L, respectively). A liver biopsy stained with period acid-Schiff (PAS) reagent and diastase digestion is shown in the image. This patient has which of the following genetic diseases?

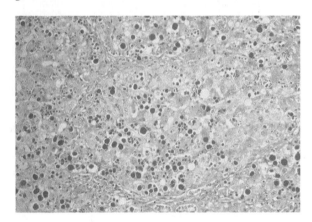

(A) α_1-Antitrypsin deficiency
(B) Glycogen storage disease
(C) Hereditary hemochromatosis
(D) Hurler syndrome
(E) Pompe syndrome

35 A 42-year-old man is brought to the emergency room with right upper quadrant pain, shaking chills, and a fever of 38.7°C (103°F). His past medical history is significant for an appendectomy 2 weeks previously. Physical examination reveals hepatomegaly and tenderness in the right upper quadrant. Laboratory studies show normal levels of serum albumin, ALT, and bilirubin, as well as increased alkaline phosphatase of 240 U/L. The WBC count is 28,000/μL. Which of the following is the most likely diagnosis?

(A) Acute cholecystitis
(B) Acute hepatitis
(C) Diffuse peritonitis
(D) Extrahepatic biliary obstruction
(E) Pyogenic liver abscess

36 A previously healthy, 24-year-old woman presents with a 1-week history of intermittent fever, lethargy, and yellow skin and sclerae. Physical examination shows jaundice. Laboratory studies reveal decreased serum albumin (2.2 g/dL), extremely high levels of AST and ALT (1,200 and 1,800 U/L, respectively), and elevated alkaline phosphatase (300 U/L). Her ceruloplasmin level is normal. She is admitted to the hospital. Her condition progressively deteriorates, and she develops hepatic encephalopathy and hepatorenal syndrome. Which of the following is the most likely diagnosis?

(A) Extrahepatic biliary obstruction
(B) Hereditary hemochromatosis
(C) Massive hepatic necrosis
(D) Primary biliary cirrhosis
(E) Sclerosing cholangitis

37 A 36-year-old, alcoholic woman presents with a 1-week history of yellow skin and sclerae. She has suffered persistent headaches. Her vital signs are normal. Physical examination reveals jaundice. Laboratory studies disclose markedly elevated levels of AST and ALT (956 and 1,400 U/L, respectively). A few days later, she develops hepatic encephalopathy and renal failure. A liver biopsy shows prominent centrilobular necrosis. Which of the following is the most likely diagnosis?

(A) Acetaminophen toxicity
(B) Fatty liver of pregnancy
(C) Metastatic carcinoma
(D) Reye syndrome
(E) Wilson disease

38 A 30-year-old man from Mexico presents with a 3-week history of constant pain in his upper right quadrant and epigastrium and persistent cough. The patient also reports a recent history of nausea, vomiting, and bloody diarrhea. Physical examination shows hepatomegaly and tenderness over the right upper quadrant. A liver biopsy displays fibroblastic proliferation and trophozoites (shown in the image). Which of the following is the most likely diagnosis?

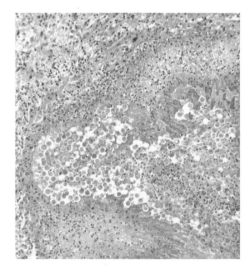

(A) Amebic liver abscess
(B) Cystic hydatid disease
(C) Hepatic malaria
(D) Pyogenic liver abscess
(E) Weil disease

39 A 69-year-old woman arrives in the emergency room complaining of weakness, abdominal pain, and a 9 kg (20 lb) weight loss during the past month. Physical examination reveals jaundice, conspicuous hepatomegaly, and ascites. The patient expires, and a section of liver is examined at autopsy (shown in the image). Which of the following is the most likely diagnosis?

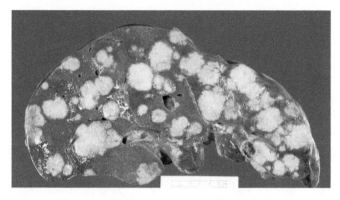

(A) Hemangiosarcoma of the liver
(B) Metastatic carcinoma of the liver
(C) Miliary tuberculosis
(D) Primary hepatocellular carcinoma
(E) Sarcoidosis

40 A 22-year-old man presents with a 3-week history of yellow skin and sclerae but is otherwise asymptomatic. He recalls a similar episode 2 years previously. Occasionally, he has noticed dark-colored urine. The serum bilirubin is 4.4 mg/dL, mostly in the conjugated form. Serum AST and ALT levels are normal. A liver biopsy is shown in the image. Which of the following is the most likely diagnosis?

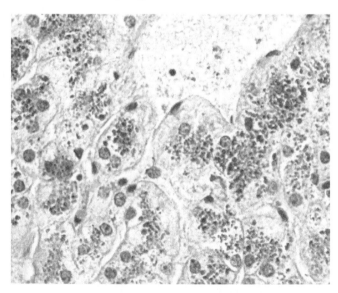

(A) α_1-Antitrypsin deficiency
(B) Crigler-Najjar syndrome
(C) Dubin-Johnson syndrome
(D) Gilbert syndrome
(E) Wilson disease

41 A 22-year-old woman from India presents with a 1-week history of fever, malaise, and nausea. The patient is 6 months pregnant. Physical examination reveals jaundice and right upper quadrant pain. Results of laboratory studies include serum bilirubin of 5.2 mg/dL (60% conjugated), AST of 400 U/L, ALT of 392 U/L, alkaline phosphatase of 70 U/L, anti-HAV antibodies negative, HBsAg negative, and IgM anti–hepatitis E virus (anti-HEV) antibodies positive. The patient is at high risk for which of the following?
(A) Diabetes mellitus
(B) Fulminant liver failure
(C) Pulmonary thromboembolism
(D) Renal failure
(E) Sclerosing cholangitis

42 A 55-year-old, obese man (BMI = 34 kg/m²) comes to the physician for a routine physical examination. His past medical history is significant for type 2 diabetes mellitus that is controlled by medication and diet. The patient neither drinks nor smokes. Physical examination shows mild hepatomegaly. Laboratory studies reveal normal serum levels of albumin and bilirubin and mildly elevated serum levels of AST and ALT (80 and 100 U/L, respectively). The serum level of alkaline phosphatase is normal (70 U/L), and total serum cholesterol is elevated to 290 mg/dL. The CBC is normal. Abdominal ultrasound reveals diffuse fatty infiltration of the liver. Which of the following is the most likely diagnosis?
(A) Autoimmune hepatitis
(B) Cirrhosis of the liver
(C) Diabetic ketoacidosis
(D) Glycogen storage disease
(E) Nonalcoholic fatty liver disease

43 A 6-month-old girl is brought to the physician by her parents, who noticed gradual enlargement of the child's abdomen. Physical examination reveals massive hepatomegaly. Laboratory studies show normal serum levels of albumin, bilirubin, and hepatic enzymes. Liver biopsy discloses enlarged hepatocytes with PAS-positive inclusions. Laboratory studies reveal the presence of amylopectin. Deposits of this abnormal glycogen are also found in a biopsy of skeletal muscle. Which of the following is the appropriate diagnosis?
(A) Andersen disease
(B) Fabry disease
(C) Gaucher disease
(D) Krabbe disease
(E) Metachromatic leukodystrophy

44 A 20-year-old woman complains of intermittent, colicky abdominal pain, fine tremors of her hands, excess sweating, and a general feeling of restlessness. Laboratory studies reveal an inherited defect in the biosynthesis of heme. This patient's genetic disease is most likely caused by deficiency of which of the following liver enzymes?
(A) Alanine aminotransferase
(B) Alkaline phosphatase
(C) Porphobilinogen deaminase
(D) Uridine diphosphate glucuronyl transferase
(E) Uroporphyrinogen decarboxylase

45 A 4-week-old infant has been evaluated for jaundice and hepatomegaly since birth. Laboratory studies reveal markedly elevated serum levels of bilirubin and alkaline phosphatase and high serum levels of AST and ALT. A liver biopsy is shown in the image. Which of the following is the most likely diagnosis?

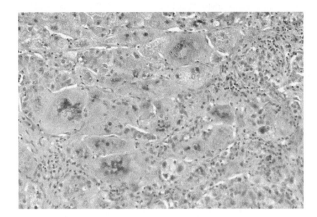

(A) Autoimmune hepatitis
(B) Dubin-Johnson syndrome
(C) Neonatal hepatitis
(D) Reye syndrome
(E) Sclerosing cholangitis

46 Which of the following is a possible cause of liver disease in the patient described in Question 45?
(A) Acute hepatitis A
(B) Annular pancreas
(C) Biliary atresia
(D) Cholelithiasis
(E) Cystic fibrosis

47 A 45-year-old, mildly obese woman presents with a 1-week history of upper abdominal pain, fever, shaking chills, and occasional vomiting. Physical examination shows severe right upper quadrant tenderness. Laboratory studies include serum bilirubin of 1.0 mg/dL, AST of 25 U/L, ALT of 35 U/L, alkaline phosphatase of 220 U/L (high), WBC of 14,000/μL, and amylase of 95 U/L (normal). An ultrasound examination of the abdomen reveals a normal-appearing liver and bile duct and thickening of the wall of the gallbladder. Which of the following is the most likely diagnosis?
(A) Acute cholecystitis
(B) Acute pancreatitis
(C) Adenocarcinoma of the gallbladder
(D) Adenocarcinoma of the pancreas
(E) Primary biliary cirrhosis

48 A 59-year-old man complains of vague abdominal pain, intermittent fever, and a 9-kg (20-lb) weight loss over the past 8 months. His past medical history is significant for drug abuse, although he claims to be drug free for the past 10 years. On physical examination, the patient shows diffuse abdominal tenderness, hepatomegaly, and mild jaundice. Serologic tests for antibodies to the hepatitis B core antigen (IgG anti-HBcAg) and surface antigen (HBsAg) were negative elsewhere. A CT scan of the abdomen reveals a diffusely nodular liver, with a

dominant mass measuring 5 cm in diameter. A liver biopsy shows neoplastic hepatocytes. Which of the following is the most likely underlying cause of this patient's neoplasm?
(A) α_1-Antitrypsin deficiency
(B) Autoimmune hepatitis
(C) Hemochromatosis
(D) Hepatitis C virus
(E) Primary biliary cirrhosis

49 A 59-year-old man complains of weakness and 5 kg (11 lb) weight loss during the past month. An abdominal CT scan suggests metastatic cancer involving the liver and the retroperitoneum. A CT-guided biopsy displays a poorly-differentiated neoplasm. Electron microscopy of the biopsy is shown. Which of the following organs is the most likely primary site for this patient's malignant neoplasm?

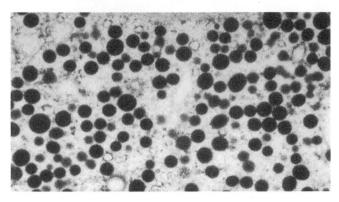

(A) Adrenals
(B) Kidneys
(C) Prostate
(D) Testes
(E) Thyroid

50 A 65-year-old man is brought to the emergency room in a disoriented state. The patient has an odor of alcohol on his breath. Physical examination reveals palmar erythema, diffuse spider angiomata on the upper trunk and face, and gynecomastia. A liver biopsy shows micronodular cirrhosis, massive steatosis, and Mallory hyaline. Serum levels of ammonia are elevated. Which of the following is the most likely underlying cause of gynecomastia in this patient?
(A) Hyperbilirubinemia
(B) Hyperestrogenism
(C) Hypersensitivity vasculitis
(D) Hypoalbuminemia
(E) Ketoacidosis

ANSWERS

1 **The answer is C: Cirrhosis.** Cirrhosis represents the end stage of chronic liver disease and is characterized by extensive fibrosis and the formation of regenerative nodules. Patients with cirrhosis often present with complications of portal hypertension, including ascites, splenomegaly, and bleeding esophageal varices. Esophageal varices arise from the opening of portal-systemic venous collaterals. Engorged collaterals in the submucosa of the lower esophagus and upper stomach, which dilate and protrude into the lumen, are susceptible to bleeding. The prognosis of patients with bleeding esophageal varices is poor, with a 40% mortality rate. Mallory-Weiss tear (choice E) is a possible cause of hematemesis, but is only seen in patients with protracted vomiting. The other choices do not present with portal hypertension or systemic signs of end-stage liver disease.

Diagnosis: Alcoholic cirrhosis, bleeding esophageal varices

2 The answer is E: Increased portal hydrostatic pressure. Ascites refers to the accumulation of fluid in the peritoneal cavity, often caused by portal hypertension. In the setting of cirrhosis, decreased intravascular oncotic pressure due to hypoalbuminemia is also an important factor in the pathogenesis of ascites (see choice D). Aldosterone secretion (choice A) is increased in cirrhotic patients. Overall, imbalances in Starling forces lead to transudation of fluid into the abdominal cavity.

Diagnosis: Alcoholic cirrhosis, portal hypertension

3 The answer is C: Gilbert syndrome. Gilbert syndrome is an inherited, mild, recurrent, unconjugated hyperbilirubinemia (<6mg/dL) that is caused by impaired clearance of bilirubin in the absence of any detectable liver disease. The syndrome tends to run in families, and both autosomal dominant and recessive patterns have been observed. Aside from jaundice, patients are asymptomatic. Factors that increase serum bilirubin concentration in normal persons, such as fasting or illness, produce an exaggerated increase in serum bilirubin levels in persons with Gilbert syndrome. Although Dubin-Johnson syndrome (choice B) is familial, it presents with conjugated hyperbilirubinemia. The other choices do not present with episodic jaundice.

Diagnosis: Gilbert syndrome

4 The answer is B: Autoimmune hemolytic anemia. Autoimmune hemolytic anemia is characterized by antibody-mediated erythrocyte destruction and may lead to severe anemia, as in this case. Intravascular hemolysis produces increased serum levels of unconjugated bilirubin, which exceed the capacity of the hepatocyte to conjugate bilirubin. In most cases, the disease is ameliorated by treatment with corticosteroids. The other choices are parenchymal liver diseases that manifest primarily as conjugated hyperbilirubinemia and are unresponsive to steroids.

Diagnosis: Autoimmune hemolytic anemia

5 The answer is A: Acute viral hepatitis A. HAV is an RNA virus that is transmitted by the fecal-oral route and may be contracted by contamination of water and food. Hepatitis A, the disease presented here, never pursues a chronic course, does not have a carrier state, and provides life-long immunity. IgM anti-HAV is identified in acute infections. The presence of serum IgG anti-HBsAg indicates prior exposure to hepatitis B virus but does not reflect active disease (choice B). Individuals with chronic hepatitis B (choice E) do not have detectable anti-HBsAg in their blood. Acute and chronic hepatitis C (choice C) are ruled out by the negative serology. Serum immunoglobulins are typically increased in patients with autoimmune hepatitis (choice D).

Diagnosis: Hepatitis A, acute

6 The answer is E: Unconjugated bilirubin. Approximately 70% of normal newborns exhibit transient unconjugated hyperbilirubinemia. Immaturity of the liver leads to inadequate conjugation of bilirubin. This physiologic jaundice is more pronounced in premature infants due to inadequate hepatic clearance of bilirubin and increased erythrocyte turnover. Fetal bilirubin levels in utero remain low because bilirubin crosses the placenta, where it is conjugated and excreted by the mother's liver. The other enzymes are unrelated to neonatal jaundice. Elevated serum levels of carotene (choice B) reflects hypervitaminosis A.

Diagnosis: Neonatal (physiologic) jaundice

7 The answer is A: Acute viral hepatitis. Pathologic changes of acute viral hepatitis include disarray of liver cell plates, ballooning degeneration of hepatocytes, intracellular and extracellular bile stasis, apoptotic (Councilman) bodies, and mononuclear inflammatory cell infiltrates. Histologic manifestations are similar in acute hepatitis A, B, and C. Liver damage in acute viral hepatitis is reflected in elevations of serum transaminases and hyperbilirubinemia. Severe liver damage leads to impaired production of serum proteins, including prothrombin and other coagulation factors. The other choices are examples of chronic liver disease.

Diagnosis: Viral hepatitis, acute

8 The answer is C: Chronic hepatitis B. Chronic hepatitis B refers to infection with hepatitis B virus (HBV) that is associated with necrosis and inflammation in the liver for more than 6 months. HBV is a DNA virus that is transmitted through blood transfusion, sexual contact, or shared needles. Most patients recover completely from acute infection, but some 10% develop chronic infection. Of the latter, 10% to 30% develop chronic hepatitis and cirrhosis. The biopsy in this case shows hepatocellular nodules and chronically-inflamed fibrous septa (see photomicrograph). Surface antigen (HBsAg) is present in the serum of patients with chronic hepatitis B, and the presence of HbeAg is often associated with progression of the disease. Choices A, B, and E do not demonstrate cirrhosis as depicted and do not show the serologic characteristics of HBV infection.

Diagnosis: Hepatitis B, chronic

9 The answer is D: Polyarteritis nodosa. Some HBV carriers manifest circulating immune complexes, which cause a variety of extrahepatic ailments, including a serum sickness-like syndrome, glomerulonephritis, cryoglobulinemia, and polyarteritis nodosa. Polyarteritis nodosa is a necrotizing arteritis of medium-sized vessels that can lead to pseudoaneurysm formation, renal thrombosis, inflammation, and hemorrhage. The other choices are not associated with chronic hepatitis.

Diagnosis: Hepatitis B, chronic; polyarteritis nodosa

10 The answer is A: Carcinoma of the gallbladder. Adenocarcinoma of the gallbladder is an incidental finding in 2% of patients who undergo gallbladder surgery due to chronic cholelithiasis. The tumor arises from the mucosal surface epithelium and may cause obstructive jaundice (as in this case) by involvement of the extrahepatic biliary tree. The other choices are not associated with a history of chronic cholecystitis and cholelithiasis and infrequently cause obstructive jaundice.

Diagnosis: Carcinoma of the gallbladder

11 **The answer is C: Ammonia.** The photomicrograph shows cirrhosis, with regenerative nodules of liver cells surrounded by fibrous septa. Hepatic encephalopathy, a syndrome frequently observed in patients with cirrhosis of the liver, is characterized by personality changes, intellectual impairment, and a depressed level of consciousness. The development of hepatic encephalopathy is caused by increased serum concentrations of neurotoxic substances, among which is ammonia. Choices A, B, and D are elevated in a variety of liver diseases but are unrelated to hepatic encephalopathy. Blood urea nitrogen (choice E) is used to assess kidney function.
Diagnosis: Hepatic encephalopathy, alcoholic cirrhosis

12 **The answer is A: Autoimmune hepatitis.** Autoimmune hepatitis is a type of chronic hepatitis, which is associated with circulating autoantibodies (e.g., antinuclear antibodies) and high levels of serum immunoglobulins. The disease typically affects young women but occasionally afflicts older women and men. It is often accompanied by other autoimmune diseases (e.g., Sjögren syndrome, systemic lupus erythematosus). None of the other choices respond to steroids. Primary biliary cirrhosis (choice C) features anti–mitochondrial antibodies. Primary biliary cirrhosis (choice C) and primary sclerosing cholangitis (choice D) do not manifest the described histologic findings.
Diagnosis: Autoimmune hepatitis

13 **The answer is B: Cholangiocarcinoma.** Carcinoma originates anywhere in the biliary tree, from the large intrahepatic ducts at the porta hepatis to the smallest bile ductules at the periphery of the hepatic lobules. Cholangiocarcinoma arising within the liver is associated with substantial fibrosis and can be confused with metastatic carcinoma and reactive fibrosis. These tumors occur at an increased frequency in persons infected with the liver fluke *C. sinensis*, which takes up residence in the biliary tree. Primary sclerosing cholangitis is another risk factor for this cancer. Patients with cholangiocarcinoma have a poor prognosis. The other choices are not associated with a history of *C. sinensis* infestation.
Diagnosis: Cholangiocarcinoma

14 **The answer is C: No histologic changes.** Hepatorenal syndrome usually occurs in the setting of cirrhosis and heralds a poor prognosis. The disorder is characterized by features of renal hypoperfusion, including oliguria, azotemia, and increased levels of serum creatinine. Microscopically, the kidney appears normal. Renal failure is caused by vasoconstriction and hypoperfusion of the kidneys, a combination mediated by various hormones and vasoactive substances, some of which may not be cleared by the cirrhotic liver. Similarly, a kidney from a patient in hepatorenal failure may be successfully transplanted into another person and assume normal functioning. The other choices are associated with direct injury to the renal parenchyma and exhibit characteristic histologic findings.
Diagnosis: Hepatorenal syndrome

15 **The answer is C: Nodular regeneration and scarring.** In about 15% of alcoholics, hepatocellular necrosis, fibrosis, and regeneration eventually lead to the formation of fibrous septa surrounding hepatocellular nodules, which are features that define cirrhosis. Morphologic changes described in the other

choices may be present in cases of alcoholic liver disease but are not directly associated with portal hypertension. Fatty liver (choice B) and Mallory hyaline are associated with alcoholism, but they are not specific indicators of cirrhosis.
Diagnosis: Alcoholic cirrhosis

16 **The answer is E: Sickle cell disease.** Black (pigmented) gallstones are irregular and measure less than 1 cm across. On cross section, the surface appears glassy. Black stones contain calcium bilirubinate, bilirubin polymers, calcium salts, and mucin. Hemolysis in patients with sickle cell disease or other chronic hemolytic anemias generates excess bilirubin, which predisposes to pigment stone formation. Cirrhosis, either through liver cell damage or hemolysis, predisposes to black stones. Gallstones can cause pancreatic duct obstruction, increasing the risk for development of acute and chronic pancreatitis (choice A). Hypercholesterolemia is a risk factor for development of cholesterol gallstones.
Diagnosis: Cholelithiasis, sickle cell disease

17 **The answer is C: Hepatitis B virus.** Massive hepatic necrosis often leads to fulminant hepatic failure. A common cause of massive hepatic necrosis is hepatitis B virus. The liver appears shrunken, the capsule is wrinkled, and the parenchymal tissue is soft and flabby. On microscopic examination, the necrotic liver lobules are hemorrhagic, and the reticulin framework has collapsed. Hepatitis A virus, C virus, and E virus (choices B, D, and E) rarely present with massive hepatic necrosis.
Diagnosis: Fulminant hepatitis B infection, hepatic failure

18 **The answer is D: Oral contraceptives.** Hepatic adenoma usually occurs as a solitary, sharply demarcated mass up to 40 cm in diameter and 3 kg in weight. On gross examination, the tumor is encapsulated and paler than the surrounding liver parenchyma. Hepatic adenoma is a complication of oral contraceptive use in women. In about 30% of patients with hepatic adenomas, the tumor tends to bleed into the peritoneal cavity, inducing hypovolemic shock that requires emergency treatment. The other choices do not induce hepatic tumors.
Diagnosis: Hepatic adenoma

19 **The answer is A: Copper.** Wilson disease is an autosomal recessive condition in which excess copper can be deposited in the liver and brain. Chronic hepatitis leads to cirrhosis in young people. Ocular lesions, so-called Kayser-Fleischer rings, represent deposition of copper in Descemet membrane in the iris (note peripheral brown color). Extrapyramidal neurologic symptoms (e.g., lack of coordination and tremor) are related to degenerative changes in the corpus striatum. Toxicity of the other elements are associated with other manifestations.
Diagnosis: Wilson disease

20 **The answer is A: Alcoholic hepatitis.** Acute alcoholic hepatitis is characterized by hepatic steatosis and hydropic swelling of hepatocytes, focal hepatocellular necrosis, neutrophilic infiltration, and cytoplasmic hyaline inclusions within the hepatocytes (Mallory bodies), which represent precipitated intermediate filament proteins. Clinically, alcoholic hepatitis presents with malaise and anorexia, fever, right upper quadrant pain, and jaundice. Mallory hyaline is seen in patients with primary biliary cirrhosis, but the other histologic findings in this patient's liver biopsy (e.g., hepatic steatosis, hydropic swelling of hepatocytes, focal hepatocellular necrosis, and neutrophilic infiltration) are not features of primary biliary cirrhosis (choice E). Mallory bodies are rare in the other choices.

Diagnosis: Alcoholic hepatitis

21 The answer is E: Xanthoma. Primary biliary cirrhosis (PBC) is a chronic progressive liver disease that is associated with many immunologic abnormalities and is, therefore, widely held to be an autoimmune disease. The hallmark of this condition is the presence in serum of antimitochondrial antibodies. These autoantibodies recognize epitopes associated with the mitochondrial pyruvate dehydrogenase complex. Despite the specificity of the antimitochondrial antibodies, they have no inhibitory effect on mitochondrial function and play no known role in the pathogenesis of the disease. The complement system is chronically activated. PBC occurs more often in women than in men (10:1 female predominance). It presents with fatigue, anorexia, jaundice, xanthomas of the skin, and pruritus. The other choices are not associated with PBC or hypercholesterolemia.

Diagnosis: Primary biliary cirrhosis

22 The answer is D: Intrahepatic bile duct damage. Primary biliary cirrhosis (nonsuppurative destructive cholangitis) is caused by chronic destruction of intrahepatic bile ducts in the portal tracts. Primary biliary cirrhosis evolves through ductal lesions, scarring, and eventually cirrhosis. Early PBC features chronic destructive cholangitis affecting intrahepatic small and medium-sized bile ducts. The bile ducts are surrounded primarily by lymphocytes (CD8+ T cells), but plasma cells and macrophages are also seen. In some portal tracts, lymphoid follicles are conspicuous. Discrete epithelioid granulomas often occur in the portal tracts and may impinge on the bile ducts. As a result of the destructive chronic inflammatory process, small bile ducts virtually disappear, and scarring of medium-sized bile ducts is common. Proliferation of bile ductules within portal tracts is common and may be florid. Collagenous septae extend from the portal tracts into the lobular parenchyma and encircle some lobules. Cholestasis, when present, may be severe and is located at the periphery of the portal tracts. The end-stage of PBC is cirrhosis, characterized by a dark green bile-stained liver that exhibits fine nodularity. The other choices do not feature destruction of intrahepatic bile ducts.

Diagnosis: Primary biliary cirrhosis

23 The answer is E: Revert to normal. Excessive alcohol consumption induces fat accumulation within hepatocytes, enlarging the liver to as much as three times the normal weight. The amount of fat deposited varies with the amount of alcohol consumed, as well as the patient's hormonal status, diet, and other factors. Triglyceride accumulation by itself is not ordinarily damaging, and the condition is fully reversible upon discontinuation of alcohol abuse (abstinence).

Diagnosis: Alcoholic fatty liver

24 The answer is E: Development of hepatocellular carcinoma. Hereditary hemochromatosis (HH) is a common, autosomal recessive, genetic disorder that is characterized by excessive iron absorption and the toxic accumulation of iron in parenchymal cells, particularly of the liver, heart, and pancreas. In the liver, HH leads to cirrhosis and a high incidence of primary hepatocellular carcinoma. The clinical hallmark of advanced HH is the presence of other diseases such as diabetes, skin pigmentation, and cardiac failure. The Prussian blue stain binds iron and provides histologic evidence for iron overload. Addison disease (choice B) presents with skin pigmentation but reflects autoimmune destruction of the adrenal glands.

Diagnosis: Hereditary hemochromatosis

25 The answer is A: Budd-Chiari syndrome. Budd-Chiari syndrome is a congestive disease of the liver caused by occlusion of the hepatic veins and their tributaries. The principal cause of Budd-Chiari syndrome is thrombosis of the hepatic veins. Intrahepatic venous thrombosis may be associated with increased blood viscosity (as in polycythemia vera or other myeloproliferative disorders) and hypercoagulable states associated with hematologic cancers, certain solid tumors, pregnancy, and paroxysmal nocturnal hemoglobinuria. However, in more than half the cases, the cause of Budd-Chiari syndrome is not apparent. Complete thrombosis of the hepatic veins presents as an acute illness characterized by abdominal pain, enlargement of the liver, ascites, and mild jaundice. Acute hepatic failure and death often occur rapidly. The needle biopsy in this case shows severe centrilobular necrosis and hemorrhage (see photomicrograph). The sinusoids of the central zone are dilated and packed with erythrocytes. The other choices do not present with centrilobular hemorrhage and are not associated with oral contraceptives.

Diagnosis: Budd-Chiari syndrome

26 The answer is E: Increased hepatic cholesterol secretion. Cholesterol stones are round or faceted, yellow to tan, and may be single or multiple. Risk factors for cholesterol stones include female sex, diabetes, pregnancy, and estrogen therapy. Solitary, yellow, hard gallstones are associated with bile that is supersaturated with cholesterol. During their reproductive years, women are up to three times more likely to develop cholesterol gallstones than men. If the bile contains excess cholesterol or is deficient in bile acids, it becomes supersaturated with cholesterol and precipitates to form stones (lithogenic bile). In obese women, cholesterol secretion by the liver is increased. Impaired gallbladder motor function is another risk factor that leads to gallstone formation. In this case, stasis permits the formation of biliary sludge, which then progresses to macroscopic stones. Choices A and B are not associated with gallstones. Choices C and D are not physiologic.

Diagnosis: Cholelithiasis, cholesterol gallstones

27 The answer is D: Extrahepatic biliary obstruction. Most complications associated with cholelithiasis are related to obstruction of the biliary tree. Passage of stones into the cystic duct often causes severe biliary colic. Lodgement of stones in the common bile duct leads to obstructive jaundice, cholangitis, and acute pancreatitis. Patients with cholelithiasis have a 25-fold increased risk of acute pancreatitis compared with the general population. Additional complications are rare and include empyema of the gallbladder, perforation, fistula formation, bile peritonitis, and gallstone ileus. In most cases, gallstones are associated with chronic cholecystitis. Choices B, C, and E are not associated with gallstones.

Diagnosis: Cholelithiasis, obstructive jaundice

28 The answer is B: Alpha-fetoprotein (AFP). AFP is a glycoprotein that is normally synthesized in the fetus by the yolk sac, liver, and gastrointestinal tract. In adults, an elevated serum level of AFP is a useful indicator of hepatocellular carcinoma and germ cell tumors of the testis. AFP levels decline rapidly after surgical resection of liver cell cancer or treatment of patients with metastatic germ cell tumors. Alkaline phosphatase (choice A) is a common indicator of hepatobiliary disease. Carcinoembryonic antigen (choice D) is principally used to monitor gastrointestinal cancers.

Diagnosis: Hepatocellular carcinoma

29 The answer is A: Liver biopsy. Microscopic examination of a liver biopsy is the best method currently available for assessing the extent of liver disease in a patient with viral hepatitis. The major histologic features of acute viral hepatitis are liver cell injury and inflammation. Microscopic examination shows ballooning degeneration of liver cells, intracellular and extracellular bile stasis, acidophilic bodies, and a mononuclear cell infiltrate. Serum alkaline phosphatase and transaminases (choices B and E) are also useful indicators of the severity of liver disease, but do not allow for an assessment of the chronicity or stage of the disease. Serum ammonia (choice C) is used to monitor patients at risk for hepatic encephalopathy and ordinarily reflects end-stage liver disease.

Diagnosis: Hepatitis C, acute

30 The answer is E: Predictable toxic liver injury. Acute, chemically induced hepatic injury spans the entire spectrum of liver disease, from transient cholestasis to massive hepatic necrosis. Drug-induced liver injury can be either direct or indirect. Indirect injury is caused by metabolites and free radicals that are produced as byproducts of xenobiotic metabolism. Immune reactions against a chemical or its metabolites are also causes of indirect liver damage. Chemically-induced hepatic injury is classified as "predictable" when toxicity is immediate and dose-dependent and as "unpredictable" or "idiosyncratic" when toxicity occurs without explanation (choice D). In this case, exposure to industrial solvents, such as carbon tetrachloride, caused predictable toxic liver injury, characterized by centrilobular necrosis and elevated serum levels of transaminases.

Diagnosis: Toxic liver injury

31 The answer is C: Chronic hepatitis B. Patients with persistent hepatitis B virus (HBV) infection have a 200-fold increased risk of developing primary hepatocellular carcinoma (HCC), the diagnosis in this case. More than 85% of cases of HCC occur in countries with a high prevalence of chronic infection with HBV. One fourth of patients with chronic hepatitis B ultimately develop HCC. Chronic hepatitis C (choice D) is associated with most cases of HCC in Europe and North America, but chronic hepatitis B remains the major global cause of HCC.

Diagnosis: Hepatitis B, chronic; hepatocellular carcinoma

32 The answer is E: Extrahepatic biliary obstruction. This patient presents with signs and symptoms of biliary obstruction due to obstruction of the biliary tree by adenocarcinoma in the head of the pancreas. Symptoms of pancreatic cancer in this patient include pain radiating to the back and weight loss. Diarrhea and steatorrhea result from fat malabsorption, which is secondary to extrahepatic obstruction to bile flow by encroachment of the tumor and metastatic lymph nodes on the common bile duct. Choices A, B, and D are incorrect because the ALT and AST were normal, which is unlikely in the setting of hepatitis. High serum alkaline phosphatase signals obstructive jaundice.

Diagnosis: Extrahepatic biliary obstruction, pancreatic carcinoma

33 The answer is B: Cholangiocarcinoma. Primary sclerosing cholangitis (PSC) is characterized by inflammation and obliterative fibrosis of intrahepatic and extrahepatic bile ducts, with dilation of preserved segments. Approximately 70% of patients with PSC have longstanding ulcerative colitis, although the prevalence of PSC in such patients is only 4%. PSC tends to occur in the third through fifth decades of life, with a significant male predominance (2:1). The clinicopathologic findings are complemented by a characteristic radiographic appearance of a beaded biliary tree, representing sporadic strictures. Cholangiocarcinoma is a late complication of PSC. The other choices are not complications of PSC.

Diagnosis: Primary sclerosing cholangitis

34 The answer is A: α_1-Antitrypsin deficiency. α_1-Antitrypsin deficiency is the most common genetic cause of liver disease in infants and children and the most frequent genetic disease for which liver transplantation is indicated. The liver may be involved with or without pulmonary disease in the form of emphysema. α_1-Antitrypsin deficiency is characterized by the presence of round-to-oval cytoplasmic globular inclusions of misfolded α_1-antitrypsin proteins in hepatocytes. These globules stain red with PAS after removing glycogen with diastase. These inclusions are not featured in the other choices.

Diagnosis: α_1-Antitrypsin deficiency

35 The answer is E: Pyogenic liver abscess. Pyogenic liver abscesses are caused by staphylococci, streptococci, and Gram-negative enterobacteria (i.e., anaerobic inhabitants of the gastrointestinal tract). The bacteria gain access to the liver by direct extension from contiguous organs or through the portal vein or hepatic artery. Extrahepatic biliary obstruction (choice D), which leads to ascending cholangitis, is the most common cause of pyogenic abscess and is usually associated with stones in the common bile duct (choledocholithiasis), benign and malignant tumors, or postsurgical strictures of the bile ducts. As in this instance of appendicitis, the infectious organisms can also originate within the abdomen and reach the liver by embolization. Other abdominal causes of pyogenic abscess in the liver include diverticulitis and inflammatory bowel diseases. Diffuse peritonitis (choice C) is a possible complication of perforated appendicitis but is not suggested by the clinical presentation described in this vignette. Acute cholecystitis (choice A) is a very unlikely complication of appendicitis.

Diagnosis: Pyogenic liver abscess

36 The answer is C: Massive hepatic necrosis. Massive hepatic necrosis is the most feared variant of acute hepatitis. The laboratory findings seen in this patient (markedly elevated ALT and AST) are characteristic for this condition. Grossly, the liver loses about one third of its normal weight, and Glisson capsule is wrinkled and mottled. Microscopic examination reveals massive death of the hepatocytes, leaving a collapsed collagenous framework. Although the other choices can lead to hepatic failure, patients are typically symptomatic prior to hepatic decompensation.

Diagnosis: Massive hepatic necrosis

37 The answer is A: Acetaminophen toxicity. Drug toxicity should be suspected in all cases of acute hepatitis. In this case, centrilobular necrosis suggests acetaminophen toxicity. The toxic dose of acetaminophen after a single acute ingestion is in the range of 150 mg/kg in children and 7 g in adults. Acetaminophen is rapidly absorbed from the stomach and small intestine and conjugated in the liver to nontoxic agents, which then are eliminated in the urine. In cases of acute overdose, normal pathways of acetaminophen metabolism become saturated. Excess acetaminophen is then metabolized in the liver via the mixed function oxidase P450 system, yielding oxidative metabolites that cause predictable, hepatocellular necrosis. The centrilobular zones are particularly affected (centrilobular necrosis). Centrilobular necrosis is not seen in the other choices. Reye syndrome (choice D) occurs in children. Fatty liver of pregnancy (choice B) features microvesicular steatosis.

Diagnosis: Acetaminophen toxicity, hepatorenal syndrome

38 The answer is A: Amebic liver abscess. Amebic liver abscess is the most common form of extraintestinal amebiasis, although fewer than 30% of patients have a history of antecedent intestinal amebiasis. The male-to-female ratio is 10:1, and the disease is rare in children. Amebic liver abscess appears with an abrupt onset of fever and dull aching abdominal pain in the right upper quadrant or epigastrium, usually lasting less than 10 days. Jaundice is unusual. The diagnosis is usually made by radiologic or ultrasound demonstration of the liver abscess, in conjunction with serologic testing for antibodies to *Entamoeba histolytica*. Cystic hydatid disease (choice B) is caused by infection with *Echinococcus granulosus* and is characterized by cyst formation in the liver over several years. Hepatic malaria (choice C) causes hepatomegaly secondary to hypertrophy and hyperplasia of Kupffer cells. Weil disease (choice E) is caused by infections with *Leptospira* spirochetes.

Diagnosis: Amebic liver abscess

39 The answer is B: Metastatic carcinoma of the liver. Liver metastasis is the most common cause of massive hepatomegaly and the most common tumor of the liver. The liver is involved in one third of all metastatic cancers, including half of those of the gastrointestinal tract, breast, and lungs. Other tumors that characteristically metastasize to the liver are pancreatic carcinoma and malignant melanoma, although any cancer may find its way to the liver. Although hemangiosarcomas of the liver (choice A) are frequently multifocal, the tumors are hemorrhagic. Primary hepatocellular carcinoma (choice D) is incorrect because it usually shows a solitary, poorly circumscribed mass, generally in the background of cirrhosis. Miliary tuberculosis (choice C) and sarcoidosis

(choice E) feature mm-sized inflammatory nodules (minute granulomas).

Diagnosis: Metastatic carcinoma of the liver

40 The answer is C: Dubin-Johnson syndrome. Dubin-Johnson syndrome is a benign autosomal recessive disease that is characterized by chronic conjugated hyperbilirubinemia and conspicuous melanin-like pigment deposition in the liver. The disease is linked to mutations that result in the complete absence of multidrug resistance protein 2 in hepatocytes. The microscopic appearance of the liver in patients with Dubin-Johnson syndrome is normal, except for the accumulation of coarse, iron-free, dark brown granules in hepatocytes and Kupffer cells. Although all of the other choices are genetic disorders that affect the liver, none present with the clinicopathologic findings seen in this case.

Diagnosis: Dubin-Johnson syndrome

41 The answer is B: Fulminant liver failure. The patient suffers from hepatitis E infection based upon antibody titers against the virus. HEV is an enteric RNA virus transmitted by the fecal-oral route. It accounts for more than half of cases of acute viral hepatitis in young to middle-aged persons in poor regions of the world. HEV is endemic in parts of Asia and South America, where there is poor sanitation. Like hepatitis A, hepatitis E usually presents as an acute self-limited illness. The average incubation period is 35 to 40 days. The symptoms (jaundice, fever, and arthralgia) usually resolve within 6 weeks. Although overall mortality rates range from 1% to 12%, the disease is especially dangerous in pregnant women due to fulminant hepatic failure, with mortality rates as high as 20% to 40%. None of the other choices are directly associated with HEV infection.

Diagnosis: Hepatitis E, acute

42 The answer is E: Nonalcoholic fatty liver disease. Nonalcoholic fatty liver is so named because it closely resembles alcoholic fatty liver. This condition represents a spectrum of liver injuries that initially display steatosis, with or without hepatitis. Nonalcoholic fatty liver not infrequently progresses to bridging fibrosis and cirrhosis of the liver. Risk factors for nonalcoholic fatty liver disease include obesity, type 2 diabetes mellitus, and hyperlipidemia. Choices A, B, and D are not fatty liver diseases. Diabetic ketoacidosis (choice C) may be associated with increased fat in the liver, but the patient clearly does not have this disorder.

Diagnosis: Nonalcoholic fatty liver disease.

43 The answer is A: Andersen disease. Andersen disease, which is also known as glycogen storage disease type IV, is an autosomal recessive genetic disease caused by deficiency of a glycogen-branching enzyme. This enzyme deficiency results in the accumulation of abnormal glycogen (amylopectin) in the liver, muscle, and other tissues. In most affected persons, the condition becomes evident in the first months of life. Clinical features of Andersen disease include failure to thrive and hepatosplenomegaly. The disease course is typically characterized by progressive hepatic fibrosis leading to cirrhosis and liver failure. None of the other choices are glycogen storage diseases.

Diagnosis: Andersen disease

44 The answer is C: Porphobilinogen deaminase. Acute intermittent porphyria is the most common genetic porphyria. This autosomal dominant genetic disease is caused by a deficiency of porphobilinogen deaminase activity in the liver. Clinical symptoms include colicky abdominal pain and neuropsychiatric symptoms. Choices A, B, and D are not involved in heme biosynthesis. Deficiency of uroporphyrinogen decarboxylase (choice E) causes a chronic hepatic porphyria that typically presents with cutaneous photosensitivity and iron overload in the middle-aged or elderly.
Diagnosis: Porphyria, acute intermittent

45 The answer is C: Neonatal hepatitis. Histologic features of neonatal hepatitis include prolonged cholestasis, inflammation, and cell injury. Giant cell transformation of hepatocytes is common. These cells contain as many as 40 nuclei and may appear detached from other cells in the liver plate. Most infants with uncomplicated neonatal hepatitis eventually recover. The other choices do not afflict newborns and do not feature multinucleation.
Diagnosis: Neonatal hepatitis

46 The answer is C: Biliary atresia. In about half of all cases of neonatal hepatitis, the cause is discernible, and about 30% of cases are assigned to α_1-antitrypsin deficiency alone. Most of the other cases with known causes can be attributed to chromosomal abnormalities or intrauterine infections. Another cause of neonatal hepatitis is biliary atresia, most often presenting with the extrahepatic form. Untreated biliary obstruction causes progressive fibrosis and may result in secondary biliary cirrhosis. The other choices are not associated with neonatal hepatitis.
Diagnosis: Biliary atresia

47 The answer is A: Acute cholecystitis. Acute cholecystitis refers to diffuse inflammation of the gallbladder, usually secondary to obstruction of the gallbladder outlet. Approximately 90% of cases of acute cholecystitis are secondary to gallstones (cholelithiasis). In patients with acute cholecystitis, the external surface of the gallbladder is intensely congested and often layered with a fibrinous exudate. Acute pancreatitis (choice B) is incorrect because the serum amylase level in this patient is normal. Unsuspected gallbladder cancer (choice C) may be discovered in cholecystectomy specimens, but such an occurrence is uncommon. Pancreatic carcinoma (choice D) often presents as painless jaundice.
Diagnosis: Acute cholecystitis

48 The answer is D: Hepatitis C virus (HCV). Although, hepatitis C has a lower global prevalence than hepatitis B, the former is associated with most cases of hepatocellular carcinoma in the United States. Most patients with HCV who develop hepatocellular carcinoma have evidence of chronic liver disease and cirrhosis. α_1-Antitrypsin (choice A) deficiency and hemochromatosis (choice C) are both associated with an elevated risk of hepatocellular carcinoma, but they are far less common than hepatitis C. Primary biliary cirrhosis (choice E) does not lead to hepatocellular carcinoma.
Diagnosis: Hepatocellular carcinoma

49 The answer is A: Adrenals. The electron micrograph of this patient's metastatic cancer shows cells with granules with dense cores. Membrane-bound dense core granules are characteristic of endocrine and neuroendocrine cells such as catecholamine-producing cells and tumors of the adrenal medulla (e.g., pheochromocytoma). None of the other organs is composed of endocrine or neuroendocrine cells. Electron microscopy can be used as an adjunct for pathologic diagnosis when other markers of cellular differentiation are lacking. Carcinomas often exhibit desmosomes and specialized junctional complexes. The presence of melanosomes signifies a melanoma.
Diagnosis: Pheochromocytoma

50 The answer is B: Hyperestrogenism. This patient is in hepatic coma and likely suffers from cirrhosis. Chronic liver failure in men leads to feminization, characterized by gynecomastia, female body habitus, and a change in pubic hair distribution. Other features of chronic liver disease include spider angiomata and palmar erythema. These findings are attributed to reduced hepatic catabolism of estrogens (i.e., hyperestrogenism). The other choices are unrelated to feminization.
Diagnosis: Alcoholic liver disease

Chapter 15

The Pancreas

QUESTIONS

Select the single best answer.

1 A 1-month-old infant is brought to the physician by her parents. She has had repeated bouts of bilious vomiting over the past month and cannot be fed adequately. She is in the 10th percentile for weight and the 50th percentile for length. An upper GI series discloses marked narrowing of the midportion of the duodenum. What is the most likely cause of this infant's GI obstruction?
(A) Annular pancreas
(B) Duodenal polyp
(C) Islet cell adenoma
(D) Pancreatic pseudocyst
(E) Pyloric stenosis

2 A 42-year-old obese woman (BMI = 32 kg/m²) presents with severe abdominal pain that radiates to the back. There is no history of alcohol or drug abuse. The blood pressure is 90/45 mm Hg, respirations are 32 per minute, and pulse is 100 per minute. Physical examination shows abdominal tenderness, guarding, and rigidity. An X-ray film of the chest shows a left pleural effusion. Laboratory studies reveal elevated serum amylase (850 U/L) and lipase (675 U/L), and hypocalcemia (7.8 mg/dL). Which of the following is the most likely diagnosis?
(A) Acute cholecystitis
(B) Acute pancreatitis
(C) Alcoholic hepatitis
(D) Chronic calcifying pancreatitis
(E) Dissecting aortic aneurysm

3 Which of the following is most likely associated with the pathogenesis of the condition of the patient described in Question 2?
(A) Carcinoid syndrome
(B) Cholelithiasis
(C) Insulinoma
(D) Pancreatic adenocarcinoma
(E) Portal hypertension

4 A 60-year-old alcoholic man presents with a 6-month history of recurrent epigastric pain, progressive weight loss, and foul-smelling diarrhea. The abdominal pain is now almost constant and intractable. An X-ray film of the abdomen reveals multiple areas of calcification in the mid-abdomen. Which of the following is the most likely diagnosis?
(A) Carcinoid syndrome
(B) Chronic pancreatitis
(C) Crohn disease
(D) Insulinoma
(E) Miliary tuberculosis

5 Which of the following findings is most likely to be encountered in the patient described in Question 4?
(A) Achlorhydria
(B) Hypoglycemia
(C) Melena
(D) Pernicious anemia
(E) Steatorrhea

6 A 50-year-old woman complains of persistent abdominal pain, anorexia, and abdominal distention. Her past medical history is significant for a previous hospitalization for acute pancreatitis. Physical examination shows jaundice and a nonpulsatile abdominal mass. Laboratory studies reveal normal serum levels of bilirubin, AST, and ALT. A CT scan of the abdomen shows a fluid-filled cavity in the head of the pancreas. What is the most likely diagnosis?
(A) Acute hemorrhagic pancreatitis
(B) Insulinoma
(C) Pancreatic cystadenoma
(D) Pancreatic islet cell tumor
(E) Pancreatic pseudocyst

7 The surgical specimen is shown in the image for the patient described in Question 6. In addition to blood and necrotic debris, which of the following best describes the contents of this cystic lesion?

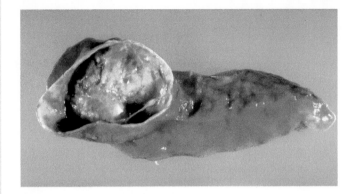

(A) Bile
(B) Chylous fluid
(C) Lymph
(D) Mucopolysaccharides
(E) Pancreatic enzymes

8 A 60-year-old man presents with a 3-week history of weight loss, vague abdominal pain, and progressive yellowing of his skin and sclerae. He also reports the recent onset of intermittent pain in the upper and lower extremities. Laboratory studies show a serum bilirubin level of 15 mg/dL, mostly in the conjugated form. A CT scan of the abdomen reveals a mass in the head of the pancreas. The patient develops sudden shortness of breath and is diagnosed with pulmonary thromboembolism. Which of the following is the most likely cause of thromboembolism in this patient?
(A) Adenocarcinoma of the ampulla of Vater
(B) Gastrinoma of the pancreas
(C) Insulinoma of the pancreas
(D) Pancreatic adenocarcinoma
(E) Pancreatic pseudocyst

9 Despite best efforts at treatment, the patient described in Question 8 subsequently dies. The gross appearance of the pancreas and liver at autopsy is shown in the image. This patient's tumor most likely arose from which of the following types of cells?

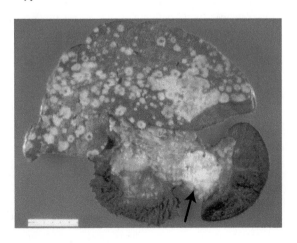

(A) Acinar cells
(B) Alpha cells
(C) Beta cells
(D) Delta cells
(E) Ductal cells

10 A 65-year-old woman presents with a 5-week history of yellow skin and sclera, anorexia, and epigastric pain. Her past medical history is significant for insulin-dependent diabetes mellitus. She smoked one pack of cigarettes a day for the past 20 years. Physical examination reveals jaundice and a palpable gallbladder. Laboratory studies show a serum bilirubin level of 10 mg/dL, mostly in the conjugated form, and an elevated alkaline phosphatase (260 U/L). A CT scan of the abdomen discloses a mass in the head of the pancreas and multiple nodules in the liver measuring up to 3 cm. Which of the following is the most likely cause of jaundice in this patient?
(A) Cholelithiasis
(B) Cirrhosis
(C) Extrahepatic biliary obstruction
(D) Hemolysis
(E) Intrahepatic cholestasis

11 Which of the following is the most important risk factor for the neoplasm arising in the patient described in Question 10?
(A) Alcohol abuse
(B) Cholelithiasis
(C) Cigarette smoking
(D) Diabetes mellitus type 1
(E) High-fat diet

12 A 47-year-old man suffers from long-standing peptic ulcer disease, which is largely unresponsive to pharmacologic therapy. Endoscopic examination reveals multiple, nonhealed ulcerations of the duodenum and jejunum. Which of the following is the most likely diagnosis?
(A) Carcinoid syndrome
(B) Insulinoma
(C) Pancreatic adenocarcinoma
(D) Verner-Morrison syndrome
(E) Zollinger-Ellison syndrome

13 A 35-year-old woman presents with 6-month history of skin rash and fatigue. Physical examination shows pallor and a necrotizing erythematous skin rash of her lower body. Laboratory studies reveal mild anemia and fasting blood glucose of 160 mg/dL. A CT scan of the abdomen demonstrates a 2-cm mass in the pancreas. Which of the following is the most likely diagnosis?
(A) Carcinoid tumor
(B) Gastrinoma
(C) Glucagonoma
(D) Insulinoma
(E) Pancreatic polypeptide-secreting tumor

14 A 40-year-old woman comes to the physician with a 6-week history of episodic hunger and fainting spells. She is currently seeing a psychiatrist because she is irritable and quarreling with her family. Laboratory studies show a serum glucose concentration of 35 mg/dL. A CT scan of the abdomen demonstrates a 1.5-cm mass in the pancreas. The gross appearance of the bisected tumor is shown in the image. What is the most likely diagnosis?

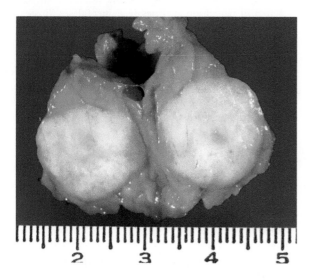

(A) Adenocarcinoma
(B) Gastrinoma
(C) Glucagonoma
(D) Insulinoma
(E) Somatostinoma

15 A 36-year-old woman complains of a 4-week history of unremitting watery diarrhea. She reports that she is always thirsty and drinks continuously. Laboratory studies show achlorhydria, hypokalemia, and mild acidosis. A CT scan of the abdomen demonstrates a 1.5-cm pancreatic mass. Which of the following is the most likely diagnosis?
(A) Carcinoid tumor
(B) Gastrinoma
(C) Pancreatic polypeptide-secreting tumor
(D) Somatostatinoma
(E) VIPoma

16 A 45-year-old woman complains of right upper quadrant abdominal pain, weight loss, dry mouth, increased urine production, and foul-smelling fatty stools. She has a recent history of mild diabetes mellitus. Abdominal ultrasound examination reveals gallstones and a solitary 1.5-cm mass in the pancreas. Which of the following hormones would most likely be elevated in the blood of this patient?
(A) Calcitonin
(B) Gastrin
(C) Insulin
(D) Somatostatin
(E) Vasoactive intestinal polypeptide

17 A 35-year-old man complains of severe acute periumbilical pain that radiates to his back and nausea. The patient recently had a heart transplant for idiopathic cardiomyopathy and is taking azathioprine for immunosuppression. Physical

examination reveals bruising of both flanks. Blood pressure is 120/70 mm Hg, pulse rate 100 per minute, and temperature 37.8°C (100°F). Laboratory studies show elevated serum levels of amylase (950 U/L) and lipase (780 U/L), normal levels of serum calcium, and a normal serum lipid profile. The patient expires, and the pancreas is examined at autopsy (shown in the image). Which of the following is the most likely underlying cause of these pathologic findings?

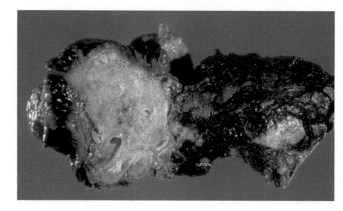

(A) Acute ischemia
(B) Drug-induced pancreatitis
(C) Graft-versus-host reaction
(D) Hypercalcemia
(E) Hyperlipidemia

18 A 63-year-old woman presents with a 6-month history of recurrent epigastric pain and nausea. Abdominal ultrasound reveals a 13-mm hypoechoic lesion in the tail of the pancreas. Physical examination shows flushing of the face, periorbital edema, and hypotension (blood pressure = 90/50 mm Hg). Laboratory studies disclose normal serum levels of gastrin, amylase, insulin, and vasoactive intestinal polypeptide. Urinalysis demonstrates elevated levels of metanephrines (10 mg per 24 hours). Which of the following is the most likely diagnosis?
(A) Adenocarcinoma of pancreas
(B) Glucagonoma
(C) Insulinoma
(D) Pancreatic carcinoid
(E) Somatostatinoma

19 A 65-year-old man with a history of acromegaly complains of recurrent epigastric pain and dark-colored tarry stools. Laboratory studies reveal moderate hypercalcemia, hyperlipidemia, and elevated serum levels of PTH and gastrin. Serum glucose is within normal limits. Abdominal ultrasound shows a mass in the tail of the pancreas. Which of the following is the most likely diagnosis?
(A) Glucagonoma
(B) Insulinoma
(C) Multiple endocrine neoplasia type 1
(D) Multiple endocrine neoplasia type 2
(E) Pancreatic carcinoid

ANSWERS

1 **The answer is A: Annular pancreas.** Annular pancreas is a congenital condition in which the head of the pancreas surrounds the second portion of the duodenum. The anomaly may be associated with duodenal atresia. Infants present with feeding disorders and growth retardation. Pyloric stenosis (choice E) involves the gastric outlet. Duodenal polyp (choice B) does not occur in infants.
Diagnosis: Annular pancreas

2 **The answer is B: Acute pancreatitis.** Acute pancreatitis is defined as an inflammatory condition of the exocrine pancreas that results from injury to acinar cells. The disease presents with a spectrum of signs and symptoms. Severe forms are characterized by the sudden onset of abdominal pain, often accompanied by signs of shock (hypotension, tachypnea, and tachycardia). The release of amylase and lipase from the injured pancreas into the serum provides a sensitive marker for monitoring injury to acinar cells. Left pleural effusion is a common finding in patients with acute pancreatitis due to local irritation below the diaphragm. The other choices do not feature increases in serum amylase and lipase.
Diagnosis: Pancreatitis, acute

3 **The answer is B: Cholelithiasis.** Some 45% of all patients with acute pancreatitis also have cholelithiasis, and the risk of developing acute pancreatitis in patients with gallstones is 25 times higher than that in the general population. Chronic alcoholism accounts for approximately one third of the cases of acute pancreatitis. Other causes include obstruction of the pancreatic duct by gallstones, intake of drugs, and viral infections. The other choices do not cause acute pancreatitis.
Diagnosis: Pancreatitis, acute; cholelithiasis

4 **The answer is B: Chronic pancreatitis.** Chronic pancreatitis is characterized by the progressive destruction of the pancreas, with accompanying irregular fibrosis and chronic inflammation. Calcification and intraductal calculi often develop. Pancreatic insufficiency results in malabsorption syndrome. Chronic pancreatitis is most commonly seen in patients with a history of alcohol abuse (70% of cases). The other choices are not associated with pancreatic calcifications. Although islets may be affected by chronic pancreatitis, hypoglycemia is an uncommon and late feature of the disease.
Diagnosis: Pancreatitis, chronic

5 **The answer is E: Steatorrhea.** Fat malabsorption in the setting of chronic pancreatitis is most often associated with steatorrhea. In patients with steatorrhea, the fecal matter is foul smelling and floats because of a high fat content. Long-standing malabsorptive disease is accompanied by nutritional deficiency, including weight loss, anemia, osteomalacia, and a tendency to bleed. Hypoglycemia (choice B) is incorrect because loss of pancreatic islet cells would be associated with hyperglycemia.
Diagnosis: Pancreatitis, chronic; steatorrhea

6 **The answer is E: Pancreatic pseudocyst.** Pancreatic pseudocyst is a late complication of acute pancreatitis, in which necrotic pancreatic tissue is liquefied through the action of pancreatic enzymes (e.g., peptidases, lipases, and amylase). The necrotic tissue becomes encapsulated by granulation tissue, which then develops into a fibrous capsule. Pseudocysts may enlarge to compress and even obstruct the duodenum. They may become secondarily infected and form an abscess. Choices B, C, and D are not consequences of acute pancreatitis.
Diagnosis: Pancreatic pseudocyst

7 **The answer is E: Pancreatic enzymes.** Pancreatic pseudocysts are lined by connective tissue and contain blood, necrotic debris, and secreted pancreatic enzymes. Reflux of bile (choice A) is not characteristic of a pancreatic pseudocyst. The other choices (B, C, and D) may be present in small quantities.
Diagnosis: Pancreatic pseudocyst

8 **The answer is D: Pancreatic adenocarcinoma.** Adenocarcinoma is the most common malignant tumor of the pancreas. Although it accounts for only 3% of all cancers in the United States, it is the fourth leading cause of cancer death in men and the fifth leading cause of cancer death in women. Migratory thrombophlebitis, which is also referred to as Trousseau syndrome, may accompany adenocarcinoma of the pancreas as well as other malignancies. The cause of migratory thrombophlebitis is not entirely understood, but it is thought that the tumor releases thrombogenic substances into the circulation (e.g., serine proteases) that initiate the coagulation cascade. The CT scan excludes adenocarcinoma of the ampulla of Vater (choice A). Endocrine tumors of the pancreas (choices B and C) are not expected to induce Trousseau syndrome.
Diagnosis: Pancreatic adenocarcinoma

9 **The answer is E: Ductal cells.** The majority of pancreatic carcinomas arise from pancreatic duct epithelium. Acinar cell carcinoma (choice A) is much less common. The other choices represent uncommon islet cell tumors.
Diagnosis: Pancreatic adenocarcinoma

10 **The answer C: Extrahepatic biliary obstruction.** Pancreatic adenocarcinomas often cause obstruction of the common bile duct due to the proximity of the duct to the head of the pancreas. Painless jaundice is a frequent initial symptom of pancreatic cancer. Dilation of the gallbladder in this setting is termed Courvoisier sign. Cirrhosis (choice B) is a late complication of extrahepatic biliary obstruction.
Diagnosis: Pancreatic adenocarcinoma

11 **The answer is C: Cigarette smoking.** Cigarette smoking is associated with a fivefold increased risk for adenocarcinoma of the pancreas. Cholelithiasis (choice B) and alcohol abuse (choice A) are associated with pancreatitis, not pancreatic adenocarcinoma.
Diagnosis: Pancreatic adenocarcinoma

12 The answer is E: Zollinger-Ellison syndrome. Zollinger-Ellison syndrome is characterized by intractable gastric hypersecretion, severe peptic ulceration of the duodenum and sometimes the jejunum, and elevated levels of gastrin in blood. The tumor responsible for Zollinger-Ellison syndrome is pancreatic gastrinoma composed of G cells. Gastrinomas are most often located in the pancreas, but they may arise in other parts of the gastrointestinal tract, notably the duodenum. Most gastrinomas are malignant. Carcinoid syndrome (choice A) is a systemic paraneoplastic disease caused by the release of hormones from carcinoid tumors into venous blood. Clinical features of carcinoid tumors (e.g., flushing, bronchial wheezing, watery diarrhea, and abdominal colic) are presumably caused by the release of serotonin, bradykinin, and histamine.

Diagnosis: Gastrinoma, Zollinger-Ellison syndrome

13 The answer is C: Glucagonoma. Necrotizing migratory erythema develops in association with the hypersecretion of glucagon by alpha cell–containing tumors (glucagonomas). These patients also have mild hyperglycemia and anemia. The other choices do not present with these clinical signs and symptoms.

Diagnosis: Glucagonoma

14 The answer is D: Insulinoma. Insulinoma is the most common islet cell tumor. These tumors of the endocrine pancreas are low-grade malignant neoplasms. Insulinomas secrete insulin and cause hypoglycemia. Symptoms of hypoglycemia include hunger, sweating, irritability, epileptic seizures, and coma. Infusion of glucose alleviates these symptoms. The other tumors do not cause marked hypoglycemia. Patients with a glucagonoma (choice C) typically present with necrotizing migratory erythema, mild hyperglycemia, and anemia. Patients with a somatostatinoma (choice E) typically present with mild diabetes mellitus, gallstones, steatorrhea, and hypochlorhydria.

Diagnosis: Insulinoma

15 The answer is E: VIPoma. Intractable diarrhea, hypokalemia, and low levels of chloride in gastric juice constitute the syndrome of "pancreatic cholera." This disorder is secondary to the secretion of vasoactive intestinal polypeptide (VIP) by an islet cell tumor. VIP stimulates adenylyl cyclase activity, which in turn leads to the production of large amounts of cAMP. The latter causes increased secretion of potassium and water into the intestinal lumen. The ensuing diarrhea results in loss of water, amounting to as much as 5 L per day. The other choices do not present with these signs and symptoms.

Diagnosis: VIPoma

16 The answer is D: Somatostatin. Delta cell tumors (somatostatinomas) produce a syndrome consisting of mild diabetes mellitus, gallstones, steatorrhea, and hypochlorhydria. These effects result from the inhibitory action of somatostatin on the secretion of hormones by cells of the endocrine pancreas, acinar cells of the pancreas, and certain hormone-secreting cells in the gastrointestinal tract. Somatostatin also inhibits the pituitary release of growth hormone. None of the other choices are associated with mild diabetes or cholelithiasis.

Diagnosis: Somatostatinoma, cholelithiasis

17 The answer is B: Drug-induced pancreatitis. Acute pancreatitis may be encountered in patients taking immunosuppressive drugs, antineoplastic agents, sulfonamides, and diuretics. Severe cases of acute pancreatitis cause retroperitoneal hemorrhage, which can track to the flank and periumbilical region (see photograph). The other choices may induce pancreatitis but are exceedingly unlikely in this clinical setting.

Diagnosis: Pancreatitis, acute

18 The answer is D: Pancreatic carcinoid. Carcinoid tumors of the pancreas are rare malignant neoplasms that closely resemble intestinal carcinoids. When confined to the pancreas, they may induce the so-called atypical carcinoid syndrome, which is associated with severe facial flushing, hypotension, periorbital edema, and tearing. Hepatic metastases cause the full blown carcinoid syndrome. Adenocarcinoma of the pancreas (choice A) does not produce hormones. The other choices lead to other endocrine syndromes.

Diagnosis: Carcinoid tumor

19 The answer is C: Multiple endocrine neoplasia type 1. The patient exhibits signs and symptoms of MEN-1 (Wermer syndrome), including adenoma of the pituitary (acromegaly), hyperplasia or adenoma of the parathyroids (hypercalcemia), and adenoma of the endocrine pancreas (gastrinoma). Gastrin-producing tumors of the pancreas may produce Zollinger-Ellison syndrome, characterized by intractable peptic ulcers. MEN-1 is caused by mutations in the *MEN1* tumor suppressor gene. MEN-2A (Sipple syndrome, choice D) features medullary thyroid carcinoma and pheochromocytoma, and is associated with *RET* protooncogene mutations.

Diagnosis: Zollinger-Ellison syndrome, multiple endocrine neoplasia

Chapter 16

The Kidney

QUESTIONS

Select the single best answer.

1 The mother of a 2-month-old child palpates a mass on the left side of the child's abdomen. Vital signs are normal. A CT-guided renal biopsy shows undifferentiated tubules surrounded by undifferentiated mesenchyme, smooth muscle, and islands of cartilage. The mass is removed (shown in the image) and displays variably sized cysts. Which of the following is the most likely diagnosis for this child's flank mass?

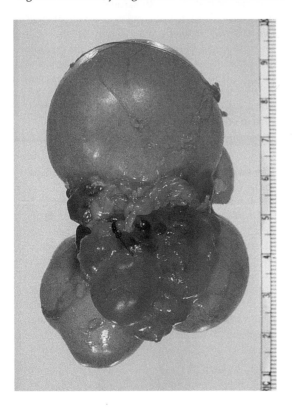

(A) Infantile polycystic disease
(B) Medullary sponge kidney
(C) Neuroblastoma
(D) Renal dysplasia
(E) Wilms tumor

2 A 38-year-old man presents with vague flank pain and describes the passage of blood clots in his urine. Physical examination reveals bilateral flank and abdominal masses. Laboratory studies show elevated blood urea nitrogen and creatinine. Urinalysis reveals hematuria, proteinuria, and oliguria. A CT scan discloses bilaterally, massively enlarged kidneys. The patient subsequently develops end-stage kidney disease and receives a renal transplant. The patient's kidneys are removed during surgery (shown in the image). What is the most likely diagnosis?

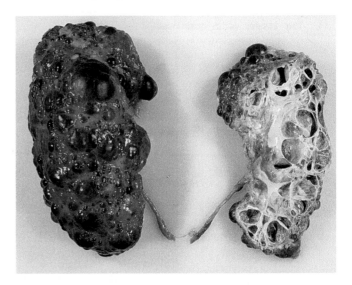

(A) Autosomal dominant polycystic kidney disease
(B) Autosomal recessive polycystic kidney disease
(C) Hydronephrosis
(D) Medullary sponge kidney
(E) Multicystic renal dysplasia

3 The patient described in Question 2 carries an increased risk for which of the following abnormalities?
(A) Hepatic cysts
(B) Horseshoe kidney
(C) Pulmonary cysts
(D) Renal cell carcinoma
(E) Transitional cell carcinoma of the bladder

4 A 46-year-old woman presents with a 6-month history of vague upper abdominal pain after fatty meals, some abdominal distension, and frequent indigestion. Physical examination shows an obese woman (BMI = 32 kg/m²) with right upper quadrant tenderness. A CT scan discloses gallstones and an ectopic kidney. Which of the following is the expected location of the ectopic kidney?
(A) Adjacent to gallbladder
(B) Attached to the left adrenal gland
(C) Fused laterally with the contralateral kidney
(D) Pelvis
(E) Posterior epigastrium

5 A 12-year-old girl complains of swelling of her eyelids, abdomen, and ankles. She had been in good health until several months ago, when she gained some weight and noted swelling of her lower legs. An X-ray film of the chest shows bilateral pleural effusions, without evidence of lung disease. Urinalysis reveals heavy proteinuria (8 g per 24 hours) without hematuria. A percutaneous needle biopsy of the kidney discloses no morphologic abnormalities by light microscopy. Which of the following best describes this patient's medical condition?
(A) Amyloid nephropathy
(B) Focal segmental glomerulosclerosis
(C) Hereditary nephritis
(D) Membranous glomerulopathy
(E) Nephrotic syndrome

6 An 8-year-old boy presents with headaches, dizziness, and malaise. He was seen for a severe sore throat 2 weeks ago. Physical examination reveals facial edema. The blood pressure is 180/110 mm Hg. A 24-hour urine collection demonstrates oliguria, and urinalysis shows hematuria. Which of the following best describes this patient's medical condition?
(A) Hereditary nephritis
(B) Membranous glomerulonephritis
(C) Minimal change nephritic syndrome
(D) Postinfectious glomerulonephritis
(E) Thin glomerular basement membrane nephropathy

7 What finding on microscopic urinalysis indicates that hematuria in the patient described in Question 6 is caused by a renal process, rather than bleeding from another site in the urinary tract?
(A) Blood clots
(B) Hemoglobin crystals
(C) Phagocytosed hemoglobin
(D) Red blood cell casts
(E) White blood cell casts

8 A 60-year-old man complains of chronic back pain and fatigue, excessive urination, and increased thirst. X-ray examination reveals numerous lytic lesions in the lumbar vertebral bodies. Laboratory studies show hypoalbuminemia, mild anemia, and thrombocytopenia. Urinalysis displays 4+ proteinuria. A monoclonal immunoglobulin light-chain peak is demonstrated by serum electrophoresis. A bone marrow biopsy discloses foci of plasma cells, which account for 20% of all hematopoietic cells. A kidney biopsy is obtained (shown in the image). Which of the following is the most likely cause of nephrotic syndrome in this patient?

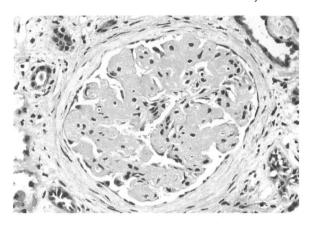

(A) Amyloid nephropathy
(B) Crescentic glomerulonephritis
(C) IgA nephropathy (Berger disease)
(D) Membranous glomerulonephritis
(E) Nodular glomerulosclerosis (Kimmelstiel-Wilson disease)

9 A 49-year-old man with a history of heavy smoking presents with a 5-year history of shortness of breath and cough and production of abundant foul-smelling sputum. A pulmonary work-up demonstrates chronic bronchiectasis. Laboratory studies reveal hypoalbuminemia and hyperlipidemia. Urinalysis shows heavy proteinuria (>4 g per day). Which of the following is the appropriate diagnosis?
(A) Amyloid nephropathy
(B) Berger disease (IgA nephropathy)
(C) Focal segmental glomerulosclerosis
(D) Minimal change glomerulopathy
(E) Wegener granulomatosis

10 A 12-year-old boy complains of swelling of his feet for the past 3 weeks. He is otherwise healthy, with no known previous illness. Vital signs are normal. Physical examination reveals pitting edema of the lower legs and a swollen abdomen. Urinalysis shows 4+ protein but no RBCs or WBCs. Which of the following are the most likely diagnoses to consider in your evaluation of this patient?
(A) Henoch-Schönlein purpura, lupus nephritis
(B) Malignant hypertension, renal vein thrombosis
(C) Minimal change disease, focal segmental glomerulosclerosis
(D) Pyelonephritis, acute tubular necrosis
(E) Wilms tumor, renal cell carcinoma

11 A 4-year-old girl presents with swelling of the legs and ankles. Physical examination reveals pitting edema of the lower extremities. Urinalysis show 2+ proteinuria. The urinary sediment contains no inflammatory cells or red blood cells. Serum levels of BUN and creatinine are normal. The patient recovers completely after a course of corticosteroids. Which of the following pathologic findings might be expected in the urine prior to treatment with corticosteroids?
(A) Amyloid casts
(B) Eosinophils
(C) Lipid droplets
(D) Red blood cell casts
(E) White blood cells casts

12 For the patient described in Question 11, electron microscopy of a renal biopsy specimen prior to treatment would most likely demonstrate which of the following abnormalities?
(A) Duplication of capillary basement membranes
(B) Electron-dense immune deposits in the capillary basement membranes
(C) Electron-dense immune deposits in the mesangium
(D) Fusion of podocyte foot processes
(E) Loss of microvilli by the tubular lining cells

13 A 44-year-old man complains of swelling of his legs and puffiness around his eyes. His abdomen has become protuberant and he feels short of breath. Physical examination reveals generalized edema and ascites. Total serum protein is 5.2 g/dL (reference = 5.5 to 8.0 g/dL), and albumin is 1.9 g/dL (reference = 3.5 to 5.5 g/dL). Serum cholesterol is elevated at 530 mg/dL. There are 5 g of protein in a 24-hour urine collection. The urinary sediment contains many hyalin casts but no RBCs or inflammatory cells. A renal biopsy stained by direct immunofluorescence for IgG is shown in the image. Which of the following is the most likely diagnosis?

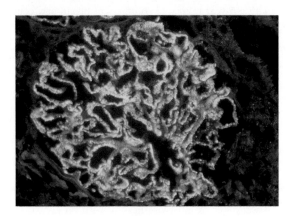

(A) Amyloid nephropathy
(B) Focal segmental glomerulosclerosis
(C) Membranoproliferative glomerulonephritis type I
(D) Membranous glomerulopathy
(E) Minimal change disease

14 The pathogenesis of nephrotic syndrome in the patient described in Question 13 is best characterized by which of the following mechanisms of disease?
(A) Deposition of antiglomerular basement membrane antibody
(B) Deposition of IgA in the mesangium
(C) Expansion of the glomerular basement membrane with PAS-positive glycoproteins
(D) Subendothelial deposits of immune complexes
(E) Subepithelial deposits of immune complexes

15 The glomerular changes in the patient described in Question 13 are frequently seen in patients with which of the following systemic diseases?
(A) Amyloid nephropathy
(B) Goodpasture syndrome
(C) Scleroderma
(D) Systemic lupus erythematosus
(E) Wegener granulomatosis

16 A 14-year-old girl presents with a 5-day history of hypertension, oliguria, and hematuria. She was seen 2 weeks earlier for a severe throat infection with group A (β-hemolytic) streptococci. A kidney biopsy displays glomerulonephritis. Immunofluorescence staining for which of the following proteins would provide the strongest evidence that this patient's glomerulonephritis is mediated by immune complexes?
(A) Complement
(B) Fibrinogen
(C) Hageman factor (clotting factor XII)
(D) Plasminogen
(E) Thrombin

17 A 28-year-old man complains of nasal obstruction, bloody nose, cough, and bloody sputum. A chest X-ray displays cavitated lesions and multiple nodules within both lung fields. Urinalysis reveals 3+ hematuria and red blood cell casts. Laboratory studies show anemia and elevated serum levels of C-ANCA (antineutrophil cytoplasmic antibody). Peripheral eosinophils are not increased. A renal biopsy exhibits focal glomerular necrosis with crescents and vasculitis affecting arterioles and venules. What is the appropriate diagnosis?
(A) Churg-Strauss syndrome
(B) Goodpasture syndrome
(C) Hypersensitivity vasculitis
(D) Polyarteritis nodosa
(E) Wegener granulomatosis

18 Which of the following best describes the renal disease of the patient described in Question 17?
(A) Chronic nephritic syndrome
(B) Nephrotic syndrome
(C) Rapidly progressive glomerulonephritis
(D) Type I membranoproliferative glomerulonephritis
(E) Type II membranoproliferative glomerulonephritis

19 A 30-year-old man with a history of drug addiction presents with a 6-month history of progressive swelling in his ankles and abdomen. Urinalysis shows heavy proteinuria (>4 g per 24 hours) but no evidence of inflammatory cells or RBCs. Laboratory studies reveal hyperlipidemia and hypoalbuminemia. Serum creatinine level is normal. The blood test for ANCA is negative. The patient responds well to treatment with corticosteroids, but edema and proteinuria recur the following year. The steroid treatment is repeated with the same results. Upon the third recurrence of edema and proteinuria, the patient becomes steroid resistant. A renal biopsy is shown in the image. Which of the following is the most likely diagnosis for this patient's glomerulopathy?

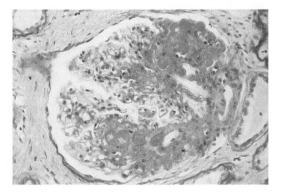

(A) Acute glomerulonephritis
(B) Amyloidosis
(C) Crescentic glomerulonephritis
(D) Diffuse proliferative glomerulonephritis
(E) Focal segmental glomerulosclerosis

20 A 20-year-old woman is involved in an automobile accident and loses a large amount of blood. In response to hypoxia, interstitial peritubular cells of the kidney would be expected to release which of the following hormones?
(A) Aldosterone
(B) Angiotensin
(C) Angiotensinogen
(D) Erythropoietin
(E) Renin

21 A 32-year-old man complains of recurrent hematuria since his youth. The hematuria typically occurs following upper respiratory tract infections. Vital signs are normal. Urinalysis shows proteinuria, hematuria, and a few red blood cell casts. Laboratory studies disclose normal levels of BUN and creatinine. The ANA and ANCA tests are negative. Which of the following is the most likely diagnosis?
(A) Amyloid nephropathy
(B) Berger disease (IgA nephropathy)
(C) Hereditary nephritis (Alport syndrome)
(D) Membranous glomerulopathy
(E) Wegener granulomatosis

22 For the patient described in Question 21, which of the following patterns of IgA immunofluorescence would be expected in the renal biopsy?
(A) Granular capillary membrane deposition
(B) Linear basement membrane staining
(C) Mesangial deposition
(D) Perivascular location
(E) Subepithelial deposits

23 A 25-year-old man complains of intermittent hematuria over the past 8 years. Urinalysis shows microscopic hematuria. Urine cultures are negative. A renal biopsy (shown in the image) displays mesangial proliferation within some glomeruli, whereas others appear normal. Immunofluorescence staining discloses mesangial deposition of IgA. Which of the following is the appropriate pathologic diagnosis?

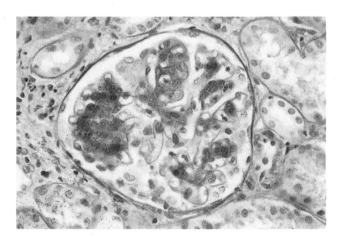

(A) Amyloid nephropathy
(B) Crescentic glomerulonephritis
(C) Focal proliferative glomerulonephritis
(D) Membranous nephropathy
(E) Nodular diabetic glomerulosclerosis

24 An 8-year-old boy presents with headaches, dizziness, and malaise approximately 2 weeks after a severe sore throat. His mother describes puffiness of his face and darkening of his urine. She also notes that her son is passing less urine and that he is becoming increasingly short of breath. On physical examination, there is anasarca, hypertension (190/130 mm Hg), and tachycardia. The urine is scanty and brownish red. Urinalysis shows 3+ proteinuria. Microscopic examination of the urine discloses numerous RBCs, as well as occasional granular and red cell casts. A renal biopsy is stained by direct immunofluorescence microscopy for complement C3, and the results are shown. Which of the following best describes the pattern of immunofluorescence observed in this renal biopsy?

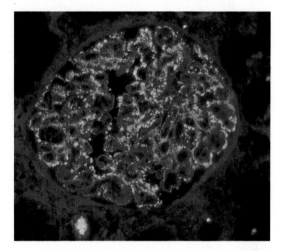

(A) Dense deposits in glomerular crescents between epithelial cells
(B) Deposits limited to the mesangium
(C) Granular deposits along the perimesangial reflections
(D) Linear staining along the glomerular basement membranes
(E) Subepithelial and subendothelial deposits

25 Which of the following is the most likely cause of acute postinfectious glomerulonephritis in the patient described in Question 24?
(A) *Escherichia coli*
(B) Epstein-Barr virus
(C) Group A (β-hemolytic) streptococci
(D) *Klebsiella* sp.
(E) *Staphylococcus* sp.

26 Which of the following is the most likely outcome of glomerulonephritis in the patient described in Question 24?
(A) Bilateral cortical necrosis
(B) Development of nephrotic syndrome
(C) Membranoproliferative glomerulonephritis
(D) Recovery without serious consequences
(E) Transition into crescentic glomerulonephritis

27 A 30-year-old woman with systemic lupus erythematosus presents with oliguria. Laboratory studies show elevated serum levels of creatinine and BUN. Urinalysis reveals 4+ proteinuria and hematuria. The renal biopsy (shown in the image) exhibits segmental endocapillary hypercellularity and thickening of capillary walls, and 90% of the glomeruli appear hypercellular. Which of the following is the appropriate pathologic diagnosis?

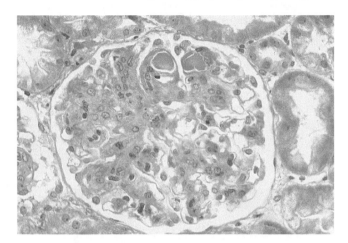

(A) Crescentic glomerulonephritis
(B) Focal segmental glomerulosclerosis
(C) Membranoproliferative glomerulonephritis, type II
(D) Membranous nephropathy
(E) Proliferative glomerulonephritis

28 A 35-year-old man with a history of smoking presents with hematuria and bloody sputum. Over the next 2 days, he develops oliguria and renal failure, after which he is placed on dialysis. A renal biopsy is stained with fluorescein-conjugated goat antihuman IgG, and the results are shown. Which of the following best describes the pattern of direct immunofluorescence observed on this photomicrograph?

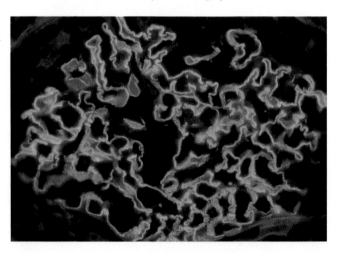

(A) Discontinuous and peripheral
(B) Finely granular along the perimesangial reflections
(C) Linear along the glomerular basement membrane
(D) Mesangial with a stalk predominance
(E) Peripheral granular humps

29 A 54-year-old woman with squamous cell carcinoma of the lung develops bilateral pitting edema of the lower extremities. Laboratory studies show hyperlipidemia, hypoalbuminemia, and 4+ proteinuria. Urinalysis reveals no inflammatory cells or RBCs. Renal biopsy in this patient would most likely show which of the following patterns of glomerulopathy?

(A) Berger disease (IgA nephropathy)
(B) Goodpasture syndrome
(C) Membranous glomerulopathy
(D) Minimal change glomerulopathy
(E) Nodular glomerulosclerosis

30 A 30-year-old man with a history of smoking suddenly develops oliguria, hematuria, and hemoptysis. Serologic studies reveal antibodies to the glomerular basement membrane (GBM). A renal biopsy is shown. Which of the following pathologic changes is visible by light microscopy in this biopsy specimen?

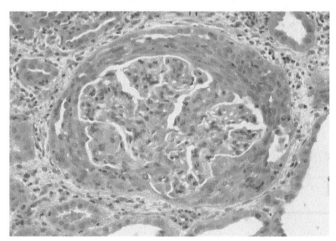

(A) Crescents in the urinary space
(B) Leukocytic infiltrates in the glomeruli
(C) Mesangial cell proliferation
(D) Thickening of the GBM
(E) Thrombi in glomerular capillaries

31 A 52-year-old woman who suffers from diabetes mellitus and frequent urinary tract infections presents with a 3-day history of flank pain, undulating fever, and general malaise. A CBC shows neutrophilic leukocytosis (16,000/μL). Urine cultures reveal more than 100,000 bacterial colonies, composed predominantly of Gram-negative microorganisms. Blood pressure is 170/100 mm Hg, BUN is 30 mg/dL, and creatinine is 2.0 mg/dL. Fasting serum glucose is 190 mg/dL. Urinalysis shows 2+ sugar and 1+ protein. Microscopic examination of the urine sediment reveals neutrophils and occasional leukocyte casts. Which of the following is the most likely diagnosis?

(A) Acute pyelonephritis
(B) Acute tubular necrosis
(C) Diabetic nephropathy
(D) Postinfectious glomerulonephritis
(E) Nephrolithiasis

32 A 22-year-old woman in the second trimester of pregnancy presents with flank pain, fever of 38.7°C (103°F), and chills. Hemoglobin is 13.4 g/dL, WBCs are elevated (13,500/μL with 78% neutrophils), and there are 265,000 platelets/μL. Physical examination reveals costovertebral angle tenderness. The urine shows numerous WBCs and WBC casts. Which of the following is the most likely diagnosis?

(A) Cystitis
(B) Endometritis
(C) Glomerulonephritis
(D) Pyelonephritis
(E) Urethritis

33 Which of the following is the most likely cause of the renal disease in the patient described in Question 32?

(A) Gram-negative bacteria
(B) Gram-positive bacteria
(C) Human papillomavirus
(D) Immune complex deposition
(E) Mycobacteria

34 A 50-year-old woman complains of severe headaches and dizziness. The patient has a history of repeated urinary tract infections. The blood pressure is 180/110 mm Hg. Laboratory studies show elevated levels of BUN (38 mg/dL) and creatinine (2.8 mg/dL). A CT scan of the lower abdomen reveals small, irregularly shaped kidneys with deep coarse scars. A percutaneous renal biopsy is shown. Which of the following is the appropriate diagnosis?

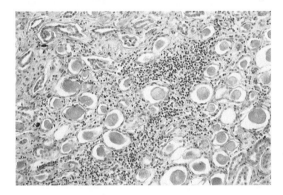

(A) Acute pyelonephritis
(B) Acute tubular necrosis
(C) Chronic pyelonephritis
(D) Nephrosclerosis
(E) Tubulointerstitial nephritis

35 The pathogenesis of the renal disease in the patient described in Question 34 is related to which of the following conditions?

(A) Amyloidosis
(B) Antiglomerular basement membrane disease
(C) Chronic hepatitis B infection
(D) Hypertension
(E) Repeated bouts of acute pyelonephritis

36 A 52-year-old woman presents with swelling of her ankles of 6 weeks in duration. Physical examination reveals an obese woman (BMI = 32 kg/m²) with pitting edema of the lower extremities

and periorbital edema. Laboratory studies show hyperlipidemia and hypoalbuminemia. Urinalysis discloses 3+ proteinuria and 3+ glucosuria but no evidence of inflammatory cells or RBCs. A kidney biopsy stained with PAS (shown in the image) displays a prominent increase in the mesangial matrix, forming nodular lesions, and thickening of capillary basement membranes. Which of the following is the most likely pathologic diagnosis?

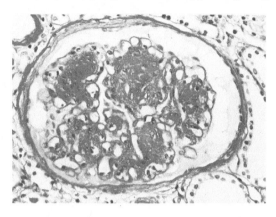

(A) Acute glomerulonephritis
(B) Amyloid nephropathy
(C) Diabetic glomerulosclerosis
(D) Malignant nephrosclerosis
(E) Membranoproliferative glomerulonephritis

37 Which of the following serum abnormalities is expected in the patient described in Question 36?

(A) Hyperbilirubinemia
(B) Hypergammaglobulinemia
(C) Hyperglycemia
(D) Hyperuricemia
(E) Hypobilirubinemia

38 A 70-year-old diabetic woman presents with sudden onset of excruciating groin and flank pain. Physical examination shows pitting edema of the lower extremities. Laboratory studies reveal decreased serum albumin and increased serum lipids. Urine cultures reveal more than 100,000 bacterial colonies composed predominantly of Gram-negative microorganisms. Which of the following is the most likely diagnosis?

(A) Acute tubular necrosis
(B) Crescentic glomerulonephritis
(C) Diabetic glomerulosclerosis
(D) Renal papillary necrosis
(E) Renal vein thrombosis

39 A 40-year-old man with Alport syndrome presents with a 3-month history of headaches. His blood pressure is 165/100 mm Hg. A urinalysis shows 3+ proteinuria and 2+ hematuria. Laboratory studies disclose elevated levels of BUN (48 mg/dL) and creatinine (3.6 mg/dL). This patient's renal disease is caused by mutation in a gene that encodes which of the following extracellular matrix proteins?

(A) Collagen
(B) Entactin
(C) Fibrillin
(D) Fibronectin
(E) Laminin

40 A 35-year-old man presents with fever and rash after beginning treatment with penicillin 2 weeks earlier for a sinus infection. Urinalysis shows 3+ hematuria, as well as mononuclear cells, neutrophils, and eosinophils. A percutaneous renal biopsy is shown. Which of the following is the most likely diagnosis?

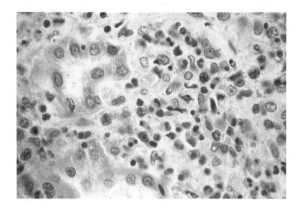

(A) Acute tubulointerstitial nephritis
(B) Chronic pyelonephritis
(C) Crescentic glomerulonephritis
(D) Focal necrotizing glomerulonephritis
(E) Focal segmental glomerulosclerosis

41 A 58-year-old man with a history of coronary artery disease, peripheral vascular disease, and a recent heart attack suddenly develops painless hematuria. He subsequently suffers a massive stroke and expires. The patient's kidney at autopsy is shown. Which of the following is the most likely diagnosis?

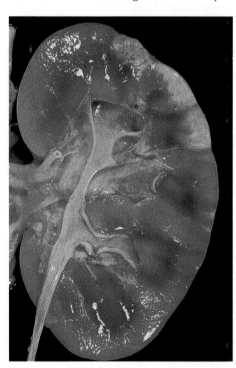

(A) Benign nephrosclerosis
(B) Chronic pyelonephritis
(C) Cortical abscess
(D) Cortical infarct
(E) Malignant nephrosclerosis

42 A 36-year-old woman in the third trimester of pregnancy (gravida II, para I) presents to the emergency room with the sudden onset of severe vaginal bleeding. Ultrasound examination of the abdomen discloses abruptio placentae. A healthy neonate is delivered; however, the mother's blood loss is uncontrollable. She becomes hypotensive and obtunded and subsequently dies of hypovolemic shock. The kidneys at autopsy are shown. Which of the following is the most likely diagnosis?

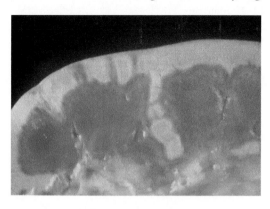

(A) Acute tubulointerstitial nephritis
(B) Bilateral renal cortical necrosis
(C) Crescentic glomerulonephritis
(D) Necrotizing glomerulonephritis
(E) Renal papillary necrosis

43 A 33-year-old woman in her third trimester of pregnancy (gravida I, para 0) is rushed to the emergency room after suffering a seizure. The patient is hypertensive and laboratory studies show that the patient manifests nephritic syndrome. What is the appropriate diagnosis?
(A) Acute tubular necrosis
(B) Crescentic glomerulonephritis
(C) Eclampsia
(D) Malignant nephrosclerosis
(E) Preeclampsia

44 A 60-year-old man undergoes resection of an abdominal aneurysm, which is complicated by massive hemorrhage. Two days after surgery, the patient develops acute renal insufficiency. He is placed on dialysis but suffers a massive heart attack and dies. Microscopic examination of the kidneys at autopsy reveals necrotic epithelial cells within the lumina of some tubules (shown in the image). The arrows identify enlarged, regenerative epithelial cells. What is the appropriate diagnosis?

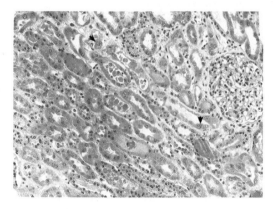

(A) Acute interstitial nephritis
(B) Acute tubular necrosis
(C) Eosinophilic interstitial nephritis
(D) Fanconi syndrome
(E) Polyarteritis nodosa

45 A 70-year-old obese woman (BMI = 34 kg/m²) presents with a 3-month history of progressive renal insufficiency. She has a longstanding history of hypertension. An intravenous pyelogram shows that both kidneys are small, and the pelves and calyces appear dilated. The patient subsequently suffers a massive stroke and expires. Examination of the kidneys at autopsy reveals symmetrically shrunken small kidneys, with a uniformly finely granular surface (shown in the image). Which of the following is the appropriate diagnosis?

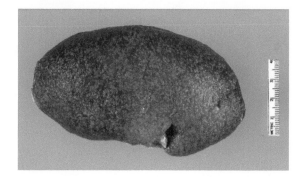

(A) Amyloidosis
(B) Hydronephrosis
(C) Ischemic acute tubular necrosis
(D) Nephrosclerosis
(E) Tubulointerstitial nephritis

46 A 60-year-old man presents with acute renal insufficiency. He treated his garden last week with a number of herbicides and insecticides, some of which may have contained heavy metals. Laboratory studies confirm oliguria and increased levels of BUN (54 mg/dL) and creatinine (3.7 mg/dL). A renal biopsy is shown. What is the most likely diagnosis?

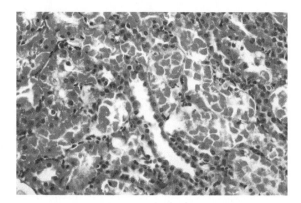

(A) Acute tubular necrosis (ATN)
(B) Bilateral cortical necrosis
(C) Papillary necrosis
(D) Rapidly progressive glomerulonephritis
(E) Tubulointerstitial nephritis

47 A 45-year-old man undergoes renal biopsy for evaluation of chronic renal failure. The patient is obese (BMI = 37 kg/m²) and admits to smoking two packs per day for 30 years. Physical examination reveals a blood pressure of 190/110 mm Hg. An echocardiogram shows conspicuous left ventricular hypertrophy. A renal biopsy discloses pathologic changes in small renal arteries, including "onion-skinning" and fibrinoid necrosis. The Congo red stain is negative. Laboratory studies show hematocrit of 40%, hemoglobin of 18.7 g/dL, serum cholesterol of 250 mg/dL, BUN of 45 mg/dL, and serum creatinine of 5.5 mg/dL. Which of the following is the most likely underlying cause of chronic renal failure in this patient?
(A) Amyloid nephropathy
(B) Chronic pyelonephritis
(C) Congestive heart failure
(D) Cushing syndrome
(E) Malignant hypertension

48 A 58-year-old man with a history of hyperlipidemia and high blood pressure presents to the emergency room for evaluation of headaches and blurred vision. His blood pressure is 200/115 mm Hg, and pulse is 95 per minute. Funduscopic examination reveals several small retinal microaneurysms and cotton-like zones of retinal edema and necrosis. Intravenous pyelography discloses small kidneys bilaterally. Renal arteriography shows stenoses of both renal arteries. Hypertension in this patient is caused by the renal release of which of the following hormones?
(A) Aldosterone
(B) Angiotensin
(C) Erythropoietin
(D) Plasminogen
(E) Renin

49 A 6-year-old child develops fever, abdominal pain, and bloody diarrhea. Several other children in the neighborhood had similar symptoms. The common feature was traced to eating hamburgers at a fast food restaurant. The clinical course is complicated by the development of acute renal failure. Which of the following is the most likely diagnosis?
(A) Acute postinfectious glomerulonephritis
(B) Churg-Strauss syndrome
(C) Hemolytic uremic syndrome
(D) Malignant hypertension
(E) Polyarteritis nodosa

50 A 5-year-old girl presents with the sudden onset of diffuse arthralgias and skin rash. Physical examination shows a violaceous maculopapular rash on the lower torso. Urinalysis discloses oliguria and 2+ hematuria. Urine cultures are negative. This child's clinical presentation is commonly associated with which of the following diseases?
(A) Berger disease
(B) Goodpasture syndrome
(C) Hemolytic uremic syndrome
(D) Henoch-Schönlein purpura
(E) Polyarteritis nodosa

51 A 50-year-old man is found to have blood in his urine during a routine checkup. He is otherwise in excellent health, except for a mild microcytic, hypochromic anemia. An enlarged right kidney is found on X-ray examination, and CT scan reveals a renal mass of irregular shape, measuring 6 cm in diameter. Which of the following is the most likely diagnosis?

(A) Angiomyolipoma
(B) Metastatic carcinoma
(C) Nephroblastoma
(D) Renal cell carcinoma
(E) Wilms tumor

52 For the patient described in Question 51, a fine-needle aspiration of the renal mass shows glycogen-rich tumor cells. Molecular studies would most likely identify mutations in which of the following growth regulatory genes?

(A) *ADPKD*
(B) *IGF-2*
(C) *PAX6*
(D) *VHL*
(E) *WT1*

53 The mother of a 12-month-old boy palpates a mass on the right side of the infant's abdomen. The surgical specimen is shown. Microscopically, the tumor is composed of multiple elements, including blastemal, stromal, and epithelial tissues. Which of the following is the most likely diagnosis?

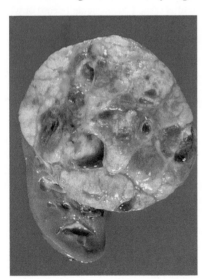

(A) Ganglioneuroma
(B) Neuroblastoma
(C) Renal cell carcinoma
(D) Teratocarcinoma
(E) Wilms tumor

54 The parents of a 6-month-old girl palpate a mass on the left side of the child's abdomen. Urinalysis shows high levels of vanillylmandelic acid. A CT scan reveals an abdominal tumor and bony metastases. Which of the following is the most likely diagnosis?

(A) Dysgerminoma
(B) Ganglioneuroma
(C) Immature teratoma
(D) Neuroblastoma
(E) Wilms tumor

55 A 50-year-old man is found to have blood in his urine during a routine checkup. A CBC shows microcytic, hypochromic anemia. An enlarged right kidney is found on X-ray examination. A CT scan reveals a renal mass of irregular shape measuring 5 cm in diameter. The nephrectomy specimen is shown. This malignant neoplasm most likely originates from which of the following tissues in the kidney?

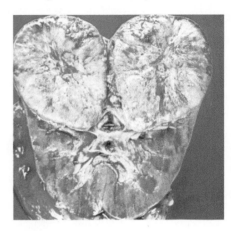

(A) Glomeruli
(B) Juxtaglomerular cells
(C) Lymphatics
(D) Renal papillae
(E) Renal tubules

56 A 56-year-old woman presents with acute renal failure. A frozen section of a renal biopsy demonstrates birefringent, intratubular deposits of uric acid crystals (shown in the image). This finding suggests that the patient has been treated recently for which of the following underlying conditions?

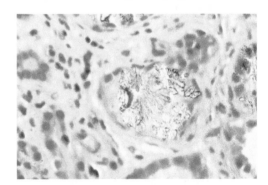

(A) Chronic hepatitis B
(B) Leukemia
(C) Porphyria
(D) Rheumatoid arthritis
(E) Ulcerative colitis

57 A 46-year-old man with no past medical history presents with excruciating episodic (colicky) right flank pain. A renal stone is passed. In the United States, this stone is most likely composed of which of the following?

(A) Calcium oxalate
(B) Calcium phosphate
(C) Cystine
(D) Magnesium ammonium phosphate
(E) Uric acid

58 A 75-year-old homeless man is brought to the emergency room in a coma. Upon admission to the hospital, the BUN is 74 mg/dL, and the creatinine is 6.5 mg/dL. He dies thereafter, and an autopsy reveals abnormal kidneys (shown in the image). The pathogenesis of this disease is most likely related to which of the following?

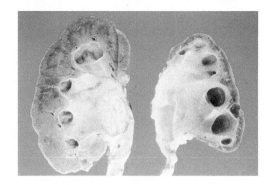

(A) Acute pyelonephritis
(B) Amyloidosis
(C) Polycystic kidney disease
(D) Systemic hypertension
(E) Urinary tract obstruction

59 A 55-year-old man dies of chronic renal failure. Examination of his kidneys at autopsy reveals a "staghorn" calculus. Which of the following best describes the pathogenesis of this renal stone?

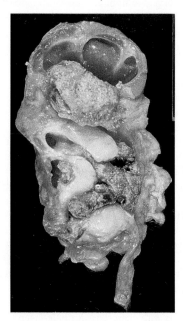

(A) Gout
(B) Hereditary cystinuria
(C) Hypercalcemia
(D) Hyperparathyroidism
(E) Infection

60 A 36-year-old woman presents with advanced cervical carcinoma, and a CT scan shows widespread pelvic spread. If this condition is not surgically corrected, the patient's kidneys will most likely develop which of the following conditions?

(A) Acute vasculitis
(B) Hydronephrosis
(C) Polycystic kidney disease
(D) Staghorn calculi
(E) Tubulointerstitial nephritis

61 A 34-year-old man undergoing cisplatin-based chemotherapy complains of a 1-week history of increasing fatigue and headaches. He also reports seeing blood in his urine. Blood pressure is 150/100 mm Hg. Physical examination reveals diffuse purpura over his upper trunk and arms. Laboratory studies show elevated levels of BUN and creatinine, and 24-hour urinalysis reveals hematuria and oliguria. Urine cultures are negative. A CBC demonstrates severe anemia (hematocrit 28%) and thrombocytopenia (50,000/μL). The direct Coombs test is negative. A peripheral blood smear reveals schistocytes. Which of the following is the most likely cause of acute renal failure in this patient?

(A) ANCA glomerulonephritis
(B) Henoch-Schönlein purpura
(C) Nephrotoxic acute tubular necrosis
(D) Polyarteritis nodosa
(E) Thrombotic microangiopathy

62 A 16-year-old black girl with sickle cell anemia presents to the emergency room because she is experiencing severe bone pain (avascular necrosis). An abdominal CT scan shows evidence of splenic infarcts. Which of the following renal diseases is a direct complication of this patient's vasoocclusive disease?

(A) Acute pyelonephritis
(B) Papillary necrosis
(C) Polycystic kidney disease
(D) Urate nephropathy
(E) Urolithiasis

63 A 35-year-old woman with end-stage renal disease of unknown etiology is transplanted with a cadaver kidney. The patient develops oliguia shortly after transplantation and a renal biopsy shows immediate (hyperacute) rejection. Immunosuppression improves renal function. Which of the following represents the principle target for immune attack directed against this patient's allograft?

(A) ABO antigens
(B) Bacterial antigens
(C) Glomerular basement membrane antigens
(D) β_2-Microglobulin
(E) Urothelium

64 A 12-year-old girl complains of headaches and blurred vision. She has a history of high blood pressure, but is not currently taking medication. Her blood pressure is 160/95 mm Hg and pulse is 95 per minute. Funduscopic examination reveals small retinal microaneurysms and cotton-like zones of retinal edema and necrosis. She is hospitalized for further evaluation. Renal arteriography shows segmental stenoses forming multiple ridges that project into the lumen. What is the most likely cause of secondary hypertension in this young patient?

(A) Buerger disease
(B) Fibromuscular dysplasia
(C) Giant cell arteritis
(D) Kawasaki disease
(E) Takayasu arteritis

ANSWERS

1 **The answer is D: Renal dysplasia.** Renal dysplasia is characterized by undifferentiated tubular structures surrounded by primitive mesenchyme, sometimes with heterotopic tissue such as smooth muscle and cartilage. Cysts often form from the abnormal tubules. Renal dysplasia results from an abnormality in metanephric differentiation. Variants of renal dysplasia include aplastic, multicystic (seen in this case), diffuse cystic, and obstructive forms. In most patients with multicystic renal dysplasia, a palpable flank mass is discovered shortly after birth. Unilateral multicystic renal dysplasia is the most common cause of an abdominal mass in newborns. Infantile polycystic disease (choice A) is invariably bilateral, and the kidneys are usually very large. Medullary sponge kidney (choice B) is characterized by multiple small cysts in the renal papillae. Wilms tumor (choice E) may contain heterologous elements but does not form large cysts.
Diagnosis: Multicystic renal dysplasia

2 **The answer is A: Autosomal dominant polycystic kidney disease.** Autosomal dominant polycystic kidney disease, which is characterized by enlarged multicystic kidneys, is the most common of a group of congenital diseases that are characterized by numerous cysts within the renal parenchyma. Most cases are caused by mutations in the polycystic kidney disease 1 gene, which encodes polycystin (function unknown). Half of all patients eventually develop end-stage renal failure. Most patients develop clinical manifestations in the fourth decade of life, which is why this condition was also called adult polycystic kidney disease. Symptoms include a sense of heaviness in the loins, bilateral flank and abdominal masses, and passage of blood clots in the urine. Azotemia is common and, in half of patients, progresses to uremia (clinical renal failure) over a period of several years. Autosomal recessive polycystic kidney disease (choice B) occurs in infants. Hydronephrosis (choice C) does not feature multiple cysts. Medullary sponge kidney (choice D) consists of multiple small cysts. Multicystic renal dysplasia (choice E) is usually unilateral.
Diagnosis: Autosomal dominant polycystic kidney disease

3 **The answer is A: Hepatic cysts.** One third of patients with autosomal dominant polycystic kidney disease (ADPKD) also have hepatic cysts, whose lining resembles bile duct epithelium. The other choices do not arise in ADPKD.
Diagnosis: Autosomal dominant polycystic kidney disease

4 **The answer is D: Pelvis.** Most ectopic kidneys are located along the pathway of renal migration during fetal development and are caudal to their normal lumbar position. During fetal life, the kidneys are initially located in the lower abdomen. As development progresses, they normally move upward toward their permanent position. Kidneys that do not reach the lumbar area but remain in the pelvis or presacral area are considered ectopic. Fusion of both kidneys results in so-called "horseshoe" kidney.
Diagnosis: Ectopic kidney

5 **The answer is E: Nephrotic syndrome.** This patient has minimal change glomerulopathy with nephrotic syndrome. The nephrotic syndrome is characterized by heavy proteinuria (>3.5 g protein per 24 hours), hypoalbuminemia, hyperlipidemia, and edema. In minimal change glomerulopathy, there is effacement of visceral epithelial cell (podocyte) foot processes, which allows protein to be lost from the plasma into the urine (proteinuria). The other choices are characterized by morphologic changes in glomeruli.
Diagnosis: Nephrotic syndrome, minimal change disease

6 **The answer is D: Postinfectious glomerulonephritis.** This case is illustrative of nephritic syndrome in the setting of poststreptococcal glomerulonephritis. Nephritic syndrome is characterized by hematuria (either microscopic or visible grossly), variable degrees of proteinuria, and decreased glomerular filtratio. It results in elevations of serum blood urea nitrogen and creatinine, as well as oliguria, salt and water retention, edema, and hypertension. Glomerular diseases associated with the nephritic syndrome are caused by inflammatory changes in glomeruli, such as infiltration by leukocytes, hyperplasia of glomerular cells, and, in severe lesions, necrosis. The other choices are not related to streptococcal pharyngitis. Choices B, C, and E do not present with hematuria.
Diagnosis: Postinfectious glomerulonephritis, nephritic syndrome

7 **The answer is D: Red blood cell casts.** Injury to the glomerular capillaries results in spillage of protein and blood cells into the urine. Hematuria is also seen in patients with bleeding from the lower urinary tract. However, RBC casts in the urine sediment originate from erythrocytes compacted during passage through the renal tubules and denote a renal origin of hematuria.
Diagnosis: Postinfectious glomerulonephritis, nephritic syndrome

8 **The answer is A: Amyloid nephropathy.** The clinicopathologic findings establish a diagnosis of multiple myeloma. The neoplastic plasma cells typically secrete a homogeneous immunoglobulin chain, which can be detected in serum or urine by electrophoresis. Amyloid nephropathy is caused by the deposition of secreted lambda or kappa light chains in the glomerular basement membranes and mesangial matrix. Amorphous acellular material expands the mesangium and obstructs the glomerular capillaries. Deposits of AL amyloid may also appear in the tubular basement membranes and in the walls of renal vessels. Renal amyloidosis usually presents with nephrotic syndrome. The deposits of amyloid may take on a nodular appearance, reminiscent of the Kimmelstiel-Wilson lesion of diabetic glomerulosclerosis (choice E). However, amyloid deposits are not PAS positive and are identifiable by Congo red staining with characteristic apple-green birefringence. IgA nephropathy (choice C) and membranous glomerulonephritis (choice D) are unrelated to light-chain disease.
Diagnosis: Amyloid nephropathy, multiple myeloma

9 **The answer is A: Amyloid nephropathy.** Amyloidosis is a well-known complication of chronic inflammatory disorders, such as chronic suppurative bronchiectasis, rheumatoid arthritis, or osteomyelitis. These conditions stimulate the production of amyloid from the serum amyloid A (SAA) protein, an acute-phase reactant secreted by the liver. The kidneys, liver, spleen, and adrenals are the most common organs involved. Renal amyloidosis leads to nephrotic syndrome (as in this case) and renal failure. Nephrotic syndrome caused by deposition of SAA amyloid is clinically indistinguishable from that related to AL amyloid. The other choices have not been linked to chronic inflammatory conditions. Wegener granulomatosis (choice E) affects the lungs and kidneys, but bronchiectasis is not a feature of this disease.

Diagnosis: Amyloid nephropathy, bronchiectasis

10 The answer is C: Minimal change disease, focal segmental glomerulosclerosis. Minimal change glomerulopathy causes 90% of the nephrotic syndrome in young children and 15% in adults. Proteinuria is generally more selective (albumin > globulins) than in the nephrotic syndrome caused by other diseases, but there is too much overlap for this selectivity to be used as a diagnostic criterion. This disease is characterized pathologically by fusion (effacement) of visceral epithelial foot processes; however, this can be visualized only by electron microscopy. Minimal change glomerulopathy is successfully treated with corticosteroids and does not progress to renal failure. Focal segmental glomerulosclerosis (FSGS) is the cause of nephrotic syndrome in 10% of children and 30% of adults. FSGS is the term applied to a heterogeneous group of glomerular diseases that have different causes, including mutations, viruses, drugs, and serum factors. Henoch-Schönlein purpura and lupus nephritis (choice A) generally present with nephritic syndrome and rash, among other signs and symptoms. Wilms tumor (choice E) is not a cause of nephrotic syndrome.

Diagnosis: Minimal change nephrotic syndrome

11 The answer is C: Lipid droplets. The loss of protein in the urine in patients with nephrotic syndrome leads to hypoalbuminemia. A compensatory increase in lipoprotein secretion by the liver results in hyperlipidemia, which is reflected in the presence of lipid droplets in the urine. For this reason, minimal change disease is also referred to as lipoid nephrosis. Eosinophils (choice B) may be observed in allergic nephritis. White blood cell casts (choice E) are features of pyelonephritis.

Diagnosis: Minimal change nephrotic syndrome

12 The answer is D: Fusion of podocyte foot processes. The light microscopic appearance of glomeruli in minimal change glomerulopathy is essentially normal. However, electron microscopic examination of glomeruli reveals total effacement of visceral epithelial cell foot processes. This retraction presumably results from extensive cell swelling and occurs in virtually all cases of proteinuria in the nephrotic range. It is not a specific marker, but is characteristic of minimal change glomerulopathy. Minimal change disease is not characterized by deposits of immune complexes (choices B and C) and does not reflect changes in the basement membrane (choice A). Choice E is incorrect because minimal change disease involves changes in glomeruli, not renal tubules.

Diagnosis: Minimal change nephrotic syndrome

13 The answer is D: Membranous glomerulopathy. Membranous glomerulopathy is a frequent cause of the nephrotic syndrome in adults and is caused by the accumulation of immune complexes in the subepithelial zone of glomerular capillaries. Immunofluorescence microscopy shows granular deposits of IgG outlining the glomerular capillary loops. The course

of membranous glomerulopathy is highly variable, with a range of possible outcomes, including spontaneous remission (25%), persistent proteinuria and stable or only partial loss of renal function (50%), and renal failure (25%). Membranoproliferative glomerulonephritis type I (choice C) is a chronic immune complex disease that features granular deposition of immunoglobulin and complement in glomerular capillary loops and mesangium.

Diagnosis: Membranous glomerulopathy

14 The answer is E: Subepithelial deposits of immune complexes. Membranous glomerulopathy exhibits localization of immune complexes in the subepithelial zone (between the visceral epithelial cell and the glomerular basement membrane) as a result of immune complex formation in situ or the deposition of circulating immune complexes. Granular deposits of IgG outlining the glomerular capillary loops are identified by immunofluorescence microscopy. Deposition of antiglomerular basement membrane antibody (choice A) is a feature of Goodpasture syndrome. Deposition of IgA in the mesangium (choice B) occurs in Berger disease. Subendothelial deposits of immune complexes (choice D) are encountered in lupus nephritis and membranoproliferative glomerulonephritis.

Diagnosis: Membranous nephropathy

15 The answer is D: Systemic lupus erythematosus. Immune complexes formed against DNA, RNA, and autologous proteins in patients with systemic lupus erythematosus may be deposited along the basement membrane of the glomeruli to form a pattern that may be indistinguishable from that of idiopathic membranous nephropathy. However, membranous nephropathy of lupus also features mesangial and subendothelial deposits of immunoglobulins. Immune complex deposition does not occur in the other choices.

Diagnosis: Systemic lupus erythematosus

16 The answer is A: Complement. In acute postinfectious glomerulonephritis, immune complexes localize in glomeruli by deposition from the circulation or by formation in situ as bacterial antigens bind circulating antibodies. The renal biopsy shows complement fixation. Complement activation is so extensive that over 90% of patients with postinfectious glomerulonephritis develop hypocomplementemia. Complement and other inflammatory mediators attract and activate neutrophils and monocytes, which stimulate the proliferation of mesangial and endothelial cells, resulting in diffuse proliferative glomerulonephritis. Typically, the level of serum C3 is depressed during the acute syndrome but returns to normal within 1 to 2 weeks. The other choices involve the coagulation system and are not components of immune complexes.

Diagnosis: Postinfectious glomerulonephritis, nephritic syndrome

17 The answer is E: Wegener granulomatosis. Wegener granulomatosis is a systemic necrotizing vasculitis of unknown etiology that is characterized by granulomatous lesions of the nose, sinuses, and lungs and is associated with renal glomerular disease. Lesions associated with this condition feature parenchymal necrosis, vasculitis, and a granulomatous inflammation composed of neutrophils, plasma cells, and macrophages. More than 90% of patients with Wegener granulomatosis exhibit ANCA, of whom 75% have C-ANCA. ANCA glomerulonephritis is an aggressive, neutrophil-mediated disease that is characterized by glomerular necrosis and crescents. Goodpasture syndrome (choice B) is characterized by both kidney and pulmonary involvement but does not display ANCA. Churg-Strauss syndrome (choice A) features eosinophilia and asthma.

Diagnosis: Wegener granulomatosis

18 **The answer is C: Rapidly progressive glomerulonephritis (RPGN).** Focal necrotizing glomerulonephritis is one of the early features of Wegener granulomatosis. The pathogenesis of this renal disease is not known, but it is thought to be immune mediated because most patients have antibodies to neutrophils (ANCA). These autoantibodies activate neutrophils and cause them to adhere to endothelial cells, release toxic oxygen metabolites, degranulate, and kill the endothelial cells. Exudation of inflammatory cells through the disrupted, segmentally necrotic basement membrane leads to the formation of crescents. Clinically, the disease presents as RPGN, a clinical term that is used to denote the rapid onset of renal failure caused by severe glomerular injury. Wegener granulomatosis does not cause membranoproliferative glomerulonephritis (choices D and E).

Diagnosis: Wegener granulomatosis, crescentic glomerulonephritis

19 **The answer is E: Focal segmental glomerulosclerosis.** Focal segmental glomerulosclerosis (FSGS) is characterized by glomerular scarring (sclerosis) that affects some (focal), but not all, glomeruli and initially involves only part of an affected glomerular tuft (segmental). By light microscopy, varying numbers of glomeruli show segmental obliteration of capillary loops by increased collagen and the accumulation of lipid or proteinaceous material. FSGS is the cause of the nephrotic syndrome in 30% of adults and 10% of children. It is also the most common renal complication of intravenous drug abuse. Clinically, it presents with proteinuria, which occasionally may be so massive as to produce nephrotic syndrome. Nephropathy associated with HIV infection is a severe and rapidly progressive collapsing form of FSGS. Patients typically progress to end-stage renal disease in less than a year. The other choices involve glomeruli diffusely. Crescents (choice C) are not observed in the photomicrograph shown.

Diagnosis: Focal segmental glomerulosclerosis

20 **The answer is D: Erythropoietin.** Erythropoietin is released by the interstitial peritubular cells of the kidney in response to hypoxia and activates specific receptors on the cell membrane of erythroid progenitor cells in the bone marrow. This effect rescues progenitor cells from programmed cell death, promotes colony growth, and restores normal red blood cell mass. Renin (choice E) is released by the juxtaglomerular apparatus.

Diagnosis: Anemia, hypoxia

21 **The answer is B: Berger disease (IgA nephropathy).** Berger disease is the most common form of glomerulonephritis in adults. Deposition of IgA-dominant immune complexes is the cause of the nephropathy, but the constituent antigens and the mechanism of accumulation have not been determined.

Exacerbations of IgA nephropathy are often initiated by infections of the respiratory or gastrointestinal tracts. The diagnostic finding on renal biopsy is intense mesangial staining for IgA, which is almost always accompanied by staining for C3. IgA nephropathy manifests a continuum of glomerulopathies, ranging from no discernible light microscopic changes to chronic sclerosing glomerulonephritis. Patients frequently present with hematuria and proteinuria, and 20% of patients develop renal failure after 10 years. Neither amyloid nephropathy (choice A) nor membranous nephropathy (choice D) features RBC casts. Hereditary nephritis (Alport syndrome; choice C) reflects abnormal type IV collagen in the glomerular basement membrane. Hematuria is present early in life; proteinuria, progressive renal failure, and hypertension develop later in the course of the disease. Wegener granulomatosis (choice E) is usually positive for ANCA.

Diagnosis: Berger disease, IgA nephropathy

22 **The answer is C: Mesangial deposition.** IgA nephropathy (Berger disease) is caused by immune complexes of IgA, which are located within the mesangium, where they most likely activate complement through the alternative pathway. The diagnostic finding is mesangial staining that is more intense for IgA than for IgG or IgM.

Diagnosis: Berger disease, IgA nephropathy

23 **The answer is C: Focal proliferative glomerulonephritis.** Focal proliferative glomerulonephritis typically presents with pathologic changes in some glomeruli, whereas others remain normal. This group of diseases includes lupus nephritis, nephritis that accompanies several vasculitides, Henoch-Schönlein purpura, and several other disorders. It also includes IgA nephropathy (Berger disease), which, as in this case, presents with mesangial deposits of IgA and mesangial cell proliferation. The clinical presentation is variable, which reflects the varied pathologic severity of disease.

Diagnosis: Berger disease, IgA nephropathy

24 **The answer is E: Subepithelial and subendothelial deposits.** The most distinctive ultrastructural features of acute postinfectious glomerulonephritis are subepithelial dense deposits that are shaped like "humps." These deposits are invariably accompanied by mesangial and subendothelial deposits, which may be more difficult to find but are probably more important in pathogenesis because of their proximity to inflammatory mediator systems in the blood. Choices A, B, and C describe limited deposition of immune complexes, whereas choice D is a feature of antiglomerular basement membrane disease (Goodpasture syndrome).

Diagnosis: Postinfectious glomerulonephritis, nephritic syndrome

25 **The answer is C: Group A (β-hemolytic) streptococci.** Acute postinfectious glomerulonephritis is an immune complex disease of childhood, which occurs after an infection with group A (β-hemolytic) streptococci and is caused by the deposition of immune complexes in glomeruli. Occasional examples are caused by staphylococcal infection (e.g., acute staphylococcal endocarditis, staphylococcal abscess), and rare cases result from viral (e.g., hepatitis B) or parasitic (e.g., malaria) infections. The primary infection involves the pharynx or, in hot and humid environments, the skin. In recent years, the proportion of cases of acute postinfectious glomerulonephritis caused by staphylococcal infection (choice E) has been increasing.

Diagnosis: Nephritic syndrome, acute postinfectious glomerulonephritis

26 The answer is D: Recovery without serious consequences. Overt nephritis after postinfectious glomerulonephritis usually resolves after several weeks, although hematuria and especially proteinuria may persist for several months.

Diagnosis: Nephritic syndrome, acute postinfectious glomerulonephritis

27 The answer is E: Proliferative glomerulonephritis. Systemic lupus erythematosus (SLE) is an autoimmune disease characterized by a generalized dysregulation and hyperactivity of B cells, with production of autoantibodies to a variety of nuclear and nonnuclear antigens. Nephritis is one of the most common complications of SLE. Immune complexes may localize in glomeruli by deposition from the circulation, formation in situ, or both. Diffuse proliferative glomerulonephritis is a severe form of lupus nephritis, characterized by widespread involvement of glomeruli and diffuse proliferation of mesangial and endothelial cells and even of epithelial cells. Deposits of immune complexes, visible by electron microscopy or immunofluorescence microscopy, are present on both sides of the basement membrane, in the mesangial areas, and even inside the capillary loops. The thickened basement membranes of the glomeruli are colloquially known as "wire loop" lesions. Membranous nephropathy (choice D) may occur in SLE, but the current biopsy displays hypercellularity. SLE is not a cause of membranoproliferative glomerulonephritis, type II (choice C).

Diagnosis: Systemic lupus erythematosus

28 The answer is C: Linear along the glomerular basement membrane (GBM). Anti-GBM antibody glomerulonephritis is an uncommon but aggressive form of glomerulonephritis that occurs as a renal limited disease or is combined with pulmonary hemorrhage (Goodpasture syndrome). The disease is mediated by an autoimmune response against a component of the GBM that is located within the noncollagenous domain of type IV collagen. A characteristic feature of anti-GBM glomerulonephritis is the presence of diffuse linear staining of GBMs for IgG, which indicates autoantibodies bound to the basement membrane. By light microscopy, over 90% of patients with anti-GBM glomerulonephritis have glomerular crescents (crescentic glomerulonephritis). Linear immunofluorescence for IgG is seen along the GBM. Anti-GBM glomerulonephritis typically presents with rapidly progressive renal failure and nephritic signs and symptoms.

Diagnosis: Goodpasture syndrome

29 The answer is C: Membranous glomerulopathy. Many malignant neoplasms may be accompanied by a variety of paraneoplastic syndromes, among which is membranous nephropathy. Other causes of secondary membranous nephropathy include autoimmune diseases (e.g., systemic lupus erythematosus), infectious diseases (e.g., hepatitis B), and therapeutic agents (e.g., penicillamine). Immune complex deposition is found in all of these conditions. IgA nephropathy and Goodpasture syndrome (choices A and B) are not paraneoplastic disorders.

Minimal change glomerulopathy (choice D) is usually found in children and is not a paraneoplastic disorder. Nodular glomerulosclerosis (choice E) reflects diabetic lesions.

Diagnosis: Membranous nephropathy, paraneoplastic syndrome

30 The answer is A: Crescents in the urinary space. Crescentic glomerulonephritis is the morphologic equivalent of acute renal failure, which may develop in rapidly progressive glomerulonephritis of Goodpasture syndrome. This disease is mediated by antibodies to collagen type IV, which attack the GBM. The same antibodies attack the lung and cause hemoptysis. Rupture of the GBM and extravasation of blood and inflammatory cells into the urinary space (i.e., the space between Bowman capsule and the glomerular capillary tufts) leads to the appearance of hypercellular, crescent-like tissue. These structures are composed of proliferating parietal epithelial cells, as well as visceral epithelial cells and macrophages. Crescentic glomerulonephritis can be caused by other diseases, such as Wegener granulomatosis or polyarteritis nodosa, which are also diseases that damage the capillary loops of the glomeruli and allow an inflammatory exudate to accumulate in the urinary space. The other choices are not representative of epithelial crescents.

Diagnosis: Goodpasture syndrome

31 The answer is A: Acute pyelonephritis. Pyelonephritis refers to bacterial infection of the kidney parenchyma. Gram-negative bacteria, most commonly *Escherichia coli*, cause 80% of acute pyelonephritis. The infection reaches the kidney by ascending through the urinary tract, a process that depends on the following several factors: (1) bacterial infection of the urine, (2) reflux of the infected urine up the ureters into the renal pelves and calyces, and (3) entry of the bacteria through the papillae into the renal parenchyma. Bacteriuria is a typical finding in patients with acute pyelonephritis. Diabetic patients with glucosuria are at increased risk for developing acute pyelonephritis. Acute bacterial infection is not a typical feature of the other choices.

Diagnosis: Acute pyelonephritis

32 The answer is D: Pyelonephritis. Symptoms of pyelonephritis include fever, chills, malaise, and flank pain. There is an increased incidence of pyelonephritis in pregnancy. On gross examination, the kidneys of acute pyelonephritis may have small white abscesses on the subcapsular surface. The urothelium of the pelvices and calyces may be hyperemic and covered by a purulent exudate. Acute pyelonephritis is often a focal disease, and much of the kidney often appears normal. Renal biopsy shows an extensive infiltrate of neutrophils in the collecting tubules and interstitial tissue. Cystitis (choice A) and urethritis (choice E) are incorrect because the finding of leukocyte casts in urine supports the diagnosis of an upper urinary tract infection.

Diagnosis: Acute pyelonephritis

33 The answer is A: Gram-negative bacteria. Acute pyelonephritis and chronic pyelonephritis are bacterial diseases that usually develop from ascending infections related to the reflux of infected urine from the lower urinary tract. Gram-negative bacteria from the feces, most commonly *E. coli*, cause 80% of cases of acute pyelonephritis. Infection of the bladder often precedes acute pyelonephritis. Bladder infection is more common in females because of a short urethra, lack of antibacterial prostatic secretions, and facilitation of bacterial migration by sexual intercourse. Hematogenous dissemination of organisms may lead to urosepsis. Infection with Gram-positive bacteria (choice B) can occur but is not common. Viruses (choice C) and mycobacteria (choice E) do not ordinarily cause renal disease. Choice D (immune complex deposition) is associated with glomerular disease.

Diagnosis: Acute pyelonephritis

34   **The answer is C: Chronic pyelonephritis.**   Patients with chronic pyelonephritis suffer episodic manifestations of urinary tract infection or acute pyelonephritis, such as recurrent fever and flank pain. Urinalysis demonstrates leukocytes, and imaging studies reveal cortical scarring. The microscopic appearance of chronic pyelonephritis is nonspecific. In this case, the biopsy shows tubular dilation and atrophy. Many tubules contain eosinophilic hyaline casts resembling the colloid of thyroid follicles (so-called thyroidization). The interstitium is scarred and contains a chronic inflammatory cell infiltrate (see photomicrograph). With the exception of acute pyelonephritis, the other choices are not related to bacterial infections. Acute pyelonephritis (choice A) is not characterized by scarred and shrunken kidneys.

Diagnosis: Chronic pyelonephritis

35   **The answer is E: Repeated bouts of acute pyelonephritis.**   Chronic pyelonephritis is caused by recurrent and persistent bacterial infection secondary to urinary tract obstruction, urine reflux, or both. Choices A, B, and C cause glomerular disease, and choice D (hypertension) is a vascular disorder that is not associated with deep cortical scarring.

Diagnosis: Chronic pyelonephritis

36   **The answer is C: Diabetic glomerulosclerosis.**   Diabetes mellitus, a complex metabolic disease associated with glucosuria and polyuria, is the leading cause of end-stage renal disease in the United States, accounting for a third of all patients with chronic renal failure. Diabetic glomerulosclerosis is a component of the vascular sclerosis that involves many small vessels throughout the body. In this condition, the glomeruli show diffuse mesangial matrix expansion with focal, segmental, nodular, and sclerotic lesions. Nodular widening of the mesangial areas is associated with hyalinization of arterioles and focal hyaline changes of Bowman capsule. Diabetic glomerulosclerosis eventually results in progressive renal failure. The other choices are not associated with diabetes and glucosuria.

Diagnosis: Diabetic nephropathy, diabetes mellitus

37   **The answer is C: Hyperglycemia.**   The cardinal sign of diabetes mellitus is increased levels of blood glucose (hyperglycemia). Abnormal nonenzymatic glycosylation of serum and matrix proteins, including those of the glomerular basement membrane and mesangial matrix, may induce binding of plasma proteins, such as immunoglobulins and, thereby, stimulate excessive matrix production. As a result, the GBMs are thickened and hyperpermeable to albumin, which leads to proteinuria. Overt proteinuria occurs 10 to 15 years after the onset of diabetes and often becomes severe enough to cause nephrotic syndrome. The other choices are not characteristic of diabetes.

Diagnosis: Diabetes mellitus, diabetic glomerulosclerosis

38   **The answer is D: Renal papillary necrosis.**   Glucosuria of diabetes predisposes to acute pyelonephritis by providing a rich medium for bacterial growth. Necrosis of the papillary tips may occur in severe cases. Symptoms include fever, urinary colic, and severe groin and flank pain. The other choices are not complications of pyelonephritits.

Diagnosis: Papillary necrosis, diabetes mellitus

39   **The answer is A: Collagen.**   Hereditary nephritis (Alport syndrome) reflects abnormal type IV collagen in the glomerular basement membrane. The syndrome is a proliferative and sclerosing glomerular disease, often accompanied by defects of the ear or the eyes, which is caused by a genetic abnormality in type IV collagen. Hematuria is present early in life in males with X-linked disease and in both sexes with autosomal recessive disease. Proteinuria, progressive renal failure, and hypertension develop later in the course of the disease. Virtually all men with the X-linked syndrome and both sexes with autosomal recessive disease develop end-stage renal disease by ages 40 to 50 years. Patients with Marfan syndrome have mutations in the fibrillin gene (choice C).

Diagnosis: Hereditary nephritis, Alport syndrome

40   **The answer is A: Acute tubulointerstitial nephritis.**   Drug-induced (hypersensitivity) acute tubulointerstitial nephritis reflects a cell-mediated immune response. It is characterized histologically by infiltrates of activated lymphocytes (T lymphocytes) and admixed eosinophils, a pattern that indicates a type IV cell-mediated immune reaction. Although eosinophils may be present, they are not essential for the diagnosis of drug-induced nephropathy. Acute tubulointerstitial nephritis typically presents as rapidly progressive renal failure, beginning approximately 2 weeks after drug administration is started. Most patients recover fully if the drug is discontinued. The other choices are not associated with an eosinophilic response and are not related to drug hypersensitivity.

Diagnosis: Acute tubulointerstitial nephritis

41   **The answer is D: Cortical infarct.**   Renal cortical infarcts are, for the most part, caused by arterial obstruction, and most represent embolization to the interlobar or larger branches of the renal artery. Common sources of emboli include mural thrombi, infected valves, and complicated atherosclerotic plaques. A cross section of the kidney shows a peripheral infarct, characterized by marked pallor extending to the subcapsular surface. Choices A and E (benign and malignant nephrosclerosis) are vascular disorders that are general rather than localized. Choices B and C do not cause ischemic lesions.

Diagnosis: Renal cortical infarct

42   **The answer is B: Bilateral renal cortical necrosis.**   Bilateral renal cortical necrosis is a syndrome characterized by massive tubular necrosis involving large portions of the cortex of both kidneys. Massive bilateral renal cortical necrosis typically occurs in the setting of hypovolemia and endotoxic shock. The term infarct is used when there is one area (or a few areas) of necrosis caused by occlusion of arteries, whereas cortical necrosis implies more widespread ischemic necrosis. The other choices are not associated with grossly visible cortical necrosis.

Diagnosis: Renal cortical necrosis

43 The answer is C: Eclampsia. Preeclampsia, which is characterized by the triad of hypertension, proteinuria, and edema, complicates the third trimester of pregnancy (choice E). When these features are complicated by convulsions, the term eclampsia is applied. On histologic examination, the glomeruli are uniformly enlarged and the endothelial cells are swollen, an appearance that results in an apparently bloodless glomerular tuft. The other choices are not ordinarily seen as complications of pregnancy.

Diagnosis: Eclampsia

44 The answer is B: Acute tubular necrosis (ATN). ATN is a severe, but potentially reversible, impairment of tubular epithelial function caused by ischemia or toxic injury, which results in acute renal failure. Ischemic ATN results from reduced renal perfusion, usually associated with hypotension. Tubular epithelial cells, with their high rate of energy-consuming metabolic activity and numerous organelles, are particularly sensitive to hypoxia and anoxia. Ischemic ATN is characterized by swollen kidneys that have a pale cortex and a congested medulla. No pathologic changes are seen in the glomeruli or blood vessels. Necrosis of individual tubular epithelial cells is evident both from focal denudation of the tubular basement membrane and from the individual necrotic epithelial cells present in some tubular lumina. Acute interstitial nephritis (choice A) and eosinophilic interstitial nephritis (choice C) feature interstitial inflammation, which is not seen in this case.

Diagnosis: Acute tubular necrosis

45 The answer is D: Nephrosclerosis. Hypertensive nephrosclerosis (so-called benign nephrosclerosis) leads to obliteration of glomeruli and may lead to end-stage kidney disease. Hypertensive nephrosclerosis is identified in approximately 15% of patients with benign hypertension. Even mild-to-moderate hypertension causes hypertensive nephrosclerosis. On histologic examination, most glomeruli are hyalinized, and the tubules are either atrophic or replaced by fibrous tissue. Arterioles exhibit concentric hyaline thickening of the wall, often with the loss of smooth muscle cells or their displacement to the periphery. This arteriolar change is termed hyaline arteriolosclerosis. The other choices are not related to hypertension.

Diagnosis: Nephrosclerosis, benign; systemic hypertension

46 The answer is A: Acute tubular necrosis (ATN). Nephrotoxic ATN is caused by chemically induced injury to epithelial cells. Because they absorb and concentrate the chemicals, tubular epithelial cells are preferred targets for certain toxins, including some antibiotics, radiographic contrast agents, heavy metals (e.g., mercury), and organic solvents. The photomicrograph shows widespread necrosis of proximal tubular epithelial cells with sparing of distal and collecting tubules. Tubulointerstitial nephritis (choice E) may be a response to certain drugs but features interstitial inflammation.

Diagnosis: Acute tubular necrosis

47 The answer is E: Malignant hypertension. The term malignant hypertension refers to a severely elevated blood pressure that results in rapidly progressive vascular disease, affecting the brain, heart, and kidney. Malignant hypertension injures endothelial cells and causes increased vascular permeability, which leads to the insudation of plasma proteins into the vessel wall and morphologic evidence of fibrinoid necrosis. Acute injury is rapidly followed by smooth muscle proliferation and a concentric increase in the number of layers of smooth muscle cells, yielding the so-called "onion skin" appearance. This form of smooth muscle cell hyperplasia may be a response to the release of growth factors derived from platelets and other inflammatory cells at the site of vascular injury. Amyloid nephropathy (choice A) is ruled out by the absence of Congo red staining. The other choices do not cause malignant nephrosclerosis.

Diagnosis: Malignant hypertension

48 The answer is E: Renin. Renal artery stenosis causes cells of the juxtaglomerular apparatus to release renin, which induces aldosterone-mediated retention of sodium and water by the kidney (renovascular hypertension). In cases of unilateral renal artery stenosis, the level of renin in the renal vein of the ischemic kidney is elevated, whereas it is normal in the contralateral kidney. Renal artery stenosis is caused by atherosclerosis in adults, but in children it reflects fibromuscular dysplasia of the renal artery. Aldosterone (choice A), angiotensin (choice B), and plasminogen (choice D) are not synthesized in the kidney. Erythropoietin (choice C) influences the production of red blood cells.

Diagnosis: Renovascular hypertension

49 The answer is C: Hemolytic uremic syndrome (HUS). HUS features microangiopathic hemolytic anemia and acute renal failure, with little or no evidence for significant vascular disease outside the kidneys. It is the most common cause of acute renal failure in children. Major causes for HUS are Shiga toxin–producing strains of *Escherichia coli*, which are ingested in contaminated food. The toxin injures endothelial cells, thereby setting in motion the sequence of events that produces thrombotic microangiopathy. Patients present with hemorrhagic diarrhea and rapidly progressive renal failure. Postinfectious glomerulonephritis (choice A) follows streptococcal infections and is not characterized by acute renal failure.

Diagnosis: Hemolytic uremic syndrome

50 The answer is D: Henoch-Schönlein purpura. Henoch-Schönlein purpura is the most common type of childhood vasculitis and is caused by vascular localization of immune complexes containing predominantly IgA. The glomerular lesion is identical with that of IgA nephropathy. Hemolytic uremic syndrome (choice C) is caused by exposure to Shiga toxin-producing strains of *Escherichia coli* and is not associated with angiopathy outside of the kidney. The other choices are not typically associated with rash.

Diagnosis: Henoch-Schönlein purpura

51 The answer is D: Renal cell carcinoma (RCC). RCC is the most common cancer of the kidney, accounting for 90% of kidney cancers. Most cases of RCC are sporadic, but about 5% are inherited. The 5-year survival is 90% if the RCC has not extended beyond the renal capsule; survival drops to 30% if there are distant metastases. The tumor spreads most frequently to the lung and the bones. Oncocytoma and angiomyolipoma (choice A) are often difficult to differentiate from RCC by imaging techniques.

Tumors such as nephroblastoma (choice C) and Wilms tumor (choice E) occur in the pediatric age group.

Diagnosis: Renal cell carcinoma

52 **The answer is D: *VHL.*** Clear cell carcinoma is the most common type of RCC. The cytoplasm appears clear because it is rich in glycogen and fat, which are washed out during histologic processing of the tissue. Loss of one allele of the *VHL* gene occurs in virtually all (98%) of sporadic clear cell RCC, and mutations in the gene are found in more than half of these tumors. Thus, the evidence strongly suggests that loss of the tumor suppressor function of the *VHL* gene product is an important event in the genesis of clear cell RCC. *WT1* is also a tumor suppressor gene, but it is implicated in the development of Wilms tumor (choice E).

Diagnosis: Renal cell carcinoma

53 **The answer is E: Wilms tumor.** This malignant neoplasm of embryonal nephrogenic elements is composed of elements that resemble normal fetal tissue, including (1) metanephric blastema, (2) immature stroma (mesenchymal tissue), and (3) immature epithelial elements. It is the most frequent abdominal solid tumor in children, with a prevalence of 1 in 10,000. Wilms tumor usually presents between 1 and 3 years of age, and 98% occur before 10 years of age. In most instances of Wilms tumor, the neoplasm is sporadic and unilateral. However, in 5% of cases, it arises in the context of several congenital syndromes. Choices A, B, and D are not renal tumors. Renal cell carcinoma (choice C) is a tumor of adults.

Diagnosis: Wilms tumor

54 **The answer is D: Neuroblastoma.** Abdominal masses in children include Wilms tumor (choice E), neuroblastoma, and multicystic renal dysplasia. Of these, only neuroblastoma secretes catecholamines and causes elevation of vanillylmandelic acid in the urine.

Diagnosis: Neuroblastoma

55 **The answer is E: Renal tubules.** Renal cell carcinoma originates from renal tubules or ductal epithelial cells. The tumor is composed of cuboidal cells that form either tubules or solid nests. It accounts for 90% of all renal cancers and more than 11,000 cases a year in the United States. Most of these tumors are of the clear cell type and almost all show loss of one allele of the von Hipple-Lindau (*VHL*) gene.

Diagnosis: Renal cell carcinoma

56 **The answer is B: Leukemia.** Any condition associated with elevated levels of uric acid in the blood may cause tubular deposits of uric acid crystals (see photomicrograph). The classic chronic disease in this category is primary gout. Chronic urate nephropathy caused by gout is characterized by tubular and interstitial deposition of crystalline monosodium urate. Acute urate nephropathy can also be caused by increased cell turnover. For example, leukemic patients who undergo chemotherapy develop hyperuricemia due to the increased formation of uric acid from nucleic acids released from destroyed leukemic cells. This oversupply of urates may cause renal changes similar to those of gout or other forms of hyperuricemia. The other choices are not associated with hyperuricemia.

Diagnosis: Acute renal failure, urate nephropathy

57 **The answer is A: Calcium oxalate.** Nephrolithiasis and urolithiasis are stones within the collecting system of the kidney (nephrolithiasis) or elsewhere in the collecting system of the urinary tract (urolithiasis). The pelves and calyces of the kidney are common sites for the formation and accumulation of calculi. Calcium oxalate stones are the most common (80%) form of kidney stones in the United States, whereas calcium phosphate stones (choice B) are more common in England. Both are usually related to idiopathic calciuria and increased absorption of calcium in the intestine. Magnesium ammonium phosphate stones (choice D) are typically formed in urine made alkaline by urea-splitting bacteria. Uric acid stones, found in 25% of patients with gout, are smooth, yellow, hard, and radiolucent. Cystine stones (choice C) occur in children with hereditary cystinuria, an inborn error of amino acid metabolism marked by an excess of cystine in the urine.

Diagnosis: Nephrolithiasis

58 **The answer is E: Urinary tract obstruction.** Obstructive uropathy is caused by structural or functional abnormalities in the urinary tract that impede urine flow, which may cause renal dysfunction (obstructive nephropathy) and dilation of the collecting system (hydronephrosis). In this neglected patient, severe prostatic hyperplasia caused urinary tract obstruction. In early hydronephrosis, the most prominent microscopic finding is dilation of the collecting ducts, followed by dilation of the proximal and distal convoluted tubules. Grossly, progressive dilation of the renal pelves and calyces occurs, and atrophy of the renal parenchyma ensues. The other choices do not cause bilateral hydronephrosis.

Diagnosis: Hydronephrosis

59 **The answer is E: Infection.** In most cases, the presence of a urinary stone is associated with an increased blood level and urinary excretion of its principal component. Most kidney stones contain calcium complexed with oxalate or phosphate, or a mixture of these anions. However, some 15% of stones result from infection. In the presence of urea-splitting bacteria, the resulting alkaline urine favors the precipitation of magnesium ammonium phosphate (struvite) and calcium phosphate (apatite). They form the so-called staghorn calculi that fill the entire pelvis and calices. Whereas the other choices may by associated with nephrolithiasis; they do not appear as staghorn calculi.

Diagnosis: Nephrolithiasis

60 **The answer is B: Hydronephrosis.** Obstructive uropathy is caused by structural or functional abnormalities in the urinary tract that impede urine flow, which may cause renal dysfunction (obstructive nephropathy) and dilation of the collecting system (hydronephrosis). Metastatic cervical cancer is a frequent cause of bilateral ureteral obstruction and resulting hydronephrosis. Polycystic kidney disease (choice C) is a congenital disease. The other choices are not related to obstruction of the lower urinary tract.

Diagnosis: Hydronephrosis

61 **The answer is E: Thrombotic microangiopathy.** Thrombotic microangiopathy has a variety of causes, all of which cause endothelial damage that initiates a final common pathway of vascular changes. Injured endothelial surfaces promote thrombosis, which may cause focal ischemic necrosis. Pathologic changes in the kidney are comparable to those seen in malignant hypertensive nephropathy. These lesions include arteriolar fibrinoid necrosis, arterial edematous intimal expansion, glomerular congestion, and vascular thrombosis. Patients typically present with thrombocytopenia, hypertension, and renal failure. The causes of thrombotic microangiopathy include infections, drugs (e.g., cisplatin chemotherapy), autoimmune diseases, malignant hypertension, and pregnancy. Alterations in blood flow lead to mechanical fragmentation of erythrocytes (schistocytes). Henoch-Schönlein purpura (choice B) does not have microangiopathic features that lead to anemia or thrombocytopenia.

Diagnosis: Thrombotic microangiopathy

62   **The answer is B: Papillary necrosis.** Patients with sickle cell disease develop painful, episodic crises. The rigidity of sickled erythrocytes results in obstruction of the microcirculation, with subsequent hypoxia and ischemic injury in many organs. Patients experience severe pain, especially in the chest, abdomen, and bones. Sickle cell nephropathy is the most common organ manifestation of sickle cell disease. The interstitial tissue in which the vasa recta course has a low oxygen tension. As a result, in patients with sickle cell disease, erythrocytes in the vasa recta tend to sickle and occlude the lumina. Infarcts in the medulla and papillae ensue, sometimes severe enough to cause renal papillary necrosis. The glomeruli are conspicuously congested with sickle cells. None of the other choices are direct complications of sickle cell anemia. Choices C, D, and E do not cause papillary necrosis, and acute pyelonephritis (choice A) does so only rarely.

Diagnosis: Sickle cell disease, papillary necrosis

63   **The answer is A: ABO antigens.** Incompatible ABO histo-blood group antigens, which are expressed on endothelial cells and erythrocytes, are absolute barriers to a successful transplant. ABO-incompatible grafts encounter preformed circulating antibodies, which bind to endothelial cells and cause immediate (hyperacute) rejection. By contrast, the most common patterns of acute and chronic rejection are caused primarily by donor-recipient differences in HLA molecules encoded by the major histocompatibility complex. These molecules are expressed on most cell surface membranes. Other causes of transplant rejection tend to be chronic, because they do not involve preformed antibodies. None of the other choices mediates hyperacute graft rejection.

Diagnosis: Graft-versus-host disease

64   **The answer is B: Fibromuscular dysplasia.** The most frequent cause of renovascular hypertension in children is fibromuscular dysplasia. This disease is characterized by fibrous and muscular stenosis of the renal artery. Areas of medial thickening alternate with areas of atrophy producing a "string of beads" pattern in angiograms. Stenosis or total occlusion of a main renal artery produces hypertension that is potentially curable by reconstitution of the arterial lumen. Buerger disease (choice A) and Kawasaki disease (choice D) do not typically affect the renal arteries. Giant cell arteritis (choice C) and Takayasu arteritis (choice E) may cause secondary hypertension by producing sclerotic thickening of the renal arteries; however, these vascular diseases are distinctly uncommon in children.

Diagnosis: Fibromuscular dysplasia

Chapter 17

The Lower Urinary Tract and Male Reproductive System

QUESTIONS

Select the single best answer.

1 A baby girl has an open defect of the lower abdominal wall (patient shown in the image). Which of the following best describes the pathogenesis of this congenital birth defect?

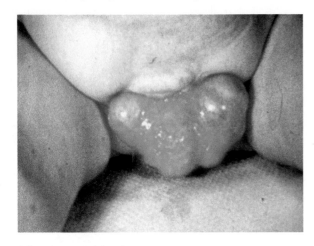

(A) Cystic renal dysplasia
(B) Development of bifid ureter
(C) Exstrophy of urinary bladder
(D) Failure of the urachus to involute
(E) Formation of Meckel diverticulum

2 The abdominal wall defect in the patient described in Question 1 is repaired surgically. Despite this corrective surgery, the child is at increased risk for developing which of the following neoplasms?
(A) Bladder carcinoma
(B) Endometrial carcinoma
(C) Cervical carcinoma
(D) Renal cell carcinoma
(E) Ureteral carcinoma

3 A 64-year-old man presents with a 4-day history of dysuria and hematuria. He has a history of repeated bouts of acute cystitis. Urine cultures are positive for *E. coli*. Ultrasound examination reveals an echogenic object in a bladder diverticulum. Which of the following conditions most likely contributed to the formation of a bladder diverticulum in this patient?
(A) Diabetes mellitus
(B) Malakoplakia
(C) Nephrolithiasis
(D) Nodular prostatic hyperplasia
(E) Urothelial cell carcinoma

4 A 20-year-old pregnant woman (gravida II, para I) complains of lower pelvic discomfort, fever, and pain during urination for the past 2 days. She also reports seeing blood in her urine. Which of the following is the most likely cause of hematuria in this patient?
(A) Acute cystitis
(B) Acute pyelonephritis
(C) Bladder calculi
(D) Postinfectious glomerulonephritis
(E) Urothelial cell carcinoma of the bladder

5 In the patient described in Question 4, which of the following would be the most likely etiologic agent?
(A) *Enterobacter* sp.
(B) *Escherichia coli*
(C) *Proteus vulgaris*
(D) *Pseudomonas aeruginosa*
(E) *Streptococcus pyogenes*

6 A 65-year-old man presents with a recent episode of painless hematuria. Vital signs are normal. All blood tests and urinalysis are normal, except for the presence of blood in the urine. The patient smokes cigarettes but does not drink alcoholic beverages. Which of the following is the most likely cause of hematuria in this patient?

(A) Acute cystitis
(B) Acute pyelonephritis
(C) Bladder calculi
(D) Carcinoma of the bladder
(E) Prostatic carcinoma

7 A 67-year-old man complains of frequency of urination, pain on urination, and pelvic discomfort. The patient had a transurethral resection of the prostate 3 months ago, which required an indwelling catheter (both before and after surgery). Urine cultures are negative. Cytoscopy reveals multiple areas of hemorrhage on the bladder wall. Biopsy shows fibrosis of the lamina propria and a predominance of lymphocytes (shown in the image). Which of the following is the most likely cause of urinary symptoms in this patient?

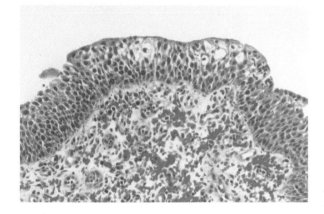

(A) Acute cystitis
(B) Bladder diverticulum
(C) Chronic cystitis
(D) Malakoplakia
(E) Malignant lymphoma

8 A 72-year-old man presents with a sudden episode of painless hematuria. Cystoscopy reveals a solitary, 2-cm papillary tumor in the posterior bladder wall. The biopsy is shown in the image. Which of the following is the most likely diagnosis?

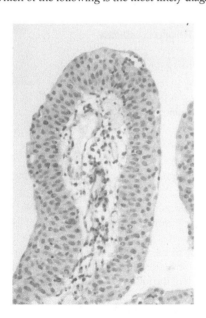

(A) Adenocarcinoma
(B) Exophytic papilloma
(C) Papillary urothelial cell carcinoma, high-grade
(D) Tubular adenoma
(E) Villous adenoma

9 A 62-year-old man presents with a 1-month history of intermittent painless hematuria. Cystoscopy reveals multiple, red, velvety flat patches in the bladder mucosa. A biopsy is shown in the image. Which of the following is the appropriate diagnosis?

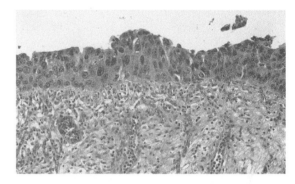

(A) Chronic interstitial cystitis
(B) Invasive urothelial cell carcinoma
(C) Malakoplakia
(D) Urothelial cell carcinoma in situ
(E) Urothelial cell papilloma

10 A 68-year-old man presents with a 4-week history of painless hematuria. Cytoscopy reveals a large exophytic tumor near the neck of the bladder. The cystectomy specimen is shown in the image. In addition to cigarette smoking, which of the following is the most significant risk factor for the development of this patient's malignant neoplasm?

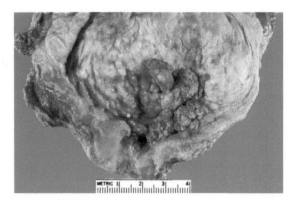

(A) Bladder calculi
(B) Chronic human papillomavirus infection
(C) Diabetes mellitus
(D) Exposure to aromatic amines and azo dyes
(E) Previous catheterization

11 A 9-month-old boy is brought to the physician by his mother, who noticed that her son had developed scrotal swelling. Physical examination reveals a scrotal mass. The lesion can be transilluminated and is composed of clear serous fluid. What is the appropriate diagnosis?

(A) Epididymitis
(B) Hematocele
(C) Hydrocele
(D) Spermatocele
(E) Varicocele

12 A 50-year-old man presents with painless hematuria. A CT scan of the abdomen reveals a mass in the left ureter, which almost completely obliterates the lumen and has resulted in mild hydronephrosis. The surgical specimen is shown in the image. Which of the following is the most likely histologic diagnosis for this malignant neoplasm?

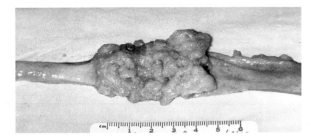

(A) Adenocarcinoma
(B) Neuroblastoma
(C) Pheochromocytoma
(D) Renal cell carcinoma
(E) Urothelial cell carcinoma

13 A 4-year-old girl is brought to the physician by her parents who report seeing blood in the child's urine. A CT scan reveals a neoplasm of the urinary bladder. Which of the following is the most likely diagnosis?
(A) Angiosarcoma
(B) Embryonal rhabdomyosarcoma
(C) Leiomyosarcoma
(D) Liposarcoma
(E) Malignant fibrous histiocytoma

14 A 55-year-old woman presents with a 2-week history of pain and bleeding near the urethral meatus. Urine cultures are negative. Biopsy of the affected tissue shows chronic inflammation, granulation tissue, and epithelial hyperplasia. Which of the following is the most likely diagnosis?
(A) Adenomatous polyp
(B) Carcinoma of the urethra
(C) Urothelial cell carcinoma
(D) Urothelial cell papilloma
(E) Urethral caruncle

15 A 40-year-old Egyptian fisherman presents with painless hematuria. The patient's past medical history is significant for chronic schistosomiasis, which is endemic in his country of origin. Urinalysis shows malignant cells and cystoscopy reveals a mass in the wall of the urinary bladder. Which of the following is the most likely diagnosis?
(A) Adenocarcinoma
(B) Leiomyosarcoma
(C) Papillary urothelial cell carcinoma
(D) Squamous cell carcinoma
(E) Urothelial cell carcinoma in situ

16 A 28-year-old man presents with multiple, raised lesions on the shaft of his penis. Physical examination shows condyloma acuminata. Biopsy of the lesion is shown in the image. This benign lesion is caused by infection with which of the following pathogens?

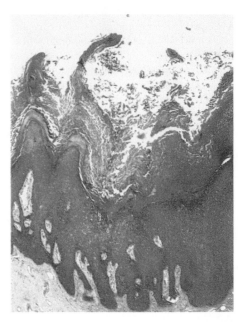

(A) *Chlamydia trachomatis*
(B) *Haemophilus ducreyi*
(C) Herpes simplex virus type 2
(D) Human papillomavirus
(E) *Treponema pallidum*

17 A 20-year-old man presents with dysuria, urgency, and urethral discharge. Physical examination shows suppurative urethritis, with redness and swelling at the urethral meatus. Which of the following is the most likely etiology of urethritis in this patient?
(A) *Borrelia recurrentis*
(B) *Chlamydia trachomatis*
(C) *Haemophilus ducreyi*
(D) *Neisseria gonorrhoeae*
(E) *Treponema pallidum*

18 A 27-year-old man presents with acute and chronic inflammation of his glans penis. Which of the following is the most likely complication of chronic balanitis in this patient?
(A) Carcinoma
(B) Epididymitis
(C) Epispadias
(D) Hypospadias
(E) Phimosis

19 A 65-year-old man presents with multiple lesions on his penis that he has had for 2 months. Physical examination reveals shiny, soft, erythematous plaques on the glans and foreskin. Biopsy of lesional skin shows neoplastic epithelial cells, connected by intercellular bridges, with invasion into the dermis. Which of the following is the appropriate histologic diagnosis for this patient's penile neoplasm?

(A) Adenocarcinoma
(B) Lichen planus
(C) Melanoma
(D) Squamous cell carcinoma
(E) Urothelial cell carcinoma

20 A 67-year-old man complains of increased urgency to void. He could not completely empty his bladder and felt "distended" and "irritated" all the time. Rectal digital examination reveals an enlarged nodular prostate. A biopsy discloses hyperplastic prostatic glands (shown in the image). If this patient's prostate continues to enlarge, which of the following is a possible complication?

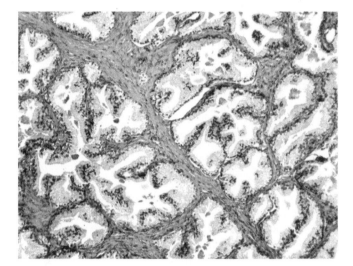

(A) Adenocarcinoma of prostate
(B) Hydroureter and hydronephrosis
(C) Intratubular germ cell neoplasia
(D) Malakoplakia of the bladder wall
(E) Urothelial cell carcinoma of bladder

21 A 60-year-old man with a history of nodular prostatic hyperplasia and recurrent cystitis presents with pain in the scrotum. His temperature is 38°C (101°F). Physical examination reveals a small, tender nodule attached to the testis. Which of the following is the most likely diagnosis?
(A) Epididymitis
(B) Orchitis
(C) Spermatocele
(D) Urethritis
(E) Varicocele

22 A 20-year-old woman presents for questions regarding fertility. Laboratory studies previously identified a 21-hydroxylase deficiency and adrenogenital syndrome. Physical examination reveals virilization of the vulva and an enlarged clitoris. What is the most likely karyotype of this patient?
(A) 45,XO
(B) 46,XX
(C) 46,XY
(D) 47,XXY
(E) 47,XXX

23 A 20-year-old intersex woman presents with questions regarding her sexual differentiation. Physical examination reveals ambiguous female external genital organs with signs of virilization. Cytogenetic studies show a normal 46,XY karyotype. Which of the following is the most likely diagnosis for this patient's medical condition?
(A) Congenital adrenal hyperplasia
(B) Cryptorchidism
(C) Klinefelter syndrome
(D) Testicular feminization syndrome
(E) Turner syndrome

24 An 8-year-old boy is brought to the physician because his parents noticed a mass on his left testicle. Physical examination reveals a solid mass that cannot be transilluminated, and biopsy shows a haphazard arrangement of benign differentiated tissues, including squamous epithelium, glandular epithelium, cartilage, and neural tissue. The left testicle was removed surgically, and the patient is symptom free 5 years later. Which of the following is the most likely diagnosis?
(A) Embryonal carcinoma
(B) Mature teratoma
(C) Mixed germ cell tumor
(D) Seminoma
(E) Teratocarcinoma

25 A 2-year-old boy is brought to the physician because his parents noticed a mass on his right testicle. Physical examination confirms the parents' observation. An orchiectomy is performed. Microscopic examination of the surgical specimen shows neoplastic cells forming glomeruloid Schiller-Duval bodies. Which of the following serum markers is most useful for monitoring the recurrence of tumor in this patient?
(A) CA-125
(B) Carcinoembryonic antigen
(C) Estrogen
(D) α-Fetoprotein
(E) Human chorionic gonadotropin

26 A 32-year-old man presents with a testicular mass that he first noticed 2 weeks ago. The mass cannot be transilluminated and appears solid and homogeneous on ultrasound examination. No tumor markers are detected on serologic testing. An orchiectomy is performed, and the surgical specimen is shown in the image. Which of the following is the most likely diagnosis?

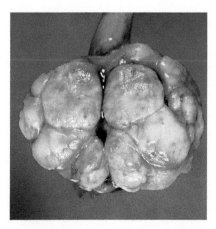

(A) Choriocarcinoma
(B) Embryonal carcinoma
(C) Lymphoma
(D) Seminoma
(E) Yolk sac carcinoma

27 A 38-year-old man presents with a 10-month history of a painless testicular mass. Physical examination reveals a small nodule of the left testis. The mass cannot be transilluminated and appears to be solid on ultrasound examination. A testicular biopsy is shown in the image. The multinucleated giant cells in this neoplasm are derived from which of the following cell types?

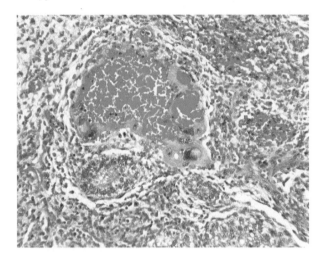

(A) Chondrocytes
(B) Leydig cells
(C) Oligodendrocytes
(D) Smooth muscle cells
(E) Trophoblastic cells

28 A left orchiectomy is performed in the patient described in Question 27. Which of the following serum markers would be most useful for monitoring tumor recurrence of this neoplasm following surgery?
(A) CA-125
(B) Carcinoembryonic antigen
(C) α-Fetoprotein
(D) Human chorionic gonadotropin
(E) Placental alkaline phosphatase

29 A 3-month-old boy is brought to the physician because his parents cannot find one of his testicles. Physical examination confirms the parents' observation. Which of the following is the most likely diagnosis?
(A) Anorchia
(B) Cryptorchidism
(C) Klinefelter syndrome
(D) Macroorchidism
(E) Male pseudohermaphroditism

30 The patient described in Question 29 develops a urogenital tumor 30 years later. An abdominal-pelvic CT scan reveals metastases to lumbar periaortic lymph nodes. Which of the following is the most likely pathologic diagnosis?

(A) Leydig cell tumor
(B) Malignant lymphoma
(C) Renal cell carcinoma
(D) Seminoma
(E) Urothelial cell carcinoma of the bladder

31 A 65-year-old man presents with a 4-month history of a scrotal mass. Which of the following is the most likely diagnosis?
(A) Choriocarcinoma
(B) Embryonal carcinoma
(C) Leydig cell tumor
(D) Malignant lymphoma
(E) Seminoma

32 An 8-year-old boy is brought to the physician by his parents who have begun to notice the onset of puberty in their child. Physical examination reveals enlargement of the external male genitalia and facial hair. Which of the following neoplasms is the most likely cause of precocious puberty in this patient?
(A) Craniopharyngioma
(B) Leydig cell tumor
(C) Pheochromocytoma
(D) Seminoma
(E) Yolk sac carcinoma

33 A 16-year-old boy from Africa presents with a 5-day history of fever and testicular pain. Physical examination shows swollen, tender parotid glands and testes. Which of the following is the most likely responsible pathogen?
(A) *Haemophilus ducreyi*
(B) Human immunodeficiency virus
(C) Human papillomavirus
(D) Mumps virus
(E) *Streptococcus pyogenes*

34 A tall and slender 16-year-old boy presents with breast enlargement. Cytogenetic studies reveal a 47,XXY karyotype. Which of the following urogenital disorders is anticipated in this patient?
(A) Anorchidism
(B) Cryptorchidism
(C) Hyperandrogenism
(D) Polyorchidism
(E) Testicular atrophy

35 A 78-year-old man was admitted to the hospital due to acute urinary tract obstruction. For the past few years, he has had recurrent bouts of cystitis. Two days before being admitted to the hospital, he could not urinate at all. What is the probable cause of bladder outlet obstruction in this patient?
(A) Nephrogenic metaplasia
(B) Nodular prostatic hyperplasia
(C) Prostatic adenocarcinoma
(D) Urothelial cell carcinoma of the bladder
(E) Urethral stricture

36 A 68-year-old man is found to have an elevated serum PSA level (9.5 ng/mL, normal = 0 to 4 ng/mL). Biopsy of the prostate gland reveals a poorly differentiated adenocarcinoma.

Which of the following best describes the putative precursor of this malignant neoplasm?

(A) Basal cell hyperplasia
(B) Chronic epididymitis
(C) Chronic prostatitis
(D) Nodular hyperplasia of the prostate
(E) Prostatic intraepithelial neoplasia

37 A 55-year-old man presents with urinary symptoms of urgency and frequency. Rectal examination reveals an enlarged prostate. Laboratory studies show an elevated serum PSA level of 4.9 ng/mL. The patient subsequently undergoes a prostate needle biopsy series, which demonstrates two cancer-positive needle cores: Gleason grades 2+2(4) and 3+2(5). Which of the following is the appropriate diagnosis?

(A) Adenocarcinoma
(B) Nodular prostatic hyperplasia
(C) Prostate intraepithelial neoplasia
(D) Squamous cell carcinoma
(E) Urothelial cell carcinoma

38 A 70-year-old man presents with pain in his back. Relevant clinical findings include a rock-hard, enlarged prostate palpated on rectal examination. Radiologic studies show multicentric, osteoblastic lesions of the lumbar vertebral bodies. The patient is treated with leuprolide acetate (lupron), an inhibitor of gonadotropin release by the pituitary. Which of the following statements best summarizes the rationale for this treatment?

(A) Leydig cells release tumor chemotactic factors.
(B) Prostate carcinomas frequently metastasize to the gonads.
(C) Sertoli cells release tumor chemotactic factors.
(D) The tumor is well known to invade the testes.
(E) Tumor cells exhibit androgen-dependent growth.

39 A 52-year-old woman complains of dysuria, frequency, and urgency. She has a long history of urinary tract infections. Urine cultures are positive for *E. coli*. Cystoscopy reveals soft yellow plaques on the mucosal surface. Histologic examination shows mucosal chronic inflammatory cells with numerous macrophages (shown in the image). The arrow (see inset) identifies small intracytoplasmic, calcium-rich spherical structures (Michaelis-Gutmann bodies). Which of the following is the appropriate diagnosis?

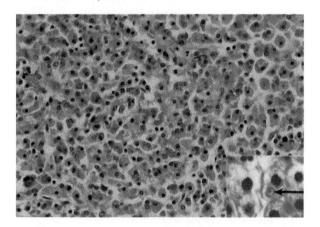

(A) Cystitis cystica
(B) Eosinophilic cystitis
(C) Malakoplakia
(D) Polypoid cystitis
(E) Urothelial cell carcinoma

40 A 60-year-old woman with a history of chronic cystitis is referred to a urologist because of hematuria. Cystoscopy reveals a mass in the dome of the bladder. Biopsy shows tumor cells arranged as gland-like structures. Special stains demonstrate mucin in the cytoplasm of the tumor cells. What is the appropriate diagnosis?

(A) Adenocarcinoma
(B) Inverted papilloma
(C) Squamous cell carcinoma
(D) Urothelial cell carcinoma
(E) Urothelial cell carcinoma in situ

41 A 65-year-old woman suffers a massive stroke and expires. At autopsy, the bladder appears edematous with a prominent central ulcer (shown in the image). Histologic examination reveals lymphocytes and mast cells, as well as extensive fibrosis within the bladder mucosa and muscularis. Which of the following is the most likely diagnosis?

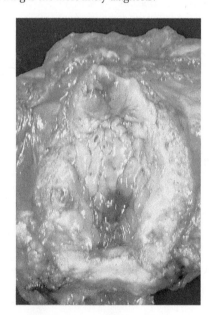

(A) Chronic interstitial cystitis
(B) Invasive urothelial cell carcinoma
(C) Malakoplakia
(D) Polypoid cystitis
(E) Urothelial cell carcinoma in situ

42 During the physical examination of a newborn boy, the pediatrician notices that the urethral meatus is positioned on the lower side of the penile shaft. What is the appropriate diagnosis for this congenital birth defect?

(A) Epispadias
(B) Hydroureter
(C) Hypospadias
(D) Peyronie disease
(E) Phimosis

43 An 18-year-old man presents with a 3-week history of scrotal swelling. The affected area can be transilluminated and is found to contain a clear, milky fluid. Microscopic examination of the aspirated fluid reveals degenerating spermatozoa. What is the appropriate diagnosis?

(A) Hematocele
(B) Hydrocele
(C) Scrotal edema
(D) Spermatocele
(E) Varicocele

44 A 48-year-old man presents for a routine physical examination. The patient has a history of hyperlipidemia and nodular prostatic hyperplasia. Physical examination reveals a large mass on the lateral side of the scrotum, which can be transilluminated. It is found to be composed of dilated blood vessels draining the left testicle. What is the appropriate diagnosis?

(A) Epididymitis
(B) Hematocele
(C) Hydrocele
(D) Spermatocele
(E) Varicocele

45 The patient described in Question 44 is at increased risk for which of the following complications?

(A) Adenocarcinoma
(B) Embryonal carcinoma
(C) Infertility
(D) Nodular prostatic hyperplasia
(E) Seminoma

46 A 25-year-old man presents with a 4-week history of a painless mass in the scrotum. Physical examination reveals a testicular mass that cannot be transilluminated. Serum levels of AFP and hCG are normal. A hemiorchiectomy is performed. On gross examination, the testicular tumor shows foci of hemorrhage and necrosis. Microscopic examination of the tumor is shown in the image. The patient was cured by orchiectomy followed by chemotherapy. Which of the following is the most likely diagnosis?

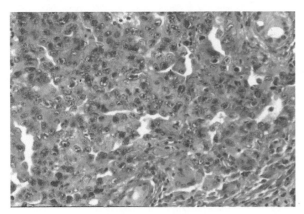

(A) Choriocarcinoma
(B) Embryonal carcinoma
(C) Lymphoma
(D) Mature teratoma
(E) Yolk sac carcinoma

ANSWERS

1 **The answer is C: Exstrophy of urinary bladder.** Exstrophy of the bladder is a serious developmental abnormality characterized by the absence of the anterior abdominal wall. In some male infants, it is associated with epispadias (incomplete formation of the penile urethra). Exstrophy of the bladder develops from incomplete resorption of the anterior cloacal membrane. In normal embryogenesis, this thin membrane is replaced by smooth muscle. Developmental anomalies of the renal pelvis and ureters are found in 2% to 3% of all persons. Bifid ureters (choice B) are of no clinical significance. Failure of the urachus to involute (choice D) may result in a vesicle-umbilical fistula or urachal diverticulum.
Diagnosis: Exstrophy of the urinary bladder

2 **The answer is A: Bladder carcinoma.** In patients with exstrophy of the bladder, the posterior wall of the bladder is continuously exposed to mechanical injury and undergoes squamous or glandular metaplasia, thereby rendering it prone to frequent infections. Despite surgical repair, the metaplastic bladder mucosa remains at an increased risk for malignant transformation. A greater than expected incidence of bladder cancer occurs 50 to 60 years after surgical repair of exstrophy. Due to squamous metaplasia of the exposed bladder mucosa, squamous carcinoma develops rather than the usual urothelial cell carcinoma. The other choices do not involve tissue that has been exposed to the external environment and do not reflect metaplastic change.
Diagnosis: Exstrophy of the urinary bladder

3 **The answer is D: Nodular prostatic hyperplasia.** Nodular hyperplasia of the prostate is a common disorder characterized clinically by enlargement of the gland and obstruction to the flow of urine through the bladder outlet and pathologically by the proliferation of glands and stroma. Nodular prostatic hyperplasia results in the retention of urine in the bladder and urinary tract infections. Structural changes develop in the bladder wall, including bladder diverticula, which are solitary or multiple saclike outpouchings of the bladder wall. Urine retained inside a diverticulum is often infected, a complication that may lead to the formation of bladder stones. The other choices do not cause structural changes in the bladder wall.
Diagnosis: Bladder diverticulum, nodular prostatic hyperplasia

4 **The answer is A: Acute cystitis.** Acute cystitis is an inflammation of the urinary bladder that is particularly common in women and is a frequent nosocomial infection in hospitalized patients. In most cases, cystitis reflects ascending infection of the lower urinary tract. Factors related to bladder infection include bladder calculi, bladder outlet obstruction, diabetes mellitus, immunodeficiency, prior instrumentation or catheterization, radiation therapy, and chemotherapy. The risk of cystitis in females is increased because of a short urethra, especially during pregnancy. Examination of the urine usually reveals inflammatory cells, and the causative agent can be identified by urine culture. Acute pyelonephritis (choice B) is more likely to present with flank pain, without gross hematuria. Bladder calculi (choice C) and urothelial cell carcinoma of the bladder (choice E) would be unlikely causes of gross hematuria in this patient's age group.
Diagnosis: Cystitis, acute

5   The answer is B: *Escherichia coli.* Gram-negative bacteria from the feces, most commonly *E. coli*, cause 80% of upper and lower urinary tract infections in females. Asymptomatic bacteriuria occurs in 10% of pregnant women, one fourth of whom go on to develop acute pyelonephritis. Less common causes of acute cystitis include *Proteus vulgaris* (choice C), *Pseudomonas aeruginosa* (choice D), and *Enterobacter* sp. (choice A). Most cases of cystitis respond well to treatment with antimicrobial agents. Stromal edema, hemorrhage, and a neutrophilic infiltrate of variable intensity are typical of acute cystitis.
Diagnosis: Cystitis, acute

6   The answer is D: Carcinoma of the bladder. Bladder cancer accounts for 3% to 5% of all cancer-related deaths. Urothelial cell carcinoma of the bladder typically manifests as sudden hematuria and, less frequently, manifests as dysuria. Bladder cancer may be encountered at any age, but most patients (80%) are 50 to 80 years old. Men are affected three times more often than women. Smoking is a known risk factor for bladder cancer. Choices A, B, and C are most often symptomatic. Prostatic carcinoma (choice E) is an uncommon cause of hematuria.
Diagnosis: Urothelial cell carcinoma of the bladder

7   The answer is C: Chronic cystitis. Virtually all patients with acute or chronic cystitis complain of excessive frequency of urination, pain on urination (dysuria), and lower abdominal or pelvic discomfort. Introduction of pathogens into the bladder may occur during instrumentation (e.g., cystoscopy) and is particularly common in patients in whom indwelling catheters remain for prolonged periods. Lack of resolution of the inflammatory reaction is associated with the hallmarks of chronic cystitis, including a predominance of lymphocytes and fibrosis of the lamina propria. Acute cystitis (choice A) is characterized by acute inflammation and hemorrhage. Bladder diverticuli (choice B), malakoplakia (choice D), and malignant lymphoma of the bladder (choice E) are uncommon.
Diagnosis: Cystitis, chronic

8   The answer is B: Exophytic papilloma. Epithelial tumors, most of which are urothelial cell carcinomas, constitute more than 98% of all primary tumors of the bladder. These lesions comprise a spectrum that includes, at one end, benign papillomas and low-grade exophytic papillary carcinomas and, at the other end, invasive urothelial cell carcinomas and other highly malignant tumors. Urothelial cell papilloma of the urinary bladder is often encountered incidentally or after painless hematuria. Benign exophytic papillomas make up 2% to 3% of bladder epithelial tumors and occur most frequently in men above the age of 50 years. These tumors feature papillary fronds that are lined by urothelial epithelium, which are virtually indistinguishable from normal urothelium. On cystoscopy, most patients show single lesions, 2 to 5 cm in diameter, although multiple papillomas are not unusual. Papillary urothelial carcinoma, high-grade (choice C) is incorrect because the lesion shown has minimal cytologic atypia.
Diagnosis: Papillary urothelial cell carcinoma of the bladder

9   The answer is D: Urothelial cell carcinoma in situ. The term carcinoma in situ is reserved for malignant changes confined to flat urothelium in nonpapillary bladder mucosa. The lesion is characterized by a urothelium that exhibits cellular atypia of the entire mucosa, from the basal layer to the surface. Invasive urothelial cell carcinoma (choice B) is incorrect because there is no invasion of the lamina propria. In one third of cases, bladder carcinoma in situ is associated with subsequent invasive carcinoma. Most invasive urothelial cell carcinomas arise from carcinoma in situ rather than from papillary urothelial cell cancers. Confined to the mucosal surface, the in situ lesion is most frequently observed endoscopically as multiple, red, velvety, flat patches, which are close to exophytic papillary urothelial cell carcinoma. Urothelial cell papilloma (choice E) does not exhibit atypia as shown in the photomicrograph.
Diagnosis: Urothelial cell carcinoma in situ

10   The answer is D: Exposure to aromatic amines and azo dyes. The most important risk factors for bladder cancer are cigarette smoking (fourfold increased risk), industrial exposure to azo dyes, infection with *Schistosoma haematobium*, drugs such as cyclophosphamide and analgesics, and radiation therapy (cervical, prostate, or rectal cancer). The other choices do not increase the risk for bladder carcinoma.
Diagnosis: Urothelial cell carcinoma of the bladder

11   The answer is C: Hydrocele. The term hydrocele refers to a collection of serous fluid in the scrotal sac between the two layers of the tunica vaginalis. The cavity is lined by mesothelium. Congenital hydrocele reflects a patent processus vaginalis testis or its incomplete obliteration. It is the most common cause of scrotal swelling in infants and is often associated with inguinal hernia. Acquired hydrocele in adults is secondary to some other disease affecting the scrotum, such as infection, tumor, or trauma. The diagnosis may be made by ultrasound examination or by transilluminating the fluid in the cavity. Hematocele (choice B) is caused by an accumulation of blood between the layers of tunica vaginalis. It may develop after trauma or hemorrhage into hydrocele. Testicular tumors and infections may also lead to a hematocele. Spermatocele (choice D) contains milky fluid and does not occur in this age group.
Diagnosis: Congenital hydrocele

12   The answer is E: Urothelial cell carcinoma. Tumors of the renal pelvis and ureter resemble those of the urinary bladder but are much less common. The etiologic factors associated with epithelial tumors of the renal pelvis and ureter are similar to those observed in bladder cancer, suggesting a field effect. Patients most frequently present with hematuria and flank pain. Excision of the entire ureter is necessary because of the high frequency of concurrent and subsequent carcinomas. The other choices do not derive from urothelial cells.
Diagnosis: Urothelial cell carcinoma of the ureter

13   The answer is B: Embryonal rhabdomyosarcoma. Rhabdomyosarcoma, typically of the embryonal type, manifests most commonly in children as sarcoma botryoides. These edematous, mucosal, polypoid masses have been likened to a "cluster of grapes." Combined treatment with radiation therapy and chemotherapy has greatly increased survival rates for children with this neoplasm. The other choices are rarely, if ever, encountered in children.
Diagnosis: Rhabdomyosarcoma, sarcoma botryoides

14 The answer is E: Urethral caruncle. Urethral caruncles are polypoid inflammatory lesions near the urethral meatus that produce pain and bleeding. They occur exclusively in women, most frequently after menopause. Urethral caruncle presents as an exophytic, often ulcerated, polypoid mass of 1 to 2 cm in diameter at or near the urethral meatus. Microscopically, the lesion exhibits acutely and chronically inflamed granulation tissue, ulceration, and hyperplasia of urothelial or squamous epithelium. Carcinoma (choices B and C) is unlikely given the lack of cellular atypia.
Diagnosis: Urethral caruncle

15 The answer is D: Squamous cell carcinoma. A high incidence of bladder cancer in Egypt, Sudan, and other African countries is attributed to endemic schistosomiasis. Parasitic infestation of the bladder causes squamous metaplasia of the bladder epithelium. Squamous cell carcinoma of the bladder then develops in foci of squamous metaplasia. Virtually all patients with this tumor demonstrate invasion of the bladder wall at the time of initial presentation and have a poor prognosis. The other choices do not reflect squamous metaplasia.
Diagnosis: Squamous cell carcinoma of the bladder

16 The answer is D: Human papillomavirus (HPV). HPV is a DNA virus that infects a variety of skin and mucosal surfaces to produce wart-like lesions, referred to as verrucae and condylomata. Microscopically, the lesion shows epidermal hyperkeratosis, parakeratosis, acanthosis, and papillomatosis. Carcinoma of the penis is also a complication of infection with HPV. Although the other choices represent sexually-transmitted diseases, they are not involved in neoplastic transformation.
Diagnosis: Condyloma acuminatum of the penis

17 The answer is D: _Neisseria gonorrhoeae._ Urethritis is the most common manifestation of sexually transmitted diseases in men, in whom it typically presents with urethral discharge. Both gonococcal and nongonococcal urethritis have an acute onset and are related to recent sexual intercourse. The infection manifests with urethral discharge, typically purulent and greenish yellow. Symptoms include pain or tingling at the meatus of the urethra and pain on micturition (dysuria). Redness and swelling of the urethral meatus are usually seen in both sexes. In gonococcal urethritis, the urethral discharge contains _N. gonorrhoeae_, which can be identified microscopically in smears of the urethral exudates. The other choices do not present with urethral suppurative discharge.
Diagnosis: Gonorrhea, urethritis

18 The answer is E: Phimosis. Balanitis usually extends from the glans of the penis to the foreskin and is called balanoposthitis. Most often, it is caused by bacterial infection, but in immunosuppressed persons and in diabetics, it can also be caused by fungi. Typically, balanitis is a consequence of poor hygiene in uncircumcised men. Significant complications of chronic balanoposthitis are stricture of the meatus, phimosis, and paraphimosis. The orifice of the prepuce may be too narrow to allow retraction over the glans penis, in which case the condition is referred to as phimosis. If the narrow prepuce is forcefully retracted, it may strangulate the glans and impede the outflow of venous blood, a disorder known as paraphimosis.

Epispadias (choice C) and hypospadias (choice D) are congenital anomalies. Epididymitis (choice B) does not reside in the penis. Carcinoma (choice A) is possible but not likely.
Diagnosis: Phimosis, balanitis

19 The answer is D: Squamous cell carcinoma. Penile carcinoma occurs as a preinvasive form (carcinoma in situ or erythroplasia of Queyrat) or invasive squamous cell carcinoma. Erythroplasia of Queyrat manifests as solitary or multiple, shiny, soft, erythematous plaques on the glans and foreskin. The other choices feature neither intracellular bridges nor these characteristic physical signs.
Diagnosis: Squamous cell carcinoma of the penis

20 The answer is B: Hydroureter and hydronephrosis. The biopsy shows hyperplastic prostatic glands embedded in enlarged, fibrovascular stroma. Immunoperoxidase staining of the hyperplastic epithelium is consistently positive for prostate-specific antigen and prostatic acid phosphatase. Approximately 75% of men 80 years of age or older have some degree of benign prostatic hyperplasia (BPH). The pathogenesis of BPH appears to be related to age-related changes in circulating levels of testosterone and dihydrotestosterone. The clinical symptoms of this disorder result from compression of the prostatic urethra and consequent obstruction to the bladder outlet. A history of decreased vigor of the urinary stream and increasing urinary frequency is typical. If severe obstruction is untreated, back pressure results in hydroureter, hydronephrosis, and ultimately renal failure and death. The other choices are not complications of BPH.
Diagnosis: Hydroureter, nodular prostatic hyperplasia

21 The answer is A: Epididymitis. Epididymitis is an inflammation of the epididymis, usually caused by bacteria, which may be acute or chronic. Bacterial epididymitis in young men most often occurs in an acute form as a complication of gonorrhea or as a sexually acquired infection with _Chlamydia._ It is characterized by suppurative inflammation. In older men, _E. coli_ from associated urinary tract infections is the most common causative agent. Patients present with intrascrotal pain and tenderness, with or without associated fever. Varicocele (choice E) is incorrect because it does not typically present with pain and fever. Neither orchitis (choice B) nor urethritis (choice D) would present with a nodular scrotal mass.
Diagnosis: Epididymitis

22 The answer is B: 46,XX. Female pseudohermaphroditism is associated with virilization of the external genital organs and may occur in genetic females (46,XX) who have normal ovaries and internal female genital organs. Virilization of the vulva, which may show fusion into scrotal folds and is associated with clitoromegaly, is most often found in the adrenogenital syndrome caused by 21-hydroxylase deficiency. Lack of this enzyme leads to overproduction of androgens in the adrenal gland during fetal life. Adrenal hyperplasia and ambiguous genitalia are seen at birth. The other choices are not associated with virilization of the external genital organs.
Diagnosis: Female pseudohermaphroditism, adrenogenital syndrome

23 The answer is D: Testicular feminization syndrome. Male pseudohermaphroditism represents a spectrum of congenital disorders that affects genetic males who have a normal 46,XY karyotype. The gonads are cryptorchid testes, but the external genital organs appear feminine or ambiguously female, with signs of virilization. Male pseudohermaphroditism is most often encountered in androgen-insensitivity syndromes due to a congenital deficiency of the androgen receptor, also known as testicular feminization syndrome. Patients with congenital adrenal hyperplasia (choice A) have a normal 46,XX karyotype.

Diagnosis: Male pseudohermaphroditism, androgen insensitivity syndrome, testicular feminization syndrome

24 The answer is B: Mature teratoma. Teratomas are the most common testicular tumor in the age group between 4 and 12 years. They are believed to be derived from primordial germ cells. Benign teratomas in the prepubertal testes are composed of mature somatic tissues representing the three embryonic germ layers (ectoderm, mesoderm, and endoderm). The other choices represent malignant tumors that would be uncommon in this patient's age group.

Diagnosis: Mature teratoma

25 The answer is D: α-Fetoprotein. Most testicular neoplasms in the first 4 years of life are classified as yolk sac tumors. Microscopic examination of a yolk sac tumor shows interlacing strands of epithelial cells surrounded by loose connective stroma. The lobular arrangement of cells, surrounded by empty spaces, leads to the formation of glomeruloid structures referred to as Schiller-Duval bodies. Although yolk sac tumors are malignant, timely orchiectomy results in a 95% cure rate. These tumors produce α-fetoprotein, which can be used for monitoring the recurrence of disease following surgery. Human chorionic gonadotropin (choice E) is secreted by choriocarcinoma.

Diagnosis: Yolk sac tumor

26 The answer is D: Seminoma. Malignant germ cells that retain the phenotypic features of spermatogonia give rise to seminomas, the most common testicular cancer, which accounts for 40% of all germ cells tumors in that organ. The peak incidence occurs in men between 30 and 40 years of age. The only consistent cytogenetic abnormality in testicular germ cell tumors is an additional fragment of chromosome 12 (isochromosome p12). On gross examination, seminomas appear as solid, rubbery-firm masses (see photograph). Neoplastic cells are arranged as nests or sheets that are separated by fibrous septae and infiltrated with chronic inflammatory cells (lymphocytes, plasma cells, and macrophages). Seminomas are exquisitely sensitive to radiation and the cure rate is over 90%. The other choices are much less common than seminoma. Moreover, choriocarcinoma (choice A) and yolk sac carcinoma (choice E) release tumor markers that can be identified in blood.

Diagnosis: Seminoma

27 The answer is E: Trophoblastic cells. Nonseminomatous germ cell tumors are derived from embryonal cells that can give rise to clones of malignant cytotrophoblastic and syncytiotrophoblastic cells, as well as other differentiated elements.

Syncytiotrophoblastic cells are multinucleated. Tumors composed exclusively of malignant chorionic epithelium are termed choriocarcinomas. The photomicrograph shows syncytiotrophoblastic giant cells and mononuclear cytotrophoblastic cells. The invasive growth of trophoblastic cells in these tumors is associated with hemorrhage. The other choices do not give rise to multinucleated giant cells in testicular cancers.

Diagnosis: Choriocarcinoma

28 The answer is D: Human chorionic gonadotropin (hCG). Syncytiotrophoblast cells in choriocarcinomas release hCG, a hormone of pregnancy that is not ordinarily found in males. This marker is useful in the postoperative follow-up of patients who have been treated for nonseminomatous germ cell tumors (NSGCTs). α-Fetoprotein (choice C) is secreted by yolk sac tumors (a common component of NSGCTs). Placental alkaline phosphatase (choice E) is a membrane-associated histochemical marker for seminoma and testicular carcinoma in situ (i.e., intratubular germ cell neoplasia).

Diagnosis: Choriocarcinoma

29 The answer is B: Cryptorchidism. Cryptorchidism, clinically known as undescended testis, is a congenital abnormality in which one or both testes are not found in their normal position in the scrotum. It is the most common urologic condition requiring surgical treatment in infants. In 5% of male infants born at term and 30% of those born prematurely, the testes are not located in the scrotum or are easily retracted. In the large majority of these infants, the testis will descend into the scrotum during the first year of life. The descent of the testis may be arrested at any point from the abdominal cavity to the upper scrotum. According to their location, the cryptorchid testes can be classified as abdominal, inguinal, or upper scrotal. Anorchia (choice A) refers to congenital absence of testes. Macroorchidism (choice D) is a pathologic finding in adult patients with fragile X syndrome.

Diagnosis: Cryptorchidism

30 The answer is D: Seminoma. The clinical significance of undescended testes is not related to the abnormal position of the gonad (patients are asymptomatic) but to an increased incidence of infertility and germ cell neoplasia. All men with untreated bilateral cryptorchid testes have azoospermia and are infertile. Unilateral cryptorchidism is associated in 40% of cases with oligospermia. Cryptorchidism is associated with a 20- to 40-fold greater than normal risk for testicular cancer. Conversely, 10% of patients with germ cell neoplasia have cryptorchid testes. Seminoma is the most common germ cell malignancy. The other choices are not complications of cryptorchidism.

Diagnosis: Seminoma

31 The answer is D: Malignant lymphoma. Malignant lymphoma is the most frequently encountered neoplasm in the testes of men older than 60 years. It usually occurs in the context of systemic disease, but a few cases of primary lymphoma of the testis have been reported. Most patients with lymphomatous involvement of the testis have a poor prognosis. The other testicular tumors tend to occur in younger men.

Diagnosis: Malignant lymphoma

32 The answer is B: Leydig cell tumor. Sex cord tumors comprise approximately 5% of testicular tumors. Leydig cell tumors are rare gonadal stromal/sex cord tumors composed of cells resembling interstitial (Leydig) cells of the testis. They can be hormonally active and secrete androgens, estrogens, or both. Leydig cell tumors can occur at any age, with two distinct peaks, one in childhood and one in adults from the third to the sixth decade. The androgenic effects of testicular Leydig cell tumors in prepubertal boys lead to precocious physical and sexual development. By contrast, feminization and gynecomastia are observed in some adults with this tumor. The other choices do not induce precocious puberty.
Diagnosis: Leydig cell tumor

33 The answer is D: Mumps virus. Orchitis occurs in 20% of adult males with mumps, but widespread immunization against mumps has reduced the incidence of the disorder in the United States. Viral infection is characterized by testicular pain and gonadal swelling, most commonly unilateral. The other choices do not involve either the parotid gland or the testis.
Diagnosis: Mumps orchitis

34 The answer is E: Testicular atrophy. Testicular atrophy is typically found in patients with Klinefelter syndrome (47,XXY). The most common cause of Klinefelter syndrome is meiotic nondisjunction during oogenesis. However, a 46,XX karyotype is found in 1 of 25 patients with classical signs of Klinefelter syndrome. Patients with Klinefelter syndrome are infertile, and the testes reveal atrophy and loss of meiotic and postmeiotic germ cells. Cryptorchidism (choice B) occurs in normal males and persons with Klinefelter syndrome display hypoandrogenism (opposite of choice C). Although the paired testicles are atrophic, they are nevertheless present (opposite of choices A and D).
Diagnosis: Testicular atrophy, Klinefelter syndrome

35 The answer is B: Nodular prostatic hyperplasia. The clinical symptoms of nodular hyperplasia result from compression of the prostatic urethra and the consequent obstruction to the bladder outlet. A history of decreased vigor of the urinary stream and increased urinary frequency is typical. Rectal examination reveals a firm, enlarged, nodular prostate. Early nodular hyperplasia of the prostate begins in the region of the proximal urethra (the urothelial zone). The developing prostatic nodules compress the centrally located urethral lumen and the more peripherally located normal prostate. In well-developed cases, the normal prostate gland is limited to an attenuated rim of tissue beneath the capsule. The other choices are much less frequent causes of bladder obstruction.
Diagnosis: Nodular prostatic hyperplasia

36 The answer is E: Prostatic intraepithelial neoplasia (PIN). In 1990, prostatic adenocarcinoma became the cancer most frequently diagnosed in American men, surpassing the incidence of lung cancer for the first time. PIN refers to prostatic ducts lined by atypical (dysplastic) epithelial cells and a *diminution* in the number of basal cells (see choice A). It is generally accepted that PIN lesions progress to invasive prostatic adenocarcinoma. There is no evidence that prostatic

adenocarcinoma originates from hyperplastic nodules seen in patients with nodular prostatic hyperplasia (choice D). The other choices are unrelated to the pathogenesis of invasive adenocarcinoma of the prostate.
Diagnosis: Prostate intraepithelial neoplasia

37 The answer is A: Adenocarcinoma. Prostatic adenocarcinomas, which account for 98% of all prostatic tumors, are commonly multicentric and located in the peripheral zones. The cut surface of the prostate shows irregular, yellow-white, indurated subcapsular nodules. One tenth of all cases of prostate cancer are initially discovered in the fragments of tissue obtained at the time of transurethral resection for prostatic hyperplasia. The aggressiveness of prostatic carcinoma correlates with the Gleason grade. Squamous (choice D) and urothelial cell carcinomas (choice E) involving the prostate are rare.
Diagnosis: Prostate adenocarcinoma

38 The answer is E: Tumor cells exhibit androgen-dependent growth. The androgenic control of normal prostatic growth and the responsiveness of prostate cancer to castration and exogenous estrogens support a role for male hormones. Chemical castration by the administration of androgenic antagonists (e.g., leuprolide) is used in the treatment of prostate cancer. Chemotactic factors (choices A and C) are not involved in bone metastases of prostatic cancer, and invasion of the gonads (choices B and D) has no influence on the growth of these metastases.
Diagnosis: Prostate adenocarcinoma

39 The answer is C: Malakoplakia. Malakoplakia is an uncommon inflammatory disorder of unknown etiology characterized by the accumulation of macrophages. It is often associated with an infection of the urinary tract by *E. coli*, although a direct causal relationship is dubious. A clinical background of immunosuppression, chronic infections, or cancer is common. Malakoplakia is characterized by soft, yellow plaques on the mucosal surface of the bladder. Histologically, the most striking feature is a chronic inflammatory cell infiltrate composed predominantly of large macrophages with abundant eosinophilic cytoplasm containing PAS-positive granules. Some of these macrophages exhibit laminated, basophilic calcospherites termed Michaelis-Gutmann bodies. None of the other choices exhibit the described histopathologic features.
Diagnosis: Malakoplakia

40 The answer is A: Adenocarcinoma. Adenocarcinoma of the bladder accounts for only 1% of all malignant tumors of the bladder. It originates from foci of cystitis glandularis or intestinal metaplasia or from remnants of urachal epithelium in the bladder dome. Most bladder adenocarcinomas are deeply invasive at the time of initial presentation and are not curable. The other choices do not feature mucin production. Squamous cell carcinoma of the bladder (choice C) develops in foci of squamous metaplasia, usually due to schistosomiasis.
Diagnosis: Adenocarcinoma of bladder

41 The answer is A: Chronic interstitial cystitis. Chronic interstitial cystitis typically affects middle-aged women and features transmural inflammation of the bladder wall, which is occasionally associated with mucosal ulceration (Hunner ulcer). The cause is unknown. Chronic inflammation, including an increased number of mast cells and fibrosis, is commonly observed within the mucosa and the muscularis. A Hunner ulcer displays an intense acute inflammatory reaction. The most common symptoms of chronic interstitial cystitis are long-standing suprapubic pain, frequency, and urgency, with or without hematuria. The other choices do not demonstrate these histologic findings.

Diagnosis: Cystitis, chronic interstitial; Hunner ulcer

42 **The answer is C: Hypospadias.** Hypospadias refers to a congenital anomaly in which the urethra opens on the underside (ventral surface) of the penis so that the meatus is proximal to its normal glandular location. The condition results from incomplete closure of the urethral folds of the urogenital sinus. Hypospadias has a frequency of 1 in 350 male neonates. Most cases are sporadic, but a familial occurrence has been noted. Surgical repair is usually uncomplicated. Epispadias (choice A) refers to a congenital anomaly in which the urethra opens on the upper side (dorsal surface) of the penis. In phimosis (choice E), the orifice of the prepuce may be too narrow to allow retraction over the glans penis.

Diagnosis: Hypospadias

43 **The answer is D: Spermatocele.** Scrotal masses and conditions that lead to swelling or enlargement of the scrotum often reflect abnormalities of testicular, epididymal, or scrotal development. Clinical problems related to these pathologic conditions are most often encountered in children but may be found in adults. A spermatocele is a cyst formed from the protrusions of widened efferent ducts of the rete testis or epididymis. It manifests as a hilar paratesticular nodule or as a fluctuating mass filled with milky fluid containing spermatozoa in various stages of degeneration. Hydrocele (choice B) is incorrect because it does not contain spermatozoa.

Diagnosis: Spermatocele

44 **The answer is E: Varicocele.** Varicocele represents a local dilation of testicular veins and presents as nodularity on the lateral side of the scrotum. Most varicoceles are asymptomatic and are discovered during routine physical examination. Massive varicoceles occur and have been likened to a "bag of worms." Hematocele, hydrocele, and spermatocele (choices B, C, and D) involve the scrotum but do not exhibit dilated blood vessels. Epididymitis (choice A) is an inflammatory condition located outside the scrotum.

Diagnosis: Varicocele

45 **The answer is C: Infertility.** Varicocele is considered a common cause of male infertility and oligospermia, although it is not clear why the dilation of veins should have such consequences. Testicular atrophy is found only rarely and only in long-standing disease. Surgical resection of varicocele by ligation of the internal spermatic vein often improves reproductive function. Varicocele is not associated with neoplasia (choices A, B, and E) or prostatic hyperplasia (choice D).

Diagnosis: Varicocele

46 **The answer is B: Embryonal carcinoma.** Nonseminomatous germ cell tumors (NSGCTs) constitute 55% of all testicular germ cell tumors. Teratocarcinoma accounts for two thirds of all NSGCTs, followed by mixed germ cell tumors (which contain seminoma) and pure embryonal carcinomas. In pure embryonal carcinoma, the tumor is composed exclusively of undifferentiated embryonal carcinoma cells that are similar to cells from early embryos. Embryonal carcinoma invades the testis, epididymis, and blood vessels and metastasizes to abdominal lymph nodes, lungs, and other organs. These malignant cells are highly sensitive to chemotherapy, and the cure rates are now over 90%. The pathologic findings in this case show undifferentiated neoplastic cells, forming sheets and chords, surrounded by dilated vascular channels filled with red blood cells. Choriocarcinoma (choice A) secretes hCG. Lymphoma (choice C) is more common in older men and does not have the morphology shown. Mature teratoma (choice D) features heterologous elements. Yolk sac carcinoma (choice E) secretes AFP.

Diagnosis: Embryonal carcinoma

Chapter 18

The Female Reproductive System

QUESTIONS

Select the single best answer.

1 A 36-year-old woman presents with infertility. She complains of having had dull pelvic pain for 9 months, which is accentuated during menstruation. Physical examination and endocrinologic studies are normal. Laparoscopy reveals multiple, small hemorrhagic lesions over the surface of both ovaries and fallopian tubes and abundant pelvic scarring. Which of the following is the most likely diagnosis?

(A) Borderline serous tumor
(B) Ectopic pregnancy
(C) Endometriosis
(D) Metastatic cervical carcinoma
(E) Pelvic inflammatory disease

2 A 58-year-old woman complains of recent swelling in her vagina. There is a past medical history of prenatal exposure to diethylstilbestrol. Physical examination reveals a 3-cm firm mass in the anterior wall of the upper vagina. Biopsy of the vaginal mass will most likely show which of the following pathologic findings?

(A) Clear cell adenocarcinoma
(B) Endodermal sinus tumor
(C) Granular cell tumor
(D) Mucinous adenocarcinoma
(E) Squamous cell carcinoma

3 A 60-year-old woman presents with a 3-week history of a painful genital lesion and bleeding. Physical examination reveals an exophytic, ulcerated 1-cm polypoid mass near the external end of the urethra. What is the most likely diagnosis?

(A) Bartholin gland cyst
(B) Caruncle
(C) Condyloma acuminatum
(D) Lichen sclerosis
(E) Lymphogranuloma venereum

4 A 30-year-old woman presents with a 5-month history of increasing abdominal girth and pelvic discomfort. Imaging studies reveal a mass replacing the left ovary. A multilocular tumor filled with thick, viscous fluid is removed (shown in the image). Tumor spaces are lined by mucinous, columnar epithelial cells, showing no evidence of atypia. There are no

papillary structures and no evidence of stromal invasion. Which of the following is the appropriate pathologic diagnosis?

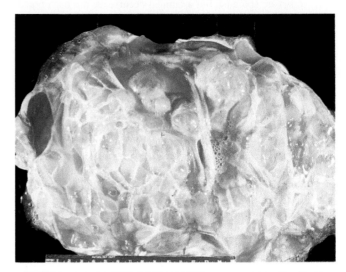

(A) Endometrioid adenoma of ovary
(B) Granulosa cell tumor
(C) Mucinous cystadenocarcinoma
(D) Mucinous cystadenoma
(E) Serous cystadenocarcinoma

5 The ovarian tumor described in Question 4 most closely resembles which of the following patterns of müllerian-type differentiation?

(A) Endometrial glands in pregnancy
(B) Epithelium of the fallopian tube
(C) Glandular epithelium of the endometrium
(D) Mucosa of the bladder
(E) Mucosa of the endocervix

6 A 19-year-old student presents to the university health service with lower abdominal pain and a painful swollen right knee. She denies any trauma to the knee. Pelvic examination is exquisitely painful and reveals an ill-defined thickening in the right and left adnexae. A vaginal discharge is noted. The patient is febrile (38.7°C/103°F). Examination of her right knee reveals an enlarged, tender, and warm joint. The WBC count is 18,500/μL (normal = 4,000 to 11,000/μL). If untreated, which of the following would be the most likely complication in this patient?

(A) Bronchopneumonia
(B) Lung abscess
(C) Meningitis
(D) Tubo-ovarian abscess
(E) Vaginal ulceration

7 A 59-year-old woman presents with a 2-year history of vulvar itching and burning. Physical examination reveals a red, moist lesion of the labium major. Biopsy reveals clusters of pale vacuolated cells within the epidermis that stain positively for periodic acid-Schiff (PAS) and carcinoembryonic antigen (CEA). Which of the following is the most likely diagnosis?
(A) Extramammary Paget disease
(B) HPV-induced papilloma
(C) Verrucous carcinoma
(D) Vulvar intraepithelial neoplasia
(E) Vulvar melanoma

8 A 52-year-old woman with hypothyroidism presents with a 2-year history of vulvar itching and painful intercourse. Physical examination reveals vulval white plaques, atrophic skin, and a parchment-like appearance. Biopsy of the lesion (shown in the image) demonstrates hyperkeratosis, loss of rete ridges, and a homogeneous, acellular zone in the upper dermis. This patient's vulvar dermatitis is most commonly associated with which of the following underlying conditions?

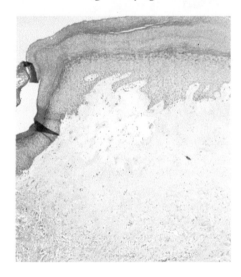

(A) Amyloidosis
(B) Autoimmune disease
(C) Diabetes mellitus
(D) Hyperlipidemia
(E) Prenatal exposure to diethylstilbestrol

9 A 29-year-old woman is evaluated for an abnormal cervical Pap smear. Colposcopy reveals condyloma acuminatum of the exocervix. A biopsy of the cervix is shown in the image. PCR amplification of this biopsy specimen will most likely demonstrate evidence of which of the following infectious agents?

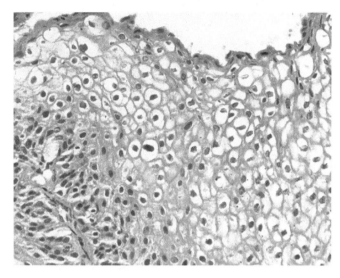

(A) Cytomegalovirus
(B) Herpes simplex virus
(C) Human papillomavirus
(D) *Molluscum contagiosum*
(E) *Treponema pallidum*

10 A 31-year-old Haitian woman is evaluated for infertility. Pelvic examination shows a markedly enlarged vulva, inguinal lymph node enlargement, and rectal stricture. Biopsy of an inguinal lymph node reveals necrotizing granulomas, neutrophilic infiltrates, and inclusion bodies within macrophages. Which of the following is the most likely etiology of infertility in this patient?
(A) *Chlamydia trachomatis*
(B) *Gardnerella vaginalis*
(C) *Molluscum contagiosum*
(D) *Mycobacterium tuberculosis*
(E) *Treponema pallidum*

11 A 35-year-old woman in Africa presents with fever, chills, and malaise. She further complains of a painful genital sore. She had sexual intercourse 5 days previously. Physical examination reveals vesiculopustular lesions on the labium major and cervix. There is bilateral inguinal lymphadenopathy. A lymph node biopsy reveals granulomatous inflammation. Which of the following is the most likely etiology of this constellation of signs and symptoms?
(A) Cytomegalovirus
(B) *Gardnerella vaginalis*
(C) *Haemophilus ducreyi*
(D) *Mycobacterium tuberculosis*
(E) *Neisseria gonorrhoeae*

12 A routine cervical Pap smear taken during a gynecologic examination of a 31-year-old woman shows numerous, loosely arranged cells with high nuclear-to-cytoplasmic ratio. Colposcopy shows white epithelium, punctation, and a mosaic pattern in the transformation zone (shown in the image). Which of the following is the most likely diagnosis?

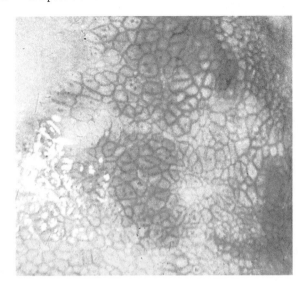

(A) Adenocarcinoma of endocervix
(B) Chronic cervicitis
(C) Clear cell adenocarcinoma
(D) Dysplasia of the cervix
(E) Herpes simplex virus infection

13 A 36-year-old woman is evaluated for an abnormal Pap smear. A cervical biopsy shows atypical squamous cells throughout the entire thickness of the epithelium, with no evidence of epithelial maturation (shown in the image). The basal membrane appears intact. What is the appropriate diagnosis?

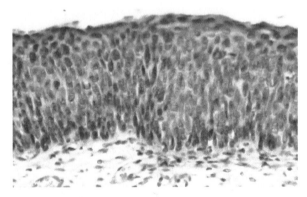

(A) Clear cell adenocarcinoma
(B) Invasive squamous cell carcinoma
(C) Mild dysplasia (cervical intraepithelial neoplasia [CIN]-1)
(D) Severe dysplasia (CIN-3)
(E) Squamous metaplasia of the transformation zone

14 A 35-year-old woman presents with a 6-week history of vaginal discharge, which is occasionally blood tinged. Pelvic examination reveals a 2-cm pedunculated, lobulated, and smooth cervical growth; it is excised. Histologic examination of the specimen would most likely reveal which of the following?
(A) Condyloma acuminatum
(B) Embryonal rhabdomyosarcoma
(C) Endocervical polyp
(D) Leiomyosarcoma
(E) Microglandular hyperplasia

15 A 28-year-old woman, who is 28 weeks pregnant, presents with vaginal bleeding. She does not have a history of uterine contractions. Pelvic examination reveals bright red blood in the endocervical canal. An ulcerated exophytic mass is identified on the left side of the cervix. There is no evidence of direct tumor extension into the parametrium. The pelvic lymph nodes are slightly enlarged, raising the possibility of nodal involvement by the tumor. A Caesarian section is performed, followed by a radical hysterectomy. The cervix is shown in the image. Which of the following is the best prognostic indicator of survival in this patient?

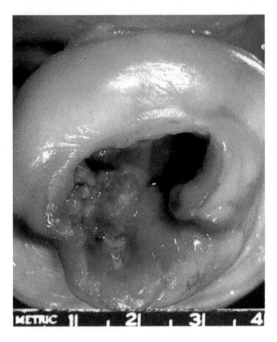

(A) *BRCA* gene mutation
(B) Degree of keratinization
(C) Nodal involvement
(D) Presence of carcinoembryonic antigen (CEA) in serum
(E) Small cell rather than large cell carcinoma

16 Imaging studies establish a diagnosis of stage IV cervical cancer. If untreated, which of the following will be the most likely cause of death in the patient described in Question 15?
(A) Adrenal cortical failure
(B) Brain metastases
(C) Lung metastases
(D) Renal failure
(E) Vertebral fractures

17 A 50-year-old nulliparous woman with a history of diabetes complains that her menstrual blood flow is more abundant than usual. During the last two menstrual cycles, she noticed spotting throughout the entire cycle. The patient is obese (BMI = 32 kg/m²), and her blood pressure is 160/100 mm Hg. An ultrasound examination reveals a thickened endometrial stripe with a polypoid mass in the uterine fundus. The patient undergoes a hysterectomy. The uterus is opened to reveal a partially necrotic mass (shown in the image). A biopsy of the mass shows moderately differentiated adenocarcinoma. Which of the following represents the most likely precursor of this patient's malignant disease?

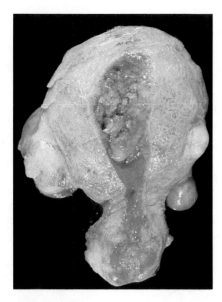

(A) Adenomyosis
(B) Atypical hyperplasia
(C) Chronic endometritis
(D) Complex hyperplasia
(E) Glandular metaplasia

18 Neoplastic cells obtained from the patient described in Question 17 would most likely show loss of function of which of the following cell cycle control proteins?
(A) p53
(B) PTEN
(C) Rb
(D) RET
(E) WT-1

19 A 45-year-old obese woman (BMI = 32 kg/m²) with a history of diabetes and poorly controlled hypertension complains of increased menstrual blood flow of 3 months in duration. An endometrial biopsy is shown in the image. Which of the following most likely accounts for the pathogenesis of endometrial hyperplasia in this patient?

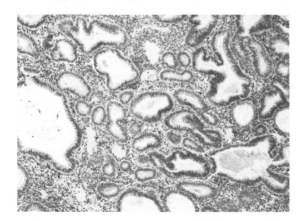

(A) Excess estrogen stimulation
(B) Exposure to exogenous progestational agents
(C) History of chronic endometritis
(D) History of oral contraceptive use
(E) Prenatal exposure to diethylstilbestrol

20 A 33-year-old woman with a history of menorrhagia presents with a 6-month history of increasing fatigue. A CBC reveals a hypochromic, microcytic anemia (hemoglobin = 8 g/dL). Bimanual pelvic examination reveals an enlarged uterus with multiple, irregular masses. A hysterectomy is performed, and a sharply circumscribed fleshy tumor is found within the uterine wall (shown in the image). Which of the following is the most likely cause of vaginal bleeding and anemia in this patient?

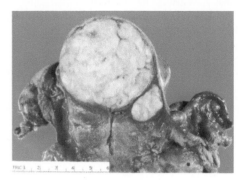

(A) Adenomyosis
(B) Cervical cancer
(C) Endometrial carcinoma
(D) Endometriosis
(E) Uterine leiomyoma

21 A 52-year-old woman presents with chronic pelvic discomfort. A CT scan of the pelvis shows a 10-cm, well-circumscribed uterine mass. A hysterectomy is performed. On gross examination, the mass is soft with areas of necrosis and irregular borders extending into the myometrium. Histologic examination demonstrates large zones of necrosis surrounded by a rim of disorganized spindle cells that display numerous mitoses. Immunohistochemical staining for smooth muscle actin is positive. Which of the following is the most likely diagnosis?
(A) Adenomyosis
(B) Carcinosarcoma
(C) Endometrial stromal sarcoma
(D) Leiomyoma
(E) Leiomyosarcoma

22 A 50-year-old woman complains of having intermenstrual bleeding for 4 months. A Pap smear is normal. An ultrasound examination shows a mass in the endometrial cavity. The patient elects to undergo a hysterectomy. A large polyp is found upon opening the endometrial cavity (shown in the image). Histologic examination of this polyp will most likely show which of the following pathologic findings?

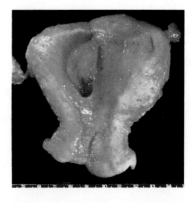

(A)   Atypical endometrial hyperplasia

(B)   Chronic endometritis

(C)   Complex endometrial hyperplasia

(D)   Endometrial glands and fibrous stroma

(E)   Multiple foci of squamous metaplasia

23   A 40-year-old woman presents with a 5-year history of dysmenorrhea. Physical examination and endocrine studies are normal. A hysterectomy is performed. Histologic examination of the uterine wall reveals areas of extensive adenomyosis. Which of the following best describes this patient's uterine pathology?

(A)   Benign neoplasm of glandular epithelial cells

(B)   Displacement of endometrial glands and stroma

(C)   Endometrial intraepithelial neoplasia

(D)   Hyperplasia of trophoblast as a sequel of incomplete abortion

(E)   Premalignant uterine lesion composed of smooth muscle

24   A 60-year-old women presents with a 2-week history of uterine bleeding. Gynecologic examination reveals an enlarged uterus. The hysterectomy specimen shows a large polypoid mass involving the endometrium and myometrium. Histologic examination reveals malignant glands and malignant stromal elements, including striated muscle and cartilage. What is the appropriate diagnosis?

(A)   Carcinosarcoma

(B)   Endometrioid adenocarcinoma

(C)   Leiomyosarcoma

(D)   Pleomorphic adenoma

(E)   Rhabdomyosarcoma

25   A 25-year-old woman is referred to the gynecologist for treatment of infertility. The patient is obese (BMI = 32 kg/m²) and has pronounced facial hair. She states that she has always had irregular menstrual periods. On gynecologic examination, both ovaries are found to be symmetrically enlarged. This patient's ovaries would likely show which of the following pathologic findings?

(A)   Bilateral endometriomas

(B)   Cystic teratoma

(C)   Mucinous cystadenoma

(D)   Serous cystadenoma

(E)   Subcapsular cysts

26   Endocrine studies of the woman described in Question 25 would most likely show which of the following results in the serum?

(A)   High levels of corticosteroids

(B)   High levels of follicle-stimulating hormone

(C)   High levels of luteinizing hormone

(D)   Low levels of estrogens

(E)   Low levels of corticosteroids

27   A 50-year-old woman who has a family history of breast cancer presents with a 6-month history of increasing abdominal girth. On close questioning, she volunteers a history of vague abdominal pain dating back 1 year. She has no children and has never been pregnant. Bimanual pelvic examination reveals a 10-cm right adnexal mass. Percussion of the abdomen indicates ascites. Aspiration cytology of the ascites fluid reveals malignant papillary structures with psammoma bodies. A mutation in which of the following genes is most likely associated with this patient's malignant disease?

(A)   *BRCA1*

(B)   *p53*

(C)   *Rb*

(D)   *VHL*

(E)   *WT-1*

28   The patient described in Question 27 undergoes surgery to have the mass removed. Histologic examination of the surgical specimen is shown in the image. The arrow points to a calcified focus (psammoma body). This neoplasm most likely originated from which of the following ovarian cells/tissues?

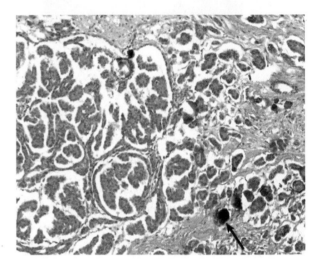

(A)   Germ cells

(B)   Granulosa cells

(C)   Sertoli-Leydig cells

(D)   Surface epithelium

(E)   Theca cells

29   Which of the following statements best characterizes the endocrine status of the malignant cells in the patient described in Questions 27 and 28?

(A)   They are hormonally inactive.

(B)   They cause arterial hypertension.

(C)   They cause polyuria and polydipsia.

(D)   They secrete polypeptide hormones.

(E)   They secrete steroid hormones.

30   A 50-year-old woman presents with a 1-month history of intermittent vaginal bleeding. A Pap smear is normal. Pelvic examination reveals a left adnexal mass. A uterine curettage shows complex endometrial hyperplasia without atypia. A CT scan of the abdomen reveals a 5-cm mass replacing the left ovary. The patient undergoes hysterectomy and bilateral salpingo-oophorectomy. Histologic examination of the ovarian mass is shown in the image. Which of the following is the appropriate pathologic diagnosis?

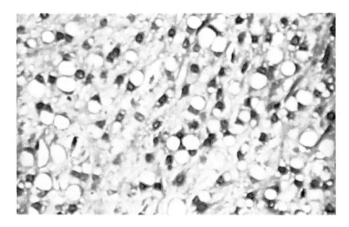

(A) Dysgerminoma
(B) Endometrioid carcinoma
(C) Granulosa cell tumor
(D) Mucinous cystadenocarcinoma
(E) Sertoli-Leydig cell tumor

31 A 40-year-old woman presents with 6 months of increasing abdominal girth. Gynecologic examination reveals large bilateral ovarian masses. The patient undergoes bilateral oophorectomy. The pathology report reads "Krukenberg tumor," and the histopathologic findings are shown in the image. Which of the following tests would likely provide the highest diagnostic yield?

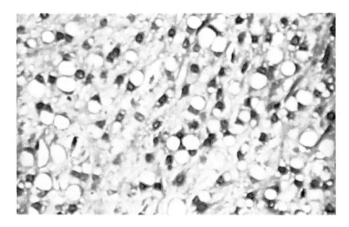

(A) Serum AFP level
(B) Biopsy of the cervix and endometrial curettage
(C) Laparoscopy
(D) Serum hCG level
(E) Gastric endoscopy

32 A 15-year-old girl presents with left lower abdominal pain. She has noted recent enlargement of her breasts. Her last menstrual period was 10 weeks ago. She denies having had sexual intercourse. Serum levels of hCG are markedly elevated. Which of the following is the most likely diagnosis?

(A) Choriocarcinoma
(B) Hydatidiform mole
(C) Mature cystic teratoma
(D) Serous cystadenocarcinoma
(E) Yolk sac carcinoma

33 A 20-year-old woman presents with increasing abdominal girth of 3 months in duration. Physical examination reveals ascites. A pelvic examination discloses a right ovarian mass. A 7-cm ovarian mass is removed at surgery. The histologic appearance of this ovarian neoplasm (shown in the image) most closely resembles which of the following malignant neoplasms seen in males?

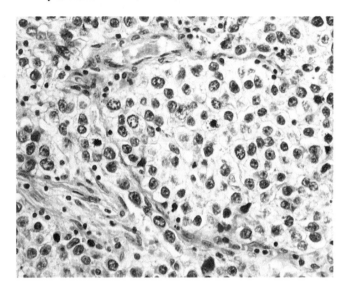

(A) Choriocarcinoma
(B) Embryonal carcinoma
(C) Immature teratoma
(D) Seminoma
(E) Sertoli cell tumor

34 A 60-year-old woman presents with a 1-year history of vulvar itching, bleeding, and inflammation. Physical examination reveals a 1-cm exophytic mass on the labium major. Biopsy of the mass is shown in the image. These neoplastic cells would most likely express which of the following tumor markers?

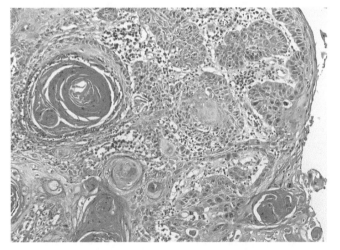

(A) Alpha-fetoprotein
(B) Carcinoembryonic antigen
(C) Cytokeratins
(D) Estrogen/progesterone receptors
(E) Her2/neu polypeptides

35   A 22-year-old woman presents to the emergency room with a 2-hour history of acute abdominal pain and vaginal bleeding. Her vital signs are normal. Physical examination reveals blood oozing from the vaginal opening. Laparotomy shows an enlarged right fallopian tube with hemorrhage and rupture. What is the most likely cause of hemorrhage in this patient?

(A)   Choriocarcinoma
(B)   Ectopic pregnancy
(C)   Infarcted tubal polyp
(D)   Intramural leiomyoma
(E)   Tubal adenocarcinoma

36   A 25-year-old woman in the last trimester of her first pregnancy presents for a routine obstetric evaluation. Her blood pressure is 160/100 mm Hg, and her pulse is 75 per minute. Physical examination shows pitting edema of the extremities. Urinalysis demonstrates 3+ proteinuria. Which of the following is the most dangerous complication of preeclampsia in this patient?

(A)   Amniotic fluid embolism
(B)   Chorioamnionitis
(C)   Choriocarcinoma
(D)   Disseminated intravascular coagulation
(E)   Rupture of the fallopian tube

37   A 17-year-old woman presents to her gynecologist with a 5-day history of vaginal bleeding. A home pregnancy test had been positive 1 week previously. This morning, the patient passed tissue with the appearance of small grapes. An ultrasound shows a dilated endometrial cavity but no evidence of a fetus. Endometrial evacuation of the uterus by suction curettage reveals grapelike clusters, with individual units measuring up to 5 mm in diameter (shown in the image). Cytogenetic examination of this tissue will most likely demonstrate which of the following genetic patterns?

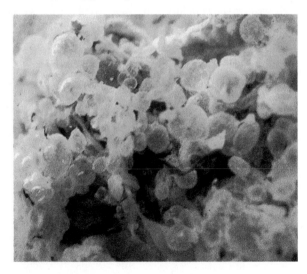

(A)   Aneuploidy
(B)   Diploidy
(C)   Haploidy
(D)   Polyploidy
(E)   Triploidy

38   A 41-year-old immigrant woman from Asia presents for prenatal care. Her uterus is significantly larger than expected, and her serum hCG level is much higher than expected for her due date. No fetus is found on ultrasound examination. The abnormal placenta is removed. One month later, this patient presents to the emergency room with abdominal pain. Exploratory laparotomy reveals rupture of the posterior uterine fundus with grape-like tissue extruding from the defect. Two liters of blood are present in the abdominal cavity. Histologic examination of the uterine mass is shown in the image. The arrows point to syncytial cells. Which of the following is the most likely diagnosis?

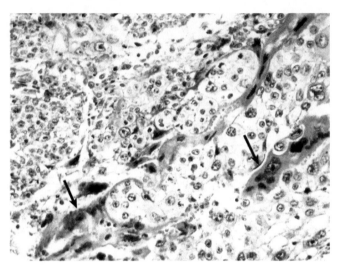

(A)   Carcinosarcoma
(B)   Choriocarcinoma
(C)   Embryonal carcinoma
(D)   Endometrial adenocarcinoma
(E)   Yolk sac carcinoma

39   A 34-year-old woman in the third trimester of her second pregnancy presents with a 1-week history of vaginal bleeding. The patient subsequently gives birth to a healthy female at 35 weeks of gestation. Immediately after delivery, the patient begins to hemorrhage transvaginally. The bleeding cannot be controlled, and the patient undergoes emergency hysterectomy. Examination of the hysterectomy specimen reveals penetration of chorionic villi deep into the myometrium, causing failure of the placental tissue to fully separate from the uterine wall. Which of the following best describes the uteroplacental abnormality seen in this patient?

(A)   Gestational choriocarcinoma
(B)   Abruptio placentae
(C)   Placenta increta
(D)   Placenta previa
(E)   Preeclampsia

40   A 30-year-old pregnant woman asks for information regarding mechanisms of sex determination during development. You explain that the Y chromosome determines male phenotype and that specific genital organs are inhibited from developing by hormones secreted by the developing testes. For example, müllerian-inhibiting substance released by Sertoli cells causes the involution of which of the following urogenital organs?

(A) Breast
(B) Clitoris
(C) Ovary
(D) Uterus
(E) Vulva

41 A 33-year-old woman presents after 3 weeks of a painful genital lesion. Physical examination reveals a tender, erythematous, submucosal lesion of the labium minor (shown in the image). Which of the following is the most likely diagnosis?

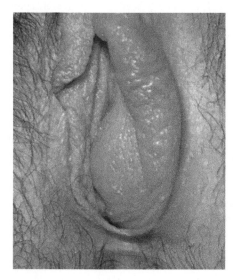

(A) Bartholin gland cyst
(B) Caruncle
(C) Condyloma acuminatum
(D) Extramammary Paget disease
(E) Lichen sclerosis

42 A 22-year-old woman presents to the emergency room with an 8-hour history of high fever, vomiting, diarrhea, and night sweats. Her temperature on admission is 38.7°C (103°F), blood pressure 100/60 mm Hg, and respirations 24 per minute. She has a diffuse desquamative erythematous rash. Upon pelvic examination, the patient is found to be menstruating, and a tampon is in place. A purulent exudate is found within the vagina, which is cultured and grows *Staphylococcus aureus*. The hemoglobin is 12 g/dL, and the platelet count is 40,000/μL. Which of the following represents the most common life-threatening complication of this patient's systemic disorder?
(A) Acute tubular necrosis
(B) Anemia
(C) Cardiac arrhythmia
(D) Disseminated intravascular coagulation
(E) Pulmonary thromboembolism

43 A 35-year-old woman complains of vaginal discomfort for 2 weeks. Physical examination reveals a scanty vaginal discharge. The fluid develops a "fishy" odor after treatment with 10% potassium hydroxide. A Pap smear taken during the pelvic examination shows squamous cells covered by coccobacilli ("clue" cells). Which of the following is the most likely etiology of vaginal discomfort in this patient?

(A) *Chlamydia trachomatis*
(B) *Gardnerella vaginalis*
(C) Herpes simplex virus
(D) Human papillomavirus
(E) *Trichomonas vaginalis*

44 A 56-year-old woman presents with a 3-month history of vaginal bleeding. A cervical Pap smear reveals malignant, glandular epithelial cells. This patient most likely has a neoplasm originating in which of the following anatomic locations?
(A) Cervix
(B) Endometrium
(C) Ovary
(D) Vagina
(E) Vulva

45 A 20-year-old woman presents for a complete physical examination. During the pelvic examination, a 5-cm cystic mass is found in the region of the right ovary. Radiographs show focal calcifications in the mass. The tumor is removed, and the surgical specimen is shown in the image. Which of the following is the most likely diagnosis?

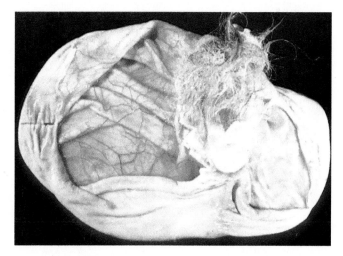

(A) Dysgerminoma
(B) Mature teratoma
(C) Mucinous cystadenoma
(D) Serous cystadenocarcinoma
(E) Teratocarcinoma

46 A 43-year-old woman presents with a 6-month history of increasing abdominal girth. On physical examination, there is pronounced ascites. Pelvic examination reveals a left adnexal mass. A 6-cm ovarian tumor is removed. The tumor is solid and white. Histologically, it is composed of cells resembling normal ovarian stroma surrounded by collagen fibers. Which of the following is the appropriate diagnosis?
(A) Fibroma
(B) Granulosa cell tumor
(C) Leiomyosarcoma
(D) Papillary cystadenoma
(E) Sertoli-Leydig cell tumor

47 A 25-year-old woman presents with a 6-month history of increasing facial hair, deepened voice, and amenorrhea.

Physical examination confirms virilization. A CT scan reveals a left ovarian mass. The tumor is surgically removed. It measures 10 cm in diameter and has a yellowish-tan appearance on cross section. The tumor is malignant and consists of two distinct cell populations. Some cells form solid nests, whereas others are arranged in trabecular and gland-like structures. Which of the following is the appropriate diagnosis?

(A) Brenner tumor
(B) Dysgerminoma
(C) Granulosa cell tumor
(D) Mature cystic teratoma
(E) Sertoli-Leydig cell tumor

48 A 25-year-old woman presents with a 6-month history of breast enlargement and menstrual irregularities. An endometrial biopsy 3 months previously showed complex hyperplasia without atypia. A CT scan of the pelvis reveals a left ovarian mass, which is subsequently removed. The surgical specimen is solid and yellow, and measures 8 cm in diameter. Histologically, it is composed of lipid-laden theca cells. Following removal of this neoplasm, a marked decrease in serum levels of which of the following hormones would be expected in this patient?

(A) Chorionic gonadotropin
(B) Estrogen
(C) Progesterone
(D) Prolactin
(E) Testosterone

49 A 34-year-old woman presents with increasing abdominal girth of 3 months in duration. Physical examination reveals a left ovarian mass and mild ascites. The ovarian mass is removed, and the pathology report states "yolk sac carcinoma." Which of the following provides the best serologic marker to monitor the course of disease in this patient after surgery?

(A) Alkaline phosphatase
(B) Alpha-fetoprotein
(C) Carcinoembryonic antigen
(D) Human chorionic gonadotropin
(E) Sex hormones (estrogen/progesterone)

50 A 20-year-old woman presents to her gynecologist with a 3-day history of vaginal bleeding. An ultrasound shows a dilated endometrial cavity. Evacuation of the uterus by suction curettage reveals grapelike clusters and fetal parts. Cytogenetic examination of this tissue will most likely demonstrate which of the following genetic patterns?

(A) Aneuploidy
(B) Diploidy
(C) Euploidy
(D) Haploidy
(E) Triploidy

51 A 55-year-old nulliparous woman presents for a physical examination. The patient is obese (BMI = 33 kg/m²) and has mild, adult-onset diabetes. Compared with multiparous women, this patient is at increased risk of developing a neoplasm in which of the following anatomic locations?

(A) Cervix
(B) Endometrium
(C) Endosalpinx
(D) Vagina
(E) Vulva

ANSWERS

1 **The answer is C: Endometriosis.** Endometriosis refers to the presence of benign endometrial glands and stroma outside the uterus. It afflicts 5% to 10% of women of reproductive age and regresses following menopause. The sites most frequently involved are the ovaries (>60%); other uterine adnexae; and the pelvic peritoneum covering the uterus, fallopian tubes, rectosigmoid colon, and bladder. With repeated cycles, hemorrhage, and the onset of fibrosis, the affected surface may take on a grossly brown discoloration ("powder burns") and form cysts up to 15 cm in diameter, which contain chocolate-colored material ("chocolate cysts"). The other choices do not present as small hemorrhagic lesions in these anatomic sites.
Diagnosis: Endometriosis

2 **The answer is A: Clear cell adenocarcinoma.** Of women exposed in utero to diethylstilbestrol, 0.1% develop clear cell adenocarcinoma. The tumor is most common between ages 17 and 22 years and is most frequent on the anterior wall of the upper third of the vagina. Almost all clear cell adenocarcinomas are associated with vaginal adenosis, but very few women with adenosis develop this cancer. The abundant clear cytoplasm, reflecting the presence of glycogen, accounts for the name "clear cell." The other choices are not associated with prenatal exposure to diethylstilbestrol.
Diagnosis: Clear cell adenocarcinoma of vagina

3 **The answer is B: Caruncle.** This polypoid inflammatory lesion near the female urethral meatus elicits pain and bleeding. It occurs exclusively in women, most frequently after menopause. Urethral caruncle presents as an exophytic, often ulcerated, polypoid mass of 1 to 2 cm in diameter. Microscopically, the lesion exhibits acutely and chronically inflamed granulation tissue and ulceration and hyperplasia of transitional-cell or squamous epithelium. The other choices do not typically involve the urethral meatus.
Diagnosis: Caruncle

4 **The answer is D: Mucinous cystadenoma.** Benign common epithelial tumors of the ovary are almost always serous or mucinous adenomas and generally arise in women between the ages of 20 and 60 years. The neoplasms are frequently large and often 15 to 30 cm in diameter. Some of these tumors, particularly the mucinous variety, reach truly massive proportion, exceeding 50 cm in diameter. As opposed to their malignant counterparts, benign ovarian epithelial tumors tend to have thin walls and lack solid areas. Lack of stromal invasion and atypia in this case exclude mucinous cystadenocarcinoma (choice C).
Diagnosis: Mucinous cystadenoma of the ovary

5 **The answer is E: Mucosa of the endocervix.** During embryonic life, the celomic cavity is lined by a mesothelium. This mesothelial lining gives rise to müllerian ducts, from which the fallopian tubes, uterus, and vagina arise. Common epithelial tumors of the ovary, in order of decreasing frequency, include: serous tumors that resemble the epithelium of the fallopian tube (choice B); mucinous tumors that mimic the mucosa of the endocervix (choice E); endometrioid tumors that are similar to glands of the endometrium (choice C); clear cell tumors that display glycogen-rich cells that resemble endometrial glands in pregnancy (choice A); and transitional cell tumors that resemble the mucosa of the bladder (choice D). These tumors are broadly classified as benign, borderline (atypical proliferative), and malignant.

Diagnosis: Mucinous cystadenoma of the ovary

6 **The answer is D: Tubo-ovarian abscess.** Gonorrhea is caused by *Neisseria gonorrhoeae*, a Gram-negative diplococcus. The infection is a frequent cause of acute salpingitis and pelvic inflammatory disease. The organisms ascend through the cervix and the endometrial cavity, where they cause an acute endometritis. The bacteria then attach to mucosal cells in the fallopian tube and elicit an acute inflammatory reaction, which is confined to the mucosal surface (acute salpingitis). From the tubal lumen, the infection spreads to involve the ovary, sometimes resulting in a tubo-ovarian abscess. Systemic complications of gonorrhea include septicemia and septic arthritis. The healing process distorts and destroys the plicae of the fallopian tube, often leading to sterility. Infections by *N. gonorrhoeae* at other sites (choices A, B, C, and E) are rare.

Diagnosis: Gonorrhea, pelvic inflammatory disease

7 **The answer is A: Extramammary Paget disease.** Paget disease of the vulva is named after similar-appearing tumors in the nipple and extramammary sites, such as the axilla and perianal region. The typical Paget cell has a pale, vacuolated cytoplasm that contains glycosaminoglycans. It stains with PAS and mucicarmine and expresses CEA. The disorder usually occurs on the labia majora in older women. Women with Paget disease of the vulva complain of pruritus or a burning sensation for many years. The other choices do not feature these specific histologic findings.

Diagnosis: Extramammary Paget disease

8 **The answer is B: Autoimmune disease.** Lichen sclerosis is an inflammatory disease of the vulva, which is often associated with autoimmune disorders such as vitiligo, pernicious anemia, and thyroiditis (e.g., Hashimoto thyroiditis). The condition is represented by white plaques, atrophic skin, a parchment-like or crinkled appearance, and, occasionally, marked contracture of the vulvar tissues. Histologically, there is hyperkeratosis, loss of rete ridges, and a homogeneous, acellular zone in the upper dermis. A band of chronic inflammatory cells typically lies beneath this layer. Itching is the most common symptom, and dyspareunia is frequent. Women with symptomatic lichen sclerosis have a 15% chance of developing squamous cell carcinoma. The other choices are not associated with lichen sclerosis.

Diagnosis: Lichen sclerosus

9 **The answer is C: Human papillomavirus (HPV).** Condyloma acuminatum is a benign, exophytic, papillomatous lesion on the skin or mucous membranes of the lower female genital tract.

HPV is a DNA virus that infects a variety of skin and mucosal surfaces to produce condylomata, which are also referred to as verrucae. The median time from infection to first detection of HPV is 3 months. HPV types 6 and 11 are detected in over 80% of macroscopically visible condylomata. Several strains of HPV are now considered the major etiologic factor in the development of squamous cell cancer in the female lower genital tract. Types 16, 18, 31, and 45 are the most representative high-risk types linked to intraepithelial neoplasia and invasive cancer. The vacuolated cells in the cervical biopsy (see photomicrograph) are typical of HPV infection and are termed koilocytes. The other pathogens do not infect the cervix and do not produce this histopathologic appearance.

Diagnosis: Condyloma acuminatum

10 **The answer is A: *Chlamydia trachomatis*.** Lymphogranuloma venereum is a sexually transmitted infection that is endemic in tropical countries but rare in developed ones. The disease is caused by *C. trachomatis*, which is a Gram-negative obligate, intracellular rickettsia. This organism has been found in the genital tract of about 8% of asymptomatic women and in 20% of women presenting with symptoms of a lower genital tract infection. After a few days to a month, a small painless vesicle forms at the site of inoculation. It heals rapidly, and in many instances, the vesicle is not even noticed. The second stage presents with bilaterally enlarged inguinal lymph nodes that may rupture and form suppurative fistulas. In some untreated patients, a third stage appears, which causes lymphatic obstruction and resulting genital elephantiasis and rectal strictures. *Mycobacterium tuberculosis* (choice D) induces granulomatous inflammation but does not feature inclusion bodies. *Gardnerella vaginalis* (choice B) causes nonspecific vaginitis. *Molluscum contagiosum* (choice C) does not involve the lymph nodes. *Treponema pallidum* (choice E) does not cause granulomas.

Diagnosis: Lymphogranuloma venaereum

11 **The answer is C: *Haemophilus ducreyi*.** Chancroid, also called soft chancre, is caused by *H. ducreyi*, a Gram-negative bacillus. This disease is rare in the United States but is common in underdeveloped countries. Usually 3 to 5 days after sexual congress with an infected partner, single or sometimes multiple small, vesiculopustular lesions appear on the cervix, vagina, vulva, or perianal region. Histologic examination reveals a granulomatous inflammatory reaction. The lesion often ruptures to form a purulent ulcer that is painful and bleeds easily. There may be associated inguinal lymphadenopathy, fever, chills, and malaise. A major complication is scar formation during the healing phase, which is an outcome that sometimes causes urethral stenosis. *Mycobacterium tuberculosis* (choice D) causes granulomatous salpingitis but is not transmitted acutely, as in this case. The other choices do not elicit granulomatous inflammation.

Diagnosis: Chancroid

12 **The answer is D: Dysplasia of the cervix.** Cervical intraepithelial neoplasia is defined as a spectrum of intraepithelial changes that begins with minimal atypia and progresses through stages of more marked intraepithelial abnormalities to invasive squamous cell carcinoma. Dysplasia and carcinoma in situ can often be detected on colposcopic examination by signs associated with their altered epithelial and vascular changes: epithelial mosaicism (irregular surface resembling inlaid woodwork) and vascular dots differentiated from the surrounding tissue surface by color and texture. The other choices do not demonstrate these gross morphologic features, although they may share dysplastic morphology.

Diagnosis: Cervical intraepithelial neoplasia

13 The answer is D: Severe dysplasia (CIN-3). The normal process by which the cervical squamous epithelium matures is disturbed in CIN, as evidenced morphologically by changes in cellularity, differentiation, polarity, nuclear features, and mitotic activity. In CIN-1 (mild dysplasia), the most pronounced changes are seen in the basal third of the epithelium. However, in this case, abnormal cells are present throughout the entire thickness of the epithelium. In CIN-2 (moderate dysplasia, choice C), most of the cellular abnormalities are in the lower and middle thirds of the epithelium. CIN-3 is synonymous with severe dysplasia and carcinoma in situ and shows abnormal cells occupying the full thickness of the epithelium, with no evidence of epithelial maturation. Invasive carcinoma (choice B) features extension of neoplastic cells through the basal membrane. Dysplasia is not synonymous with squamous metaplasia (choice E).

Diagnosis: Cervical intraepithelial neoplasia

14 The answer is C: Endocervical polyp. Endocervical polyp, the most common cervical growth, appears as a single smooth or lobulated mass, typically smaller than 3 cm in greatest dimension. It typically manifests as vaginal bleeding or discharge. The lining epithelium is mucinous, with varying degrees of squamous metaplasia, but may feature erosions and granulation tissue in women with symptoms. Simple excision or curettage is curative. Cancer rarely arises in an endocervical polyp (0.2% of cases). The other choices are rare causes of an endocervical polyp.

Diagnosis: Endocervical polyp

15 The answer is C: Nodal involvement. Squamous cell carcinoma is by far the most common type of cervical cancer. In the earliest stages of cervical cancer, patients complain most frequently of vaginal bleeding after intercourse or douching. With more advanced tumors, the symptoms are referable to the route and degree of spread. The clinical stage of cervical cancer is the best prognostic index of survival. Radical hysterectomy is favored for localized tumor, especially in younger women; radiation therapy or combinations of the two are used for more advanced tumors. Histologic or cytologic findings (choices B and E) are of secondary importance. CEA (choice D) is not typically expressed by squamous carcinoma cells.

Diagnosis: Cervical cancer

16 The answer is D: Renal failure. Cervical cancer spreads by direct extension and through lymphatic vessels and only rarely by the hematogenous route, which would result in distant metastases (choices A, B, C, and E). Local extension into surrounding tissues (parametrium) results in ureteral compression. The corresponding clinical complications of local extension are hydroureter, hydronephrosis, and renal failure, the last being the most common cause of death (50% of patients). Bladder and rectal involvement may lead to fistula formation. Metastases to regional lymph nodes involve the paracervical, hypogastric, and external iliac nodes.

Diagnosis: Cervical cancer

17 The answer is B: Atypical hyperplasia. Endometrial hyperplasia refers to a spectrum that ranges from simple glandular crowding to conspicuous proliferation of atypical glands, which are difficult to distinguish from early carcinoma. The risk of developing endometrial cancer increases with progressively higher degrees of endometrial hyperplasia. The progression from *hyperplasia free of atypia* (complex type, choice D) to invasive cancer requires some 10 years, but the corresponding time for *hyperplasia with atypia* is only 4 years. Atypical hyperplasia is characterized by cytologic atypia and marked glandular crowding, frequently as back-to-back glands. The epithelial cells are enlarged and hyperchromatic and have prominent nucleoli and an increased nuclear-to-cytoplasmic ratio. One fourth of these cases progress to adenocarcinoma. Adenomyosis (choice A) and chronic endometritis (choice C) are not premalignant conditions.

Diagnosis: Endometrial adenocarcinoma

18 The answer is B: PTEN. The *PTEN* tumor suppressor gene, which is hormonally regulated in normal endometrium, is an informative biomarker for endometrial carcinogenesis. Loss of this gene function occurs in two thirds of endometrial carcinomas. *PTEN* knockout mice uniformly develop "endometrial hyperplasia" that evolves to carcinoma in one fifth of the animals. Loss of Rb function (choice C) has been implicated in HPV-induced cervical carcinoma. Mutations in *p53* (choice A) are found in many tumors, but loss of *p53* function is not associated with endometrial carcinoma. Loss of WT-1 tumor suppressor protein (choice E) is related to Wilms tumor.

Diagnosis: Endometrial adenocarcinoma

19 The answer is A: Excess estrogen stimulation. Endometrial hyperplasia and adenocarcinoma are frequently associated with exogenous or endogenous estrogen excess. For example, endometrial hyperplasia may result from anovulatory cycles, polycystic ovary syndrome, an estrogen-producing tumor, or obesity. In such cases, therapy aimed at the primary disease may alleviate the estrogenic stimulation. Estrogenic stimulation of the endometrium beyond the 2-week interval of a normal proliferative menstrual cycle causes progressive changes that have been associated with a 2- to 10-fold increased risk of endometrial cancer. In contrast to benign hyperplasia, endometrial intraepithelial neoplasia (EIN) is recognized as monoclonal neoplastic growth of genetically altered cells. The other choices do not predispose to endometrial hyperplasia, EIN, or carcinoma.

Diagnosis: Endometrial hyperplasia

20 The answer is E: Uterine leiomyoma. Leiomyoma is a benign tumor of smooth muscle origin that is colloquially known as a fibroid. These tumors are rare before age 20 years, and most regress after the menopause. Estrogen promotes the growth of leiomyomas, although it does not initiate them. Grossly, leiomyomas are firm, pale gray, whorled, and without encapsulation. Most leiomyomas are intramural, but some are submucosal, subserosal, or pedunculated. Submucosal leiomyomas may cause bleeding, which is an effect due to ulceration of the thinned, overlying endometrium. Adenomyosis (choice A) does not present as a discrete mass. Endometrial carcinoma (choice C) is much less common than leiomyoma.

Diagnosis: Leiomyoma of the uterus

21 **The answer is E: Leiomyosarcoma.** Leiomyosarcoma is a malignant tumor of smooth muscle cell origin. It should be suspected if an apparent leiomyoma is soft, shows areas of necrosis on gross examination, has irregular borders, or does not bulge above the surface when cut. The following features are considered evidence for the diagnosis of leiomyosarcoma: (1) ten or more mitoses per high-powered field (HPF); (2) five or more mitoses per 10 HPFs, with nuclear atypia and necrosis; and (3) myxoid and epithelioid smooth muscle tumors with five or more mitoses per 10 HPFs. Adenomyosis (choice A) refers to the presence of benign endometrial glands and stroma in the myometrium. Carcinosarcoma (choice B) is a mixed tumor with malignant epithelial and stromal components. Endometrial stromal sarcomas (choice C) show a vascular supporting framework with neoplastic cells concentrically arranged around blood vessel; they are much rarer than leiomyosarcoma.
Diagnosis: Leiomyosarcoma of the uterus

22 **The answer is D: Endometrial glands and fibrous stroma.** Endometrial polyps occur most commonly in the perimenopausal period and are virtually unknown before menarche. They are thought to arise from endometrial foci that are hypersensitive to estrogenic stimulation or unresponsive to progesterone. In either case such foci do not slough during menstruation and continue to grow. Microscopically, the core of a polyp is composed of (1) endometrial glands, which often are cystically dilated and hyperplastic; (2) a fibrous endometrial stroma; and (3) thick-walled, coiled, dilated blood vessels. The other choices may be observed occasionally in an endometrial polyp.
Diagnosis: Endometrial polyp

23 **The answer is B: Displacement of endometrial glands and stroma.** Adenomyosis refers to the presence of endometrial glands and stroma within the myometrium. One fifth of all uteri removed at surgery show some adenomyosis. Microscopic examination of these lesions reveals glands lined by mildly proliferative to inactive endometrium and surrounded by endometrial stroma with varying degrees of fibrosis. Many patients with adenomyosis are asymptomatic; however, it is not uncommon for patients to exhibit varying degrees of pelvic pain, dysfunctional uterine bleeding, dysmenorrhea, and dyspareunia. Adenomyosis does not represent a neoplastic process (choices A, C, and E).
Diagnosis: Adenomyosis

24 **The answer is A: Carcinosarcoma.** Carcinosarcoma is an aggressive, mixed mesodermal tumor, in which the epithelial and stromal components are both highly malignant. These neoplasms are derived from multipotential stromal cells. The overall 5-year rate survival is 25%. Pleomorphic adenoma (choice D) is a mixed tumor of salivary gland. The other choices do not feature biphasic components.
Diagnosis: Carcinosarcoma

25 **The answer is E: Subcapsular cysts.** Polycystic ovary syndrome, also known as Stein-Leventhal syndrome, describes (1) clinical manifestations related to the secretion of excess androgenic hormones, (2) persistent anovulation, and (3) ovaries containing many small subcapsular cysts. It was described initially as a syndrome of secondary amenorrhea, hirsutism, and obesity. The clinical presentation is now recognized to be far more variable and includes amenorrheic women who appear otherwise normal and, even rarely, have ovaries lacking polycystic features. Up to 7% of women experience the polycystic ovary syndrome, making this condition a common cause of infertility. Unopposed acyclic estrogen secretion in women with polycystic ovary syndrome results in an increased incidence of endometrial hyperplasia and adenocarcinoma. On gross examination, both ovaries are enlarged. On cut section, the cortex is thickened and discloses numerous cysts (typically 2 to 8 mm in diameter) arranged peripherally around a dense core of stroma. The other choices are not typically associated with Stein-Leventhal syndrome.
Diagnosis: Polycystic ovary syndrome

26 **The answer is C: High levels of luteinizing hormone.** Polycystic ovary syndrome represents a state of functional ovarian hyperandrogenism associated with increased levels of luteinizing hormone (LH), although the increase in LH is probably a result rather than a cause of the ovarian dysfunction. The central abnormality is thought to be increased ovarian production of androgens, but adrenal hypersecretion of androgens may also contribute to the clinical manifestations.
Diagnosis: Polycystic ovary syndrome

27 **The answer is A: *BRCA1*.** Malignant papillary structures and psammoma bodies (laminated calcified concretions) in a patient with ascites is most compatible with the diagnosis of papillary serous cystadenocarcinoma of the ovary. The same gene implicated in hereditary breast cancers, namely *BRCA1*, has been incriminated in the pathogenesis of familial ovarian cancer. Women who bear *BRCA1* gene mutations tend to develop ovarian cancer considerably earlier than women who have sporadic ovarian cancer, but their prognosis is considerably better. Mutations in the *WT-1* tumor suppressor gene (choice E) are related to Wilms tumor.
Diagnosis: Ovarian cancer, papillary serous cystadenocarcinoma

28 **The answer is D: Surface epithelium.** The tumor depicted is a papillary serous cystadenocarcinoma. The most frequently encountered ovarian tumors (e.g., benign and malignant serous and mucinous neoplasms) arise from the surface epithelium and are termed common epithelial tumors. Epidemiologic studies suggest that common epithelial neoplasms are related to repeated disruption and repair of the epithelial surface during normal cyclic ovulation. Thus, these tumors most commonly afflict women who are nulliparous and, conversely, occur least often in women in whom ovulation has been suppressed (e.g., by pregnancy or oral contraceptives). Germ cells (choice A) give rise to benign teratomas and a variety of malignant tumors. The other cells give rise to sex cord/stromal tumors.
Diagnosis: Ovarian cancer, papillary serous cystadenocarcinoma

29 **The answer is A: They are hormonally inactive.** Ovarian tumors that arise from the surface (germinal or celomic) epithelium are hormonally inactive and do not produce endocrine syndromes. Ovarian masses rarely cause symptoms until they are large. When they distend the abdomen, they cause pain, pelvic pressure, or compression of regional organs. By the time ovarian cancers are diagnosed, many have metastasized to the surfaces of the pelvis, abdominal organs, or bladder. Overall 5-year survival is only 35%.

Diagnosis: Ovarian cancer

30 **The answer is C: Granulosa cell tumor.** Granulosa cell tumor is the prototypical functional neoplasm of the ovary associated with estrogen secretion. The tumor is derived from sex cord stromal cells. Most granulosa cell tumors occur after the menopause. A juvenile form occurs in children and young women and has distinct clinical and pathologic features (hyperestrogenism and precocious puberty). Microscopically, granulosa cell tumors display haphazard orientation of the nuclei about a central degenerative space (Call-Exner bodies), which results in a characteristic follicular histologic pattern. Three fourths of granulosa cell tumors secrete estrogens. Consequently, endometrial hyperplasia is a common presenting sign. Hyperplasia may progress to endometrial adenocarcinoma if the functioning granulosa cell tumor remains undetected. Sertoli-Leydig cell tumors (choice E) typically secrete weak androgens. The other choices do not secrete hormones.

Diagnosis: Granulosa cell tumor of the ovary

31 **The answer is E: Gastric endoscopy.** Krukenberg tumors are ovarian metastases in which the tumor appears as nests of mucin-filled "signet ring" cells within a cellular stroma derived from the ovary. The stomach is the primary site in 75% of cases, and most of the other Krukenberg tumors are from the colon. Bilateral ovarian involvement and multinodularity are important clues to the diagnosis of metastatic carcinoma.

Diagnosis: Krukenberg tumor of the ovary, gastric adenocarcinoma

32 **The answer is A: Choriocarcinoma.** Choriocarcinoma of the ovary is a rare tumor that mimics the epithelial covering of placental villi (cytotrophoblast and syncytiotrophoblast). Choriocarcinoma of germ cell origin manifests in young girls as precocious sexual development, menstrual irregularities, and rapid breast enlargement. In women of reproductive age, ovarian choriocarcinoma may represent metastasis from an intrauterine gestational tumor. Microscopically, it displays an admixture of malignant cytotrophoblast and syncytiotrophoblast. The syncytial cells of choriocarcinoma secrete hCG, which accounts for the frequent finding of a positive pregnancy test result. The tumor is highly aggressive but responds to chemotherapy. Hydatidiform mole secretes hCG but is a gestational trophoblastic disease. The other choices do not secrete hCG.

Diagnosis: Choriocarcinoma of the ovary

33 **The answer is D: Seminoma.** Dysgerminoma is the ovarian counterpart of testicular seminoma and is composed of activated germ cells. The neoplasm demonstrates large nests of monotonously uniform cells, which have a clear glycogen-filled cytoplasm and irregularly flattened central nuclei. Fibrous septa containing lymphocytes traverse the tumor. The other choices are also found in both sexes but do not show this histologic appearance.

Diagnosis: Dysgerminoma

34 **The answer is C: Cytokeratins.** The tumor depicted is a well-differentiated squamous cell carcinoma with keratin pearls. Squamous cell carcinoma is the most common primary malignant neoplasm of the vulva, and these tumors commonly express cytokeratins. Squamous cell carcinoma of the vulva is the end result of a multistep process that has its origin in vulvar intraepithelial neoplasia. Two thirds of larger tumors are exophytic; the others are ulcerative and endophytic. The tumors grow slowly and then extend to the contiguous skin, vagina, and rectum. They metastasize to the superficial inguinal and then the deep inguinal, femoral, and pelvic lymph nodes. The other tumor markers are not expressed by vulvar squamous cell carcinoma.

Diagnosis: Squamous cell carcinoma

35 **The answer is B: Ectopic pregnancy.** Over 95% of ectopic pregnancies occur in the fallopian tube. Ectopic pregnancy results when the passage of the conceptus along the fallopian tube is impeded, for example, by mucosal adhesions or abnormal tubal motility secondary to inflammatory disease or endometriosis. The trophoblast readily penetrates the mucosa and tubal wall. The thin tubal wall usually ruptures by the 12th week of gestation. Tubal rupture is life threatening because it can result in rapid exsanguination. The other choices are rare.

Diagnosis: Ectopic pregnancy

36 **The answer is D: Disseminated intravascular coagulation.** Preeclampsia usually begins insidiously after the 20th week of pregnancy with (1) excessive weight gain occasioned by fluid retention, (2) increased maternal blood pressure, and (3) the appearance of proteinuria. As the disease progresses from mild to severe preeclampsia, the diastolic pressure persistently exceeds 110 mm Hg. Proteinuria is greater than 3 g per day, and renal function declines. Disseminated intravascular coagulation (DIC) often supervenes. DIC is a prominent feature of preeclampsia, manifested as fibrin thrombi in the liver, brain, and kidneys. The definitive therapy is the removal of the placenta, hopefully by normal delivery. The other choices are not complications of preeclampsia.

Diagnosis: Preeclampsia

37 **The answer is B: Diploidy.** The term gestational trophoblastic disease embraces the spectrum of trophoblastic disorders that exhibit abnormal proliferation and maturation of trophoblast, as well as neoplasms derived from the trophoblast. Complete hydatidiform mole is a placenta that has grossly swollen chorionic villi, resembling bunches of grapes, in which there are varying degrees of trophoblastic proliferation. Complete mole results from the fertilization of an empty ovum that lacks functional DNA. The haploid (23,X) set of paternal chromosomes duplicates to 46,XX. Hence, most complete moles are homozygous 46,XX, but all of the chromosomes are of paternal origin. Since the embryo dies at a very early stage, fetal parts are absent. Malignant transformation (choriocarcinoma) develops in about 2% of cases. Triploidy (choice E) is encountered in partial hydatidiform mole, but this diagnosis is ruled out by the absence of fetal tissue.

Diagnosis: Complete hydatidiform mole

38 **The answer is B: Choriocarcinoma.** Choriocarcinoma occurs in 1 in 30,000 pregnancies in the United States. In Asia, the frequency is far greater. Choriocarcinoma develops in about 2% of patients after a complete hydatidiform mole has been evacuated. Abnormal uterine bleeding is the most frequent initial indication that heralds choriocarcinoma. Occasionally, the first sign relates to metastases to the lungs or brain. In some cases, choriocarcinoma only becomes evident 10 or more years after the last pregnancy. The other choices are not sequelae of gestational trophoblastic disease.

Diagnosis: Choriocarcinoma

39 The answer is C: Placenta increta. Abnormal adherence of the placenta to the underlying uterine wall is subclassified according to the depth of villous invasion into the myometrium. Placenta *accreta* refers to the attachment of villi to the myometrium without further invasion. Placenta *increta* (correct answer) defines villi invading the underlying myometrium. Placenta *percreta* describes villi penetrating the full thickness of the uterine wall. Most patients with placenta acreta have a normal pregnancy and delivery. However, bleeding in the third trimester is the most common presenting sign before delivery. In patients with placenta increta and percreta, substantial fragments of placenta may remain adherent to the uterine wall after delivery and are a source of postpartum hemorrhage. Abruptio placentae (choice B) refers to retroplacental hemorrhage in the absence of clinical hemorrhage. A deficiency of decidua at the implantation site may result from implantation of the placenta close to or over the cervix (placenta previa, choice D).

Diagnosis: Placenta increta

40 The answer is D: Uterus. A central tenet of genital tract development in both sexes holds that the müllerian tubes will develop along female lines unless specifically impeded by embryonic testicular factors. In males, Sertoli cells in the developing testis produce müllerian-inhibiting substance, a protein that causes the müllerian ducts to regress. These ducts are the precursors of the fallopian ducts, uterus, and upper third of the vagina. Formation of the ovary (choice C) and vulva (choice E) is not affected by this hormone.

Diagnosis: Sex determination, müllerian-inhibiting substance

41 The answer is A: Bartholin gland cyst. The Bartholin glands produce a clear mucoid secretion that continuously lubricates the vestibular surface. The ducts are prone to obstruction and cyst formation. Infection of the cyst leads to abscess formation. Bartholin gland abscess was formerly associated with gonorrhea, but staphylococci, chlamydia, and anaerobes are now more frequently the cause. The other choices do not present as discrete submucosal nodules.

Diagnosis: Bartholin gland abscess

42 The answer is D: Disseminated intravascular coagulation. Toxic shock syndrome is an acute, sometimes fatal disorder characterized by fever, shock, and a desquamative erythematous rash. In addition, vomiting, diarrhea, myalgias, neurologic signs, and thrombocytopenia are common. Certain strains of *Staphylococcus aureus* release an exotoxin called toxic shock syndrome toxin-1. In addition to the pathologic alterations characteristic of shock, the lesions of disseminated intravascular coagulation (DIC) are usually prominent. The disease was first recognized when long-acting tampons were first introduced, providing sufficient time for the staphylococcal

organisms to proliferate. The other choices are less common and may be secondary to DIC.

Diagnosis: Toxic shock syndrome

43 The answer is B: *Gardnerella vaginalis*. Sexual transmission of *G. vaginalis*, a Gram-negative coccobacillus, causes a substantial proportion of cases classified as nonspecific vaginitis. The diagnosis of *Gardnerella* infection is best established by identifying the organisms either in a wet mount specimen of a vaginal discharge or in a Papanicolaou-stained smear. The "clue cell" is pathognomonic and shows squamous cells covered by coccobacilli. Other aids to the diagnosis are a thin, homogeneous, milk-like vaginal discharge, a vaginal pH above 4.5, and the presence of a "fishy" odor from the discharge once alkalinized with 10% potassium hydroxide. Viruses (choices C and D) do not produce vaginal discharge. Choices A and E are not associated with "clue" cells.

Diagnosis: Vaginitis, cervicitis

44 The answer is A: Cervix. Adenocarcinoma of the endocervix accounts for 20% of malignant cervical tumors. An increased incidence of cervical adenocarcinoma has been reported recently, with a mean age at presentation of 56 years. Most of the tumors are of the endocervical cell (mucinous) type, but the various subtypes have little importance for overall survival. Adenocarcinoma shares epidemiologic factors with squamous cell carcinoma of the cervix and spreads similarly. The tumors are often associated with adenocarcinoma in situ and are frequently infected with HPV types 16 and 18. Malignant cells derived from endometrial carcinoma (choice B) may be identified occasionally by cervical Pap smear.

Diagnosis: Adenocarcinoma of the exocervix

45 The answer is B: Mature teratoma. Mature teratoma is a tumor of germ cell origin that differentiates toward somatic structures. More than 90% contain skin, sebaceous glands, and hair follicles. Half of the tumors exhibit smooth muscle, sweat glands, cartilage, bone, teeth, and respiratory tract epithelium. Tissues such as gut, thyroid, and brain are encountered less frequently. Haploid (postmeiotic) germ cells are believed to auto-fertilize, yielding diploid tumor cells that are genetically female (46,XX). Teratocarcinoma (choice E) features immature embryonic tissues and malignant stem cells.

Diagnosis: Mature cystic teratoma of the ovary

46 The diagnosis is A: Fibroma. Fibromas are the most common ovarian stromal tumors, accounting for 75% of all stromal tumors and 7% of all ovarian tumors. They occur at all ages, with a peak in the perimenopausal period, and are virtually always benign. The tumors are solid, firm, and white. Microscopically, the cells resemble the stroma of the normal ovarian cortex, being composed of well-differentiated fibroblasts and variable amounts of collagen. Half of the larger tumors are associated with ascites and, rarely, with ascites and pleural effusions. Ascites is not a typical clinical feature of the other choices.

Diagnosis: Fibroma of the ovary

47 The answer is E: Sertoli-Leydig cell tumor. Sertoli-Leydig cell tumor is a rare mesenchymal neoplasm of the ovary of low malignant potential that resembles the embryonic testis. It is the prototypical functional tumor associated with androgen secretion. The neoplastic cells typically secrete weak androgens (dehydroepiandrosterone), which accounts for the large tumor size required to achieve masculinizing signs. Sertoli-Leydig cell tumor occurs at all ages but is most common in young women of childbearing age. Nearly half of all patients with Sertoli-Leydig cell tumors exhibit androgenic effects (i.e., signs of virilization, evidenced by hirsutism, male escutcheon, enlarged clitoris, and deepened voice). The initial sign is often defeminization, which is manifested as breast atrophy, amenorrhea, and loss of hip fat. Once the tumor is removed, the signs disappear or are at least ameliorated. The other choices are not associated with virilization.

Diagnosis: Sertoli-Leydig cell tumor

48   The answer is B: Estrogen. Thecomas are functional ovarian tumors that arise in postmenopausal women. In most cases, they produce signs of estrogen production. Thecomas are solid tumors of 5 to 10 cm in diameter. The cut section is yellow, owing to the presence of many lipid-laden theca cells. Microscopically, the cells are large and oblong to round, with a vacuolated cytoplasm that contains lipid. Bands of hyalinized collagen separate nests of theca cells. Thecomas are almost always benign. Because of estrogen output by the tumor, thecomas in premenopausal women commonly cause irregularity in menstrual cycles and breast enlargement. Endometrial hyperplasia and cancer are well-recognized complications. The other choices do not produce endometrial hyperplasia.

Diagnosis: Thecoma

49   The answer is B: Alpha-fetoprotein. Yolk sac tumor is a highly malignant tumor of women under the age of 30 years that histologically resembles mesenchyme of the primitive yolk sac. The tumor secretes alpha-fetoprotein (AFP), which can be demonstrated histochemically within eosinophilic droplets. Detection of AFP in the blood is useful both for diagnosis and for monitoring the effectiveness of therapy. The hormone human chorionic gonadotropin (choice D) is secreted by choriocarcinoma. Estrogen (choice E) is secreted by sex cord tumors.

Diagnosis: Yolk sac carcinoma

50   The answer is E: Triploidy. Cytogenetic examination of a partial hydatidiform mole will reveal triploidy. This abnormal chromosomal complement results from the fertilization of a normal ovum (23,X) by two normal spermatozoa, each carrying 23 chromosomes, or a single spermatozoon that has not undergone meiotic reduction and bears 46 chromosomes. The fetus associated with a partial mole usually dies after 10 weeks of gestation, and the mole is aborted shortly thereafter. In contrast to a complete mole, which exhibits diploidy (choice B), fetal parts are commonly present in a partial hydatidiform mole.

Diagnosis: Partial hydatidiform mole

51   The answer is B: Endometrium. The major form of endometrial cancer, endometrioid adenocarcinoma, is linked to prolonged estrogenic stimulation of the endometrium. In addition to treatment with exogenous estrogens, the most common risk factors are obesity, diabetes, nulliparity, early menarche, and late menopause. Each risk factor points to relative hyperestrinism. A high frequency of endometrial cancer is also found in women with estrogen-secreting granulosa cell tumors. In the case of obesity, the incidence correlates with body weight, with the risk being increased 10-fold for women who are more than 23 kg (50 lb) overweight. This effect of obesity is related to the enhanced aromatization of androstenedione to estrone in adipocytes. Cancers of the other organs are not related to estrogenic stimulation.

Diagnosis: Endometrial adenocarcinoma

Chapter 19

The Breast

QUESTIONS

Select the single best answer.

1 A 30-year-old woman suffers traumatic injury to her breast while playing soccer. Physical examination reveals a 3-cm area of ecchymosis on the left breast. Two weeks later, the patient palpates a firm lump beneath the area where the bruise had been located. Which of the following is the most likely pathologic diagnosis?
(A) Duct ectasia
(B) Fat necrosis
(C) Fibrocystic change
(D) Granulomatous mastitis
(E) Intraductal papillomatosis

2 A 50-year-old woman presents with a mass in her left breast that she first detected 6 months earlier. A firm 4-cm mass is palpated on breast examination. Excisional biopsy reveals malignant cuboidal cells that form gland-like structures and solid nests, surrounded by dense collagenous stroma. Which of the following terms best describes the adaptive response of this patient's normal breast tissue to the tumor?
(A) Anaplasia
(B) Desmoplasia
(C) Fibrinolysis
(D) Lipohyalinosis
(E) Metaplasia

3 A 54-year-old woman complains of bloody discharge from her left nipple. Physical examination reveals a 0.5-cm nodule in the subareolar breast tissue, which is surgically excised. Histologic examination (shown in the image) reveals cuboidal and myoepithelial cell–lined vascular connective tissue cores, which project into the lumen of a major lactiferous duct. Which of the following is the appropriate diagnosis?

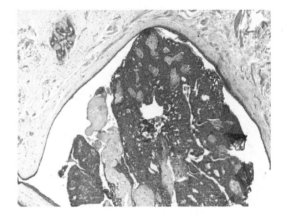

(A) Ductal carcinoma in situ
(B) Intraductal papilloma
(C) Lobular carcinoma in situ
(D) Medullary carcinoma
(E) Paget disease

4 A 53-year-old woman discovers a lump in her breast and physical examination confirms a mass in the lower, outer quadrant of the left breast. Mammography demonstrates an ill-defined, stellate density measuring 1 cm. Needle aspiration reveals malignant ductal epithelial cells. A modified radical mastectomy is performed. The surgical specimen reveals a firm irregular mass (arrows). Which of the following cellular markers would be the most useful to evaluate before considering therapeutic options for this patient?

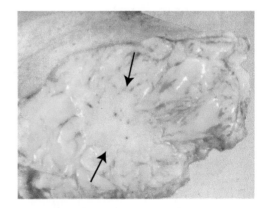

225

(A) Collagenase
(B) Estrogen receptors
(C) Galactosyltransferase
(D) Lysosomal acid hydrolases
(E) Myeloperoxidase

5 A 35-year-old nulliparous woman complains that her breasts are swollen and nodular upon palpation. A mammogram discloses foci of calcification in both breasts. A breast biopsy reveals cystic duct dilation and ductal epithelial hyperplasia without atypia (shown in the image). What is the appropriate diagnosis?

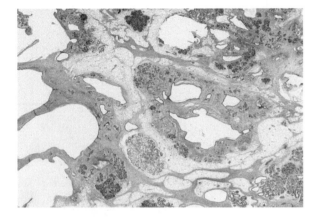

(A) Ductal carcinoma in situ
(B) Fibroadenoma
(C) Fibrocystic change
(D) Granulomatous mastitis
(E) Intraductal papilloma

6 A 24-year-old woman delivers a 3.5-kg baby and begins breastfeeding her infant. The patient presents 2 weeks later with a fever of 38°C (101°F). Physical examination shows no abnormal vaginal discharge or evidence of pelvic pain but does reveal redness on the lower side of the left breast. The patient stops nursing the infant temporarily, but the symptoms persist, and the entire breast becomes swollen and painful. What is the most likely diagnosis?
(A) Acute mastitis
(B) Chronic mastitis
(C) Duct ectasia
(D) Granulomatous mastitis
(E) Lactating adenoma

7 A 35-year-old woman consults her family physician because of painful swelling of her breasts, particularly as she approaches the end of her menstrual cycle. On self-examination she recently felt a tender nodule in the right breast. Physical examination reveals an irregular nodularity of both breasts with diffuse tenderness. Examination of the axilla is negative. A mammogram demonstrates irregular areas of density in the lower, outer quadrants of both breasts. Which of the following histopathologic features is considered to be a risk factor for the development of carcinoma in this patient?

(A) Apocrine metaplasia
(B) Cystic change
(C) Duct ectasia
(D) Papillomatosis
(E) Stromal fibrosis

8 A 60-year-old man presents with painless, bilateral enlargement of both breasts. The patient has a history of nodular prostatic hyperplasia and is taking medication for hypercholesterolemia. Physical examination reveals no discrete breast masses or axillary lymph node enlargement. Which of the following is the most likely underlying cause of breast enlargement in this patient?
(A) Chronic glomerulonephritis
(B) Cirrhosis
(C) Nonseminomatous germ cell neoplasm
(D) Parathyroid adenoma
(E) Progressive systemic sclerosis

9 A 30-year-old woman presents with nipple discharge of 3 weeks in duration. Physical examination reveals a white discharge from both nipples. The patient has not menstruated for the past 4 months, and she is not pregnant. The breasts are firm and nontender. A cytologic smear of the discharge shows no evidence of acute or chronic inflammatory cells. Which of the following is the most likely cause of galactorrhea in this patient?
(A) Adrenal cortical adenoma
(B) Fibroadenoma of the breast
(C) Fibrocystic change of the breast
(D) Pituitary adenoma
(E) Sheehan syndrome

10 A woman consults her physician because of painful swelling of her breasts. Physical examination reveals nodularity of both breasts. Mammography shows irregular areas of increased density in the lower, outer quadrants of both breasts. A breast biopsy reveals increased fibrous stoma, cystic dilation of the terminal ducts, and varying degrees of apocrine metaplasia. This patient's condition is most commonly seen in which of the following groups?
(A) Patients with testicular feminization syndrome
(B) Postmenopausal women
(C) Pubertal girls
(D) Women of reproductive age
(E) Women treated with oral contraceptives

11 A 22-year-old woman presents with a painless nodule in the lower outer aspect of her right breast that she has had for 2 months. The nodule appears to be freely movable, sharply demarcated from the surrounding parenchyma, and firm. A mammogram demonstrates a circumscribed, homogeneous density. A biopsy of the breast mass is shown in the image. Which of the following best estimates the risk of subsequent invasive breast cancer developing in this patient?

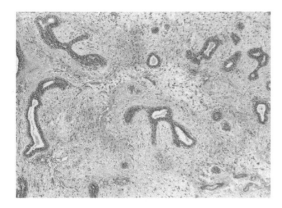

(A) Greater than 90% lifetime risk

(B) Greater than 50% lifetime risk

(C) Risk is doubled

(D) Risk is halved

(E) No risk at all

12 A 20-year-old woman asks for your advice regarding her risk of developing breast cancer. Her mother, maternal aunt, and maternal grandmother all developed breast cancer. She would like to know if she has a genetic predisposition. Laboratory tests for mutations in which of the following genes would be most likely to answer your patient's question?

(A) BRCA1

(B) C-myc

(C) Estrogen receptor

(D) HER2/neu

(E) Rb-1

13 A 26-year-old woman presents with a breast mass that was detected on self-examination 1 week earlier. Mammography reveals a round, sharply demarcated 1-cm nodule in the right breast (shown in the image). Biopsy of the breast mass shows neoplastic epithelial ductal structures situated within a fibro-myxoid stroma. The patient refuses further treatment and informs you that she wishes to become pregnant. Which of the following is the most likely effect of pregnancy on this breast lesion?

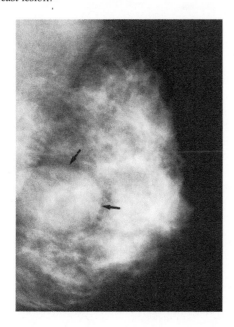

(A) Development of invasive ductal carcinoma within the lesion

(B) Fibrocystic change with sclerosing adenosis

(C) Formation of intraductal papilloma

(D) Metastasis to regional lymph nodes

(E) Rapid growth

14 Upon self-examination, a 53-year-old woman discovers a lump in her left breast. Physical examination reveals a palpable lump about 1 cm in diameter in the outer quadrant of the left breast. No palpable lymph nodes are found in the axilla. Mammography reveals an ill-defined, stellate density measuring 1 cm in the left breast. Fine-needle aspiration of the mass discloses malignant epithelial cells. A partial mastectomy is performed and shows invasive ductal adenocarcinoma. Which of the following is the most important prognostic factor for this patient?

(A) Estrogen receptor status of the tumor tissue

(B) Histologic grade of the tumor

(C) Inherited BRCA1 gene mutation

(D) Somatic mutation of the p53 tumor suppressor gene

(E) Status of the axillary lymph nodes

15 A mammogram of a 52-year-old woman demonstrates calcifications in her left breast. No axillary lymph node enlargement is detected on physical examination. An excisional biopsy is shown in the image. If this patient foregoes further treatment, which of the following best estimates her risk of developing invasive carcinoma in this breast over the next 20 years?

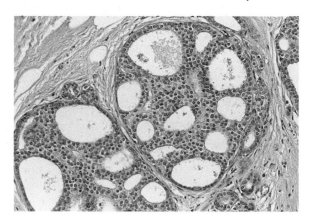

(A) 1%

(B) 5%

(C) 30%

(D) 90%

(E) 100%

16 A 54-year-old woman presents with a mass in her right breast that she first palpated 5 days before. A breast biopsy reveals malignant cells, and a mastectomy is performed. Immunohistochemical staining is performed for HER2/neu (shown in the image). Which of the following genetic mechanisms best accounts for the intensity of staining in this specimen?

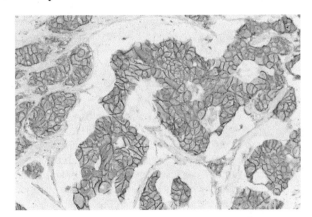

(A) Gene amplification
(B) Insertional mutagenesis
(C) Chromosomal nonhomologous crossing over
(D) Polyploidy
(E) Single nucleotide polymorphism

17 A 45-year-old woman discovers a solitary, freely movable mass in her right breast on self-examination, which is confirmed on physical examination. Mammography demonstrates focal calcification, with a linear configuration in the region of the breast mass. A breast biopsy (shown in the image) reveals large, pleomorphic epithelial cells confined to dilated ducts, with central zones of necrosis. What is the appropriate pathologic diagnosis?

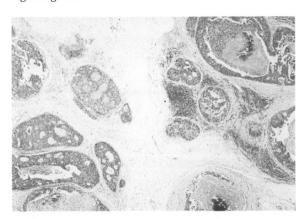

(A) Colloid carcinoma
(B) Ductal carcinoma in situ, comedocarcinoma type
(C) Medullary carcinoma
(D) Phyllodes tumor
(E) Tubular carcinoma

18 A 50-year-old woman has been aware of a mass in her left breast for the past 6 months. A 4-cm mass is palpated on examination. The mass is hard, tender, and fixed to the overlying skin. A lumpectomy is performed. The surgical specimen is firm, has poorly defined margins, and cuts with a gritty sensation. The cut surface is gray, opaque, and slightly depressed. Streaks of gray connective tissue extend into the surrounding fibroadipose tissue. The tumor histology is shown in the image. Which of the following risk factors has the strongest association with this patient's tumor?

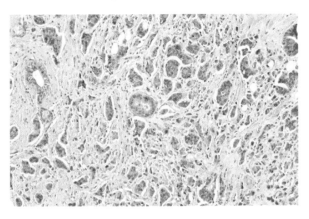

(A) Exposure to carcinogens
(B) Family history
(C) Fibrocystic change
(D) Obesity
(E) Smoking

19 A 58-year-old woman presents with an irregular nodularity that has developed in her right breast over the past 3 months. Mammography demonstrates irregular densities in both breasts. A needle biopsy of one breast lesion is shown. An excisional biopsy of the contralateral breast shows similar histology. Which of the following is the most likely pathologic diagnosis?

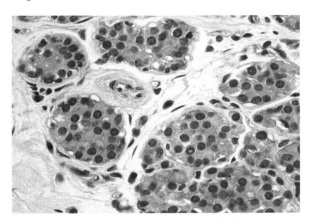

(A) Colloid carcinoma
(B) Lobular carcinoma in situ
(C) Malignant phyllodes tumor
(D) Medullary carcinoma
(E) Tubular carcinoma

20 A 22-year-old woman nursing her newborn develops a tender erythematous area around the nipple of her left breast. On physical examination, a purulent exudate is observed to drain from an open fissure. Culture of this exudate will most likely grow which of the following microorganisms?

(A) *Candida albicans*
(B) *Escherichia coli*
(C) *Haemophilus influenzae*
(D) *Lactobacillus acidophilus*
(E) *Staphylococcus aureus*

21 A 52-year-old woman presents with a 3-month history of a palpable breast mass. Physical examination confirms a 1-cm nodule in the upper outer quadrant of the right breast. A biopsy reveals small cuboidal cells, with round nuclei and prominent nucleoli. The cells are arranged in single cell columns, between strands of connective tissue (shown in the image). Which of the following is the appropriate diagnosis?

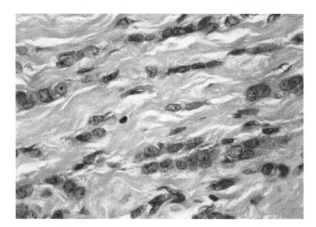

(A) Ductal carcinoma in situ
(B) Invasive ductal carcinoma, tubular type
(C) Invasive lobular carcinoma
(D) Lobular carcinoma in situ
(E) Medullary carcinoma

22 A 58-year-old woman has a screening mammography and is found to have a 4-cm circumscribed mass, without calcifications, in her left breast. An excisional biopsy shows solid nests and sheets of highly pleomorphic cells, with many mitotic figures, surrounded by a dense infiltrate of lymphocytes. Which of the following is the most likely diagnosis?

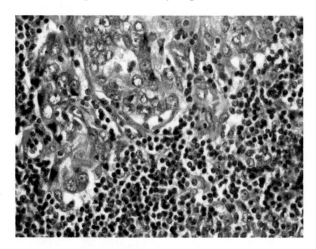

(A) Invasive ductal carcinoma
(B) Invasive lobular carcinoma
(C) Medullary carcinoma
(D) Paget disease
(E) Phyllodes tumor

23 A 45-year-old woman presents with an oozing, reddish patch on her left nipple (patient shown in the image). The patient has a history of skin rashes and food allergies and believes this condition is due to an allergic reaction to her bra. Cytologic examination of fluid oozing from the skin lesion reveals neoplastic cells. Excisional biopsy shows large clear malignant cells in the epidermis of the areola. Which of the following is the most likely diagnosis?

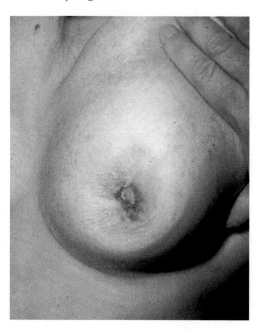

(A) Chronic dermatitis
(B) Colloid carcinoma
(C) Intraductal papilloma
(D) Paget disease
(E) Phyllodes tumor

24 A 60-year-old woman presents with a large breast mass that she first detected 3 months ago. Mammography reveals a well-circumscribed mass measuring 8 cm in diameter. A breast biopsy shows loose fibroconnective tissue with a sarcomatous stroma, abundant mitoses, and nodules and ridges lined by cuboidal epithelial cells. Which of the following is the appropriate diagnosis?
(A) Fibroadenoma
(B) Medullary carcinoma
(C) Paget disease
(D) Phyllodes tumor
(E) Tubular carcinoma

25 A 65-year-old woman presents with a palpable breast mass that she palpated 1 month earlier. Physical examination reveals a soft, jelly-like tumor measuring 5 cm in diameter. Histologic examination of a breast biopsy is shown in the image. What is the appropriate diagnosis?

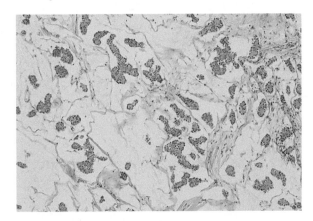

(A) Colloid carcinoma
(B) Lobular carcinoma
(C) Medullary carcinoma
(D) Paget disease
(E) Phyllodes tumor

26 A 55-year-old man presents with a solitary breast mass and biopsy reveals malignant cells. Immunohistochemical staining experiments show that the tumor cells are positive for HER2/neu and cytokeratins 4 and 11 and negative for estrogen receptors. What is the most likely diagnosis?
(A) Basal cell carcinoma
(B) Invasive ductal carcinoma
(C) Invasive lobular carcinoma
(D) Medullary carcinoma
(E) Tubular adenoma

27 Which of the following is thought to play a role in the development of cancer in the patient described in Question 26?
(A) *BRCA2* mutation
(B) Chronic alcoholism
(C) Gynecomastia
(D) Hyperestrinism
(E) *PTEN* mutation

ANSWERS

1 **The answer is B: Fat necrosis.** A history of trauma can usually be elicited in cases of fat necrosis occurring in the breast. Initially, the lesion consists of necrosis of adipocytes and hemorrhage, after which phagocytic cells remove the lipid debris. Fibroblastic proliferation during healing leads to fingers of fibrous scar tissue that extend into the adjacent breast tissue. As a result, an irregular, fixed, hard mass may ensue and clinically resemble breast cancer. Dystrophic calcification, a common feature of breast cancer, may also be detected radiographically in areas of fat necrosis. Thus, the lesions often require biopsy to establish their benign character. The other choices are not associated with trauma.
Diagnosis: Fat necrosis of the breast

2 **The answer is B: Desmoplasia.** Breast cancer is the most common malignancy of women in the United States, and the mortality from this disease among women is second only to that of lung cancer. Invasive, or infiltrating, ductal car-

cinoma is the most common form of breast cancer. In this cancer stromal invasion by malignant cells usually incites a pronounced fibroblastic proliferation. This "desmoplasia" creates a palpable mass, which is the most common initial sign of ductal carcinoma. Invasive ductal carcinoma usually manifests as a hard, fixed mass, which is often referred to as scirrhous carcinoma. On gross examination, the tumor is typically firm and shows irregular margins. The cut surface is pale gray and gritty and flecked with yellow, chalky streaks. Microscopically, invasive ductal carcinoma grows as irregular nests and cords of epithelial cells, usually within a dense fibrous stroma. Metaplasia (choice E) is the conversion of one differentiated cell type to another. Lipohyalinosis (choice D) is a particular form of fibrosis associated with fat deposition. Fibrinolysis (choice C) is related to clot dissolution.
Diagnosis: Invasive ductal carcinoma of the breast

3 **The answer is B: Intraductal papilloma.** Intraductal papilloma is a benign breast tumor that usually causes nipple discharge (serous or hemorrhagic) and occurs in the lactiferous ducts of middle-aged and older women. Because intraductal papilloma is situated in the large, subareolar ducts, the lesion may be associated with a serous or bloody nipple discharge. This lesion must be distinguished from papillomatosis, which occurs in the peripheral ducts as a component of proliferative fibrocystic change. Intraductal papillomas are attached to the wall of the duct by a fibrovascular stalk. The papillomatous portion consists of a double layer of epithelial cells, an outer layer of cuboidal or columnar cells, and an inner layer of more rounded myoepithelial cells. Solitary intraductal papilloma is not a premalignant lesion or a marker for increased risk of cancer in the breast. Ductal carcinoma in situ (choice A) and lobular carcinoma in situ (choice C) feature neoplastic cells confined to ducts and lobules, respectively, and typically lack myoepithelial cells. Paget disease (choice E) is a form of carcinoma that involves the epidermis of the nipple and areola.
Diagnosis: Intraductal papilloma

4 **The answer is B: Estrogen receptors.** Over half of breast cancers exhibit nuclear estrogen receptor protein. A slightly smaller proportion also has progesterone receptors. Women whose cancers possess hormone receptors have a longer disease-free survival and overall survival than those with early-stage cancers who are negative for these receptors. The beneficial effects of oophorectomy on survival in patients with breast cancer led to the use of estrogen antagonists in the treatment of breast cancer. In general, antiestrogen therapy seems to prolong disease-free survival, particularly in postmenopausal and node-positive women. It also lowers the risk of cancer in the contralateral breast. The latter discovery has led to the use of antiestrogens as chemoprevention in women at high risk for developing breast cancer. None of the other choices are related prognostically to breast carcinoma.
Diagnosis: Invasive ductal carcinoma of the breast

5 **The answer is C: Fibrocystic change.** Fibrocystic change of the breast refers to a constellation of morphologic features characterized by (1) cystic dilation of terminal ducts, (2) relative increase in fibrous stroma, and (3) variable proliferation of terminal duct epithelial elements. Some of the florid manifestations appear to be indicators for an increased risk for breast cancer. Such lesions are designated proliferative fibrocystic change. Forms of fibrocystic change that do not carry an increased risk for the development of cancer, termed nonproliferative fibrocystic change, are far more prevalent. Ductal carcinoma in situ (choice A) features apparently malignant epithelial cells that have not penetrated the basement membrane. Intraductal papilloma (choice E) occurs in the subareolar lactiferous ducts. None of the remaining incorrect choices feature cystic duct dilation.

Diagnosis: Fibrocystic change, proliferative

6 **The answer is A: Acute mastitis.** Acute mastitis is a bacterial infection of the breast. It may be seen at any age, but by far the most frequent setting is in the postpartum lactating or involuting breast. This disorder is usually secondary to obstruction of the duct system by inspissated secretions. The other choices are not typically associated with fever.

Diagnosis: Acute mastitis

7 **The answer is D: Papillomatosis.** Proliferative fibrocystic change increases the risk of cancer. The most common proliferative change is an increase in the number of cells lining the dilated terminal ducts, described as ductal epithelial hyperplasia. Proliferative fibrocystic change can, at times, become exuberant and form papillary structures within the lumen of the distended ductule (papillomatosis). The morphologic spectrum of ductal hyperplasia in patients with proliferative fibrocystic change includes (1) minor degrees of hyperplasia; (2) florid, but cytologically benign hyperplasia; (3) hyperplasia with cytologic atypia not sufficient to warrant a diagnosis of malignancy; and (4) ductal carcinoma in situ. The other choices do not increase the risk of breast cancer.

Diagnosis: Fibrocystic change, proliferative

8 **The answer is B: Cirrhosis.** Gynecomastia refers to an enlargement of the adult male breast and is morphologically similar to juvenile hypertrophy of the female breast. In the adult man, gynecomastia is caused by an absolute increase in circulating estrogens or by a relative increase in the estrogen/androgen ratio. Gynecomastia associated with excess estrogens occurs with (1) the intake of exogenous estrogens, (2) the presence of hormone-secreting adrenal or testicular tumors, (3) the paraneoplastic production of gonadotropins by cancers, and (4) metabolic disorders, such as liver disease and hyperthyroidism, which are characterized by increased conversion of androstenedione into estrogens. Gynecomastia is often idiopathic, in which case it is commonly unilateral. The other choices are not associated with gynecomastia.

Diagnosis: Gynecomastia

9 **The answer is D: Pituitary adenoma.** Pituitary adenomas are benign neoplasms of the anterior lobe of the pituitary, which are often associated with excess secretion of pituitary hormones and evidence of corresponding endocrine hyperfunction. They occur in both sexes at almost any age but are more common in men between the ages of 20 to 50 years. Small, nonfunctioning pituitary adenomas are found incidentally in as many as 25% of adult autopsies. Hyperprolactinemia is the most common endocrinopathy associated with pituitary adenomas. Prolactin secreted by pituitary lactotrophic adenomas

may cause galactorrhea, most often in young women. Galactorrhea is not associated with the other choices.

Diagnosis: Prolactinoma

10 **The answer is D: Women of reproductive age.** Fibrocystic change is most often diagnosed in women from their late 20s to the time of menopause, and some fibrocystic change occurs in 75% of adult women in the United States. The morphologic hallmarks of nonproliferative fibrocystic change seen in this patient are an increase in fibrous stroma and cystic dilation of the terminal ducts. Fibrocystic change occurs in multiple areas of both breasts. A dominant cyst or aggregate of fibrous connective tissue containing smaller cysts may manifest as a discrete mass, prompting biopsy to exclude the possibility of cancer. The large cysts often contain dark fluid that imparts a blue color—the so-called "blue-domed cysts of Bloodgood." Aspiration of a large cyst will usually cause it to collapse and the mass to disappear. A frequent concomitant of nonproliferative fibrocystic change is an alteration of the epithelial lining, termed apocrine metaplasia. The metaplastic cells are larger and more eosinophilic than the cells that usually line the ducts and resemble apocrine sweat gland epithelium. The frequency of fibrocystic change decreases progressively after menopause (choice B). Fibrocystic change is not encountered during puberty (choice C). Oral contraceptives (choice E) do not increase the frequency of fibrocystic change.

Diagnosis: Fibrocystic change, nonproliferative

11 **The answer is C: Risk is doubled.** Fibroadenoma is the most common benign neoplasm of the breast and is composed of epithelial and stromal elements that originate from the terminal duct lobular unit. Fibroadenomas are usually found in women between the ages of 20 and 35, although they may occur in adolescent girls. The tumor is round and rubbery, is sharply demarcated from the surrounding breast, and thus, is freely movable. The cut surface appears glistening gray-white. On microscopic examination, fibroadenomas are composed of a mixture of fibrous connective tissue and elongated epithelial ducts (see photomicrograph). This connective tissue, which forms most of the tumor, often compresses the proliferated ducts, reducing them to curvilinear slits. The risk of subsequent invasive cancer in a breast from which a fibroadenoma has been removed is doubled. Surgical removal is curative. Choices A and B are principally associated with *BRCA* mutations.

Diagnosis: Fibroadenoma

12 **The answer is A: *BRCA1*.** *BRCA1* is a tumor suppressor gene that has been implicated in the pathogenesis of hereditary breast and ovarian cancers. Mutations in this tumor suppressor gene are thought carried by 1 in 200 to 400 people in the United States. Germline point mutations and deletions in *BRCA1* place a woman at a remarkable 60% to 85% lifetime risk for breast cancer. Moreover, breast cancer develops in more than half of these women before the age of 50 years. It is currently suspected that mutated *BRCA1* is responsible for 20% of all cases of inherited breast cancer (about 3% of all breast cancers). Somatic mutations in *BRCA1* are uncommon in sporadic (nonfamilial) breast cancers. Women with *BRCA1* mutations are also at greater lifetime risk of ovarian cancer. Estrogen receptor expression (choice C) is often increased in breast cancer cells, but the gene for the estrogen receptor is not mutated. Neither estrogen receptor status nor *HER2/neu* expression (choice D) predict genetic predisposition.

Diagnosis: Breast cancer

13 **The answer is E: Rapid growth.** Fibroadenomas commonly enlarge more rapidly during pregnancy and cease to grow after the menopause. Although they are hormonally responsive, a causal relationship between hormones and the pathogenesis of fibroadenoma has not been established. Development of invasive ductal carcinoma (choice A) in a fibroadenoma is rare.

Diagnosis: Fibroadenoma

14 **The answer is E: Status of the axillary lymph nodes.** Although all of the choices are prognostic indicators for breast cancer, the most important prognostic factor at the time of diagnosis is stage. A sentinel node assessment often is performed intra-operatively to assess the status of the ipsilateral lymph nodes. The sentinel lymph node is the most proximate lymph node and is assumed to be the initial site of nodal metastasis. It is identified with a dye or radioactive material. An axillary lymph node dissection is performed if metastatic tumor is identified in the sentinel lymph node. The presence of invasion indicates that tumor cells have access to lymphatic and blood vascular channels in the stroma, increasing the possibility of metasta-ses to regional lymph nodes and distant sites. The prognosis for women with distant metastases (stage IV) is poor in terms of survival, but palliative treatment may significantly prolong life. With the expanding use of screening mammography, more than half of the breast cancers currently diagnosed in the United States manifest as stage I disease, and almost all of these women will be cured by surgery.

Diagnosis: Invasive ductal carcinoma of the breast

15 **The answer is C: 30%.** The biopsy reveals intraductal carcinoma in situ, which arises in the terminal duct lobular unit, greatly distorting the ducts by its growth. Intraductal carcinoma in situ has two main histologic types, namely come-docarcinoma and noncomedocarcinoma. Noncomedocarcino-mas exhibit a spectrum of cytologic atypia. The patterns are classified as micropapillary, cribriform (shown in the image), and solid. The tumor cells and nuclei are smaller and more regular than those of the comedo type. Noncomedo intraduc-tal carcinoma in situ is less likely than the comedo type to incite a desmoplastic response in the surrounding tissue. Duc-tal carcinoma in situ, treated only by biopsy, carries a 20% to 30% risk of developing invasive carcinoma in the same breast over the ensuing 20 years. The risk of cancer in the contral-ateral breast is also increased. Choices A and B are incorrect because they suggest that the risk of invasive carcinoma is very small, whereas choices D and E are far too great.

Diagnosis: Ductal carcinoma in situ

16 **The answer is A: Gene amplification.** Overexpression of *HER2/neu* is identified in 10% to 35% of primary breast tumors and is mostly attributable to gene amplification. Amplification or overexpression of *HER2/neu* has also been described in cancers of the lung, ovary, and stomach. Overexpression can be deter-mined by immunohistologic detection of the c-erbB2 protein

on the cell membrane or by analysis of the *HER2/neu* gene using fluorescent in situ hybridization. Patients whose tumors demonstrate *HER2* gene amplification benefit from therapy with a monoclonal antibody (Herceptin) that selectively binds to the extracellular domain of the protein. Although the other genetic processes occur in some cancers, they are unrelated to *HER2/neu* expression.

Diagnosis: Breast cancer

17 **The answer is B: Ductal carcinoma in situ, comedocarcinoma type.** Intraductal carcinoma in situ of the comedo type is composed of very large, pleomorphic cells that have abundant eosinophilic cytoplasm and irregular nuclei, commonly with prominent nucleoli, and typically grows in a solid pattern. Central necrosis is a prominent factor. The necrotic debris may undergo dystrophic calcification. On gross examination, the cut surface shows distended ducts containing pasty necrotic debris resembling comedos, hence the term comedocarci-noma. Although the malignant cells do not invade through the basement membrane of the ducts, this form of carcinoma in situ commonly incites a chronic inflammatory and fibro-blastic response in the surrounding stroma. The cancer may extend within the duct system beyond the clinically detect-able tumor growth. The consequent difficulties in obtaining complete excision of the primary tumor frequently necessi-tate mastectomy rather than "lumpectomy." The chances of local recurrence as either in situ or invasive cancer are sub-stantially greater in the case of the comedo subtype than the noncomedo subtype. Colloid carcinoma (choice A) features abundant mucin production. Medullary carcinoma (choice C) is composed of sheets of invasive and pleomorphic cells. Phyl-lodes tumor (choice D) demonstrates proliferation of spindly stromal cells. Tubular carcinoma (choice E) is an invasive well-differentiated carcinoma with well-formed small duct structures.

Diagnosis: Comedocarcinoma, ductal carcinoma in situ

18 **The answer is B: Family history.** The strongest association with an increased risk for breast cancer is a family history, spe-cifically breast cancer in first-degree relatives (mother, sister, or daughter). The risk is greater when the relative is afflicted at a young age or with bilateral breast cancer. A woman who has two sisters with breast cancer, one of whom had bilateral tumors, or a mother and sister who show the same pattern has a greater than 25% chance of developing breast cancer by age 70 years. Fibrocystic change (choice C) also has an increased risk of breast cancer (proliferative lesions), but the relative risk does not approach that of family history.

Diagnosis: Invasive ductal carcinoma of the breast

19 **The answer is B: Lobular carcinoma in situ.** Lobular carcinoma in situ arises in the terminal duct lobular unit. Malignant cells appear as solid clusters that pack and distend the terminal ducts but not to the extent of ductal carcinoma in situ. The lesion does not usually incite the dense fibrosis and chronic inflammation so characteristic of intraductal carcinoma in situ and is, therefore, less likely to cause a detectable mass. It is not uncommon for lobular carcinoma in situ to be an "incidental" finding in a biopsy that was prompted by benign changes. As with intraductal carcinoma in situ, 20% to 30% of women with lobular carcinoma in situ receiving no further treatment after biopsy will develop invasive cancer within 20 years of diagnosis. However, about half of these invasive cancers will arise in the contralateral breast and may be either lobular or ductal cancers. Thus, lobular carcinoma in situ, more than ductal carcinoma in situ, serves as a marker for an enhanced risk of subsequent invasive cancer in both breasts. The histologic appearance is not consistent with any of the other choices.

Diagnosis: Lobular carcinoma in situ

20   The answer is E: *Staphylococcus aureus*.   This lactating patient has developed acute mastitis. The most common organisms isolated are *Staphylococcus* and *Streptococcus*. Untreated, the infection may progress to abscess formation, which is a complication that necessitates surgical intervention. A firm, walled-off, nontender abscess may be mistaken for cancer. Acute bacterial mastitis may be treated successfully by aggressive mechanical suction, with frequent emptying of the breasts, and by the administration of antibiotics. None of the other pathogens are ordinarily seen in acute mastitis.

Diagnosis: Acute mastitis

21   The answer is C: Invasive lobular carcinoma.   Invasive lobular carcinoma is the second most common form of invasive breast cancer. Because the amount of fibrosis is variable, the clinical presentation of invasive lobular carcinoma varies from a discrete firm mass, similar to ductal carcinoma, to a more subtle, diffuse, indurated area. Microscopically, classic invasive lobular carcinoma consists of single strands of malignant cells infiltrating between stromal fibers, which is a feature termed "Indian filing" (see photomicrograph). Despite the innocuous cytologic characteristics of this form of invasive carcinoma, it is biologically as aggressive as the invasive ductal type. Twenty-five percent of invasive carcinomas have features of both ductal and lobular carcinoma. Lobular carcinoma in situ (choice D) is confined to the lobule. Invasive ductal carcinoma may share features of invasive lobular carcinoma, but it usually forms glands, particularly the tubular type (choice B).

Diagnosis: Invasive lobular carcinoma

22   The answer is C: Medullary carcinoma.   Medullary carcinomas present as fleshy, bulky tumors measuring 5 to 10 cm in diameter. They are generally larger at the time they are detected than infiltrating ductal carcinomas (average size, 2 to 3 cm). This invasive tumor presents as a circumscribed mass that lacks calcifications. On gross examination, medullary carcinoma appears as a well-circumscribed, fleshy, pale gray mass. Microscopically, it is composed of sheets of cells that are highly pleomorphic and have a high mitotic index. The pathologic definition of medullary carcinoma includes a lymphoid infiltrate encompassing the periphery of the tumor. Despite the highly malignant histologic appearance of this neoplasm, it has a distinctly better prognosis than infiltrating ductal or lobular carcinoma. A dense lymphoid infiltrate is not characteristic of the other choices.

Diagnosis: Medullary carcinoma of the breast

23   The answer is D: Paget disease.   Paget disease of the nipple refers to an uncommon variant of ductal carcinoma, either in situ or invasive, that extends to involve the epidermis of the nipple and areola. This condition usually comes to medical attention because of an eczematous change in the skin of the nipple and areola. Microscopically, large cells with clear cytoplasm (Paget cells) are found singly or in groups within the epidermis. The prognosis of Paget disease is related to that of the underlying ductal cancer. Eczematous change in the skin of the nipple and areola are not features of the other choices.

Diagnosis: Paget disease of the breast

24   The answer is D: Phyllodes tumor.   Phyllodes tumor of the breast is a proliferation of stromal elements accompanied by a benign growth of ductal structures. These tumors usually occur in women between 30 and 70 years of age. Phyllodes tumors resemble fibroadenomas in their overall architecture and the presence of glandular and stromal elements. Like fibroadenoma, benign phyllodes tumor is sharply circumscribed, and the cut surface is firm, glistening, and grayish white. Microscopically, the stroma of a benign phyllodes tumor is hypercellular and has mitotic activity. The distinction from fibroadenoma is made not on the size, but on the histologic and cytologic characteristics of the stromal component. Malignant phyllodes tumors have an obviously sarcomatous stroma with abundant mitotic activity, and the stromal component is increased out of proportion to the benign duct elements. They are usually poorly circumscribed, with invasion into the surrounding breast tissue. Sarcomatous elements are not features of the other choices.

Diagnosis: Phyllodes tumor of the breast

25   The answer is A: Colloid carcinoma.   Colloid (mucinous) carcinoma is an invasive variant that tends to occur in older women. On cut section colloid carcinoma has a glistening surface and mucoid consistency. Histologically, it is composed of small clusters of epithelial cells, occasionally forming glands, floating in pools of extracellular mucin. In its pure form, colloid carcinoma has a considerably better prognosis than infiltrating ductal or lobular carcinoma. However, it is often admixed with infiltrating ductal carcinoma, in which circumstance the prognosis is determined by the ductal component. Abundant mucin production is not a feature of the other choices.

Diagnosis: Mucinous carcinoma of the breast

26   The answer is B: Invasive ductal carcinoma.   Cancer in the male breast is uncommon and accounts for less than 1% of all cases of breast cancer. The most common subtype is infiltrating (invasive) ductal carcinoma. Because there is less fat in the male breast, invasion of chest wall muscles is more frequent at the time of diagnosis. For tumors of the same stage, however, the prognosis for male breast cancer is similar to that of female breast cancer. Choice A is a skin tumor and the other choices (C, D, and E) are rare in the male breast.

Diagnosis: Male breast cancer, invasive ductal carcinoma of the breast

27   The answer is A: *BRCA2* mutation.   Predisposing factors for the development of breast cancer in men are largely unknown, although mutations in the *BRCA2* gene increase the risk of this tumor. Choices B, C, and D are not risk factors for breast cancer in men. *PTEN* mutations (choice E) are associated with endometrial intraepithelial neoplasia and endometrial adenocarcinoma.

Diagnosis: Male breast cancer

Chapter 20

Hematopathology

QUESTIONS

Select the single best answer.

1 An 18-year-old man moves from sea level to an elevation of 2,400 m to train as a skier. The increased requirement for oxygen delivery to tissues at the higher elevation stimulates the synthesis of a renal hormone (erythropoietin), which targets hematopoietic stem cells in the bone marrow. Erythropoietin promotes the survival of early erythroid progenitor cells primarily through which of the following mechanisms?
(A) Altered cell-matrix adhesion
(B) Downregulation of p53
(C) Enhanced glucose uptake
(D) Inhibition of apoptosis
(E) Stimulation of globin biosynthesis

2 A 6-year-old girl is brought into the emergency room after an automobile accident. Physical examination shows bleeding from multiple wounds, and a CBC reveals a normocytic, normochromic anemia. Which of the following indices is most helpful in defining this patient's anemia as normocytic?
(A) Hematocrit
(B) Hemoglobin
(C) Mean corpuscular hemoglobin concentration
(D) Mean corpuscular volume
(E) Red blood cell count

3 A 60-year-old man presents with a 6-month history of increasing fatigue. Physical examination reveals marked pallor, and a CBC shows a macrocytic anemia. Which of the following is the most likely cause of anemia in this patient?
(A) Alcoholism
(B) Chronic disease
(C) Iron deficiency
(D) Renal disease
(E) Thalassemia

4 A 43-year-old woman of Scandinavian descent complains of constant tiredness, light-headedness, and occasional palpitations and shortness of breath while ascending the stairs. Physical examination shows pallor of the oral mucosa and a raspberry-red tongue (glossitis). Neurologic examination reveals paresthesias, numbness, decreased vibration sensation, and loss of deep tendon reflexes. The results of laboratory studies include hemoglobin of 7.2 g/dL, WBC of 4,500/μL, platelets of 140,000/μL, erythrocyte folate of 220 ng/mL, serum vitamin B_{12} of 40 pg/mL (normal >200 pg/mL), serum anti-intrinsic factor of 1:128, and serum anti–parietal cell antibody of 1:64. Examination of peripheral blood shows macrocytic anemia, with poikilocytosis of RBCs and hypersegmented neutrophils. Atrophic gastritis is diagnosed by gastric biopsy. Bone marrow examination in this patient will reveal which of the following pathologic findings?
(A) Absent stainable bone marrow iron
(B) Atypical megakaryocytes with fibrosis
(C) Hypercellularity with megaloblastic erythroid maturation
(D) Hypocellularity with absence of erythroid precursors
(E) Myeloid hyperplasia with increased basophils

5 Which of the following mechanisms of disease best describes the pathogenesis of anemia in the patient described in Question 4?
(A) Bone marrow fibrosis
(B) Clonal stem cell abnormality
(C) Defective heme synthesis
(D) Immune destruction of circulating erythrocytes
(E) Impaired DNA synthesis

6 A 30-year-old woman complains of recent easy fatigability, bruising, and recurrent throat infections. Physical examination reveals numerous petechiae over her body and mouth. Abnormal laboratory findings include hemoglobin of 6 g/dL, WBC of 1,500/μL, and platelets of 20,000/μL. The bone marrow is hypocellular and displays increased fat. What is the appropriate diagnosis?
(A) Aplastic anemia
(B) Iron-deficiency anemia
(C) Megaloblastic anemia
(D) Myelofibrosis with myeloid metaplasia
(E) Pure red cell aplasia

7 A 20-year-old thin fashion model complains that she cannot concentrate and is always tired. She has heavy menstrual bleeding every month but is otherwise healthy. The peripheral blood smear is shown in the image. Which of the following laboratory findings would be expected in this patient?

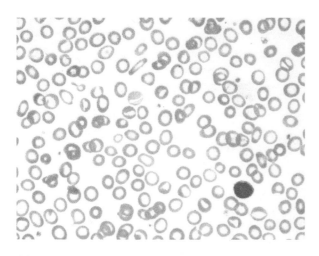

(A) Hyperbilirubinemia
(B) Increased serum ferritin
(C) Low plasma iron saturation
(D) Positive direct Coombs test
(E) Vitamin B$_{12}$ deficiency

8 A 39-year-old woman presents with a 2-month history of upper abdominal pain, weakness, and fatigue. Physical examination reveals marked pallor. Laboratory studies show microcytic, hypochromic anemia (hemoglobin = 8.5 g/dL) and mild thrombocytosis. Gastroscopy discloses a mucosal defect in the antrum measuring 1.5 cm in diameter. Which of the following best describes the pathogenesis of anemia in this patient?
(A) Defective globin chain synthesis
(B) Impaired heme synthesis
(C) Poor utilization of iron stores
(D) Synthesis of structurally abnormal hemoglobin molecules
(E) Toxic damage to bone marrow stem cells

9 A 10-year-old boy presents with chronic fatigue. Physical examination reveals slight jaundice and splenomegaly. The results of laboratory studies include hemoglobin of 11.7 g/dL, hematocrit of 32%, total bilirubin of 2.6 mg/dL, and conjugated bilirubin of 0.8 mg/dL. The peripheral blood smear is shown in the image. The osmotic fragility of the patient's RBCs is increased, but the Coombs test is negative. Defects in which of the following are involved in the pathogenesis of this disorder?

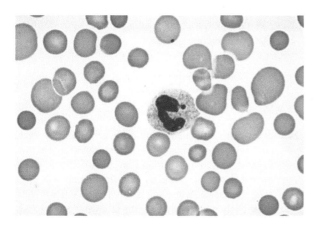

(A) DNA synthesis
(B) Erythrocyte cytoskeleton
(C) Erythrocyte maturation
(D) Glucose-6-phosphate dehydrogenase (G6PD)
(E) Hemoglobin synthesis

10 The patient described in Question 9 is at increased risk for development of which of the following conditions?
(A) Acute renal tubular necrosis
(B) Cholelithiasis
(C) Cirrhosis
(D) Nephrolithiasis
(E) Portal hypertension

11 A 27-year-old pregnant woman comes to the obstetrician for a prenatal check-up. Routine laboratory testing reveals a mild normocytic anemia. The peripheral blood smear is shown in the image. Which of the following best explains the pathogenesis of anemia seen in this patient?

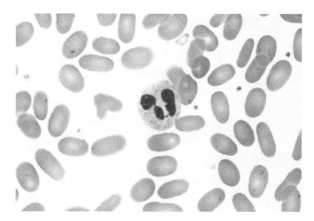

(A) Abnormal membrane lipoprotein molecules
(B) Abnormal polymerization of spectrin molecules
(C) Decreased iron release in the bone marrow
(D) Destabilization of the lipid bilayer of the RBC membrane
(E) Oxidative denaturation of hemoglobin

12 A 10-month-old boy of Arabic extraction is brought to the physician by his parents who complain that their child is failing to thrive. Physical examination reveals splenomegaly and jaundice. A CBC shows a microcytic, hypochromic anemia (hemoglobin = 7.4 g/dL). Fetal hemoglobin accounts for most of the hemoglobin. A peripheral blood smear is shown in the image. Which of the following is the appropriate diagnosis?

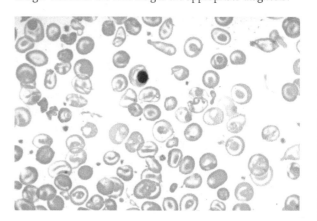

(A) G6PD deficiency
(B) Hereditary elliptocytosis
(C) Hereditary spherocytosis
(D) Iron deficiency anemia
(E) β-Thalassemia

13 Which of the following best describes the pathogenesis of splenomegaly seen in the patient described in Question 12?
(A) Amyloidosis
(B) Chronic malaria
(C) Extramedullary hematopoiesis
(D) Infectious mononucleosis
(E) Splenic vein thrombosis

14 A 22-year-old woman from a large Italian family is screened for a familial blood disorder. The results of laboratory studies include a hemoglobin of 9.5 g/dL and a smear displaying mild microcytosis, hypochromia, and a few target cells. Hemoglobin electrophoresis shows a mild increase in hemoglobin A2 (7.5%). What is the appropriate diagnosis?
(A) Anemia of chronic disease
(B) G6PD deficiency
(C) Heterozygous β-thalassemia
(D) Homozygous β-thalassemia
(E) Silent carrier α-thalassemia

15 A 28-year-old woman delivers a male neonate at 36 weeks of gestation. The mother has a history of poor prenatal care and several previous miscarriages. Examination of the neonate reveals marked pallor and generalized edema (anasarca), and the peripheral blood smear is shown in the image. The nucleated cells in this blood smear are which of the following?

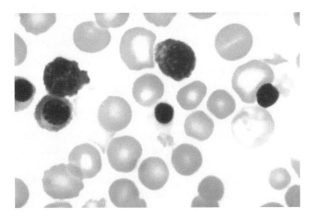

(A) B lymphocytes
(B) Eosinophils
(C) Erythroblasts
(D) Monocytes
(E) T lymphocytes

16 A 60-year-old man presents with headaches and pruritis. Physical examination reveals splenomegaly but no lymphadenopathy. A CBC demonstrates elevated hemoglobin of 19.5 g/dL, WBC of 12,800/μL, and platelets of 550,000/μL. The bone marrow displays hypercellularity of all lineages and depletion of marrow iron stores. Which of the following is the most likely diagnosis?

(A) Acute myelogenous leukemia
(B) Essential thrombocythemia
(C) Idiopathic myelofibrosis
(D) Occult infection
(E) Polycythemia vera

17 The patient described in Question 16 is at increased risk of developing which of the following conditions?
(A) Cerebral aneurysm
(B) Cerebrovascular accident
(C) Cholelithiasis
(D) Osteogenic sarcoma
(E) Raynaud phenomenon

18 A 10-year-old black girl is brought to the emergency room. She complains of severe pain in her chest, abdomen, and bones. Physical examination reveals jaundice and anemia. Her parents state that she has been anemic since birth. A CBC shows normocytic anemia with marked poikilocytosis. A peripheral blood smear is shown in the image. Hemoglobin electrophoresis demonstrates hemoglobin S. This child's chest and bone pain is most likely caused by which of the following mechanisms?

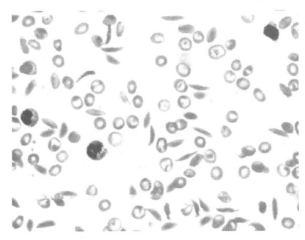

(A) Amyloidosis
(B) Coagulopathy
(C) Infection
(D) Ischemia
(E) Vasculitis

19 Over the next 6 years, the patient described in Question 18 develops multiple splenic infarcts. Which of the following is a common complication of autosplenectomy in this patient?
(A) Autoimmune gastritis
(B) Cholelithiasis
(C) Megaloblastic anemia
(D) Membranous nephropathy
(E) Pneumonia

20 A 24-year-old woman with sickle cell disease is seen in the emergency room for an acute upper respiratory tract infection. Laboratory findings include a severe, normocytic anemia. The patient develops a rapid drop in the hemoglobin level. However, the reticulocyte count is very low (<0.01%). This finding most likely reflects which of the following conditions?

(A) Bone marrow failure due to repeated infarction
(B) Expected result for the patient's underlying anemia
(C) Parvovirus B19 infection
(D) Retroperitoneal hemorrhage
(E) Vitamin B$_{12}$ deficiency

21 A 36-year-old man from China presents with increasing fatigue. He has a 3-year history of tuberculosis, and CBC shows a mild microcytic anemia. Blood work-up demonstrates low serum iron, low iron-binding capacity, and increased serum ferritin. The pathogenesis of anemia in this patient is most likely caused by which of the following mechanisms?
(A) Clonal stem cell defect
(B) Hypoxemia
(C) Impaired utilization of iron from storage sites
(D) Synthesis of structurally abnormal globin chains
(E) Toxic damage to bone marrow stem cells

22 A 45-year-old chronic alcoholic man presents with mental confusion. The peripheral blood smear is shown in the image. The morphologic abnormalities demonstrated in this blood smear are most likely associated with which of the following conditions?

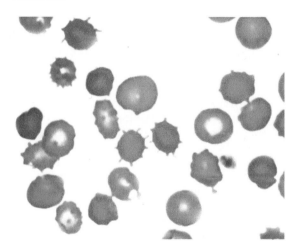

(A) Abnormal spectrin in red cell membranes
(B) Chronic liver disease
(C) Chronic renal failure
(D) Microthrombi in capillaries
(E) Vitamin B$_{12}$ deficiency

23 A 78-year-old man presents with increasing fatigue. A CBC shows pancytopenia, with moderate anemia (hemoglobin = 10.5 g/dL) and normochromic, hypochromic RBCs. Mild neutropenia and thrombocytopenia are noted. A bone marrow evaluation reveals erythroid hyperplasia with increased iron. A Prussian blue–stained bone marrow aspirate is shown in the image. Which of the following is the appropriate diagnosis?

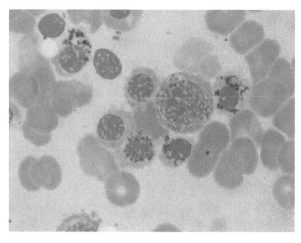

(A) Hairy cell leukemia
(B) Multiple myeloma
(C) Myelodysplastic syndrome
(D) Polycythemia vera
(E) Promyelocytic leukemia

24 Which of the following best describes the pathogenesis of the hematologic disorder seen in the patient described in Question 23?
(A) Clonal stem cell defect
(B) C-*myc* translocation
(C) Deletion of a portion of the β-globin gene
(D) Functional asplenia
(E) Mutation of the T-cell receptor gene

25 A 32-year-old man presents with mild fever and increasing fatigue. He is an immigrant from Russia and worked in a benzene factory. Physical examination does not reveal lymphadenopathy or splenomegaly, but petechial skin lesions are noted. A CBC demonstrates severe pancytopenia, with normocytic red cell indices. A bone marrow biopsy is shown in the image. Which of the following is the most likely underlying mechanism in the development of this patient's anemia?

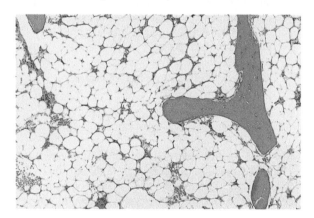

(A) Damage to stem cells
(B) Decreased erythropoietin production by the kidneys
(C) Folate deficiency
(D) Impaired globin chain synthesis
(E) Neoplastic proliferation of committed stem cells

26 A patient with a history of chronic alcoholism presents with a macrocytic anemia and thrombocytopenia. Blood smear examination demonstrates numerous oval macrocytes and hypersegmented neutrophils (results shown in the image). A Schilling test is normal. Which of the following is the most likely diagnosis?

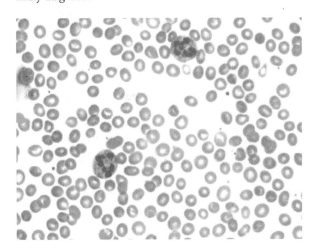

(A) Anemia of chronic disease
(B) Folic acid deficiency
(C) G6PD deficiency
(D) Iron deficiency anemia
(E) Sickle cell anemia

27 A 23-year-old, previously healthy man of Italian origin develops moderate to severe hemolytic anemia. The previous evening he had celebrated a Saint's day with a feast of beans and pasta. Urinalysis shows free hemoglobin, and the direct Coombs test is negative. Supravital staining of the blood smear demonstrates numerous membrane-bound inclusions (Heinz bodies) within erythrocytes. Which of the following is the most likely diagnosis?
(A) G6PD deficiency
(B) Paroxysmal nocturnal hemoglobinuria
(C) Sickle cell anemia
(D) β-Thalassemia minor
(E) Warm antibody autoimmune hemolytic anemia

28 A 60-year-old man complains of night sweats, weight loss, easy fatigability, and discomfort in the left upper abdominal quadrant. Physical examination reveals splenomegaly. Laboratory studies show leukocytosis (40,000/μL). A peripheral blood smear demonstrates mature and maturing granulocytes, myelocytes, basophils, and occasional myeloblasts. The bone marrow is hypercellular and dominated by WBC precursors. Megakaryocytes are numerous, and RBC precursors are less prominent. A smear of the bone marrow aspirate is shown in the image. Cytogenetic studies disclose a monoclonal population of abnormal cells with a t(9;22)(q34;q11) chromosomal translocation. What is the appropriate diagnosis?

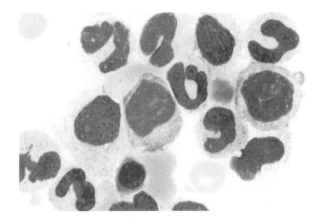

(A) Acute lymphoblastic leukemia
(B) Acute myeloid leukemia
(C) Chronic lymphocytic leukemia
(D) Chronic myelogenous leukemia
(E) Myelodysplastic syndrome

29 Which oncogene is located at the t(9;22) chromosomal breakpoint in the patient described in Question 28?
(A) *abl*
(B) *erb*
(C) *myb*
(D) *myc*
(E) *neu*

30 A 40-year-old woman complains of fatigue and nausea of 3 months in duration. Physical examination reveals numerous pustules on the face, as well as splenomegaly and hepatomegaly. Laboratory studies show hemoglobin of 6.3 g/dL and platelets of 50,000/μL. A peripheral smear shows malignant cells with Auer rods (arrow). The patient develops diffuse purpura, bleeding from the gums, and laboratory features of disseminated intravascular coagulation (DIC). Which of the following is the appropriate diagnosis?

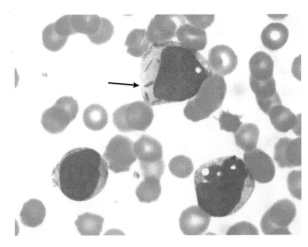

(A) Acute lymphoblastic leukemia
(B) Acute megakaryocytic leukemia
(C) Acute promyelocytic leukemia
(D) Chronic myelogenous leukemia
(E) Monocytic leukemia

31 Cytogenetic studies in malignant cells from the patient described in Question 30 demonstrate a chromosomal translocation. Which of the following genes is most likely found at the translocation site?

(A) *abl*
(B) *bcl-1*
(C) *bcl-2*
(D) *myc*
(E) Retinoic acid receptor

32 A 60-year-old man presents with a 3-week history of lymph node enlargement in his neck and axillae. A CBC reveals mild anemia, with a leukocytosis of 20,000/μL. The peripheral blood smear is shown in the image. More than 80% of WBCs are small lymphocytes, but there are also prominent "smudge cells." Examination of a bone marrow biopsy shows nodular and interstitial infiltrates of lymphocytes, which demonstrate clonal rearrangement of the IgG light-chain gene. Which of the following is the appropriate diagnosis?

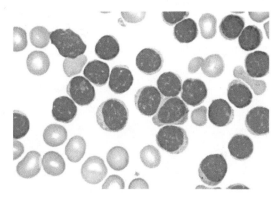

(A) Acute lymphoblastic lymphoma
(B) Chronic lymphocytic leukemia
(C) Chronic myelogenous leukemia with lymphoid blast crisis
(D) Multiple myeloma
(E) Waldenström macroglobulinemia

33 A 6-year-old boy presents with fatigue, fever, and night sweats. Physical examination reveals marked pallor. Palpation of his sternum demonstrates diffuse tenderness. Laboratory studies disclose anemia, thrombocytopenia, and leukocytosis. The WBC differential count shows that 90% blasts. A bone marrow biopsy stained immunohistochemically for terminal deoxynucleotidyl transferase (TdT) is shown in the image. Which of the following is the appropriate diagnosis?

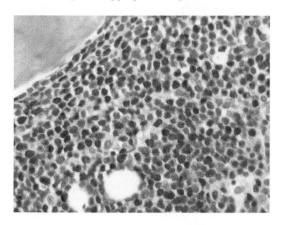

(A) Acute lymphoblastic leukemia
(B) Acute myelogenous leukemia
(C) Acute promyelocytic leukemia
(D) Chronic lymphocytic leukemia
(E) Chronic myelogenous leukemia

34 A 27-year-old man presents with an 8-week history of fevers, chills, pruritis, and night sweats. Two months ago, he experienced a flu-like illness. A nagging cough with occasional hemoptysis persisted for several weeks following resolution of his other symptoms. Physical examination reveals moderately enlarged, firm, nontender lymph nodes located in the right supraclavicular region. A lymph node biopsy is shown in the image. What is the appropriate diagnosis?

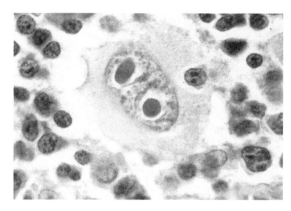

(A) Acute myelogenous leukemia
(B) Burkitt lymphoma
(C) Hodgkin lymphoma
(D) Infectious mononucleosis
(E) Lymphoblastic lymphoma

35 Which of the following is the most common histologic subtype of the disease in the patient described in Question 34?
(A) Lymphocyte depleted
(B) Lymphocyte predominant
(C) Lymphocyte rich
(D) Mixed cellularity
(E) Nodular sclerosis

36 A 55-year-old man complains of pain in his back, fatigue and occasional confusion. He admits to polyuria and polydipsia. An X-ray examination reveals numerous lytic lesions in the lumbar vertebral bodies. Laboratory studies disclose hypoalbuminemia, mild anemia, and thrombocytopenia. A monoclonal Igκ peak is demonstrated by serum electrophoresis. Urinalysis shows 4+ proteinuria. A bone marrow biopsy discloses foci of plasma cells, which account for 18% of all hematopoietic cells. What is the appropriate diagnosis?
(A) Acute lymphoblastic lymphoma
(B) Chronic lymphocytic leukemia
(C) Extramedullary plasmacytoma
(D) Multiple myeloma
(E) Waldenström macroglobulinemia

37 For the patient described in Question 36, which of the following is the most common, and ultimately lethal, extramedullary complication?

(A) Dementia
(B) Hepatic failure
(C) Pericarditis
(D) Peritonitis
(E) Renal failure

38 A 62-year-old man presents with a history of several months of vague abdominal pain and fatigue. Physical examination reveals marked splenomegaly but no evidence of lymphadenopathy. The patient subsequently develops bacterial sepsis and expires. A bone marrow biopsy at autopsy shows numerous atypical megakaryocytes and marked marrow fibrosis (results shown in the image). Which of the following is the most likely diagnosis?

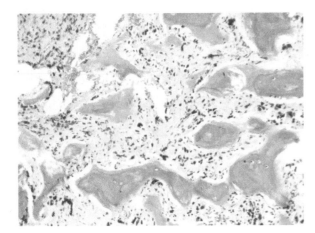

(A) Acute myelogenous leukemia
(B) Acute promyelocytic leukemia
(C) Chronic idiopathic myelofibrosis
(D) Chronic lymphocytic leukemia
(E) Chronic myelogenous leukemia

39 A 57-year-old man is admitted to the hospital with inguinal and cervical lymphadenopathy. He had noticed the first palpable nodule about 6 months ago. Upon physical examination, more palpable lymph nodes are found in the axillary and supraclavicular regions. Laboratory data show the serum proteins to be within normal limits, whereas the WBC count is 25,000/µL with many small abnormal lymphocytes. A cervical lymph node biopsy is shown in the image. The histologic features are most consistent with which of the following hematologic disorders?

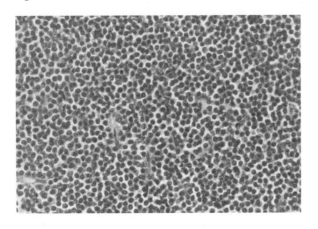

(A) Burkitt lymphoma
(B) Hodgkin lymphoma
(C) Plasmacytoma
(D) Reactive follicular hyperplasia
(E) Small lymphocytic lymphoma

40 A 50-year-old man presents with fever and diffuse lymphadenopathy. A lymph node biopsy reveals non-Hodgkin follicular lymphoma. Immunohistochemical staining of neoplastic lymphoid cells within the nodular areas of the lymph node would be expected to stain positively for which of the following protein markers?

(A) Abl
(B) Bax
(C) Bcl-2
(D) Myc
(E) Retinoic acid receptor

41 A 12-year-old girl presents with a fever of 38°C (101°F) and a swollen lymph node of 6 days in duration. The CBC is normal. Biopsy of the swollen lymph node shows benign follicular hyperplasia (shown in the image). This pathologic finding is best interpreted as which of the following?

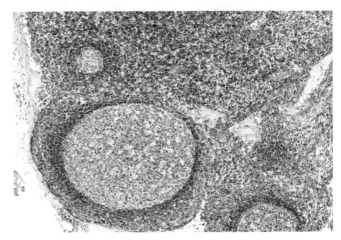

(A) Proliferation in B-cell areas
(B) Proliferation of dendritic cells
(C) Proliferation of plasma cells
(D) Proliferation in T-cell areas
(E) Proliferation of marginal-zone lymphocytes

42 A 4-year-old boy from Kenya presents with a 3-week history of a rapidly expanding jaw. A biopsy of an enlarged cervical lymph node is shown in the image. Histologic examination reveals numerous mitotic figures and many macrophages containing nuclear and cytoplasmic debris. The cells express surface IgM and are positive for common B-cell antigens. Which of the following is the appropriate diagnosis?

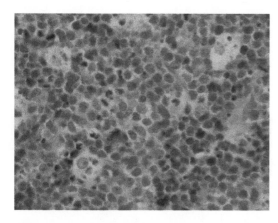

(A) Acute myelogenous leukemia
(B) Burkitt lymphoma
(C) Plasmacytoma
(D) Reactive follicular hyperplasia
(E) Small lymphocytic lymphoma

43 A 24-year-old woman presents with an earache of 4 days in duration. She also reports increased urine production, a skin rash, and bone pain on her scalp. Physical examination reveals otitis media, dermatitis, and exophthalmos. An X-ray of the scalp shows calvarial bone defects. A fine-needle aspirate displays numerous eosinophils. Which of the following is the most likely diagnosis?
(A) Hodgkin lymphoma
(B) Langerhans cell histiocytosis
(C) Malignant melanoma
(D) Metastatic breast carcinoma
(E) Multiple myeloma

44 A 42-year-old woman presents with an enlarged supraclavicular lymph node. The patient is HIV positive and takes antiviral medications. A lymph node biopsy is shown in the image. The tumor cells express B cell antigens and are positive for Epstein-Barr virus (EBV). Which of the following is the most likely diagnosis?

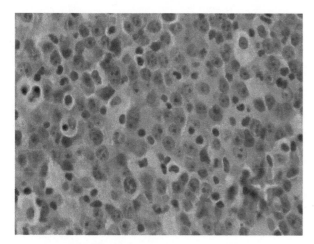

(A) Follicular lymphoma
(B) Hodgkin lymphoma
(C) Large B-cell lymphoma
(D) MALT lymphoma
(E) Mantle cell lymphoma

45 A 55-year-old man presents with a 3-week history of abdominal discomfort. Physical examination demonstrates splenomegaly but no lymphadenopathy. A CBC shows pancytopenia. Examination of a peripheral blood smear reveals atypical lymphoid cells that exhibit tartrate-resistant acid phosphatase activity. Which of the following is the appropriate diagnosis?
(A) Acute lymphocytic leukemia
(B) Chronic lymphocytic leukemia
(C) Chronic myelogenous leukemia
(D) Hairy cell leukemia
(E) Hodgkin disease

46 A 55-year-old man presents with recurrent epigastric pain. Upper GI endoscopy and gastric biopsy reveal a neoplastic, lymphocytic infiltrate invading glandular tissue. Giemsa staining is positive for *Helicobacter pylori*. Which of the following is the most likely diagnosis?
(A) Burkitt lymphoma
(B) Follicular lymphoma
(C) Hodgkin lymphoma
(D) Mantle cell lymphoma
(E) Marginal zone lymphoma

47 A 58-year-old man presents with a 2-month history of erythematous, scaly plaques over his trunk and upper extremities. Biopsy of these lesions reveals an atypical lymphocytic infiltrate in the dermis, which extends into the overlying epidermis. Immunohistochemical staining demonstrates positive staining for CD4. Which of the following is the most likely diagnosis?
(A) Acute lymphoblastic lymphoma
(B) Chronic lymphoid leukemia
(C) Extramedullary plasmacytoma
(D) Hairy cell leukemia
(E) Mycosis fungoides

48 A 56-year-old man presents with enlarged lymph nodes. Physical examination reveals mild hepatosplenomegaly. A lymph node biopsy shows small lymphocytes, as well as plasmacytoid lymphocytes containing Dutcher and Russell bodies. Immunohistochemical studies demonstrate cytoplasmic accumulation of IgM. What is the appropriate diagnosis?
(A) Burkitt lymphoma
(B) Hodgkin lymphoma
(C) Richter syndrome
(D) Sézary syndrome
(E) Waldenström disease

49 A 9-year-old girl develops widespread pinpoint skin hemorrhages. She recovered from a flu-like illness 1 week earlier. Laboratory findings reveal a platelet count of 20,000/μL but no other abnormalities. Her bone marrow shows an increased number of megakaryocytes. The platelet count is normal after 2 months. Which of the following is the appropriate diagnosis?
(A) Antiphospholipid antibody syndrome
(B) Disseminated intravascular coagulation
(C) Hemolytic-uremic syndrome
(D) Idiopathic thrombocytopenic purpura
(E) Thrombotic thrombocytopenic purpura

50 A 25-year-old woman with a history of systemic lupus erythematosus presents with diffuse petechiae and fatigue. Physical examination demonstrates lymphadenopathy and splenomegaly. Laboratory findings include normocytic anemia (hemoglobin = 6.1 g/dL) and thrombocytopenia (30,000/μL). Which of the following is the most likely underlying mechanism in the development of thrombocytopenia in this patient?

(A) Antibody-mediated platelet destruction
(B) Clonal plasma cell circulating paraprotein
(C) Decreased susceptibility to complement-mediated lysis
(D) Defect in the platelet cytoskeleton
(E) Increased activity of an enzyme in the glycolytic pathway

51 For the patient described in Question 50, a peripheral blood smear shows polychromasia with 10% reticulocytes. This patient most likely has which of the following hematologic diseases?

(A) Anemia of chronic renal failure
(B) Aplastic anemia
(C) Hemolytic anemia
(D) Iron deficiency anemia
(E) Myelophthisic anemia

52 A 22-year-old man presents with a 6-day history of sore throat, fever, and general malaise. Physical examination reveals generalized lymphadenopathy, which is most prominent in the cervical lymph nodes. A CBC demonstrates atypical lymphocytes. The monospot test is positive. Two weeks later, the patient complains of intermittent pain and tingling in the tips of his fingers. A CBC discloses a mild, macrocytic anemia. The peripheral blood smear is shown in the image. Which of the following is the most likely cause of anemia in this patient?

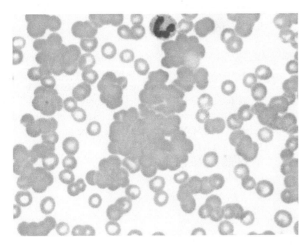

(A) Autoantibodies directed against the erythrocyte membrane
(B) Clonal plasma cell dyscrasia with circulating paraprotein
(C) Decreased activity of an enzyme in the glycolytic pathway
(D) Defect in the erythrocyte cytoskeleton
(E) Increased susceptibility to complement-mediated hemolysis

53 A 25-year-old previously healthy woman develops spontaneous vaginal bleeding. The following day, she experiences a tonic-clonic seizure. On physical examination, she is febrile and jaundiced and has widespread purpura. Laboratory findings include a hemoglobin of 5.3 g/dL with 8% reticulocytes, a platelet count of 10,000/μL, and a BUN of 48 mg/dL. The peripheral blood smear is shown in the image. Which of the following is the appropriate diagnosis?

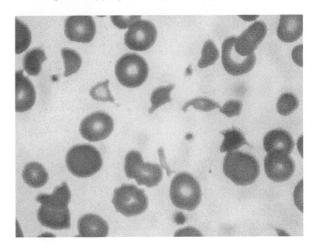

(A) Drug-induced thrombocytopenia
(B) Henoch-Schönlein purpura
(C) Idiopathic thrombocytopenic purpura
(D) Thrombotic thrombocytopenic purpura
(E) von Willebrand disease

54 A 45-year-old man suffers severe third-degree burns in an industrial accident. During his hospital stay, the patient develops anemia, thrombocytopenia, and widespread purpura. Blood oozes from venipuncture sites. Laboratory studies show that fibrin split products are elevated. The peripheral blood smear is shown in the image. What is the appropriate diagnosis?

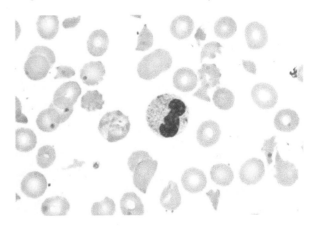

(A) Acanthocytosis
(B) Henoch-Schönlein purpura
(C) Idiopathic thrombocytopenic purpura
(D) Microangiopathic hemolytic anemia
(E) Paroxysmal nocturnal hemoglobinuria

55 A 67-year-old woman with a prosthetic aortic valve develops progressive anemia. Examination of a peripheral blood smear reveals reticulocytosis and schistocytes. What is the appropriate diagnosis?

(A) Acanthocytosis

(B) Henoch-Schönlein purpura

(C) Idiopathic thrombocytopenic purpura

(D) Macroangiopathic hemolytic anemia

(E) Microangiopathic hemolytic anemia

56 A 14-year-old boy presents with acute onset of right flank pain, which developed after he helped his father paint the ceiling of his bedroom. Physical examination demonstrates an area of ecchymosis in the right flank that is tender to palpation. The patient has a lifelong history of easy bruising. His brother shows the same tendency. The serum level of clotting factor VIII is less than 2% of normal. Which of the following is the most likely underlying mechanism for bleeding tendency in this patient?

(A) Circulating antibodies directed against factor VIII

(B) Decreased hepatic synthesis of multiple coagulation factors

(C) Deficiency of vitamin K

(D) Genetic defect involving the factor VIII gene

(E) Nonimmune peripheral consumption of coagulation proteins

57 A 4-year-old boy develops severe bleeding into the knee joint. Laboratory studies show that serum levels of factor IX are reduced, but levels of factor VIII are normal. What is the appropriate diagnosis?

(A) Hemophilia A

(B) Hemophilia B

(C) Henoch-Schönlein purpura

(D) Idiopathic thrombocytopenic purpura

(E) von Willebrand disease

58 A 39-year-old man reports seeing red-colored urine in the morning. The CBC reveals anemia, low serum iron, and an elevated reticulocyte count. Laboratory studies show increased lysis of erythrocytes when incubated with either sucrose or acidified serum. Which of the following is the appropriate diagnosis?

(A) Anemia of chronic renal failure

(B) Hereditary spherocytosis

(C) Microangiopathic hemolytic anemia

(D) Paroxysmal nocturnal hemoglobinuria

(E) Vitamin B_{12} deficiency

59 A 46-year-old man presents with ataxia. MRI shows a cerebellar infarct. The platelet count is discovered to be 955,000/μL. The bone marrow biopsy reveals increased megakaryocytes with absent fibrosis (shown in the image). Cytogenetic studies are normal. Which of the following is the most likely diagnosis?

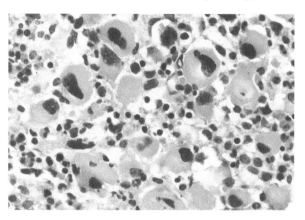

(A) Chronic myelogenous leukemia

(B) Essential thrombocythemia

(C) Myelofibrosis with myeloid metaplasia

(D) Polycythemia vera

(E) Thrombotic thrombocytopenic purpura

60 An 18-year-old man is rushed to the emergency room in shock following a motor vehicle accident. He is transfused with 5 U of blood. Following the transfusion the patient complains of fever, nausea, vomiting, and chest pain. Laboratory data show elevated indirect serum bilirubin, decreased serum haptoglobin, and a positive Coombs test. Which of the following is the most likely diagnosis?

(A) Autoimmune hemolytic anemia

(B) Disseminated intravascular coagulation

(C) Hemolytic transfusion reaction

(D) Hemolytic uremic syndrome

(E) Microangiopathic hemolysis

61 A 60-year-old woman complains of weakness and hematuria. Physical examination shows marked pallor, hepatosplenomegaly, and numerous ecchymoses of the upper and lower extremities. A CBC reveals a normocytic normochromic anemia, thrombocytopenia, neutropenia, and a marked leukocytosis, which is composed mainly of myeloblasts. The major clinical problems associated with this patient's condition are most directly related to which of the following?

(A) Avascular necrosis of bone

(B) Disseminated intravascular coagulation

(C) Hypersplenism

(D) Microangiopathic hemolytic anemia

(E) Suppression of hematopoiesis

62 A 69-year-old man is scheduled for surgery, but the procedure is canceled because of abnormal findings in the preoperative blood work. A CBC shows leukocytosis (WBC = 124,000/μL), consisting mainly of maturing neutrophils. Basophilia and eosinophilia are also observed. The platelet count is 820,000/μL. A t(9;22)(q34;q11) translocation is documented. A bone marrow biopsy is shown in the image. Which of the following best characterizes the pathogenesis of the hematologic condition encountered in this patient?

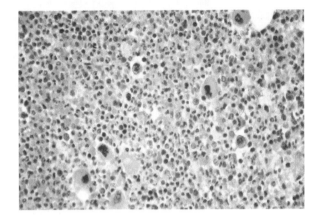

(A) Blocked differentiation of pre-B cells
(B) Blocked differentiation of pre-T cells
(C) Maturational arrest of lymphoid progenitor stem cells
(D) Transformation of a lymphoplasmacytic cell
(E) Transformation of a pluripotent bone marrow stem cell

63 A 48-year-old alcoholic man presents with a 6-day history of productive cough and fever. The temperature is 38.7°C (103°F), respirations are 32 per minute, and blood pressure is 125/85 mm Hg. The patient's cough worsens, and he begins expectorating large amounts of foul-smelling sputum. A chest X-ray shows a right upper and middle lobe infiltrate. A CBC demonstrates leukocytosis (WBC = 38,000/μL), with 80% slightly immature neutrophils and toxic granulation. Laboratory studies reveal elevated leukocyte alkaline phosphatase. Which of the following best describes this patient's hematologic condition?
(A) Acute myelogenous leukemia
(B) Chronic lymphocytic leukemia
(C) Chronic myelogenous leukemia
(D) Leukemoid reaction
(E) Richter syndrome

64 A 20-year-old carpenter with a wound infection on his left thumb presents with an enlarged and tender lymph node in the axilla. A lymph node biopsy shows follicular enlargement and hyperemia. The sinuses are filled with neutrophils. Which of the following is the most likely diagnosis?
(A) Castleman disease
(B) Histiocytosis X
(C) Interfollicular hyperplasia
(D) Sinus histiocytosis
(E) Suppurative lymphadenitis

65 A 56-year-old man with 3-year history of B-cell chronic lymphocytic leukemia complains of the recent onset of fever, weight loss, abdominal pain, and enlargement of lymph nodes. Physical examination reveals hepatosplenomegaly and generalized lymphadenopathy. A lymph node biopsy shows a high-grade, large-cell lymphoma. This patient has which of the following diseases?

(A) Acute lymphoblastic lymphoma
(B) Chronic myelogenous leukemia
(C) Hodgkin lymphoma
(D) Leukemoid reaction
(E) Richter syndrome

66 A 21-year-old woman complains of generalized weakness, blurred vision, and difficulty swallowing. Physical examination shows bilateral ptosis and facial muscle weakness. A CT scan of the chest reveals a mass in the anterior mediastinum. The patient's mass is surgically removed (shown in the image). A microscopic examination demonstrates epithelial cells and normal lymphocytes. What is the most likely diagnosis?

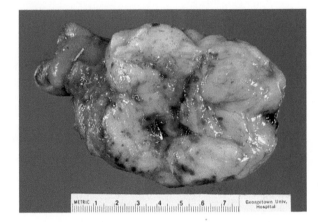

(A) Carcinoid tumor
(B) Hodgkin lymphoma
(C) Lymphocytic lymphoma
(D) Squamous cell carcinoma
(E) Thymoma

67 A 47-year-old man with a history of a heart-lung transplant 3 years ago complains of fever, malaise, and abdominal pain. The patient has been taking cyclosporine for immunosuppression. Physical examination reveals an abdominal mass. A CT-guided biopsy of the mass shows atypical lymphocytes that are positive for latent membrane proteins of Epstein-Barr virus (EBV). What is the most likely diagnosis?
(A) Acute suppurative lymphadenitis
(B) Burkitt lymphoma
(C) Graft-versus-host disease
(D) Infectious mononucleosis
(E) Posttransplant lymphoproliferative disorder

68 A 56-year-old man presents with a 2-week history of fatigue. The patient's past medical history is significant for aortic and mitral valve replacement 5 months ago. A CBC shows moderate anemia with an increased reticulocyte count. Which of the following best explains the pathogenesis of anemia in this patient?
(A) Complement-mediated hemolysis
(B) Decreased blood flow
(C) Direct red cell trauma
(D) Sludging of erythrocytes
(E) Thrombin activation

69 A 46-year-old man is rushed to the hospital after suffering massive trauma in an automobile accident. Two days later the patient suffers a clonic-tonic seizure. Blood cultures are positive for Gram-negative bacteria, and the patient is started on intravenous antibiotics. Laboratory studies show prolonged prothrombin time (PT) and partial thromboplastin time (PTT), low levels of fibrinogen, a positive D-dimer test, and thrombocytopenia. The patient develops renal failure and expires. A section of the kidney at autopsy is stained with phosphotungstic acid hematoxylin (shown in the image). The dark purple objects within the glomeruli are best identified as which of the following?

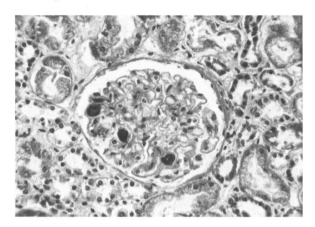

(A) Arteriovenous malformations
(B) Fat emboli
(C) Fibrin thrombi
(D) Psammoma bodies
(E) Vascular calcifications

ANSWERS

1 **The answer is D: Inhibition of apoptosis.** Recent studies indicate that erythropoietin promotes the survival of early erythroid progenitor cells through an inhibition of the default apoptosis pathway. Thus, this hormone rescues stem cells that are otherwise fated to undergo programmed cell death. None of the other choices are known to control the expansion of hematopoietic stem cell colonies in the bone marrow.
Diagnosis: Erythropoiesis

2 **The answer is D: Mean corpuscular volume (MCV).** MCV is the index used to measure the volume of a red blood cell. It categorizes RBCs by size. Cells with normal size are called normocytic, smaller cells are termed microcytic, and larger cells are referred to as macrocytic. Mean corpuscular hemoglobin concentration (choice C) measures hemoglobin content.
Diagnosis: Anemia

3 **The answer is A: Alcoholism.** Macrocytic anemia may be caused by impaired DNA synthesis due to a deficiency of folic acid or vitamin B_{12}. This results in abnormal nuclear development, which, in turn, leads to ineffective erythrocyte maturation and macrocytic anemia. Folic acid deficiency is most commonly due to inadequate dietary intake, which often develops in patients with poorly balanced diets (e.g., alcoholics). Other

possible causes of macrocytic anemia include liver disease, hypothyroidism, and primary bone marrow disease. None of the other choices are associated with macrocytic anemia. Chronic disease (choice B) and renal disease (choice D) cause normochromic, normocytic anemia. Iron deficiency (choice C) and thalassemia (choice E) are microcytic anemias.
Diagnosis: Macrocytic anemia

4 **The answer is C: Hypercellularity with megaloblastic erythroid maturation.** Pernicious anemia is an autoimmune disorder in which patients develop antibodies directed against gastric parietal cells and intrinsic factor. Parietal cell antibodies lead to atrophic gastritis with achlorhydria. Deficiency of vitamin B_{12} or folic acid results in megaloblastic anemia. The peripheral blood smear shows macrocytosis and hypersegmentation of neutrophils. Megaloblastic maturation, characterized by cellular enlargement with asynchronous maturation between the nucleus and cytoplasm, is noted in bone marrow precursors from all lineages. Although the bone marrow tends to be hypercellular, the blood demonstrates pancytopenia because of ineffective hematopoiesis. Neurologic symptoms develop in vitamin B_{12} deficiency, secondary to degeneration of the posterior and lateral columns of the spinal cord. The other choices are not seen in pernicious anemia.
Diagnosis: Megaloblastic anemia, pernicious anemia

5 **The answer is E: Impaired DNA synthesis.** Megaloblastic anemias are caused by impaired DNA synthesis, usually due to a deficiency of either vitamin B_{12} or folic acid. In the face of defective DNA synthesis, nuclear development is impaired, whereas cytoplasmic maturation proceeds normally. This situation, termed nuclear to cytoplasmic asynchrony, results in the formation of megaloblasts. Because the megaloblastic precursors do not mature enough to be released into the blood, they undergo intramedullary destruction. Pernicious anemia is not related to any of the other choices.
Diagnosis: Megaloblastic anemia

6 **The answer is A: Aplastic anemia.** Aplastic anemia is a disorder of pluripotential stem cells that leads to bone marrow failure. The disorder features hypocellular bone marrow and pancytopenia (decreased circulating levels of all formed elements in the blood). Most cases are idiopathic. The bone marrow in aplastic anemia shows variably reduced cellularity, depending on the clinical stage of the disease. There is a decrease in the number of cells of myeloid, erythroid, and megakaryocytic lineages, with a relative increase in lymphocytes and plasma cells. As the cellularity decreases, there is a corresponding increase in bone marrow fat. Anemia, leukopenia (primarily granulocytopenia), and thrombocytopenia characterize aplastic anemia. Patients with aplastic anemia present with weakness, fatigue, infection, and bleeding. Iron-deficiency anemia (choice B) and megaloblastic anemia (choice C) are not characterized by a hypoplastic bone marrow. Myelofibrosis (choice D) shows increased connective tissue. Megakaryocytes and myeloid cells are not decreased in pure red cell aplasia (choice E).
Diagnosis: Aplastic anemia

7 **The answer is C: Low plasma iron saturation.** The blood smear reveals microcytic, hypochromic erythrocytes, characteristic of iron deficiency anemia caused by inadequate uptake or, more often, excessive loss of iron. Women who have menorrhagia, especially those who consume restricted diets, are especially prone to iron deficiency anemia. Iron stores of the body are reduced, as evidenced by reduced levels of serum ferritin (not increased ferritin, choice B) and low iron saturation (iron/total iron binding capacity). None of the other laboratory findings would be expected in a patient with iron deficiency anemia.

Diagnosis: Iron deficiency anemia

8 **The answer is B: Impaired heme synthesis.** The presence of a peptic ulcer incriminates gastrointestinal bleeding as the cause of anemia. The resulting iron deficiency interferes with heme synthesis and thus leads to impaired hemoglobin production and anemia. Defective globin chain synthesis (choice A) and synthesis of structurally abnormal hemoglobin molecules (choice D) are hemoglobinopathies. Poor utilization of iron stores (choice C) reflects sideroblastic anemia and anemia of chronic disease.

Diagnosis: Iron deficiency anemia, peptic ulcer disease

9 **The answer is B: Erythrocyte cytoskeleton.** The smear shows many RBCs to be spherocytes, with decreased diameter and no central pallor. Hereditary spherocytosis (HS) represents a heterogeneous group of inherited disorders of the erythrocyte cytoskeleton, characterized by a deficiency of spectrin or other cytoskeletal components (ankyrin, protein 4.2, band 3). Most forms of HS are inherited as autosomal dominant traits, and most patients have a moderate normocytic anemia. The bone marrow demonstrates erythroid hyperplasia (erythroid maturation is not affected). The deficiency of a cytoskeletal protein in HS leads to uncoupling of the lipid bilayer from the underlying cytoskeleton. The defect results in progressive loss of membrane surface area and formation of spherocytes, which show increased osmotic fragility and are susceptible to chronic extravascular hemolysis. The osmotic fragility test is not abnormal in G6PD deficiency (choice D).

Diagnosis: Hereditary spherocytosis

10 **The answer is B: Cholelithiasis.** While circulating through the spleen, spherocytes lose additional surface membrane before they ultimately succumb to extravascular hemolysis and produce hyperbilirubinemia. Up to 50% of patients with spherocytosis develop cholelithiasis, with pigmented (bilirubin) gallstones due to the increased supply of bilirubin. Kidney stones (choice D) do not contain bilirubin. The liver (choices C and E) and kidney (choice A) are not affected by hereditary spherocytosis.

Diagnosis: Hereditary spherocytosis

11 **The answer is B: Abnormal polymerization of spectrin molecules.** The smear displays elliptical erythrocytes. Hereditary elliptocytosis (HE) refers to a heterogeneous group of inherited disorders involving the erythrocyte cytoskeleton, all of which feature a horizontal abnormality within the cytoskeleton. Variants of HE include defects in self-assembly of spectrin, spectrin-ankyrin binding, protein 4.1, and glycophorin C.

Diagnosis: Hereditary elliptocytosis

12 **The answer is E: β-Thalassemia.** The β-thalassemias are a heterogeneous group of disorders that most often arise sec-ondary to point mutations affecting the β-globin gene. Accordingly, hemoglobin A (α2 β2) is not formed. Unpaired α-chains precipitate in red blood cells, accounting for ineffective erythropoiesis and increased hemolysis. The blood smear shows features characteristic of thalassemia, including hypochromic and microcytic RBCs, with anisocytosis, poikilocytosis, and target cells. In homozygous β-thalassemia, fetal hemoglobin (hemoglobin F) accounts for most of the hemoglobin, although increased levels of hemoglobin A2 are also present. Symptoms of the disease appear early in life, and affected children require constant transfusions. A heterozygous state for thalassemia may provide a protective effect against malaria and increase the reproductive potential of heterozygotes, thereby explaining the persistence of thalassemic disorders. Hemoglobin F is not increased in choices A, B, or C.

Diagnosis: Homozygous β-thalassemia

13 **The answer is C: Extramedullary hematopoiesis.** Increased oxygen affinity of hemoglobin F and the underlying anemia impair oxygen delivery and lead to marked bone marrow erythroid hyperplasia. The marrow space is expanded, causing facial and cranial bone deformities. Extramedullary hematopoiesis contributes to splenomegaly and the formation of soft tissue masses. Excess erythropoiesis leads to increased iron absorption, which, together with repeated transfusions, creates iron overload. Excess iron deposition in tissues is a major cause of morbidity and mortality in thalassemic patients. The other choices may cause splenomegaly, but they are not related to β-thalassemia.

Diagnosis: Homozygous β-thalassemia, splenomegaly

14 **The answer is C: Heterozygous β-thalassemia.** A normal hemoglobin molecule contains four globin chains, consisting of two α- and two non–α-chains. Three normal variants of hemoglobin are encountered, based on the nature of the non–α-chains. Hemoglobin A (α2 β2) accounts for 95% to 98% of the total hemoglobin in adults; only minor amounts of hemoglobin F (α2 γ2) and hemoglobin A2 (α2 δ2) are present. Heterozygous β-thalassemia is associated with microcytosis and hypochromia, and the degree of microcytosis is disproportionate to the severity of the anemia, which is generally mild. Target cells, basophilic stippling, and a mild increase in hemoglobin A2 are present. Most patients are asymptomatic. Choice D (homozygous β-thalassemia) is a more serious disease and choice E (silent carrier for α-thalassemia) is asymptomatic.

Diagnosis: Heterozygous β-thalassemia

15 **The answer is C: Erythroblasts.** The peripheral blood smear displays erythroid precursors, which are normally confined to the bone marrow. Hemolytic disease of the newborn reflects a histoincompatibility between the mother and the developing fetus. The mother lacks an antigen that is expressed by the fetus. Maternal IgG alloantibodies cross the placenta, causing complement-mediated hemolysis of fetal erythrocytes and resulting in the release of numerous erythroid precursors (erythroblasts). The other choices represent normal immune cells.

Diagnosis: Hemolytic disease of newborn, erythroblastosis fetalis

16 The answer is E: Polycythemia vera (PV). PV is a myeloproliferative disease that arises from a single clonal hematopoietic stem cell and results in uncontrolled production of RBCs. The increase in erythrocytes in PV is autonomous and is not regulated by erythropoietin. PV derives from the malignant transformation of a single, hematopoietic stem cell with primary commitment to the erythroid lineage. Proliferation of the neoplastic clone occurs predominantly in the bone marrow but may involve extramedullary sites including the spleen, lymph nodes, and liver (myeloid metaplasia). The bone marrow is hypercellular with hyperplasia of all elements. The spleen is moderately enlarged, and its cut surface is uniformly dark red, with expansion of the red pulp and obliteration of the white pulp. Acute myelogenous leukemia (choice A) and essential thrombocythemia (choice B) involve the myeloid and megakaryocytic lines, respectively. Idiopathic myelofibrosis (choice C) features marrow collagen deposition (fibrosis).

Diagnosis: Polycythemia vera

17 The answer is B: Cerebrovascular accident. The patient has polycythemia vera (PV). Hyperviscosity associated with PV increases the risk for thrombotic stroke. The other choices are not associated with PV.

Diagnosis: Polycythemia vera

18 The answer is D: Ischemia. Sickle cell disease is characterized by the presence of an abnormal hemoglobin (hemoglobin S). Erythrocyte sickling is initially reversible with reoxygenation, but after several cycles of sickling and unsickling, the process becomes irreversible. Irreversibly sickled cells display a rearrangement of phospholipids between the outer and inner monolayers of the cell membrane. The erythrocytes are no longer deformable and are more adherent to endothelial cells, which are properties that predispose to thrombosis of small blood vessels. The resulting vascular occlusions lead to widespread ischemic complications, which are associated with severe pain, especially in the chest, abdomen, and bones.

Diagnosis: Sickle cell disease

19 The answer is E: Pneumonia. The asplenic state associated with sickle cell anemia renders the patient susceptible to infections by encapsulated bacteria, especially *Streptococcus pneumoniae*. In addtion to splenic infarcts, patients with sickle cell disease frequently develop renal papillary necrosis due to conditions of low oxygen, low pH, and high osmolality in the renal medulla. None of the other choices represent complications of splenectomy.

Diagnosis: Sickle cell disease

20 The answer is C: Parvovirus B19 infection. Patients with sickle cell anemia may undergo an aplastic crisis because of infection of the bone marrow by parvovirus B19, which suppresses erythrocyte production. None of the other choices are complications of sickle cell anemia.

Diagnosis: Sickle cell anemia, aplastic crisis

21 The answer is C: Impaired utilization of iron from storage sites. Anemia of chronic disease arises in association with chronic inflammatory diseases (e.g., tuberculosis and rheumatoid arthritis) and malignant conditions. Chronic disease leads to ineffective use of iron from macrophage stores in the bone marrow, resulting in a functional iron deficiency, although storage iron is normal or even increased. The anemia of chronic disease is mild to moderate, and the red cells are often microcytic. Serum iron levels tend to be reduced. However, in contrast to iron deficiency anemia, total iron-binding capacity also tends to be decreased (as is the serum albumin level). The other choices are not related to anemia of chronic disease.

Diagnosis: Anemia of chronic disease

22 The answer is B: Chronic liver disease. Acanthocytosis (shown in the photomicrograph) results from a defect within the lipid bilayer of the red cell membrane and features spiny projections of the surface, which may be associated with hemolysis. The most common cause of acanthocytosis is chronic liver disease, in which increased free cholesterol is deposited within the cell membrane. Abnormalities in the lipid membrane cause erythrocytes to become deformed and develop irregular spiny surface projections and centrally dense cytoplasm (acanthocytes or spur cells). Chronic renal failure (choice C) features burr cells. Abnormal spectrin (choice A) causes hereditary spherocytosis.

Diagnosis: Acanthocytosis

23 The answer is C: Myelodysplastic syndrome (MDS). MDS exhibits dysplastic morphologic features in one or more hematopoietic lineages and is accompanied by ineffective hematopoiesis. The disease is most common in the elderly and presents with anemia, neutropenia, and thrombocytopenia. The morphologic classification of MDS is based on the presence of abnormally shaped hematopoietic cells and an increased proportion of myeloblasts. Dysplastic features may be present in one or more hematopoietic lineages. Ringed sideroblasts are common. In this case, a smear of a bone marrow aspirate stained with Prussian blue shows erythroid precursor cells containing iron-laden mitochondria that encircle the nuclei. Ringed sideroblasts are not a feature of the other choices.

Diagnosis: Myelodysplastic syndrome

24 The answer is A: Clonal stem cell defect. Myelodysplastic syndromes (MDS) are hematopoietic stem cell disorders that are characterized by a discrepancy between the paucity of peripheral blood elements and marked hyperplasia in the bone marrow. MDS may be either primary (de novo) or secondary (therapy related). Patients with secondary myelodysplasia usually have a history of chemotherapy, especially alkylating agents, or radiation therapy for the treatment of cancer. Other risk factors for MDS include viruses, benzene exposure, cigarette smoking, and Fanconi anemia.

Diagnosis: Myelodysplasia

25 The answer is A: Damage to stem cells. The bone marrow is aplastic, consisting largely of fat cells and lacking normal hematopoietic activity. Patients with aplastic anemia present with severe pancytopenia and clinical symptoms related to the various cytopenias, including fatigue (anemia), fever (neutropenia), and petechiae (thrombocytopenia). The lack of an appropriate reticulocyte response to the anemia indicates decreased or ineffective hematopoiesis as the mechanism for the pancytopenia. Injury to bone marrow stem cells is idiopathic (two thirds of cases), toxic (as in this case), immunologic, or hereditary (Fanconi anemia).

Diagnosis: Aplastic anemia

26 **The answer is B: Folic acid deficiency.** Folic acid deficiency commonly occurs in alcoholics who have poor nutrition. Macrocytosis, hypersegmented neutrophils, and a normal Schilling test (vitamin B_{12} absorption) point to folic acid deficiency. Folic acid and vitamin B_{12} are required for synthesis of DNA, and deficiency of either factor leads to megaloblastic transformation of hematopoietic cells. Macrocytosis and hypersegmented neutrophils are not features of the other choices.

Diagnosis: Megaloblastic anemia

27 **The answer is A: G6PD deficiency.** G6PD deficiency is an X-linked disorder that causes a hemolytic anemia characterized by abnormal sensitivity of red cells to oxidative stress. The highest prevalence is in Africa and the Mediterranean region. Because of the role of G6PD in recycling reduced glutathione, red cells deficient in this enzyme are susceptible to oxidative stress, which, in this case, is fava bean ingestion (favism). In quiescent periods, the erythrocytes of G6PD deficiency appear normal. However, during a hemolytic episode precipitated by oxidative stress, Heinz bodies can be demonstrated by supravital staining. Full expression of G6PD deficiency is seen only in males, with females being asymptomatic carriers. Heinz bodies are not characteristic of the other choices.

Diagnosis: Glucose-6-phosphate dehydrogenase deficiency

28 **The answer is D: Chronic myelogenous leukemia (CML).** Chronic myeloproliferative diseases are defined as clonal hematogenous stem cell disorders with increased proliferation of one or more myeloid lineages. CML is derived from an abnormal pluripotent bone marrow stem cell and results in prominent neutrophilic leukocytosis over the full range of myeloid maturation. CML is the most common myeloproliferative disease and accounts for 15% to 20% of all cases of leukemia. It affects middle-aged or older adults. Replacement of the bone marrow by neoplastic cells causes anemia and thrombocytopenia and a predisposition to infections. In 95% of all CML cases, the Philadelphia chromosome can be demonstrated by conventional cytogenetics. The initial symptoms are nonspecific and include weakness, malaise, fever, and splenomegaly. Acute lymphoblastic leukemia (choice A) and acute myeloid leukemia (choice B) feature clonal expansion of lymphoblasts and myeloblasts, respectively. Although myelodysplastic syndrome (choice E) features hyperplastic bone marrow, the Philadelphia chromosome does not occur, and there is peripheral cytopenia in various cell lines.

Diagnosis: Chronic myelogenous leukemia

29 **The answer is A: abl.** Presence of the Philadelphia chromosome or molecular demonstration of the *bcr/abl* fusion gene is required to establish the diagnosis of chronic myelogenous leukemia (CML). The *bcr/abl* gene encodes a fusion protein, p210, which acts as a constitutively activated tyrosine kinase. The other choices may be involved in malignant transformations but they are not related to CML.

Diagnosis: Chronic myelogenous leukemia

30 **The answer is C: Acute promyelocytic leukemia (APL).** In APL, the bone marrow is packed with tumor cells that have promyelocytic features, with abundant Auer rods. Patients with APL frequently present with DIC. Senescent leukemic cells degranulate and activate the coagulation cascade. The presence of Auer rods excludes acute lymphoblastic leukemia (choice A), acute megakaryocytic leukemia (choice B), and chronic myelogenous leukemia (choice D). DIC is not characteristic of the other choices.

Diagnosis: Acute promyelocytic leukemia

31 **The answer is E: Retinoic acid receptor (RAR).** The underlying genetic defect in acute promyelocytic leukemia is a translocation involving the *PML* gene on chromosome 15 and the RAR (*RARα*) gene on chromosome 17. The resulting *PML/RARα* fusion gene encodes a functional RAR. The receptor can be targeted by all-*trans*-retinoic acid, which mediates maturation of the tumor cells. Complete remissions have been obtained in some patients. The other choices may be involved in other translocations.

Diagnosis: Acute promyelocytic leukemia

32 **The answer is B: Chronic lymphocytic leukemia (CLL).** CLL is characterized by clonal proliferation of small, mature-appearing lymphocytes in the bone marrow, lymph nodes, and spleen, with an expression in the peripheral blood. In most instances, the leukemic cells belong to B-cell lineage and show clonal Ig gene rearrangements and activation of the *bcl* protooncogene. Most patients are over 50 years of age. The symptoms tend to be nonspecific, but 80% of patients have lymph node enlargement, and 50% show splenomegaly. CLL usually has an indolent and protracted course. Acute lymphoblastic lymphoma (choice A) is principally a leukemia of childhood. Multiple myeloma (choice D) is a neoplasm of plasma cells. Waldenström macroglobulinemia (choice E) is a neoplasm of small lymphocytes and a variable number of IgM-secreting plasma cells of the same malignant clone.

Diagnosis: Chronic lymphocytic leukemia

33 **The answer is A: Acute lymphoblastic leukemia (ALL).** Most precursor B-cell malignances involve primarily bone marrow and peripheral blood and are termed B-cell acute lymphoblastic leukemias (B-ALL). Only 15% of childhood ALLs) are derived from T cells, and 75% of B-ALL cases occur in children under the age of 6 years. B-ALL features numerical aberrations and chromosomal translocations, including the Philadelphia chromosome. In childhood ALL, a *bcr/abl* fusion protein, P190, is produced. B-ALLs are positive for nuclear expression of TdT. The demonstration of TdT activity suggests that a leukemic blast is of lymphoid rather than myeloid lineage. The other choices are rarely, if ever, encountered in this age group.

Diagnosis: Acute lymphocytic leukemia

34 **The answer is C: Hodgkin lymphoma (HL).** The lymph node biopsy shows a Reed-Sternberg cell. These large atypical mononuclear or multinucleated tumor cells in an inflammatory background are the diagnostic hallmark of HL. HL is the most common malignant neoplasm of Americans between the ages of 10 and 30 years. There is a distinctive bimodal

age distribution in developed countries. Most patients with HL present with lymphadenopathy. Constitutional symptoms include night sweats, fever, and weight loss exceeding 10% of body weight. Pruritus may occur with disease progression. Reed-Sternberg cells do not occur in the other choices.
Diagnosis: Hodgkin lymphoma

35   The answer is E: Nodular sclerosis. Nodular sclerosis accounts for 70% of classical Hodgkin lymphoma, with most cases occurring between the ages of 20 and 30 years. Histologic examination shows dense, band-like collagenous fibrosis that envelops cellular aggregates of lymphoid and inflammatory cells, as well as the specific lacunar cell variant of the Reed-Sternberg cell.
Diagnosis: Hodgkin lymphoma, nodular sclerosis subtype

36   The answer is D: Multiple myeloma. Plasma cell myeloma (multiple myeloma) is characterized by a multifocal infiltration of malignant plasma cells in the bone marrow. There are typically multiple destructive lytic lesions or diffuse demineralization of bone. Major diagnostic criteria for plasma cell myeloma include marrow plasmacytosis (>30%), plasmacytoma on biopsy, and immunoglobulin paraprotein (M-component). Neoplastic cells typically secrete a homogeneous complete or partial immunoglobulin chain, which can be seen in serum or urine electrophoresis. In this patient, the neoplastic clone secretes excess kappa light chains. Waldenström macroglobulinemia (choice E) is a neoplastic disorder of small lymphocytes that secrete IgM.
Diagnosis: Multiple myeloma

37   The answer is E: Renal failure. The most common and important extramedullary complication of multiple myeloma is amyloid nephropathy, which accounts for more than half of all deaths. Other complications include bone fractures and infection.
Diagnosis: Multiple myeloma

38   The answer is C: Chronic idiopathic myelofibrosis. Chronic idiopathic myelofibrosis is a clonal myeloproliferative disease in which marrow fibrosis is accompanied by prominent megakaryopoiesis and granulopoiesis. A prefibrotic stage is recognized wherein the bone marrow is hypercellular, with predominant neutrophilic and megakaryocytic proliferation. In the fibrotic stage, the peripheral blood shows either leukopenia or marked leukocytosis, and myeloid precursors and nucleated RBCs are usually present. Conspicuous reticulin or collagen fibrosis in the marrow defines this stage. Transformation to acute myelogenous leukemia (choice A) occurs in 15% of cases. The other choices do not feature marrow fibrosis.
Diagnosis: Myelofibrosis

39   The answer is E: Small lymphocytic lymphoma (SLLs). Chronic lymphocytic leukemias (CLLs) as well as SLLs are malignant B-cell proliferations of small, mature-appearing lymphocytes and a variable number of large cells. A diagnosis of CLL is made if bone marrow and peripheral blood are primarily involved. If the tumor cells give rise to lymphadenopathy or solid tumor masses, the term small lymphocytic lymphoma is used. Reactive follicular hyperplasia (choice D) is excluded

in this case by the peripheral lymphocytosis and by the lack of reactive follicles in the lymph node biopsy. Hodgkin lymphoma (choice B) features Reed-Sternberg cells.
Diagnosis: Small lymphocytic lymphoma

40   The answer is C: Bcl-2. Follicular lymphoma is a clonal lymphoid proliferation derived from germinal-center B cells. The most common cytogenetic translocation in follicular lymphoma is t(14;18)(q32;q21), with *IgH* and *bcl-2* as partner genes. The bcl-2 protein, expressed in follicular lymphoma, is localized in the mitochondrial membrane and functions as an apoptosis inhibitor. Choices A, D, and E (abl, myc, and retinoic acid receptor) represent translocations in other disorders. Bax (choice B) is a pro-apoptotic protein.
Diagnosis: Follicular lymphoma

41   The answer is A: Proliferation in B-cell areas. Follicular hyperplasia refers to enlarged lymph follicles (principally in the cortex of the lymph node), which consist of B lymphocytes. Reactive follicular hyperplasia of lymph nodes represents a response to infections, inflammation, or tumors. Hyperplasia of the secondary follicles, germinal centers, and plasmacytosis of the medullary cords indicate B-lymphocyte immunoreactivity. Hyperplasia of the deep cortex or paracortex (interfollicular of diffuse hyperplasia) is characteristic of T-lymphocyte immunoreactivity (choice D).
Diagnosis: Follicular hyperplasia

42   The answer is B: Burkitt lymphoma (BL). BL, one of the most rapidly growing malignancies, is defined by a chromosomal translocation involving 8q24, which harbors the *myc* oncogene. Endemic BL is the most common childhood malignancy in Central Africa. Sporadic BL affects mainly children and young adults in the Western world, where it accounts for 1% to 2% of all lymphomas. Immunodeficiency-associated BL mainly occurs in HIV-infected persons. The cellular debris of apoptotic tumor cells is cleared by macrophages, whose scattered appearance is termed "starry sky macrophage." Most patients present with extranodal tumors that emerge in a short period of time and respond to aggressive chemotherapy. Choices A, C, and E are not endemic in Africa, and choice D (reactive follicular hyperplasia) is a nonmalignant disorder.
Diagnosis: Burkitt lymphoma

43   The answer is B: Langerhans cell histiocytosis (LCH). LCH refers to a spectrum of uncommon proliferative disorders of Langerhans cells. The disease ranges from asymptomatic involvement of a single site, such as bone or lymph nodes, to an aggressive systemic disorder that involves multiple organs. There is clinical heterogeneity of LCH; eosinophilic granuloma (75% of all cases) is a localized, usually self-limited disorder of older children and young adults; Hand-Schuller-Christian disease is a multifocal and typically indolent disorder, usually in children between 2 and 5 years of age; and Letterer-Siwe disease (fewer than 10% of cases) is an acute, disseminated variant of LCH in infants and children younger than 2 years of age. Organs involved by LCH include the skin (seborrheic or eczematoid dermatitis), lymph nodes, spleen, liver, lungs, and bone marrow. Otitis media is a common finding. Painful lytic lesions of bone are common. Proptosis may complicate infiltration of the orbit. The classic triad of diabetes insipidus, proptosis, and defects in membranous bones characterizes Hand-Schuller-Christian disease. Hodgkin lymphoma (choice A) often features eosinophils but does not have this clinical presentation.

Diagnosis: Langerhans cell histiocytosis

44   The answer is C: Large B-cell lymphoma.   Most lymphomas in patients who have AIDS are high-grade B-cell lymphomas. These aggressive, but potentially curable neoplasms include Burkitt lymphoma and diffuse large-cell B-cell lymphoma. As in follicular lymphoma, *bcl2* gene rearrangements are often seen, suggesting a potential germinal center origin. Diffuse large-cell B-cell lymphomas associated with immunodeficiency are usually positive for EBV. The other choices are not complications of HIV infection.

Diagnosis: Large B-cell lymphoma

45   The answer is D: Hairy cell leukemia.   Hairy cell leukemia is a clonal B-cell proliferation of small- to medium-sized lymphocytes that display abundant cytoplasm and hair-like protrusions of the cell membrane. The disease involves primarily the monocyte/macrophage system of the bone marrow, spleen, and liver. Hairy cell leukemia is rare and affects mainly middle-aged to elderly persons, with a markedly increased male-to-female ratio of 5:1. Unlike the other choices, hairy cell leukemia expresses tartrate-resistant acid phosphatase.

Diagnosis: Hairy cell leukemia

46   The answer is E: Marginal zone lymphoma.   Extranodal marginal-zone B-cell lymphomas that originate in mucosa-associated lymphoid tissue are referred to as MALT lymphomas. MALT lymphomas are indolent, malignant lymphocyte proliferations that consist of small- to medium-sized lymphocytes with frequent monocytoid features and variable admixtures of plasma cells. The malignant lymphocytes appear to originate from marginal-zone B cells. Most primary gastric lymphomas are MALT lymphomas. MALT lymphomas occur either in granular organs or along mucosal surfaces. They commonly arise in the context of a chronic inflammatory process or autoimmune disease. The other choices may rarely affect organs such as the stomach, but unlike MALT lymphoma, they are unrelated to *H. pylori* infection.

Diagnosis: Marginal zone lymphoma, MALT lymphoma

47   The answer is E: Mycosis fungoides.   Mycosis fungoides represents a cutaneous T-cell lymphoma, composed of mature, postthymic T-helper (CD4+) lymphocytes. Mycosis fungoides displays lymphocytic infiltrates at the dermal-epidermal junction and, in some cases, intraepidermal accumulations of tumor cells (Pautrier microabscesses). The other choices are not characteristically seen as skin lesions.

Diagnosis: Mycosis fungoides

48   The answer is E: Waldenström disease.   Waldenström disease (lymphoplasmacytic lymphoma) is a neoplastic proliferation of small lymphocytes and a variable number of IgM-secreting plasma cells of the same malignant clone. Waldenström disease is not a variant of multiple myeloma, but rather, is an indolent malignant lymphoma that mainly affects the elderly. Eighty percent of patients with Waldenström macroglobulinemia present with a monoclonal IgM spike on serum electrophoresis (>3 g/dL). Many of the clinical symptoms are associated with hyperviscosity of the blood. The other choices do not feature IgM-producing lymphocytes.

Diagnosis: Waldenström macroglobulinemia

49   The answer is D: Idiopathic thrombocytopenic purpura (ITP).   ITP is a quantitative disorder of platelets caused by antibodies directed against platelet or megakaryocytic antigens. Similar to autoimmune hemolytic anemia, the etiology of ITP is related to antibody-mediated immune destruction of platelets or their precursors. In adults with acute ITP, the platelet count is typically less than 20,000/μL. In chronic adult ITP, the platelet count varies from a few thousand to 100,000/μL. The peripheral blood smear in ITP exhibits numerous large platelets, and the bone marrow shows a compensatory increase in megakaryocytes. Acute ITP in children typically appears after a viral illness and presents with sudden onset of petechiae and purpura without other symptoms. Spontaneous recovery can be expected in more than 80% of cases within 6 months. Thrombocytopenia may be observed in the other choices but is usually associated with other systemic signs and symptoms.

Diagnosis: Idiopathic thrombocytopenic purpura

50   The answer is A: Antibody-mediated platelet destruction.   In common with idiopathic thrombocytopenic purpura and certain drug-induced thrombocytopenias, systemic lupus erythematosus is associated with increased platelet destruction due to immune-mediated damage and removal of circulating platelets (antibody-mediated platelet destruction). The other choices do not represent immune destruction of platelets.

Diagnosis: Idiopathic thrombocytopenic purpura, systemic lupus erythematosus

51   The answer is C: Hemolytic anemia.   Reticulocytes are non-nucleated cells that represent the last stage before mature erythrocytes. The nucleus is extruded from the orthochromatic erythroblast, leaving mitochondria and hemoglobin-producing polyribosomes in the reticulocyte. After release from the bone marrow, the reticulocyte loses its capacity for aerobic metabolism and hemoglobin synthesis, and after 1 to 2 days, it becomes a mature erythrocyte. Hemolytic anemias are characterized by a compensatory increase in production and release of red cells by the bone marrow, manifested in the blood by polychromasia of red cells and an increased reticulocyte count. Increased peripheral reticulocytes are not observed in the other choices.

Diagnosis: Hemolytic anemia, idiopathic thrombocytopenic purpura

52   The answer is A: Autoantibodies directed against the erythrocyte membrane.   The peripheral blood smear from this patient shows clumped red cells caused by cold agglutinins (autoantibodies). Cold agglutinins are mostly IgM, are directed against the I/i antigen system, and act optimally at 4°C. Cold agglutinins may be idiopathic or develop secondary to an underlying condition, most frequently infections (Epstein-Barr virus) or lymphoproliferative disorders. However, most autoimmune hemolytic anemias are mediated by IgG antibodies that exert their maximal effect at body temperature (warm agglutinins). Choices D and E are associated with hemolysis rather than clumping of red blood cells.

Diagnosis: Autoimmune hemolytic anemia

53 **The answer is D: Thrombotic thrombocytopenic purpura (TTP).** TTP occurs in acute or chronic form and presents with a pentad that includes fever, thrombocytopenia, microangiopathic hemolytic anemia, renal impairment, and neurologic symptoms. The morphologic hallmark of TTP is the deposition throughout the body of PAS-positive hyaline microthrombi in arterioles and capillaries, principally in the heart, brain, and kidneys. The microthrombi contain platelet aggregates, fibrin, and a few erythrocytes and leukocytes. The peripheral blood smear displays microangiopathic hemolytic anemia. The peripheral blood smear shows numerous schistocytes. TTP resembles hemolytic uremic syndrome, which occurs more often in children than adults. The other choices are not associated with microangiopathic changes (e.g., schistocytes).

Diagnosis: Thrombotic thrombocytopenic purpura

54 **The answer is D: Microangiopathic hemolytic anemia.** Microangiopathic hemolytic anemia results from abnormalities in the microcirculation that cause turbulent blood flow patterns. The classic examples of this type of hemolytic anemia are DIC (this case) and TTP; both of which feature generalized thrombosis of capillary vessels. Long-distance running or walking or prolonged vigorous exercise can cause repetitive trauma to red blood cells in the microcirculation leading to hemolysis. Alterations in blood flow, as are encountered in malignant hypertension or vasculitis syndromes, may also produce mechanical fragmentation of erythrocytes. Microangiopathic features are not observed in the other choices.

Diagnosis: Microangiopathic hemolytic anemia

55 **The answer is D: Macroangiopathic hemolytic anemia.** Macroangiopathic hemolytic anemia most commonly results from direct erythrocyte trauma due to an abnormal vascular surface (e.g., prosthetic heart valve, synthetic vascular graft). Anemia is mild to moderate and is accompanied by an appropriate reticulocyte response. Blood smear examination reveals fragmented red blood cells (schistocytes) and polychromasia. Although choice E (microangiopathic hemolytic anemia) results in morphologically-similar red blood cells, it reflects changes in small blood vessels.

Diagnosis: Macroangiopathic hemolytic anemia

56 **The answer is D: Genetic defect involving the factor VIII gene.** Hemophilia A is an X-linked recessive disorder of blood clotting that results in spontaneous bleeding, particularly into joints, muscles, and internal organs. Classic hemophilia results from mutations in the gene encoding factor VIII (hemophilia A). Hemophilia A is the most frequently encountered sex-linked inherited bleeding disorder (1 per 5,000 to 10,000 males). Choices C and E represent acquired disorders.

Diagnosis: Hemophilia A

57 **The answer is B: Hemophilia B.** Hemophilia B is an X-linked recessive disease caused by mutations in the gene encoding factor IX. It accounts for only 10% of all cases of hemophilia. One third of all cases represent new mutations. It is clinically indistinguishable from hemophilia A (factor VIII deficiency) (choice A). In both forms of hemophilia, the partial thromboplastin time (PTT) is prolonged. Mixing of a patient's blood with that of a normal donor normalizes the PTT.

Diagnosis: Hemophilia B

58 **The answer is D: Paroxysmal nocturnal hemoglobinuria (PNH).** Despite its name, the disorder is nocturnal in only a minority of cases. PNH is a clonal stem cell disorder characterized by episodic intravascular hemolytic anemia that is secondary to increased sensitivity of erythrocytes to complement-mediated lysis. The underlying defect involves somatic mutation of the phosphatidylinositol glycan-class A (*PIG-A*) gene. PNH may develop as a primary disorder or evolve from preexisting cases of aplastic anemia. During hemolytic episodes, patients develop normocytic or macrocytic anemia, accompanied by an appropriate reticulocyte response. The traditional diagnostic tests for PNH, hemolysis in sucrose (sucrose hemolysis test) or acidified serum (Ham test), are now more easily diagnosed by demonstrating loss of GPI-anchored proteins on blood cells by flow cytofluorometry. Choices B and C, which are hemolytic conditions, do not show increased lysis in the described laboratory studies.

Diagnosis: Paroxysmal nocturnal hemoglobinuria

59 **The answer is B: Essential thrombocythemia.** Essential thrombocythemia is an uncommon neoplastic disorder of hematopoietic stem cells that is characterized by uncontrolled proliferation of megakaryocytes. A marked increase in circulating platelets is accompanied by recurrent episodes of thrombosis and hemorrhage. The WHO criteria require a sustained platelet count above 600,000/μL and prominent megakaryocytic proliferation in the bone marrow. Essential thrombocythemia is believed to derive from the malignant transformation of a hematopoietic stem cell with principal commitment to the megakaryocytic lineage. Increased megakaryocytes are a feature of chronic myelogenous leukemia (choice A) but in the context of multilineage expansion. Megakaryocytosis is also seen in myelofibrosis (choice C), but the marrow is fibrotic.

Diagnosis: Essential thrombocythemia

60 **The answer is C: Hemolytic transfusion reaction.** An immediate hemolytic transfusion reaction occurs when grossly incompatible blood is administered to patients with preformed alloantibodies, usually because of clerical errors. Massive hemolysis of the transfused blood may be associated with severe complications, including hypotension, renal failure, and even death. Choices B, D, and E are not characterized by a positive Coombs test. Choice A is not related to blood transfusions.

Diagnosis: Acute hemolytic transfusion reaction

61 **The answer is E: Suppression of hematopoiesis.** The presence of myeloblasts in the peripheral blood is indicative of acute myelogenous leukemia (AML). In AML, there is an accumulation in the marrow of immature myeloid cells that lack the potential for further differentiation and maturation, which leads to suppression of normal hematopoiesis. As a consequence, the major clinical problems associated with AML are granulocytopenia, thrombocytopenia, and anemia. Promyelocytic leukemia causes disseminated intravascular coagulation (choice B).

Diagnosis: Acute myelogenous leukemia

62 **The answer is E: Transformation of a pluripotent bone marrow stem cell.** The patient exhibits the Philadelphia chromosome and clinicopathologic features of chronic myelogenous leukemia (CML). The neoplastic cells in CML are derived from an abnormal pluripotent bone marrow stem cell, which results in prominent neutrophilic leukocytosis over the full range of myeloid maturation. The other choices relate to cells in the lymphoid lineage.

Diagnosis: Chronic myelogenous leukemia

63 **The answer is D: Leukemoid reaction.** Neutrophilia is an absolute neutrophil count above 7,000/μL. In acute infections, neutrophilia may be so pronounced that it may be mistaken for leukemia, especially, chronic myelogenous leukemia (CML), in which case it is termed a leukemoid reaction. Clues to the benign (or reactive) nature of a leukemoid reaction include the following: (1) the cells in the peripheral blood smear are more mature than myelocytes; (2) leukocyte alkaline phosphatase activity is high in benign conditions and low in patients with CML; and (3) benign neutrophils often contain large blue cytoplasmic inclusions referred to as "Dohle bodies" or toxic granulation. The other choices are incorrect because the neutrophils in these disorders do not display these morphologic features, and they are usually associated with other hematologic abnormalities.

Diagnosis: Leukemoid reaction

64 **The answer is E: Suppurative lymphadenitis.** Acute suppurative lymphadenitis occurs in the lymph nodes that drain a site of acute bacterial infection. Suppurative lymph nodes enlarge rapidly because of edema and hyperemia and are tender due to distention of the capsule. Microscopically, infiltration of the lymph node sinuses and stroma by polymorphonuclear leukocytes and prominent follicular hyperplasia are noted. Neutrophils are not a morphologic feature of the other choices.

Diagnosis: Suppurative lymphadenitis

65 **The answer is E: Richter syndrome.** Five percent of patients with B-cell chronic lymphocytic leukemia (B-CLL) develop a large-cell lymphoma. Patients with this complication present with a rapid onset of fever, abdominal pain, and progressive lymphadenopathy and hepatosplenomegaly. Richter syndrome is aggressive and refractory to therapy, with a mean

survival of 2 months. The other choices are not associated with B-CLL.

Diagnosis: Richter syndrome, B-cell chronic lymphocytic leukemia

66 **The answer is E: Thymoma.** Thymoma is a neoplasm of thymic epithelial cells, without regard to the number of lymphocytes. This tumor of adults is usually benign, but malignant examples occur. Fifteen percent of patients with myasthenia gravis have thymoma, as in this case. Conversely, one third to one half of patients with thymoma develop myasthenia gravis. Myasthenia gravis is not associated with the other choices, although mediastinal presentations occur.

Diagnosis: Thymoma, myasthenia gravis

67 **The answer is E: Posttransplant lymphoproliferative disorder (PTLD).** PTLD results from immunosuppression and is often associated with EBV infection. In most cases, the disease is an EBV-driven, monoclonal, lymphocyte proliferation with variable morphology. The incidence of PTLD parallels the extent of immunosuppression. In this connection, liver transplant recipients have a higher incidence of PTLD than do patients who receive kidney transplants. Burkitt lymphoma (choice B) has been related to EBV infection but is not a complication of immunosuppression. Infectious mononucleosis (choice D) does not present with an abdominal mass.

Diagnosis: Posttransplant lymphoproliferative disorder

68 **The answer is C: Direct red cell trauma.** Red cell fragmentation syndromes are disorders in which erythrocytes are subjected to mechanical disruption as they circulate in the blood (intravascular hemolysis). These disorders are classified as either macroangiopathic (large vessels), as in this case, or microangiopathic (capillaries), according to the site of hemolysis. Mechanical fragmentation of red cells is primarily due either to alteration of the endothelial surface of blood vessels or disturbances in blood flow patterns that lead to turbulence and increased shear stress. Macroangiopathic hemolytic anemia most commonly results from direct red cell trauma due to an abnormal vascular surface (e.g., prosthetic heart valve). The other choices are not an expected complication of a prosthetic valve.

Diagnosis: Macroangiopathic hemolysis

69 **The answer is C: Fibrin thrombi.** Disseminated intravascular coagulation (DIC) refers to widespread ischemic changes secondary to microvascular fibrin thrombi, which are accompanied by the consumption of platelets and coagulation factors and a hemorrhagic diathesis. DIC typically occurs as a complication of massive trauma, septicemia, and obstetric emergencies. It is also associated with metastatic cancer, hematopoietic malignancies, cardiovascular and liver diseases, and numerous other conditions. The other choices are not directly associated with DIC.

Diagnosis: Disseminated intravascular coagulation

Chapter 21

The Endocrine System

QUESTIONS

Select the single best answer.

1 A 14-year-old boy presents with 3 months of lethargy, headaches, and muscle weakness. His parents note that he drinks water excessively. His vital signs are normal. A 24-hour urine collection shows polyuria. The fasting blood sugar is normal. An X-ray film of the brain reveals suprasellar calcification. An autopsy specimen of a similar case is shown in the image. Which of the following neoplasms is the most likely cause of polyuria in this patient?

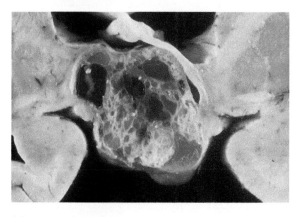

(A) Craniopharyngioma
(B) Glioblastoma multiforme
(C) Pheochromocytoma
(D) Pituitary adenoma
(E) Retinoblastoma

2 A 60-year-old man with small cell carcinoma of the lung is rushed to the emergency room in a coma after suffering a clonic-tonic seizure. The patient's temperature is 37°C (98.6°F), blood pressure 100/50 mm Hg, and pulse 88 per minute. Laboratory studies show a serum sodium of 103 mmol/L, normal serum levels of BUN and creatinine, and a dilute but otherwise normal urine. A CT scan of the head is normal. Which of the following is the most likely cause of seizures in this patient?

(A) Central diabetes insipidus
(B) Diabetes mellitus
(C) Renal metastases
(D) Sheehan syndrome
(E) Syndrome of inappropriate ADH secretion

3 A 60-year-old woman with small cell carcinoma of the lung notes rounding of her face, upper truncal obesity, and muscle weakness. Physical examination reveals thin, wrinkled skin, abdominal striae, and multiple purpuric skin lesions. The patient's blood pressure is 175/95 mm Hg. Laboratory studies will likely show elevated serum levels of which of the following hormones?

(A) Aldosterone
(B) Corticotropin
(C) Epinephrine
(D) Prolactin
(E) Thyrotropin

4 A 21-year-old woman experiences abruptio placentae with severe bleeding during the delivery of a term fetus. Five months later, she presents with profound lethargy, pallor, muscle weakness, failure of lactation, and amenorrhea. Which of the following pathologic findings is expected in this patient?

(A) Atrophy of the endocrine pancreas
(B) Autoimmune destruction of the adrenal cortex
(C) Infarction of the pituitary
(D) Pituitary prolactinoma
(E) Polycystic ovaries

5 A 25-year-old man presents with 3 months of polyuria and increased thirst. The patient suffered trauma to the base of the skull in a motorcycle accident 4 months ago. A 24-hour urine collection shows polyuria but no evidence of hematuria, glucosuria, or proteinuria. The pathogenesis of polyuria in this patient is most likely caused by a lesion in which of the following areas of the brain?

(A) Adenohypophysis
(B) Brain stem
(C) Mammillothalamic tract
(D) Neurohypophysis
(E) Subthalamic fasciculus

6 A 30-year-old woman complains of headache, visual disturbances, deepening of the voice, and generalized weakness. She reports amenorrhea for the past year and states that she recently required a larger shoe size. Laboratory studies show impaired glucose tolerance. What other procedure would be useful for establishing your diagnosis?

(A) CBC with differential count

(B) CT scan of the abdomen

(C) MRI of the sella turcica

(D) Test for serum 21-hydroxylase

(E) Test for serum androstenedione

7 A 35-year-old woman with a history of schizophrenia complains of headaches, visual disturbances, and irregular menses for 9 months. On physical examination the breasts are firm and tender. MRI shows enlargement of the anterior pituitary (arrow). Which of the following is the most likely cause of pituitary enlargement in this patient?

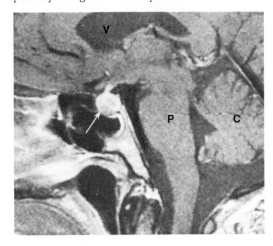

(A) Corticotrope adenoma

(B) Gonadotrope adenoma

(C) Lactotrope adenoma

(D) Null cell adenoma

(E) Somatotrope adenoma

8 A 55-year-old man complains of severe muscle weakness and drooping eyelids. He states that his symptoms worsen with repetitive movements but then resolve after a short rest. A chest X-ray reveals an anterior mediastinal mass. A biopsy of this mass would most likely reveal which of the following pathologic changes?

(A) B-cell lymphoma

(B) Hodgkin lymphoma

(C) Metastatic carcinoma

(D) Small cell carcinoma of the lung

(E) Thymic hyperplasia

9 A 45-year-old woman complains of tingling in her hands and feet, 24 hours after surgery to remove a thyroid follicular carcinoma. Her symptoms rapidly progress to severe muscle cramps, laryngeal stridor, and convulsions. Which of the following laboratory findings would be expected in this patient prior to treatment?

(A) Decreased serum calcium and decreased PTH

(B) Decreased serum calcium and increased PTH

(C) Increased serum calcium and decreased PTH

(D) Increased serum calcium and increased PTH

(E) Normal serum calcium and decreased PTH

10 A 55-year-old woman presents with a large anterior neck mass (patient shown in the image). She also complains of dysphagia and hoarseness. Physical examination reveals inspiratory stridor. Laboratory evaluation of this patient would most likely demonstrate which of the following?

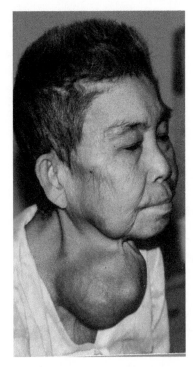

(A) Euthyroidism

(B) Hypercalcemia

(C) Hyperthyroidism

(D) Hypocalcemia

(E) Hypothyroidism

11 A 48-year-old man presents with recurrent headaches and arthritic pain in his knees of 9 months in duration. He notes that his hat size has recently increased. He also states that he suffers from erectile dysfunction. His past medical history is significant for kidney stones 2 years ago. Physical examination reveals a blood pressure of 170/100 mm Hg. The patient is observed to have coarse facial features and a goiter. Urinalysis reveals glucosuria and hypercalciuria. Which of the following is the most likely explanation for this patient's clinical presentation?

(A) Excess growth hormone secretion

(B) Excess parathyroid hormone secretion

(C) Excess prolactin secretion

(D) Hypersecretion of bone morphogenetic protein

(E) Insufficient growth hormone production

12 Why does the patient described in Question 11 suffer from erectile dysfunction?

(A) Excess cortisol secretion by the adrenal cortex

(B) Excess growth hormone secretion by the pituitary

(C) Excess prolactin secretion by the pituitary

(D) Insufficient cortisol secretion by the adrenal cortex

(E) Insufficient FSH secretion by the pituitary

13 Physical examination of a neonate shows peculiar genitalia (shown in the image). Cytogenetic studies reveal a 46, XX karyotype. Laboratory studies will most likely reveal a deficiency of which of the following?

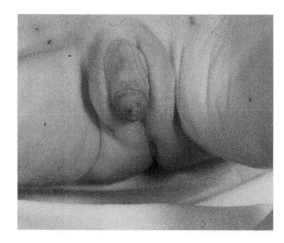

(A) Androstenedione
(B) Corticotropin
(C) 21-Hydroxylase
(D) Progesterone
(E) Prolactin

14 The infant described in Question 13 is shown to have an autosomal recessive genetic disorder. The infant is expected to manifest which of the following developmental anomalies?
(A) Adrenal hyperplasia
(B) Bladder diverticulum
(C) Cystic renal dysplasia
(D) Empty sella turcica
(E) Polycystic ovaries

15 A 7-week-old infant develops severe dehydration and hypotension and expires. The kidneys and adrenal glands at autopsy are shown in the image. Hypovolemic shock in this infant was most likely caused by inadequate synthesis of which of the following hormones?

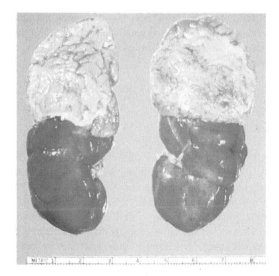

(A) Aldosterone
(B) Angiotensin
(C) Antidiuretic hormone
(D) Atrial natriuretic factor
(E) Renin

16 A 6-month-old girl with Wiskott-Aldrich syndrome is brought to the emergency room shortly after spiking a fever of 38.7°C (103°F). The infant has a history of chronic respiratory infections, gastrointestinal infections, petechiae, and eczema. This infant likely has which of the following associated birth defects?
(A) Adrenal cortical hyperplasia
(B) Cystic renal dysplasia
(C) Hypoplasia of thymus
(D) Meckel diverticulum
(E) Pituitary hypoplasia

17 A female neonate with DiGeorge syndrome develops severe muscle cramps and convulsions soon after birth. Which of the following is the cause of convulsions in this neonate?
(A) Acute hemorrhagic adrenalitis
(B) Hypocalcemia
(C) Hypoglycemia
(D) Hypokalemia
(E) Hyponatremia

18 In addition to parathyroid agenesis, the neonate described in Question 17 would be expected to have which of the following conditions?
(A) Adrenal hyperplasia
(B) Congenital goiter
(C) Extralobar sequestration of the lung
(D) Immune deficiency
(E) Pituitary hypoplasia

19 A 15-year-old boy with Albright hereditary osteodystrophy is rushed to the emergency room with severe muscle cramps and convulsions. The child has a history of mental retardation. Laboratory studies reveal hypocalcemia and elevated blood levels of PTH. Which of the following distinguishes this patient's endocrinopathy from hypoparathyroidism seen in DiGeorge syndrome?
(A) Abnormalities in cardiac conduction and contractility
(B) Accelerated degradation of PTH
(C) Decreased neuromuscular excitability
(D) End-organ unresponsiveness to PTH
(E) Increased neuromuscular excitability

20 A 50-year-old woman presents with acute right flank pain of 72 hours in duration. Physical examination is unremarkable. Her temperature is 37°C (98.6°F), blood pressure 140/85 mm Hg, and pulse 85 per minute. A CBC is normal. Urinalysis reveals hematuria and urine cultures are negative. Imaging studies show stones in the right renal pelvis and ureter. This patient's condition may be associated with which of the following endocrine disorders?
(A) Conn syndrome
(B) Cushing syndrome
(C) Hyperparathyroidism
(D) Hyperthyroidism
(E) Hypoparathyroidism

21 Laboratory evaluation of the patient described in Question 20 shows markedly elevated serum levels of calcium and PTH. A CT scan of the neck reveals a 3-cm mass on the posterior surface of the right lobe of the thyroid gland. External and cross-sectional views of the surgical specimen are shown in the image. Microscopic examination of this neck mass would most likely reveal a benign neoplasm derived from which of the following cells?

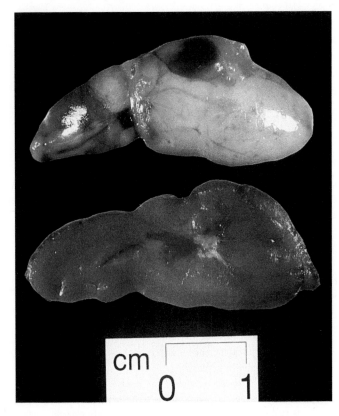

(A) Chief
(B) Clear
(C) Follicular
(D) Parafollicular
(E) Oxyphil

22 A 72-year-old woman with a long history of diabetes type 2 presents with abdominal pain. Physical examination reveals neuromuscular weakness and hypertension. Laboratory studies show markedly elevated levels of serum calcium and PTH. A surgical exploration of the patient's neck demonstrates four symmetrically enlarged parathyroid glands. This patient's endocrinopathy may be caused by which of the following underlying disorders?

(A) Adrenal insufficiency
(B) Chronic liver disease
(C) Insulin deficiency
(D) Pituitary adenoma
(E) Renal insufficiency

23 A 20-year-old woman with Hirschsprung disease presents with acute leg pain. The patient had a glioma resected 3 years ago. An X-ray film of the leg reveals a fracture of the left tibia. Laboratory studies show elevated serum levels of calcium and PTH. A CT scan of the patient's neck demonstrates a solitary parathyroid mass. Two years later, the patient presents with hypertension, and a CT scan of the abdomen displays a 4-cm mass in the right adrenal. Genetic studies conducted on this patient would likely reveal germline mutations in which of the following protooncogenes?

(A) BRCA1
(B) Rb
(C) RET
(D) VHL
(E) WT-1

24 A 40-year-old woman with a history of hyperparathyroidism presents with a 2-month history of burning epigastric pain. The pain can be relieved with antacids or food. The patient also reports a recent history of tarry stools. She denies taking aspirin or NSAIDs. Laboratory studies show a microcytic, hypochromic anemia (hemoglobin = 8.5 g/dL). Gastroscopy reveals a bleeding mucosal defect in the antrum. Which of the following best characterizes the pathogenesis of epigastric pain in this patient?

(A) Decreased calcium resorption by renal tubules
(B) Decreased serum levels of PTH
(C) Gastric nonresponsiveness to PTH
(D) Immunologic tolerance to H. pylori gastritis
(E) Increased secretion of gastrin

25 The parents of a 4-week-old girl complain that their baby is apathetic and sluggish. On physical examination, the child's abdomen is large and exhibits an umbilical hernia. The skin is pale and cold, and the temperature is 35°C (95°F). Which of the following provides a plausible explanation for the signs and symptoms of this child?

(A) Cystic fibrosis
(B) Muscular dystrophy
(C) Parathyroid hyperplasia
(D) Thyroid agenesis
(E) Vitamin D deficiency

26 A 55-year-old man who is on dialysis because of end-stage renal disease complains of pain in his jaw and left arm for 6 months. An X-ray of the left arm reveals multiple, small bone cysts and pathologic fractures. What is the appropriate diagnosis for this patient's bone lesions?

(A) Chronic osteomyelitis
(B) Marble bone disease
(C) Osteitis fibrosa cystica
(D) Osteoid osteoma
(E) Osteoporosis

27 A 46-year-old woman complains of increasing fatigue and muscle weakness over the past 6 months. She reports an inability to concentrate at work and speaks with a husky voice. The patient denies drug or alcohol abuse. Physical examination reveals cold and clammy skin, coarse and brittle hair, boggy face with puffy eyelids, and peripheral edema. There is no evidence of goiter or exophthalmos. Laboratory studies show reduced serum levels of T3 and T4. Which of the following is the most likely underlying cause of these signs and symptoms?

(A) Amyloidosis of the thyroid
(B) Autoimmune thyroiditis
(C) Thyroid follicular adenoma
(D) Multinodular goiter
(E) Papillary carcinoma of the thyroid

28 A 65-year-old woman with a history of multinodular goiter complains of increasing nervousness, insomnia, and heart palpitations. She has lost 9 kg (20 lb) over the past 6 months. Physical examination reveals a diffusely enlarged thyroid. There is no evidence of exophthalmos. Laboratory studies show elevated serum levels of T3 and T4. Serologic tests for antithyroid antibodies are negative. Which of the following is an important complication of this patient's endocrinopathy?

(A) Autoimmune hepatitis
(B) Cardiac arrhythmia
(C) Follicular carcinoma of the thyroid
(D) Medullary carcinoma of the thyroid
(E) Myxedema madness

29 A 40-year-old woman complains of chronic constipation and anovulatory cycles for the last 8 months. Her vital signs are normal. Physical examination reveals peripheral edema and a firm, diffusely enlarged thyroid gland. Serum levels of T3 and T4 are abnormally low. A thyroid biopsy is shown in the image. What is the appropriate diagnosis?

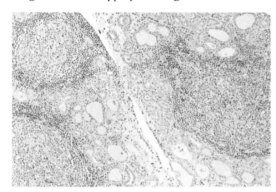

(A) Acute necrotizing thyroiditis
(B) Autoimmune thyroiditis
(C) Multinodular goiter
(D) Reidel thyroiditis
(E) Subacute (DeQuervain) thyroiditis

30 A 52-year-old woman complains of swelling in the anterior portion of her neck, which she first noticed 6 months ago. Except for some discomfort during swallowing, the patient does not report any significant symptoms. Physical examination reveals a symmetrically enlarged thyroid. A thyroid biopsy is shown in the image. Which of the following is the most likely diagnosis?

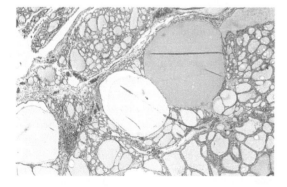

(A) Follicular adenoma
(B) Graves disease
(C) Hashimoto thyroiditis
(D) Nontoxic goiter
(E) Non-Hodgkin lymphoma

31 Five years later, the patient described in Question 30 returns with symptoms of hyperthyroidism. Which of the following best summarizes the clinical symptoms expected in this patient?

(A) Dry skin, hypogonadism, fatigability
(B) Hyperpigmentation, weakness, hypotension
(C) Nervousness, irritability, paresthesias, tetany
(D) Pale complexion, cold intolerance, lethargy
(E) Tremor, tachycardia, weight loss

32 A 32-year-old woman presents with a solitary, nontender, firm nodule on the left side of her neck. Thyroid function tests are within normal limits. A fine-needle biopsy reveals malignant cells. The tumor is excised and examined by light microscopy (shown in the image). What is the appropriate pathologic diagnosis?

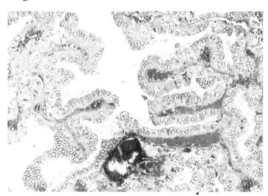

(A) Anaplastic carcinoma
(B) Follicular carcinoma
(C) Lymphoma
(D) Medullary carcinoma
(E) Papillary carcinoma

33 A 43-year-old woman complains of low-grade fever and has a 3-day history of pain in her neck. Physical examination reveals a slightly enlarged thyroid. A CBC is normal. A biopsy of the thyroid reveals granulomatous inflammation and the presence of giant cells (shown in the image). What is the appropriate diagnosis?

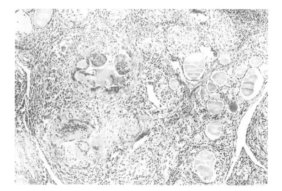

(A) Graves disease

(B) Hashimoto thyroiditis

(C) Lymphadenoid thyroiditis

(D) Nontoxic multinodular goiter

(E) Subacute (deQuervain) thyroiditis

34 A 33-year-old woman complains of swelling in the anterior portion of her neck, which she first noticed 8 months ago. Except for some discomfort during swallowing and hoarseness, the patient does not report any symptoms. Physical examination reveals a stony, hard thyroid gland that is adherent to other neck structures. A thyroid biopsy is shown in the image. The pathologist reports that the thyroid parenchyma is replaced by dense, hyalinized fibrous tissue and a chronic inflammatory infiltrate. What is the appropriate diagnosis?

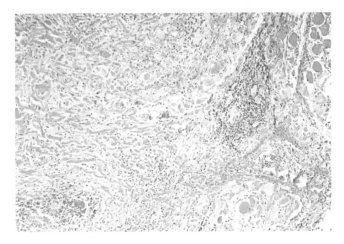

(A) Follicular adenoma

(B) Graves hyperthyroidism

(C) Multinodular goiter

(D) Papillary thyroid carcinoma

(E) Riedel thyroiditis

35 A 29-year-old woman complains of nervousness and muscle weakness of 6 months in duration. She is intolerant of heat and sweats excessively. She has lost 9 kg (20 lb) pounds over the past 6 months, despite increased caloric intake. She frequently finds her heart racing and can feel it pounding in her chest. She also states that she has missed several menstrual periods over the past few months. Physical examination reveals warm and moist skin and bulging eyes (exophthalmos). Laboratory studies will likely reveal which of the following endocrine abnormalities in this patient?

(A) Anti-thyroid DNA antibodies

(B) Anti-TSH receptor antibodies

(C) Decreased uptake of radioactive iodine in the thyroid

(D) Increased serum TSH

(E) Low serum T3

36 A thyroid biopsy obtained from the patient described in Question 35 is shown in the image. Which of the following best describes the pathologic findings?

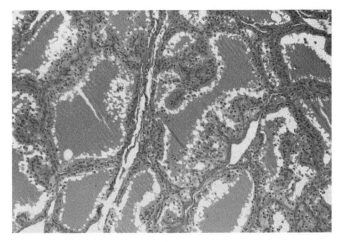

(A) Atrophy and fibrosis

(B) Dense lymphoid infiltrate with germinal centers

(C) Follicular hyperplasia with scalloping of colloid

(D) Necrotizing parenchymal granulomas

(E) Papillary hyperplasia with psammoma bodies

37 A 33-year-old woman presents with a swelling in her neck, which she first noticed 2 months ago. Physical examination reveals a solitary, nontender nodule of the thyroid gland measuring 2 cm in diameter. Thyroid function tests are within normal limits. The nodule does not accumulate ^{125}Iodine on thyroid scintiscan. A biopsy of the nodule is shown in the image. Which of the following is the most likely diagnosis?

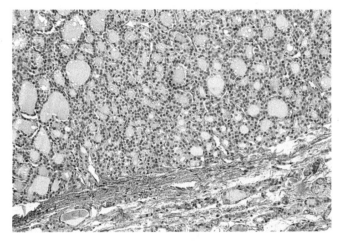

(A) Follicular adenoma

(B) Medullary thyroid carcinoma

(C) Metastatic carcinoma

(D) Multinodular goiter

(E) Papillary thyroid carcinoma

38 A 36-year-old woman presents with swelling in her neck that she first noticed 3 months ago. She also complains of intermittent watery diarrhea over the same time period. Physical examination reveals a nontender nodule in the left lobe of the thyroid. The patient's mother died of thyroid cancer 8 years ago. The thyroid nodule is found to be "cold" by radioiodine scintiscan. A needle biopsy of the nodule reveals malignant cells and homogeneous eosinophilic material (shown in the image). Laboratory studies would likely show elevated blood levels of which of the following hormones in this patient?

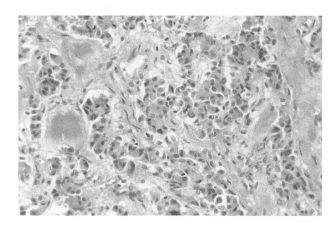

(A) Calcitonin
(B) Cortisol
(C) PTH
(D) T4
(E) TSH

39 The tumor in the patient described in Question 38 is removed, and a section stained with Congo red reveals birefringent amyloid stroma. Genetic studies show that this patient has a familial cancer syndrome. In addition to hyperparathyroidism, the patient is advised that she is at risk of developing which of the following neoplastic diseases?
(A) Craniopharyngioma
(B) Follicular adenoma of thyroid
(C) Neuroblastoma
(D) Pheochromocytoma
(E) Pituitary adenoma

40 A 45-year-old man presents with swelling in the anterior portion of his neck. Physical examination reveals an enlarged nodular thyroid. Thyroid function tests are within normal limits. A thyroid scintiscan shows a dominant "hot" nodule. A biopsy of this nodule reveals neoplastic cells with evidence of vascular and capsular invasion (shown in the image). X-rays demonstrate distant bony metastases. What is the most likely diagnosis?

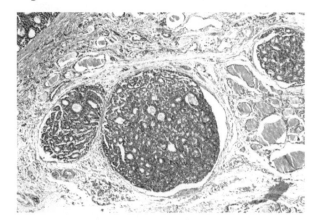

(A) Anaplastic carcinoma
(B) B-cell lymphoma
(C) Follicular carcinoma
(D) Medullary carcinoma
(E) Metastatic carcinoma

41 A 4-year-old girl is brought to the pediatric clinic by her mother who reports that her daughter has decreased appetite, lethargy, and an enlarging belly. Physical examination reveals a large, firm, irregular, nontender mass in the child's abdomen. A CT-guided biopsy reveals neoplastic "small blue cells." The child's malignant neoplasm is removed and the surgical specimen is shown in the image. Which of the following laboratory tests would be useful in monitoring this patient for recurrence of disease?

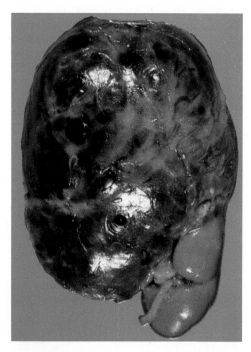

(A) Serum acetylcholine
(B) Serum α_1-antitrypsin
(C) Serum potassium
(D) Urinary angiotensin
(E) Urinary vanillylmandelic acid

42 Genetic analysis of tumor cells taken from the patient described in Question 41 may reveal which of the following mutations?
(A) C-*ras* amplification
(B) Deletion of c-*myc*
(C) N-*myc* amplification
(D) 8;21 chromosomal translocation
(E) 9;22 chromosomal translocation

43 A 45-year-old man with a recent history of bizarre behavior is seen by a psychiatrist, who recommends evaluation of his endocrine status. On physical examination, the patient appears moderately obese (BMI = 31 kg/m²), with mild hypertension, facial acne, fat accumulation in the supraclavicular fossae, and a protuberant abdomen. Laboratory studies demonstrate a neutrophilic leukocytosis, with a decrease in the percentage of lymphocytes and an absence of eosinophils. The hematocrit and hemoglobin are normal. There is a mild hypokalemia and mild metabolic alkalosis. The fasting serum glucose is within the reference range, but on a 2-hour glucose tolerance test, both the 60- and 120-minute samples had glucose concentrations greater than 200 mg/dL. Laboratory studies show free urinary cortisol of 156 mg per 24 hours (normal = 10 to

100 μg per 24 hours). Which of the following questions would be of most help in establishing a diagnosis?
(A) Are you experiencing muscle weakness?
(B) Are you experiencing shortness of breath?
(C) Are you receiving corticosteroids for some other disease?
(D) Do you have a family history of endocrine neoplasia?
(E) Have you received recent blood transfusions?

44 A 42-year-old woman presents with amenorrhea and emotional disturbances. You note upper truncal obesity and suspect Cushing syndrome. Laboratory studies reveal elevated serum levels of corticosteroids that can be lowered by administration of dexamethasone. Which of the following is the most likely cause of hypercortisolism in this patient?
(A) Adrenal cortical adenoma
(B) Adrenal cortical carcinoma
(C) Adrenal cortical hyperplasia
(D) Pheochromocytoma
(E) Pituitary adenoma

45 A 40-year-old woman with a history of diabetes complains of recent changes in her bodily appearance. A photograph of the patient is shown in the image. Laboratory studies reveal elevated serum corticosteroids and low serum corticotropin. Administration of dexamethasone does not lower serum levels of corticosteroids. This patient most likely has a tumor that originates in which of the following anatomic locations?

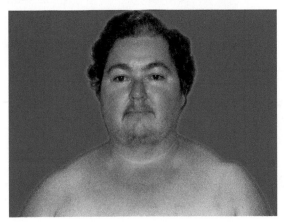

(A) Adrenal cortex, zona fasciculata
(B) Adrenal cortex, zona glomerulosa
(C) Adrenal cortex, zona reticularis
(D) Adrenal medulla
(E) Anterior pituitary

46 A 46-year-old woman with severe asthma presents with increasing weight and back pain for 9 months. The patient is taking corticosteroids for her asthma. An X-ray of the vertebrae will likely reveal which of the following pathologic findings?
(A) Bone infarct
(B) Dislocation
(C) Osteomalacia
(D) Osteomyelitis
(E) Osteoporosis

47 A 40-year-old man complains of nausea, vomiting, diarrhea, and cramping abdominal pain. His temperature is 38°C (101°F), blood pressure 90/60 mm Hg, and pulse rate 90 per minute. On physical examination, the patient appears dehydrated, with sunken eyeballs, dry tongue, and poor skin turgor. Hyperpigmentation is noted in the palmar creases and the gingival margins. Laboratory results include fasting serum glucose of 62 mg/dL (normal = 70 to 115 mg/dL), BUN of 27 mg/dL (normal = 11 to 23 mg/dL), Na of 122 mEq/L (normal = 136 to 145 mEq/L), and K of 6.5 mEq/L (normal = 3.5 to 5.0 mEq/L). Which of the following is the most likely cause of this patient's symptoms?
(A) Amyloidosis
(B) Autoimmunity
(C) Metastatic cancer
(D) Sarcoidosis
(E) Tuberculosis

48 A 50-year-old man complains of muscle weakness and dizziness of 3 months in duration. His blood pressure is 185/100 mm Hg. Laboratory studies show hypernatremia and hypokalemia. Endocrine studies reveal elevated serum aldosterone and low renin and angiotensin. BUN is 24 mg/dL, and creatinine is 1.2 mg/dL. Endocrinologic studies rule out Cushing syndrome. Which of the following is the most likely cause of hypertension in this patient?
(A) Adrenogenital syndrome
(B) Chronic adrenal failure
(C) Chronic renal failure
(D) Conn syndrome
(E) Pheochromocytoma

49 A 34-year-old man complains of sudden attacks of dizziness, blurred vision, and excruciating headaches of 4 months in duration. During one of these attacks, his blood pressure was 180/120 mm Hg. The patient's father had been treated for thyroid cancer about 15 years ago. Laboratory studies show normal serum levels of aldosterone, renin, and angiotensin. A 24-hour urinalysis reveals increased metanephrines. Episodic hypertension in this patient is most likely caused by a tumor in which of the following endocrine organs?
(A) Adrenal
(B) Kidney
(C) Parathyroid
(D) Pituitary
(E) Thyroid

ANSWERS

1 **The answer is A: Craniopharyngioma.** Central diabetes insipidus is characterized by an inability to concentrate the urine, with consequent chronic water diuresis, thirst, and polydipsia. The disease reflects a deficiency of antidiuretic hormone (ADH, arginine vasopressin), which is secreted by the posterior pituitary under the influence of the hypothalamus. One fourth of cases of central diabetes insipidus are associated with brain tumors, particularly craniopharyngioma. This tumor arises above the sella turcica from remnants of Rathke pouch and invades and compresses adjacent tissues. Destruction of the posterior lobe of the pituitary, the source of ADH, causes polyuria and diabetes insipidus. This coronal section of the brain shows a large cystic tumor mass replacing the midline structures in the region of the hypothalamus. The other choices do not occur in this location and are rarely associated with central diabetes insipidus.

Diagnosis: Craniopharyngioma, diabetes insipidus

2 The answer is E: Syndrome of inappropriate ADH secretion. The inappropriate production of ADH by a tumor may cause a paraneoplastic syndrome that features water retention, which is manifested as water intoxication with hyponatremia, resulting in altered mental status, seizures, coma, and sometimes death. This syndrome is most often related to small cell carcinoma of the lung. It is also reported with carcinomas of the prostate, gastrointestinal tract, and pancreas and with thymomas, lymphomas, and Hodgkin disease. Diabetes mellitus (choice B) may cause polyuria but features glucosuria and does not cause severe hyponatremia. Sheehan syndrome (choice D) refers to hypopituitarism caused by infarction of the anterior pituitary.

Diagnosis: Syndrome of inappropriate ADH secretion

3 The answer is B: Corticotropin. This patient most likely has a paraneoplastic condition associated with a corticotropin (ACTH)-producing small cell carcinoma of the lung. The major clinical manifestations of hypercortisolism in patients with Cushing syndrome include emotional disturbances, moon facies, osteoporosis, hypertension, upper truncal obesity (buffalo hump), amenorrhea, muscle weakness, thin wrinkled skin, purpura, glucose intolerance, poor wound healing and skin ulcers. None of the other hormones are associated with Cushing syndrome.

Diagnosis: Cushing syndrome, paraneoplastic syndrome

4 The answer is C: Infarction of the pituitary. This patient experienced postpartum ischemic necrosis of the pituitary (Sheehan syndrome). This commonly, but not exclusively, occurs after severe hypotension induced by postpartum hemorrhage. The pituitary is particularly susceptible at this time because its enlargement during pregnancy renders it vulnerable to a reduction in blood flow. Major clinical manifestations of panhypopituitarism include pallor (decreased MSH), hypothyroidism (decreased TSH), failure of lactation (decreased prolactin), adrenal insufficiency, and ovarian failure (decreased FSH and LH). None of the other choices lead to this constellation of hormone deficiencies.

Diagnosis: Sheehan syndrome

5 The answer is D: Neurohypophysis. Central diabetes insipidus may be caused by head trauma that damages the posterior lobe of the pituitary (neurohypophysis) and interrupts the secretion of ADH. One fourth of cases of central diabetes insipidus are associated with brain tumors, particularly craniopharyngioma. The other choices do not involve areas of the brain that secrete ADH. The anterior pituitary (adenohypophysis, choice A) does not secrete ADH.

Diagnosis: Diabetes insipidus

6 The answer is C: MRI of the sella turcica. This patient has clinical features of a pituitary adenoma with acromegaly. Pituitary adenomas range from small lesions that do not enlarge the gland to expansive tumors that erode the sella turcica and impinge on adjacent cranial structures. Adenomas smaller than 10 mm in diameter are referred to as microadenomas, and larger ones are termed macroadenomas. Microadenomas do not produce symptoms unless they secrete hormones. The mass effects of pituitary macroadenomas include impingement on the optic chiasm, often with bitemporal hemianopsia and loss of central vision, oculomotor palsies when the tumor invades the cavernous sinuses, and severe headaches. Large adenomas may invade the hypothalamus and lead to loss of temperature regulation, hyperphagia, and hormonal syndromes because they interfere with the normal hypothalamic input to the pituitary. Symptoms of acromegaly include characteristic facial changes, goiter, barrel chest, abnormal glucose tolerance, male sexual dysfunction, menstrual disorders in women, degenerative arthritis, peripheral neuropathy, and thickened skin. The other choices represent tests that will not provide the diagnosis of pituitary tumor.

Diagnosis: Acromegaly, pituitary adenoma

7 The answer is C: Lactotrope adenoma. Pituitary adenomas are benign neoplasms of the anterior lobe of the pituitary and are often associated with excess secretion of pituitary hormones and evidence of corresponding endocrine hyperfunction. They occur in both sexes at almost any age but are more common in men between the ages of 20 to 50 years. Hyperprolactinemia is the most common endocrinopathy associated with pituitary adenoma. Almost half of all pituitary microadenomas synthesize prolactin. Functional lactotrope adenomas lead to amenorrhea, galactorrhea, and infertility. None of the other pituitary tumors produce prolactin or lead to inappropriate lactation.

Diagnosis: Galactorrhea, pituitary adenoma

8 The answer is E: Thymic hyperplasia. Myasthenia gravis is an acquired autoimmune disease characterized by abnormal muscular fatigability and is caused by circulating antibodies to the acetylcholine receptor at the myoneural junction. In two thirds of patients, thymic hyperplasia is closely associated with myasthenia gravis, and 15% have thymoma. Conversely, one third to one half of patients with thymoma develop myasthenia gravis. Thymectomy is often an effective treatment for these patients. None of the other choices are associated with myasthenia gravis, although paraneoplastic muscle weakness can occur.

Diagnosis: Myasthenia gravis

9 The answer is A: Decreased serum calcium and decreased PTH. The most common cause of hypoparathyroidism is surgical resection of the parathyroids as a complication of thyroidectomy. Of patients undergoing surgery for primary hyperparathyroidism, 1% develop irreversible hypoparathyroidism. The symptoms of hypoparathyroidism relate to hypocalcemia, which causes increased neuromuscular excitability. This is reflected in symptoms that range from mild tingling in the hands and feet to severe muscle cramps, laryngeal stridor, and convulsions. Neuropsychiatric manifestations include depression, paranoia, and psychoses. Increased PTH in the setting of parathyroid adenoma or a paraneoplastic syndrome is associated with hypercalcemia (choice D).

Diagnosis: Hypoparathyroidism

10 The answer is A: Euthyroidism. Nontoxic goiter (also termed simple, colloid, or multinodular goiter) refers to an enlargement of the thyroid that is not associated with functional, inflammatory, or neoplastic alterations. Patients with nontoxic goiter are neither hyperthyroid nor hypothyroid and do not suffer from any form of thyroiditis. Large goiters may cause dysphagia or inspiratory stridor by compressing the esophagus or trachea. Hoarseness may result from recurrent laryngeal nerve compression. The disease is far more common in women than in men (8:1). A number of drugs and naturally occurring chemicals in foods are goitrogenic due to their suppression of thyroid hormone synthesis. The most commonly used goitrogenic drug is lithium, which is used in the management of manic-depressive states. Endemic goiter refers to the goitrous hypothyroidism of dietary iodine deficiency in locales with a high prevalence of the disease. Without sufficient iodine, thyroid hormones are not produced and the pituitary continuously secretes thyroid stimulating hormone.
Diagnosis: Nontoxic goiter

11 The answer is A: Excess growth hormone secretion. Acromegaly refers to enlargement of the terminal portions of the extremities and the jaw and is caused by growth hormone–secreting tumors of the pituitary (somatotrope adenomas). The pituitary tumor may lead to headaches and may compress the optic chiasm. These patients also have other hormonal problems, such as menstrual irregularities in women and diabetes mellitus. The excess secretion of growth hormone produces dramatic bodily changes. A somatotrope adenoma that arises in a child or adolescent before the epiphyses close results in gigantism. By contrast, after the epiphyses of the long bones have fused and adult height has been achieved, the same tumor produces enlargement of the skull (acromegaly). Most acromegalics suffer from neurologic and musculoskeletal symptoms. One third have hypertension. Diabetes occurs in as many as 20% of these patients, and hypercalciuria and renal stones are present in another fifth of the patients. None of the other choices present this wide variety of signs and symptoms.
Diagnosis: Acromegaly

12 The answer is C: Excess prolactin secretion by the pituitary. In mixed somatotroph-lactotroph adenomas the two cells types elaborate growth hormone and prolactin, respectively. In half of patients with acromegaly, hyperprolactinemia is severe enough to be symptomatic, causing loss of libido and erectile dysfunction in men. Functional lactotroph microadenomas are successfully treated with dopamine agonists (bromocriptine) to inhibit prolactin secretion. Insufficient FSH secretion by the pituitary (choice E) would inhibit spermatogenesis, but would not affect testosterone production by Leydig cells. The other choices do not halt the production of androgens that are involved in male sexual function.
Diagnosis: Acromegaly

13 The answer is C: 21-Hydroxylase. Congenital deficiency of 21-hydroxylase results in adrenogenital syndrome, which is associated with virilization of external genitalia in female infants (pseudohermaphroditism). The photograph shows a markedly virilized and hypertrophic clitoris and partial fusion of labioscrotal folds in a genetic female. The extent of the biochemical defect is highly variable, ranging from mild to complete deficiency. Male infants show normal external genitalia. Levels of adrenal androgens (choice A) and progesterone (choice D) increase in this disorder.
Diagnosis: Congenital adrenal hyperplasia, adrenogenital syndrome

14 The answer is A: Adrenal hyperplasia. Congenital adrenal hyperplasia (CAH) is a syndrome that results from a number of autosomal recessive, enzymatic defects in the biosynthesis of cortisol from cholesterol. CAH is the most common cause of ambiguous genitalia in newborn girls. Most cases of CAH (>90%) represent an inborn deficiency of 21-hydroxylase, more specifically termed P450C21. Deficiency in the synthesis of corticosteroids in the adrenal cortex results in the continuous secretion of ACTH by the anterior pituitary, resulting in congenital adrenal hyperplasia. The adrenal glands are greatly enlarged, weighing as much as 30 g (normal = 4 g). Polycystic ovary syndrome (choice E) occurs in adult women.
Diagnosis: Congenital adrenal hyperplasia, adrenogenital syndrome

15 The answer is A: Aldosterone. The autopsy specimen shows massive bilateral adrenal enlargement characteristic of congenital adrenal hyperplasia (CAH). Congenital 21-hydroxylase deficiencies may be associated with impaired aldosterone synthesis (salt-wasting CAH). Hypoaldosteronism develops within the first few weeks of life in two thirds of newborns with congenital adrenal hyperplasia, who suffer dehydration and hypotension. Laboratory studies in these neonates show hyponatremia, hyperkalemia, and increased renin secretion (choice E).
Diagnosis: Congenital 21-hydroxylase deficiency

16 The answer is C: Hypoplasia of thymus. Wiskott-Aldrich syndrome is a sex-linked, hereditary disease in which severe immunodeficiency is associated with a hypoplastic thymus, eczema, and thrombocytopenia. Alterations in the thymus vary from complete absence (agenesis) or severe hypoplasia to a situation in which the thymus is small but exhibits a normal architecture. Some small glands exhibit thymic dysplasia, characterized by an absence of thymocytes, few, if any, Hassall corpuscles, and only epithelial components. The other choices do not involve the immune system.
Diagnosis: Wiskott-Aldrich syndrome

17 The answer is B: Hypocalcemia. DiGeorge syndrome is caused by a failure in the development of the third and fourth branchial pouches, resulting in agenesis or hypoplasia of the thymus and parathyroid glands, congenital heart defects, dysmorphic facies, and a variety of other congenital anomalies. As a result of parathyroid agenesis, patients with DiGeorge syndrome exhibit hypocalcemia, which manifests as increased neuromuscular excitability. Symptoms range from mild tingling in the hands and feet to severe muscle cramps and convulsions. DiGeorge syndrome does not feature any of the other choices.
Diagnosis: DiGeorge syndrome

18 The answer is D: Immune deficiency. Thymic aplasia in patients with DiGeorge syndrome results in a congenital immune deficiency syndrome characterized by the loss of T cells. As a result, patients exhibit a deficiency of cell-mediated immunity, with a particular susceptibility to *Candida* sp. infections. None of the other choices are associated with DiGeorge syndrome.

Diagnosis: DiGeorge syndrome

19 The answer is D: End-organ unresponsiveness to PTH. Pseudohypoparathyroidism designates a group of hereditary conditions in which hypocalcemia is caused by target organ insensitivity to PTH. The defect in these patients has been traced to mutations in a gene whose product couples hormone receptors to the stimulation of adenylyl cyclase. Consequently, in the renal tubular epithelium, the production of cAMP in response to PTH is impaired, and inadequate resorption of calcium from the glomerular filtrate ensues. These patients demonstrate a characteristic phenotype (Albright hereditary osteodystrophy), including short stature, obesity, mental retardation, subcutaneous calcification, and a number of congenital anomalies of bone. Abnormalities in cardiac conduction (choice A) and increased neuromuscular excitability (choice E) are related to hypocalcemia.

Diagnosis: Pseudohypoparathyroidism, Albright hereditary osteodystrophy

20 The answer is C: Hyperparathyroidism. Primary hyperparathyroidism refers to the syndrome caused by excessive secretion of PTH by a parathyroid adenoma, primary hyperplasia of all parathyroids, or parathyroid carcinoma. Excessive PTH leads to excessive loss of calcium from the bones and enhanced calcium resorption by the renal tubules. The clinical manifestations of primary hyperparathyroidism range from asymptomatic hypercalcemia detected on routine blood analysis to florid systemic renal and skeletal disease. Hypercalcemia and hypophosphatemia lead to an increased risk of urolithiasis. Hyperparathyroidism is often accompanied by mental changes, including depression, emotional liability, poor mentation, and memory defects. The other choices are not associated with hypercalcemia or the formation of renal calculi.

Diagnosis: Urolithiasis, hyperparathyroidism

21 The answer is A: Chief. Parathyroid adenoma is the cause of 85% of all cases of primary hyperparathyroidism. The tumor arises sporadically or in the context of multiple endocrine neoplasia (MEN-1 and MEN-2A, 20% of cases). In a small minority of cases of sporadic adenoma, genetic analysis has identified rearrangement and overexpression of the cyclin D protooncogene. On gross examination, a parathyroid adenoma appears as a circumscribed, reddish brown, solitary mass, measuring 1 to 3 cm in diameter. Microscopically, these tumors show sheets of neoplastic chief cells in a rich capillary network. A rim of normal parathyroid tissue is usually evident outside the tumor capsule and distinguishes adenoma from parathyroid hyperplasia. None of the other cells secretes PTH.

Diagnosis: Hyperparathyroidism, parathyroid adenoma

22 The answer is E: Renal insufficiency. Hyperparathyroidism can be primary as a result of autonomous proliferation of chief cells or may be secondary, in which case it is a compensatory mechanism. Secondary parathyroid hyperplasia is encountered principally in patients with chronic renal failure, although the disorder also occurs in association with vitamin D deficiency, intestinal malabsorption, Fanconi syndrome, and renal tubular acidosis. Diabetic glomerulosclerosis

is a major cause of renal insufficiency. Chronic hypocalcemia due to renal retention of phosphate leads to compensatory hypersecretion of PTH. As a result, secondary hyperplasia of all parathyroid glands occurs. Enlarged parathyroid glands occasionally become independently hyperfunctional. None of the other choices are associated with hypocalcemia or secondary parathyroid hyperplasia.

Diagnosis: Hyperparathyroidism

23 The answer is C: *RET.* Patients with multiple endocrine neoplasia (MEN) syndromes types 1 and 2 have gene mutations that make them susceptible to neoplasia or hyperplasia in multiple organs. Patients with MEN-2A (Sipple syndrome) have C-cell–derived medullary thyroid carcinoma and chromaffin cell–derived pheochromocytoma. One third of patients exhibit hyperparathyroidism as a result of parathyroid hyperplasia or adenoma. Hirschsprung disease (congenital megacolon) and a variety of neural crest tumors (e.g., glioma) are also seen in patients with MEN-2A. Mutations of the *RET* protooncogene, a transmembrane receptor of the tyrosine kinase family, are responsible for MEN-2 syndromes. MEN-1 (Wermer syndrome) comprises adenoma of the pituitary, parathyroid hyperplasia or adenoma, and islet cell tumors of the pancreas (insulinoma and gastrinoma). MEN-1 is caused by mutation of the *MEN1* tumor suppressor gene. The other choices are not associated with endocrine syndromes.

Diagnosis: Parathyroid adenoma, multiple endocrine neoplasia

24 The answer is E: Increased secretion of gastrin. The incidence of peptic ulcer disease is increased in patients with hyperparathyroidism, possibly because hypercalcemia increases serum gastrin, thereby stimulating gastric acid secretion. Peptic ulcers in the context of MEN-1 may be secondary to Zollinger-Ellison syndrome (i.e., gastrinoma of the endocrine pancreas). None of the other choices are associated with gastric ulcers.

Diagnosis: Peptic ulcer disease, hyperparathyroidism

25 The answer is D: Thyroid agenesis. Cretinism denotes physical and mental insufficiency that is secondary to congenital hypothyroidism. Cretinism may be endemic, sporadic, or familial and is twice as frequent in girls as in boys. Iodination of salt has reduced the incidence of cretinism in the United States and other countries. The most common cause of neonatal hypothyroidism today is agenesis of the thyroid, which occurs at a rate of 1 in 4,000 newborns. Hypothyroidism in pregnant women also has grave neurologic consequences for the fetus, expressed after birth as cretinism. Symptoms of congenital hypothyroidism appear in the early weeks of life and include sluggishness, a large abdomen often with umbilical herniation, low body temperature, and refractory anemia. Mental retardation, stunted growth, and characteristic facies become evident. If thyroid hormone replacement therapy is not promptly provided, congenital hypothyroidism results in mentally retarded dwarfs. None of the other choices produces the listed signs and symptoms at such an early age.

Diagnosis: Congenital hypothyroidism

26 The answer is C: Osteitis fibrosa cystica. Secondary hyperparathyroidism is a complication of chronic renal insufficiency due to renal retention of phosphate and resulting hypocalcemia. Excess PTH causes renal osteodystrophy or, in severe cases, osteitis fibrosa cystica. The latter is characterized by severe bone deformities and the formation of "brown tumors" of hyperparathyroidism. Patients present with bone pain, bone cysts, pathologic fractures, and localized bone swellings (brown tumors). The other choices are not related to hypocalcemia or hyperparathyroidism.

Diagnosis: Osteitis cystica fibrosa, hyperparathyroidism

27 The answer is B: Autoimmune thyroiditis. Hypothyroidism refers to the clinical manifestations of thyroid hormone deficiency. It can be the consequence of three general processes: (1) defective synthesis of thyroid hormone; (2) inadequate function of thyroid parenchyma; and (3) inadequate secretion of TSH. Dominant clinical manifestations of hypothyroidism include muscular weakness, peripheral edema, "myxedema madness," pallor, and enlarged tongue. Women with hypothyroidism suffer ovulatory failure, progesterone deficiency, and irregular and excessive menstrual bleeding. Erectile dysfunction and oligospermia are common symptoms of hypothyroidism in men. Primary (idiopathic) hypothyroidism is often autoimmune. Three fourths of patients with primary hypothyroidism have circulating antibodies to thyroid antigens, suggesting that these cases represent the end stage of autoimmune thyroiditis. Nongoitrous hypothyroidism may also result from antibodies that block TSH itself or the TSH receptor, without activating the thyroid. Some cases of primary hypothyroidism are part of multiglandular autoimmune syndrome. The other choices present with either an enlarged thyroid or a mass and rarely present with hypothyroidism. Hypothyroidism secondary to amyloidosis of the thyroid (choice A) is rare.

Diagnosis: Hypothyroidism

28 The answer is B: Cardiac arrhythmia. Hyperthyroidism refers to the clinical consequences of an excessive amount of circulating thyroid hormone. The principal metabolic products of the thyroid gland are triiodothyronine (T3) and tetraiodothyronine (thyroxine; T4). T4 is principally a prohormone; the major effector of thyroid function is T3. These molecules are formed by the iodination of tyrosine residues of thyroglobulin within the follicular cells. Iodinated thyroglobulin is then secreted into the lumen of the follicle. Many patients with nontoxic goiter, usually over the age of 50 years, eventually develop a toxic form of the disease. Since patients with toxic goiter tend to be older, cardiac complications, including atrial fibrillation and congestive heart failure, dominate the clinical presentation.

Diagnosis: Hyperthyroidism, toxic goiter

29 The answer is B: Autoimmune thyroiditis. Chronic autoimmune thyroiditis (Hashimoto thyroiditis) is a common cause of goitrous hypothyroidism. The disease is characterized by the presence of circulating antibodies to thyroid antigens and features of cell-mediated immunity to thyroid tissue. The disorder arises most commonly in the fourth and fifth decades, and women are six times more likely to be affected than men. On gross examination, the gland in patients with Hashimoto thyroiditis is diffusely enlarged and firm, weighing 60 to 200 g. The cut surface is pale tan and fleshy and exhibits a vaguely nodular pattern. Microscopically, the thyroid displays (1) a conspicuous infiltrate of lymphocytes and plasma cells, (2) destruction and atrophy of the follicles, and (3) oxyphilic metaplasia of the follicular epithelial cells (Hürthle or Aska-

nazy cells). The inflammatory infiltrates are focally arranged in lymphoid follicles, often with germinal centers (see photomicrograph). Choice A (acute necrotizing thyroiditis) has the appearance of an infection, whereas choice C (multinodular goiter) is characterized by a nodular gland without significant inflammation. Choice D (Reidel thyroiditis) is a fibrosing condition and choice E (subacute [DeQuervain] thyroiditis) features multinucleated giant cells.

Diagnosis: Hashimoto thyroiditis, autoimmune thyroiditis

30 The answer is D: Nontoxic goiter. Nontoxic goiters range from double the size of a normal gland (40 g) to massive thyroid weighing hundreds of grams. Microscopically, nontoxic goiter exhibits hypertrophy and hyperplasia. There is marked variation in size of the follicles (see photomicrograph), fibrosis, and evidence of old hemorrhage. The diffuse form is frequent in adolescence and during pregnancy, whereas the multinodular type usually occurs in persons older than 50 years of age. Hashimoto thyroiditis (choice C) features lymphocytic infiltrates. Graves disease (choice B) demonstrates a hyperplastic and vascular thyroid.

Diagnosis: Nontoxic goiter, multinodular goiter

31 The answer is E: Tremor, tachycardia, weight loss. Some patients with nontoxic goiter, usually over the age of 50 years, eventually develop hyperthyroidism, in which case the term toxic multinodular goiter is applied. Hyperthyroidism gives rise to tremors, tachycardia, heat intolerance, and weight loss. Women may experience oligomenorrhea. The symptoms of toxic goiter are less severe than those associated with Graves disease, and patients do not develop exophthalmos. Because patients with toxic goiter tend to be older, cardiac complications are common. The other choices, which include symptoms such as hypogonadism (choice A), hyperpigmentation (choice B), tetany (choice C), and lethargy (choice D), are encountered in other endocrinopathies.

Diagnosis: Toxic goiter

32 The answer is E: Papillary carcinoma. Although thyroid nodules are found in up to 10% of the population, malignant tumors of the thyroid account for only about 1% of all cancers. Papillary carcinoma of the thyroid is the most common thyroid tumor in younger women. It has a tendency to metastasize to regional lymph nodes, but distant metastases are rare. The tumor is usually cured by surgery. As illustrated in this case, papillary carcinoma of the thyroid shows branching papillae lined by epithelial cells with clear (ground glass or Orphan Annie) nuclei and fibrovascular cores. A calcospherites (psammoma body) is also evident. These structures are virtually diagnostic of papillary thyroid carcinoma. Psammoma bodies are not a feature of the other choices.

Diagnosis: Papillary carcinoma of the thyroid

33 The answer is E: Subacute (DeQuervain) thyroiditis. Subacute thyroiditis (deQuervain, granulomatous, or giant-cell thyroiditis) is caused by a viral infection. It is an infrequent, self-limited disorder of the thyroid characterized by granulomatous inflammation. The disease typically occurs after upper respiratory tract infections, including those caused by influenza virus, adenovirus, echovirus, and coxsackievirus. The thyroid gland is enlarged to 40 to 60 g, and the cut surface is firm and pale. Initially, microscopic examination reveals an acute inflammation, often with microabscesses. This is followed by the appearance of a patchy infiltrate of lymphocytes, plasma cells, and macrophages throughout the thyroid. Destruction of follicles allows the release of colloid, which elicits a conspicuous granulomatous reaction. The other choices do not feature a granulomatous reaction.

Diagnosis: Subacute (DeQuervain) thyroiditis

34   **The answer is E: Riedel thyroiditis.**   The term thyroiditis in Riedel thyroiditis is something of a misnomer because this rare disease also affects soft tissues of the neck and is often associated with progressive fibrosis in other locations, including the retroperitoneum, mediastinum, and orbit. On gross examination, part or all of the thyroid is stony hard and is described as "woody." In most instances, the process is asymmetric and often affects only one lobe. Patients with Riedel thyroiditis notice the gradual onset of a painless goiter. Subsequently, they may suffer from the consequences of compression of the trachea (stridor), esophagus (dysphagia), and recurrent laryngeal nerve (hoarseness). The other choices do not feature extensive fibrosis.

Diagnosis: Riedel thyroiditis

35   **The answer is B: Anti-TSH receptor antibodies.**   Graves disease is the most frequent cause of hyperthyroidism in young adults. It is an autoimmune disorder characterized by diffuse goiter, hyperthyroidism, and exophthalmos. The disorder is the most prevalent autoimmune disease in the United States, affecting 0.5% to 1% of the population under 40 years of age, and is seven to ten times more frequent in women than in men. Patients with Graves disease are hyperthyroid due to the presence of stimulating IgG antibodies that bind to the TSH receptor expressed on the plasma membrane of thyrocytes. Patients note the gradual onset of nonspecific symptoms, such as nervousness, emotional lability, tremor, weakness, and weight loss. They are intolerant of heat, seek cooler environments, tend to sweat profusely, and may report heart palpitations. Anti-thyroid DNA antibodies (choice A) are not common in patients with Graves disease, and the thyroid shows *increased* uptake of radioactive iodine (see choice C). Serum levels of TSH are *low* (see choice D) and serum levels of T3 and T4 are *high* (see choice E).

Diagnosis: Graves disease

36   **The answer is C: Follicular hyperplasia with scalloping of colloid.**   In Graves disease, the follicles are lined by hyperplastic, tall columnar cells. Colloid is pink and scalloped at the periphery adjacent to the follicular cells. None of the other choices would appear in biopsy.

Diagnosis: Graves disease

37   **The answer is A: Follicular adenoma.**   A single, well-circumscribed, thyroid nodule in a young patient most likely represents a follicular adenoma, which refers to a benign neoplasm that exhibits follicular differentiation. It is the most common tumor of the thyroid and typically presents in euthyroid persons as a solitary "cold" nodule (i.e., a tumor that does not take up radiolabeled iodine). Follicular adenoma is an encapsulated neoplasm in which the cells are arranged in follicles resembling normal thyroid tissue. The other choices do not typically present as an isolated small nodule, but a biopsy

is necessary to rule out other causes. In this case, the biopsy demonstrates a benign proliferation of thyroid follicles.

Diagnosis: Follicular adenoma of the thyroid

38   **The answer is A: Calcitonin.**   Medullary thyroid carcinoma (MTC) is derived from C cells of the thyroid, which secrete the calcium-lowering hormone calcitonin. The disease represents fewer than 5% of all thyroid cancers, although the incidence is considerably higher in familial forms (e.g., MEN-2). MTC is characteristically solid and composed of polygonal, granular cells that are separated by a distinctly vascular stroma. A conspicuous feature is the presence of stromal amyloid, representing the deposition of procalcitonin. This material is eosinophilic with the hematoxylin and eosin stain and takes up the Congo red stain. MTC extends by direct invasion into soft tissues and metastasizes to the regional lymph nodes and distant organs. Patients with MTC often suffer a number of symptoms related to endocrine secretion, including carcinoid syndrome (serotonin) and Cushing syndrome (ACTH). Watery diarrhea in one third of patients is caused by the secretion of vasoactive intestinal peptide. T4 (choice D) is incorrect because the tumor does not cause hyperthyroidism and TSH (choice E) is normal because the remaining thyroid produces adequate thyroid hormone. Choices B and C (cortisol and PTH) are not thyroid hormones.

Diagnosis: Medullary carcinoma of the thyroid

39   **The answer is D: Pheochromocytoma.**   Patients with the familial form of medullary carcinoma are often affected with MEN-2, which includes pheochromocytoma of the adrenal medulla and parathyroid hyperplasia or adenoma. Somatic mutations of the *RET* protooncogene are found in patients with MEN-2A, and *RET* mutations have been detected in 25% to 70% of cases of sporadic medullary thyroid carcinoma. None of the other choices are encountered in patients with MEN-2.

Diagnosis: Multiple endocrine neoplasia

40   **The answer is C: Follicular carcinoma.**   Follicular thyroid carcinoma (FTC) is purely follicular and does not contain any papillary or other elements. Minimally invasive FTC is seen grossly as a well-defined, encapsulated tumor, which on cut section is soft and pale tan and bulges from the confines of its capsule. Microscopically, most lesions resemble follicular adenoma, although they tend more to a microfollicular or trabecular pattern. Anaplastic carcinoma of the thyroid (choice A) manifests as large masses of the gland that are poorly circumscribed and frequently extend into the soft tissues of the neck.

Diagnosis: Follicular carcinoma of the thyroid

41   **The answer is E: Urinary vanillylmandelic acid.**   Neuroblastoma is a malignant tumor of neural crest origin that is composed of neoplastic neuroblasts, and originates in the adrenal medulla or sympathetic ganglia (note the suprarenal location of the tumor). The neuroblast is derived from primitive sympathogonia and represents an intermediate stage in the development of the sympathetic ganglion neurons. On histologic examination, pseudorosettes, featuring tumor cells clustered radially around small vessels, are present. Tumor cells, like their more mature descendants in the adrenal medulla, may secrete catecholamines. These compounds are metabolized and excreted as urinary vanillylmandelic acid in the urine. Neuroblastoma is one of the most important malignant tumors of childhood, accounting for up to 10% of all childhood cancers and 15% of cancer deaths among children. The overall incidence is 1 in 7,000. The peak incidence is in the first 3 years of life. The other choices do not serve as markers for neuroblastoma or other childhood malignancies.

Diagnosis: Neuroblastoma

42 **The answer is C: N-*myc* amplification.** Neuroblastoma is characterized by extrachromosomal double minutes, and homogeneously staining regions (HSRs) are found on chromosome 2 in 30% of cases. These HSRs represent amplification of N-*myc*, an abnormality that plays a key role in determining the aggressiveness of neuroblastoma. The other genetic abnormalities are not characteristic of neuroblastoma.

Diagnosis: Neuroblastoma

43 **The answer is C: Are you receiving corticosteroids for some other disease?** The clinical features of hypercortisolism from any cause are referred to as Cushing syndrome, and the term Cushing disease is reserved for excessive secretion of corticotropin by pituitary corticotrope tumors. The most common cause of Cushing syndrome in the United States is chronic administration of corticosteroids in the treatment of immunologic and inflammatory disorders. Major clinical manifestations of Cushing syndrome include emotional disturbance, moon facies, osteoporosis, upper truncal obesity, thin and wrinkled skin, amenorrhea, muscle weakness, purpura, and skin ulcers. Half of patients exhibit absolute lymphopenia. These clinical manifestations depend on the degree and duration of excessive corticosteroid levels, as well as on the levels of adrenal androgens and mineralocorticoids. Muscle weakness (choice A) is a feature of Cushing syndrome but is nonspecific.

Diagnosis: Cushing syndrome

44 **The answer is E: Pituitary adenoma.** Cushing disease is caused by pituitary tumors that secrete ACTH and result in adrenal hyperfunction. It is five times more frequent than the type of Cushing syndrome associated with adrenal tumors. The dexamethasone suppression test is used to distinguish between ACTH-dependent and ACTH-independent forms of Cushing syndrome. Dexamethasone suppresses pituitary secretion of corticotropin and, hence, hypercortisolism, whereas it is without effect in cases of adrenal hyperplasia or functional adrenal tumors. Thus, the dexamethasone suppression test can be used to distinguish between ACTH-dependent and ACTH-independent forms of Cushing syndrome. Adrenal cortical carcinoma (choice B) is often a functioning tumor but is rare. Adrenal cortical hyperplasia (choice C) usually occurs secondary to a corticotropin-secreting pituitary tumor.

Diagnosis: Cushing disease

45 **The answer is A: Adrenal cortex, zona fasciculata.** Cushing syndrome presents with an accumulation of subcutaneous fat on the posterior neck ("buffalo hump"), striae, and diabetes mellitus. In this case, the disorder was caused by an adrenal tumor, which could have been either a cortical adenoma or carcinoma. The typical adenoma is an encapsulated, firm, yellow, slightly lobulated mass, measuring about 4 cm in diameter, which secretes glucocorticoid hormones. Tumors of the zona glomerulosa (choice B) secrete aldosterone (mineralocorticoid), and those of the adrenal medulla (choice D) are pheochromocytomas that secrete epinephrine. Lack of dexamethasone suppression rules out pituitary adenoma (choice E).

Diagnosis: Cushing syndrome

46 **The answer is E: Osteoporosis.** Long-term administration of corticosteroids causes increased bone resorption and decreased bone formation, thereby leading to osteoporosis. As many as 20% of patients with Cushing syndrome suffer compression fractures of the vertebrae. Osteomalacia (choice C) usually reflects abnormalities of vitamin D metabolism and features inadequate mineralization of newly formed bone.

Diagnosis: Cushing syndrome

47 **The answer is B: Autoimmunity.** Primary chronic adrenal insufficiency (Addison disease) most often reflects autoimmune destruction of the adrenal gland. It is a fatal wasting disorder caused by the failure of the adrenal glands to produce glucocorticoids, mineralocorticoids, and androgens. If untreated, Addison disease is characterized by weakness, weight loss, gastrointestinal symptoms, hypotension, electrolyte disturbances, and hyperpigmentation. More than 90% of the adrenal gland must be destroyed before the symptoms of chronic adrenal insufficiency surface. Less common causes of Addison disease include tuberculosis (choice E), metastatic carcinoma (choice C), amyloidosis (choice D), sarcoidosis, adrenoleukodystrophy, and congenital adrenal hypoplasia.

Diagnosis: Addison disease

48 **The answer is D: Conn syndrome.** Primary hyperaldosteronism (Conn syndrome) reflects inappropriate secretion of aldosterone by an adrenal adenoma (75%) or hyperplastic adrenal glands. Most patients with primary aldosteronism are diagnosed after the detection of asymptomatic diastolic hypertension. Muscle weakness and fatigue are produced by the effects of potassium depletion on skeletal muscle. Less Common syndrome is associated with low or normal renin levels. Chronic renal failure (choice C) is excluded by normal BUN and creatinine.

Diagnosis: Conn syndrome

49 **The answer is A: Adrenal.** Pheochromocytoma is a rare tumor of chromaffin cells of the adrenal medulla that secretes catecholamines. Such tumors also originate in extra-adrenal sites, in which case they are termed paragangliomas. The clinical features associated with pheochromocytoma are caused by the release of catecholamines. Patients with pheochromocytoma come to medical attention because of (1) asymptomatic hypertension discovered on a routine physical examination, (2) symptomatic hypertension that is resistant to antihypertensive therapy; (3) malignant hypertension (e.g., encephalopathy, papilledema, proteinuria), (4) myocardial infarction or aortic dissection, or (5) convulsions. The other choices do not include tumors that lead to episodic hypertension.

Diagnosis: Pheochromocytoma

Chapter 22

Obesity, Diabetes Mellitus, Metabolic Syndrome

QUESTIONS

Select the single best answer.

1 A 14-year-old boy presents for a presummer camp physical examination. Routine urinalysis discloses 3+ glucosuria. He admits to thirst and frequent urination, accompanied by a 4-kg (9-lb) weight loss over the past few months. His parents note that he had a flu-like illness 5 months ago. His blood glucose is 220 mg/dL. Which of the following best explains the pathogenesis of hyperglycemia in this patient?

(A) Excess dietary glucose
(B) Increased peripheral insulin uptake
(C) Irregular insulin secretion
(D) Islet cell destruction
(E) Peripheral insulin resistance

2 A 10-year-old boy with a recent onset of diabetes mellitus dies following an automobile accident. Histologic examination of the child's pancreas at autopsy is shown in the image. Injury to pancreatic islet cells in this patient was most likely mediated by which of the following mechanisms of disease?

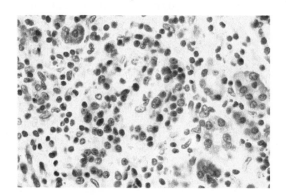

(A) Antibody-mediated islet cell destruction
(B) Cell-mediated immunity
(C) Direct viral cytopathic effects
(D) Hypovolemic shock
(E) Phagocytosis by activated macrophages

3 A 55-year-old obese woman (body mass index = 33 kg/m²) complains of declining visual acuity. Funduscopic examination shows peripheral retinal microaneurysms. Urinalysis reveals 3+ proteinuria and 3+ glucosuria. Serum albumin is 3 g/dL, and serum cholesterol is 350 mg/dL. These clinicopathologic findings are best explained by which of the following mechanisms of disease?

(A) Anti-insulin antibodies
(B) Increased peripheral insulin uptake
(C) Irregular insulin secretion
(D) Peripheral insulin resistance
(E) Secretion of insulin-like proteins

4 A 61-year-old man presents with a 5-year history of pain in both legs during exercise. He has been treated for diabetes for 8 years. His fasting blood glucose is 280 mg/dL. Which of the following best explains the pathogenesis of leg pain in this patient?

(A) Atherosclerosis
(B) Malignant hypertension
(C) Microaneurysms
(D) Peripheral neuropathy
(E) Vasculitis

5 A 60-year-old man with diabetes mellitus complains of deep burning pain and sensitivity to touch over his hands and fingers. Nerve conduction studies show slow transmission of impulses and diminished muscle stretch reflexes in the ankles and knees. Sensations to vibrations and light touch are also markedly diminished. The development of polyneuropathy in this patient correlates best with which of the following conditions?

(A) Anti-insulin antibody titer
(B) Hyperglycemia
(C) Insulin deficiency
(D) Intermittent hypoglycemia
(E) Ketoacidosis

6 A 56-year-old man with a 14-year history of diabetes mellitus presents with poor vision, peripheral vascular disease, and mild proteinuria. Which of the following is the best monitor of the control of blood sugar levels in this patient?

(A) Glycosylated hemoglobin
(B) Islet cell autoantibody
(C) Serum myoinositol
(D) Serum sorbitol
(E) Serum triglycerides

7 A 65-year-old obese man (body mass index = 32 kg/m²) presents with a 2-year history of difficulty walking. Physical examination reveals chronic ulcers in the lower extremities. Funduscopic examination reveals proliferative retinopathy. Which of the following best describes the pathogenesis of chronic ulcers on the legs of this patient?

(A) Abnormal glycosylation of hemoglobin
(B) Inadequate leukocytic response to infection
(C) Low concentrations of insulin in tissues
(D) Microvascular disease
(E) Varicose veins

8 Thickening of small vessel basement membranes in the patient described in Question 7 is most likely related to abnormalities in which of the following cellular and biochemical processes?

(A) Amyloidosis
(B) Collagenous fibrosis
(C) Glycosylation
(D) Immunoglobulin deposition
(E) Insudation of fibrin

9 A 58-year-old man with a long-standing history of type 2 diabetes mellitus suffers a massive hemorrhagic stroke and expires. Examination of the pancreas shows hyalinization of many islets of Langerhans. Which of the following characterizes the material within the islets of Langerhans?

(A) Amyloid
(B) Collagen type IV
(C) Fibrin
(D) Fibronectin
(E) Proteoglycan

10 A 50-year-old man with diabetes mellitus develops swelling in his lower extremities. Urinalysis shows 3+ proteinuria and 3+ glucosuria. Serum albumin is 3 g/dL and serum cholesterol is 350 mg/dL. A kidney biopsy is shown in the image. Which of the following glomerular changes is evident in this biopsy specimen?

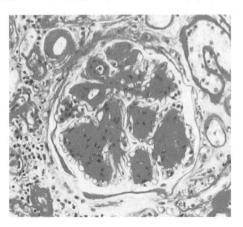

(A) Amyloidosis
(B) Deposition of basement membrane–like material
(C) Endothelial cell hyperplasia
(D) Fibrinoid necrosis
(E) Mesangial hyperplasia

11 A 75-year-old woman with well-controlled diabetes complains of poor eyesight. A grayish-white opacification of the lens is found during a comprehensive eye examination. Which of the following metabolic pathways is most likely involved in this lens abnormality?

(A) Aldose reductase pathway
(B) Amino acid degradation cycle
(C) Citric acid cycle
(D) Oxidative phosphorylation
(E) Pentose-phosphate shunt

12 A 40-year-old diabetic woman complains of flank pain and fever. Her temperature is 38.7°C (103°F), respirations are 25 per minute, and blood pressure is 150/90 mm Hg. Urinalysis reveals pyuria with WBC casts. Which of the following features of diabetes is the most important contributing factor in the development of flank pain and fever in this patient?

(A) Anti-insulin antibodies
(B) Glycosylation of hemoglobin
(C) Hyperglycemia
(D) Peripheral insulin resistance
(E) Sorbitol accumulation

13 A 32-year-old woman with diabetes mellitus delivers a child after 38 weeks of gestation. Which of the following is the most likely abnormality that might be encountered in this child at birth?

(A) Cataracts
(B) Hyperbilirubinemia
(C) Hypoglycemia
(D) Low birth weight
(E) Mental retardation

14 An obese woman (body mass index [BMI] = 32 kg/m²) presents for a routine physical examination. In reviewing your patient's health status, you mention that obesity is associated with an increased incidence of which of the following diseases?

(A) Cardiomyopathy
(B) Cervical carcinoma
(C) Chronic obstructive pulmonary disease
(D) Degenerative joint disease
(E) Diabetes mellitus type 1

ANSWERS

1 **The answer is D: Islet cell destruction.** Type 1 diabetes mellitus (T1DM) is a lifelong disorder of glucose homeostasis that results from the autoimmune destruction of the β-cells in the islets of Langerhans. The clinical onset of T1DM often coincides with another acute illness, such as a febrile viral or bacterial infection. The disease is characterized by few, if any, remaining functional cells in the islets of Langerhans and limited or absent insulin secretion. The most characteristic early lesion in the pancreas is a lymphocytic infiltrate in the islets (insulitis), sometimes accompanied by a few macrophages and neutrophils. As the disease becomes chronic, β-cells of the islets are progressively depleted. Choice E (peripheral insulin resistance) represents diabetes type 2. The other choices do not lead to hyperglycemia in normal persons.
Diagnosis: Diabetes mellitus, type 1

2 **The answer is B: Cell-mediated immunity.** Cell-mediated immune mechanisms are fundamental to the pathogenesis of type 1 diabetes mellitus (T1DM), and cytotoxic T lymphocytes sensitized to β-cells in T1DM persist indefinitely. Circulating antibodies (choice A) against components of the β-cells of the islets, including insulin itself, are identified in most newly diagnosed patients with diabetes. However, these antibodies are regarded as a response to β-cell injury, rather than the initial cause of β-cell depletion. Evidence for viral causes of diabetes mellitus type 1 (choice C) remains controversial.
Diagnosis: Diabetes mellitus, type 1

3 **The answer is D: Peripheral insulin resistance.** Type 2 diabetes mellitus results from a complex interplay between underlying resistance to the action of insulin in its metabolic target tissues (liver, skeletal muscle, and adipose tissue) and a reduction in glucose-stimulated insulin secretion, which fails to compensate for the increased demand for insulin. In obese persons, the release of inhibitory mediators from adipose tissue interferes with intracellular signaling by insulin. Hyperinsulinemia secondary to insulin resistance also downregulates the number of insulin receptors on the plasma membrane. The other choices have not been related to the pathogenesis of type 2 diabetes.
Diagnosis: Diabetes mellitus, type 2

4 **The answer is A: Atherosclerosis.** The extent and severity of atherosclerotic lesions in medium-sized and large arteries are increased in patients with long-standing diabetes. Leg pain during walking or exercise, which forces the patient to stop or limp (intermittent claudication) is typically a complication of atherosclerosis involving the major arteries of the lower extremities. Peripheral neuropathy (choice D) is a complication of diabetes but is an unlikely cause of claudication. Diabetes does not cause vasculitis (choice E).
Diagnosis: Atherosclerosis

5 **The answer is B: Hyperglycemia.** The severity and chronicity of hyperglycemia in both T1DM and T2DM are the major pathogenetic factors leading to the microvascular complications of diabetes, including retinopathy, nephropathy, and neuropathy. Thus, control of blood glucose remains the major means by which the development of microvascular diabetic complications can be minimized. Glucose binds nonenzymatically by attaching to a variety of proteins. This process, termed glycosylation, occurs roughly in proportion to the severity of hyperglycemia. Unfortunately, trials in which blood glucose levels were carefully controlled did not necessarily prevent all complications of diabetes.
Diagnosis: Diabetic neuropathy

6 **The answer is A: Glycosylated hemoglobin.** A specific fraction of glycosylated hemoglobin in circulating red blood cells (hemoglobin A1c) is measured routinely to monitor the overall degree of hyperglycemia that occurred during the preceding 6 to 8 weeks. Nonenzymatic glycosylation of hemoglobin is irreversible, and the level of hemoglobin A1c, therefore, serves as a marker for glycemic control. None of the other choices are quantitative measures of glucose levels.
Diagnosis: Diabetes mellitus

7 **The answer is D: Microvascular disease.** Microvascular disease, a characteristic complication of diabetes, causes ischemia and is, in part, responsible for the slow healing of wounds in the diabetic patient. It also results in other complications of diabetes such as renal disease. In addition to microvascular disease, aggregation of platelets in the smaller blood vessels and impaired fibrinolytic mechanisms have also been suggested to play a role in the pathogenesis of diabetic microvascular disease. The susceptibility of diabetics to infection is a complex problem, but it does not seem that the functions of polymorphonuclear leukocytes are directly affected (choice B). The tissue concentration of insulin (choice C) does not influence the healing process. Diabetes mellitus does not predispose to varicose veins (choice E).
Diagnosis: Diabetic microvascular disease

8 **The answer is C: Glycosylation.** Increased deposition and glycosylation of basement membrane proteins contribute to the pathogenesis of diabetic microvascular disease. Thus, control of blood glucose remains the major means by which the development of microvascular diabetic complications can be minimized. The other choices do not preferentially accumulate in small vessels affected by diabetes.
Diagnosis: Diabetic microvascular disease

9 **The answer is A: Amyloid.** In T2DM, amyloid is often present within the islets of Langerhans, particularly in patients over 60 years of age. This type of amyloid derives from a polypeptide molecule known as amylin, which is secreted with insulin by the β-cell. As many as 20% of aged nondiabetic persons also have amyloid deposits in the pancreas, which is a finding that has been attributed to the aging process itself. None of the other choices show Congo red staining and apple-green birefringence under polarized light.
Diagnosis: Amyloidosis

10 **The answer is B: Deposition of basement membrane–like material.** Microvascular disease is the major cause of renal failure and blindness in diabetics. Hyaline arteriolosclerosis and capillary basement membrane thickening are characteristic vascular changes in those with diabetes. The frequent occurrence of hypertension contributes to the development of the arteriolar lesions. In addition, deposition of basement membrane proteins, which may also become glycosylated, increases in diabetes. Increased mesangium results in glomerulosclerosis and, eventually, in renal failure. Eventually, the glomeruli in the diabetic kidney exhibit a unique lesion termed Kimmelstiel-Wilson disease or nodular glomerulosclerosis. Of patients with T1DM, 30% to 40% ultimately develop renal failure. A somewhat smaller proportion (up to 20%) of patients with T2DM are similarly affected. The deposited basement membrane material has a similar morphologic appearance to amyloid (choice A) but does not stain with Congo red.

Diagnosis: Diabetic glomerulopathy

11 **The answer is A: Aldose reductase pathway.** The aldose reductase pathway has been implicated in the pathogenesis of diabetic complications in some tissues, including the formation of cataracts. Glucose is converted to sorbitol (sugar alcohol), which can be cytotoxic. It is suspected to play a role in diabetic complications in a variety of tissues, including peripheral nerves, retina, lens and kidney. None of the other choices have been implicated in the pathogenesis of cataracts.

Diagnosis: Cataract

12 **The answer is C: Hyperglycemia.** Flank pain, fever, and pyuria are indicative of acute pyelonephritis, a common complication of diabetes. Glucose in the urine provides an enriched culture medium. In addition, patients with autonomic neuropathy often have a dystonic bladder that retains urine. Pyelonephritis is a constant threat for patients with diabetes, and necrotizing papillitis may be a devastating complication of renal infection. The other choices are not related to renal infection.

Diagnosis: Pyelonephritis, papillary necrosis

13 **The answer is C: Hypoglycemia.** Tight glucose control in the diabetic mother is necessary to prevent overstimulation of the fetal pancreas during gestation. Fetuses exposed to hyperglycemia in utero may develop hyperplasia of the pancreatic β-cells, which may secrete insulin autonomously and cause hypoglycemia at birth and in the early neonatal period. Infants of diabetic mothers show a 5% to 10% incidence of major development abnormalities. Increased birth weight is commonly encountered in offspring of diabetic mothers (see choice D). The incidence of mental retardation (choice E) is not specifically increased.

Diagnosis: Gestational diabetes

14 **The answer is D: Degenerative joint disease.** Degenerative joint disease (osteoarthritis) of weight-bearing joints is a common complication of obesity. The hips and knees are most commonly affected. Obesity is determined according to BMI, which is calculated as weight (kg)/height (m²). A BMI of 25 to 30 kg/m² is classed as overweight. Obesity is a risk factor for the development of adult-onset (type 2) diabetes mellitus, but not for juvenile-onset (type 1) diabetes mellitus (choice E). Obesity by itself does not cause cardiomyopathy (choice A).

Diagnosis: Obesity

Chapter 23

The Amyloidoses

QUESTIONS

Select the single best answer.

1　A 57-year-old woman presents with a 1-year history of diarrhea, increasing fatigue, and weight loss. Physical examination reveals a large tongue and induration of the anterior abdominal wall. Laboratory tests are all within normal ranges. A D-xylose absorption test is abnormal, indicating small intestinal malabsorption. A CT scan of the pelvis shows diffuse thickening of the rectal wall, retroperitoneum, and mesentery. Urinalysis documents proteinuria (0.5 g per day), without evidence of Bence-Jones protein. The plasma cell count in the bone marrow biopsy is increased by 10%, but there is no evidence of multiple myeloma. Which of the following tests would be most useful for establishing a diagnosis of primary amyloidosis?
(A) Magnetic resonance imaging
(B) Polymerase chain reaction (PCR)
(C) Protein electrophoresis
(D) Technetium scan
(E) Tissue biopsy

2　Which of the following histochemical stains is most useful for identifying amyloid in a tissue biopsy taken from the patient described in Question 1?
(A) Congo red
(B) Masson trichrome
(C) Mucicarmine
(D) Periodic acid-Schiff (PAS)
(E) Rhodanine

3　A biopsy taken from the rectum of the patient described in Questions 1 and 2 is appropriately stained and observed under polarizing light (shown in the image). Immunohistochemical assays show that this birefringent material contains kappa chains. This patient's amyloidosis belongs to which of the following categories?

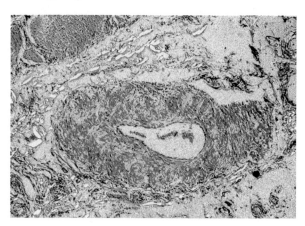

(A) AA
(B) Aβ2M
(C) AL
(D) APrP
(E) ATTR

4　A 65-year-old woman with longstanding rheumatoid arthritis complains of swelling of her eyelids, abdomen, and ankles. A chest X-ray shows bilateral pleural effusions, without evidence of pulmonary infiltration or consolidation. Urinalysis reveals heavy proteinuria (8 g per 24 hours). A percutaneous renal biopsy demonstrates glomerular deposits that are PAS-negative (shown in the image). The acellular material obstructing the glomerular capillaries in this patient is most likely derived from which of the following serum proteins?

271

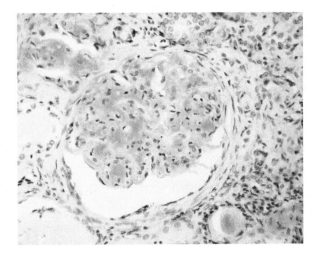

(A) Apo serum amyloid A
(B) Calcitonin
(C) Immunoglobulin light chain
(D) β-Protein precursor
(E) Transthyretin

5 The patient described in Question 4 asks for further information regarding her medical condition. You explain that "amyloid" refers to a group of extracellular protein deposits that are best defined as which of the following?
(A) Breakdown products of fibrinogen
(B) Immunoglobulin light chains
(C) Polypeptides with alpha-helical structure
(D) Proteins with common morphologic properties
(E) Substances visualized as dense deposits on electron microscopy

6 A 55-year-old man, who has smoked heavily for many years, presents with a 3-year history of persistent cough, frequent upper respiratory infections, and production of foul-smelling, mucopurulent sputum. An X-ray film of the chest shows bronchiectasis. Five years later, the patient complains of frequent diarrhea. A CT scan of the abdomen and pelvis shows diffuse thickening of the rectal wall, retroperitoneum, and mesentery. A rectal biopsy demonstrates amyloid that is most likely derived from which of the following serum proteins?
(A) Apo serum amyloid A
(B) Calcitonin
(C) Fibrinogen
(D) Immunoglobulin light chain
(E) β_2-Microglobulin

7 For the patient described in Question 6, progressive cell and organ dysfunction will develop primarily as a result of which of the following biological processes?
(A) Accumulation of abnormal protein within lysosomes
(B) Deposition of extensive collagen scar tissue
(C) Diminished blood supply to parenchymal cells
(D) Interference with inflammation and immunity
(E) Progressive DNA damage in parenchymal cells

8 A 38-year-old woman complains of tingling sensations in her hands and fingers for the past year. Neurologic studies show loss of pain and temperature sensation in the patient's

extremities. Laboratory analysis of cerebrospinal fluid shows no biochemical abnormalities. A skin biopsy reveals amyloid deposits in nerves. Based on these findings and a strong family history of a similar disorder, the patient is diagnosed with familial amyloidotic polyneuropathy. Amyloid deposits in this patient's nerves are derived from which of the following serum proteins?
(A) Apo serum amyloid A
(B) Immunoglobulin light chain
(C) β_2-Microglobulin
(D) β-Protein precursor
(E) Transthyretin

9 A 74-year-old man with a history of progressive cognitive impairment dies from complications of congestive heart failure. At the time of autopsy, his brain shows diffuse atrophy. Microscopic examination demonstrates numerous senile plaques and neurofibrillary tangles, as well as deposition of eosinophilic material in the walls of the cerebral vasculature. A section is stained with Congo red and examined under polarized light (shown in the image). The birefringent material is derived from which of the following proteins?

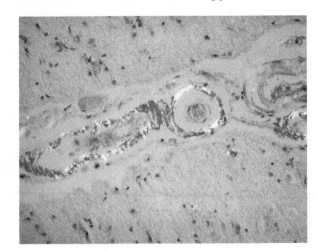

(A) Apo serum amyloid A
(B) Fibrinogen
(C) Immunoglobulin light chain
(D) β-Protein precursor
(E) Transthyretin

10 A 56-year-old woman dies of a chronic neurodegenerative disease. Autopsy reveals spongiform encephalopathy with brain amyloidosis. This patient's amyloidosis most likely belongs to which of the following categories?
(A) Aβ
(B) AA
(C) AE
(D) AH
(E) APrP

11 A 30-year-old woman with Down syndrome receives several rounds of aggressive chemotherapy for leukemia but subsequently dies of complications of septic shock. Immunohistochemical examination of this patient's brain at autopsy would most likely show cerebral deposits of which of the following amyloid proteins?

(A) Aβ
(B) AA
(C) AL
(D) ATTR
(E) β₂-Microglobulin

12 A 52-year-old man complains of pain in his back and fatigue for 6 months. He admits to polyuria and polydipsia. An X-ray film of the upper torso reveals numerous lytic lesions in the lumbar vertebral bodies. Laboratory studies show hypoalbuminemia and mild anemia and thrombocytopenia. A monoclonal immunoglobulin peak is demonstrated by serum electrophoresis, and a bone marrow aspiration demonstrates numerous atypical plasma cells. Urinalysis shows 4+ proteinuria. A renal biopsy in this patient would most likely show deposits of which of the following amyloid precursor proteins?
(A) Amylin
(B) Apo serum amyloid A
(C) Fibrinogen
(D) Immunoglobulin light chain
(E) β₂-Microglobulin

13 A 56-year-old woman with a cold thyroid nodule is admitted for fine-needle aspiration, which results in a diagnosis of medullary carcinoma. Histologic examination of a subsequent surgical specimen reveals tumor cells surrounded by extracellular, amorphous eosinophilic material (shown in the image). These amyloid deposits are most closely related to which of the following serum proteins?

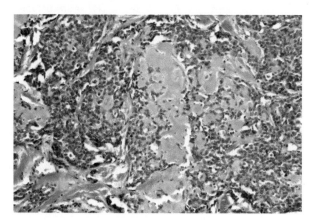

(A) Apo serum amyloid A
(B) Calcitonin
(C) Immunoglobulin light chain
(D) β₂-Microglobulin
(E) Transthyretin

14 A 45-year-old man presents with flank pain and the passage of blood clots in his urine. Physical examination reveals bilateral flank and abdominal masses. Laboratory studies show elevated BUN and creatinine. Urinalysis discloses hematuria, proteinuria, and oliguria. A CT scan shows bilaterally enlarged, polycystic kidneys. The patient undergoes weekly hemodialysis for 5 years and develops severe joint pain. The deposition of which of the following amyloid proteins best explains the pathogenesis of joint pain in this patient?

(A) Amylin
(B) Apo serum amyloid A
(C) Fibrinogen
(D) Immunoglobulin light chain
(E) β₂-Microglobulin

15 A 65-year-old woman dies of trauma suffered in an automobile accident. Examination of her pancreas at the time of autopsy reveals acellular, eosinophilic material within the pancreatic islets. This material is congophilic and has a fibrillar appearance by electron microscopy. These findings suggest that prior to her death, the patient suffered from which of the following conditions?
(A) Alcoholism
(B) Chronic pancreatitis
(C) Pancreatic cancer
(D) Diabetes mellitus type 1
(E) Diabetes mellitus type 2

16 The precursor of the pancreatic amyloid found in the patient described in Question 15 helps regulate which of the following normal cellular functions?
(A) Apoptosis
(B) DNA synthesis
(C) Glucose uptake
(D) Membrane fluidity
(E) Protein glycosylation

ANSWERS

1 **The answer is E: Tissue biopsy.** No single set of clinical signs or symptoms points unequivocally to amyloidosis. The symptoms are governed by both the underlying disease and the type of protein deposited. Even when one suspects amyloidosis, the diagnosis ultimately rests on its histologic demonstration in biopsy specimens. The staining and structural properties of amyloid allow a general definition, based primarily on morphologic characteristics. When routine stains are used, amyloid is amorphous, glassy, and has almost cartilage-like properties, which are responsible for its so-called hyaline appearance. PCR (choice B) is used to amplify DNA, generating thousands to millions of copies of a particular sequence. PCR is currently used in biomedical research laboratories for the diagnosis of hereditary and infectious diseases. Protein electrophoresis (choice C) may disclose a paraproteinemia but by itself does not inform about tissue amyloid formation.
Diagnosis: Lymphoma

2 **The answer is A: Congo red.** All forms of amyloid stain positively with Congo red and show red-green birefringence when viewed under polarized light. The fibrillary deposits organized in one plane have one color, and those organized perpendicular to that plane have the other color. Ultrastructurally, all forms of amyloid consist of interlacing bundles of parallel arrays of fibrils, which have a diameter of 7 to 13 nm. The protein in the amyloid fibrils contains a large proportion of crossed β-pleated sheet structure. Masson trichrome stain (choice B) highlights collagen. Mucicarmine (choice C) stains mucin. The PAS stain (choice D) identifies glycogen and basement membranes. Rhodanine stain (choice E) demonstrates copper.
Diagnosis: Lymphoma

3 **The answer is C: AL.** Primary amyloidosis refers to the presentation of amyloid without any preceding disease. In one third of these cases, primary amyloidosis is the harbinger of frank plasma cell neoplasia, such as multiple myeloma or other B-cell lymphomas. AL amyloid usually consists of the variable region of immunoglobulin light chains (L) and can be derived from either the kappa (κ) or lambda (λ) polypeptides. The other choices do not involve immunoglobulins.

Diagnosis: AL amyloid, lymphoma

4 **The answer is A: Apo serum amyloid A.** AA amyloid is common to a host of seemingly unrelated, persistent, inflammatory, neoplastic, and hereditary disorders that lead to so-called secondary amyloidosis. For example, patients with rheumatoid arthritis, ankylosing spondylitis, and tuberculosis may develop secondary amyloidosis. There is a spectrum of AA peptides of differing size in the deposits, all of which have the same amino-terminal sequence. This includes the intact precursor of AA, serum amyloid A (SAA). SAA is an acute-phase reactant protein that increases up to 1,000-fold during inflammatory processes. Denaturing of SAA releases a subunit termed apoSAA, which renders it amyloidogenic. In contrast to AL protein derived from immunoglobulin light chain (choice C), the amino acid sequence of AA proteins is identical in all patients, regardless of the underlying disorder. Progressive glomerular obliteration may ultimately lead to renal failure.

Diagnosis: Rheumatoid arthritis

5 **The answer is D: Proteins with common morphologic properties.** Amyloid refers to a group of diverse extracellular protein deposits that have (1) common morphologic proprieties, (2) affinities for specific dyes, and (3) a characteristic appearance under polarized light. Although the different types of amyloid vary in amino acid sequence, all amyloid proteins are folded in such as way as to share common ultrastructural and physical properties (e.g., β-pleated sheets). Thus, all amyloids have a similar ultrastructural appearance, regardless of which protein is responsible for the fibrillary components. By electron microscopy, amyloid consists of interlacing bundles of parallel arrays of fibrils, which have a diameter of 7 to 13 nm (not dense deposits, choice E). Amyloid proteins rich in alpha-helical structures (choice C) are encountered in diseases that generate AA amyloid.

Diagnosis: AA amyloid, rheumatoid arthritis

6 **The answer is A: Apo serum amyloid A.** Chronic bronchitis and bronchiectasis are chronic inflammatory conditions that may lead to the deposition of AA amyloid. Termed secondary amyloidosis, this form of amyloidosis most often affects the kidneys, liver, adrenals, and spleen. Afib (derived from fibrinogen, choice C) is encountered in hereditary renal amyloidosis. None of the other choices are associated with chronic inflammation.

Diagnosis: AA amyloid, bronchiectasis

7 **The answer is C: Diminished blood supply to parenchymal cells.** Regardless of type, amyloidosis leads eventually to cell atrophy and death. Amyloid adds interstitial material to sites of deposition, thereby increasing the size of affected organs. This increase may be counterbalanced by the deposition of amyloid in blood vessels, an effect that impairs circulation and may lead to organ atrophy and cell death.

Diagnosis: AA amyloid, bronchiectasis

8 **The answer is E: Transthyretin.** Familial amyloidotic polyneuropathy (FAP) is an autosomal dominant disorder that affects families in Sweden, Portugal, and Japan and is related to a mutation in the transthyretin gene, which encodes a thyroxine-binding protein. Amyloid in the peripheral and autonomic nerves is derived from the abnormal transthyretin. At least 60 different FAP mutations have been described, which give rise to clinical variants of the disease. The familial polyneuropathic forms of amyloid usually manifest as paresthesias, with loss of temperature and pain sensation of the extremities.

Diagnosis: Familial amyloidotic polyneuropathy

9 **The answer is D: β-Protein precursor.** This patient suffers from Alzheimer disease, the principal cause of so-called senility. Amyloid deposits in the brain and cerebral vessels of patients suffering from Alzheimer disease contain fibrils of β-amyloid ($A\beta$). The deposited protein, namely $A\beta$ protein, is a fragment of a larger $A\beta$-protein precursor ($A\beta$PP), which is a normal cell membrane constituent. The larger part of $A\beta$PP is extracellular, with the remainder traversing the cell membrane and ending in a cytoplasmic portion. None of the other choices are found in Alzheimer disease.

Diagnosis: Alzheimer disease

10 **The answer is E: APrP.** APrP amyloid is found in spongiform encephalopathies. Prion proteins (PrPs) are natural plasma membrane constituents found in a variety of cells, including the central nervous system. Their physiologic function is not yet apparent. PrP in an altered conformation serves as a template for the association of additional PrP molecules and, in so doing, confers on them a new PrP conformation (PrPsc). PrPsc and its aggregates form fibrils with the characteristic of amyloid and play a role in a group of human and animal central nervous system degenerative diseases, such as Kuru, Creutzfeldt-Jakob disease, Gerstmann-Straussler-Sheinker disease, scrapie, and bovine spongiform encephalopathy (mad cow disease). None of the other choices are seen in prion diseases.

Diagnosis: Spongiform encephalopathy

11 **The answer is A: $A\beta$.** Brains of middle-aged patients with Down syndrome show changes similar to those of Alzheimer disease. As in Alzheimer disease, the deposits of cerebral amyloid are derived from the $A\beta$ protein. The gene for the $A\beta$ protein precursor resides on chromosome 21, trisomy of which causes Down syndrome. None of the other choices are characteristic of Down syndrome.

Diagnosis: Down syndrome

12 **The answer is D: Immunoglobulin light chain.** AL amyloid usually consists of the variable region of immunoglobulin light chains and can be derived from either the kappa (κ) or lambda (λ) moieties. Since the light chains produced by the neoplastic cells in plasma cell dyscrasias are unique to each patient, AL amyloid isolated from different persons differs in its amino

acid sequence. AL protein is common to primary amyloidosis and amyloidosis associated with multiple myeloma, B-cell lymphomas, or other plasma cell dyscrasias. Multiple myeloma is accompanied by amyloidosis in 10% to 15% of cases. The other choices do not involve immunoglobulins.
Diagnosis: Multiple myeloma

13 The answer is B: Calcitonin.   Isolated amyloidosis has been described in the major arteries, lungs, heart, and various joints and in association with endocrine tumors that secrete polypeptide hormones. In endocrine tumors, the amyloid is usually part of a hormone or a prohormone. Medullary carcinoma of the thyroid originates from C cells of the thyroid, which normally secrete calcitonin. The amyloid found in this tumor is a fragment of procalcitonin. The other choices are not derived from endocrine cells.
Diagnosis: Medullary carcinoma of the thyroid

14 The answer is E: β_2-Microglobulin.   The deposition of amyloid formed from β_2-microglobulin is characterized by a destructive arthropathy due to amyloid deposition in the major joints of patients undergoing chronic renal dialysis. The other choices do not follow chronic renal dialysis.
Diagnosis: Autosomal dominant polycystic kidney disease

15 The answer is E: Diabetes mellitus type 2.   Type 2 diabetes is a heterogeneous disorder characterized by reduced tissue sensitivity to insulin and inadequate secretion of insulin from the pancreas. A variety of microscopic lesions are found in the islets of Langerhans of many patients with type 2 diabetes mellitus. Fibrous tissue may accumulate to such a degree that the islets are obliterated. Islet amyloid deposits are often present, particularly in patients over 60 years of age.
Diagnosis: Diabetes mellitus, type 2

16 The answer is C: Glucose uptake.   The amyloid deposited in the islets of Langerhans in type 2 diabetes is derived from a larger precursor, a peptide related to a variant of calcitonin termed islet amyloid polypeptide or amylin. Like insulin, this hormone is produced by β-cells of the islets and seems to have a profound effect on glucose uptake by the liver and striated muscle. These observations suggest that islet amyloid may be involved in the pathogenesis of type 2 diabetes. Amylin per se does not regulate any of the other choices.
Diagnosis: Diabetes mellitus, type 2

Chapter 24

The Skin

QUESTIONS

Select the single best answer.

1 A 55-year-old man from China presents with a 3-month history of scales on his skin. Physical examination reveals numerous scaly, pigmented plaques, which rub off easily. Biopsy of a plaque shows anastomosing cords of mature and stratified squamous epithelium, associated with small keratin cysts. This patient may have which of the following underlying conditions?
(A) Acquired immunodeficiency
(B) Basal cell nevus syndrome
(C) Familial hypercholesterolemia
(D) Human papillomavirus infection
(E) Internal malignancy

2 An 18-year-old woman notes that one of her moles has increased in size and become darker. The patient has a family history of melanoma, and she is seen by her dermatologist regularly to "follow her moles." Physical examination reveals numerous, 5 to 10 mm, darkly pigmented, variegated lesions distributed primarily on her trunk but also involving non–sun-exposed skin. This patient may harbor a germline mutation in a gene that regulates which of the following proteins?
(A) Caspase
(B) Cyclin-dependent kinase
(C) Epidermal growth factor receptor
(D) Glycogen phosphorylase
(E) Sodium-potassium ATPase

3 An 80-year-old farmer presents with a 1-cm, red, slightly raised plaque on his face. A biopsy of the lesion shows cytologic atypia and dyskeratosis limited to the basal layers of the stratum spongiosum, as well as hyperkeratosis and parakeratosis. This lesion is a precursor for which of the following dermatologic diseases?
(A) Basal cell carcinoma
(B) Erythema multiforme
(C) Lichen planus
(D) Malignant melanoma
(E) Squamous cell carcinoma

4 A 45-year-old man presents with painful, purple nodules on the dorsal surface of his left hand that he first noticed 9 months ago. A biopsy (shown in the image) discloses a poorly demarcated lesion composed of atypical spindle-shaped neoplastic cells and extravasated red cells. Similar lesions are found in the lymph nodes and liver. Which of the following viruses is associated with the pathogenesis of these skin lesions?

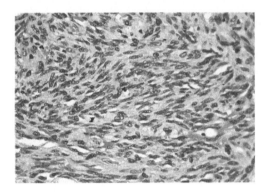

(A) Cytomegalovirus
(B) Epstein-Barr virus
(C) Herpes simplex virus type 2
(D) Human herpesvirus type 8
(E) Human papillomavirus types 16/18

5 A 36-year-old woman presents with a pigmented lesion on the posterior aspect of her left calf (shown in the image). An excisional biopsy demonstrates a superficial spreading type of melanoma. Which of the following histologic features has the most important prognostic value in your evaluation of this patient?

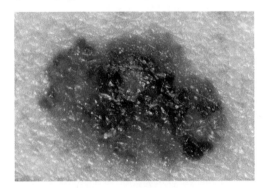

(A) Degree of melanocytic atypia
(B) Degree of vascularity
(C) Depth of dermal invasion
(D) Extent of intraepidermal invasion by melanoma cells
(E) Presence of variable melanin pigmentation

6 A 3-year-old child has numerous small, white scales covering the extensor surfaces of the extremities, trunk, and face (shown in the image). The child's mother and grandmother have the same condition. Biopsy of lesional skin shows hyperkeratosis and a thin stratum granulosum. Which of the following is the most likely diagnosis?

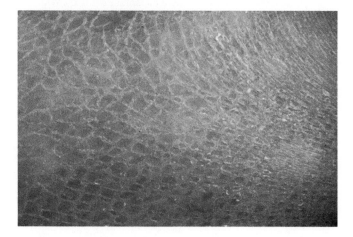

(A) Acute eczematous dermatitis
(B) Bullous pemphigoid
(C) Epidermolysis bullosa
(D) Ichthyosis vulgaris
(E) Pemphigus vulgaris

7 A 70-year-old woman presents with facial discoloration. The patient is observed to have a flat, pigmented lesion on the atrophic, sun-damaged skin (shown in the image). Which of the following is the most likely diagnosis?

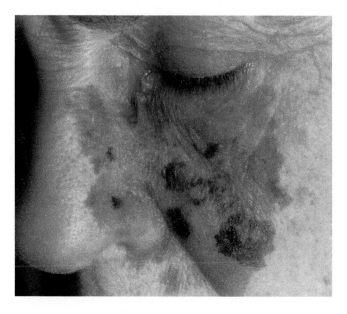

(A) Acral lentiginous melanoma
(B) Alopecia
(C) Lentigo maligna melanoma
(D) Mucosal lentiginous melanoma
(E) Nodular melanoma

8 A 25-year-old man presents with a 1-month history of fatigue, mild fever, and an erythematous scaling rash. His major concern is related to the scaling plaques distributed on his knees, buttocks, elbows, scalp, and feet. He also notes some joint pain and swelling, primarily involving the small bones of his fingers. Physical examination reveals erythematous plaques with adherent silvery scales that induce punctate bleeding points when removed. Biopsy of lesional skin would most likely show an accumulation of which of the following cells in the epidermis?

(A) B lymphocytes
(B) Mast cells
(C) Melanocytes
(D) Neutrophils
(E) T lymphocytes

9 Examination of a 2-day-old neonate reveals numerous blisters on the trunk and extremities. Skin biopsy discloses separation of the basal layer of the epidermis from its basement membrane and is devoid of inflammatory cells. No antibody deposits are identified by immunofluorescence microscopy. Which of the following is the most likely diagnosis?

(A) Bullous pemphigoid
(B) Dermatitis herpetiformis
(C) Epidermolysis bullosa
(D) Ichthyosis vulgaris
(E) Pemphigus vulgaris

10 A 25-year-old man complains of eruptions of blisters on his scalp and inner surface of the groin and in his mouth. The blisters rupture easily and leave large crusted areas. Histologically, the lesions show separation of the stratum spinosum from the basal layer. The results of direct immunofluorescence microscopy for IgG are shown. Which of the following proteins is targeted by IgG autoantibody in the skin of this patient?

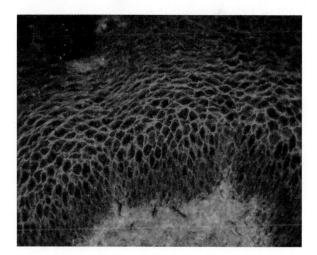

(A) Collagen type IV
(B) Desmoglein-3
(C) E-cadherin
(D) Fibronectin
(E) L-selectin

11 A 60-year-old former lifeguard presents with several small, pearly nodules on the back of her neck. A biopsy of one of the nodules (shown in the image) reveals buds of atypical, deeply-basophilic keratinocytes extending from the overlying epidermis into the papillary dermis. Which of the following is the appropriate diagnosis?

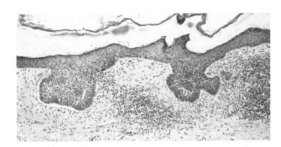

(A) Basal cell carcinoma
(B) Fibroepithelial polyp
(C) Keratoacanthoma
(D) Squamous cell carcinoma
(E) Xanthoma

12 A 10-year-old girl presents with multiple papules on the back of her hand that bleed easily. Histologic examination of a lesion reveals squamous epithelial-lined fronds with fibrovascular cores (shown in the image). Which of the following viruses is most likely responsible for the development of these skin lesions?

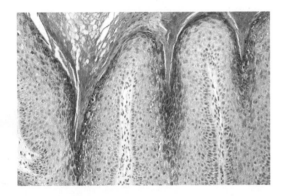

(A) Cytomegalovirus
(B) Epstein-Barr virus
(C) Herpes simplex virus type 2
(D) Human herpesvirus type 8
(E) Human papillomavirus

13 A 28-year-old woman presents with a 2-day history of dome-shaped erythematous nodules appearing on her skin. She recently had a urinary tract infection for which she was treated with trimethoprim sulfamethoxazole (Bactrim). Biopsy discloses focal hemorrhage, neutrophilic infiltrates in the subcutaneous fibrous tissue septa, and giant cells at the interface between the septa and the adipose fat tissue. No infectious agents are identified. Which of the following is the most likely diagnosis?
(A) Allergic contact dermatitis
(B) Dermatitis herpetiformis
(C) Bullous pemphigoid
(D) Erythema nodosum
(E) Lupus erythematosus

14 A 65-year-old woman complains of having an itchy rash for the past few months. She said the lesions first appeared as red swollen plaques on her abdomen and flexor aspect of her forearms. Physical examination reveals urticarial plaques, as well as large bullae on her abdomen and thighs (shown in the image). A skin biopsy shows a positive direct immunofluorescence test for IgG antibasement membrane antibody. Which of the following is the appropriate diagnosis?

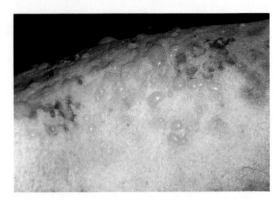

(A) Allergic contact dermatitis
(B) Bullous pemphigoid
(C) Dermatitis herpetiformis
(D) Epidermolysis bullosa
(E) Pemphigus vulgaris

15 A 15-year-old girl complains of itchy skin lesions of 6 months in duration. Physical examination reveals numerous wheal-like lesions with small vesicles over her elbows and knees. A skin biopsy demonstrates inflammation in the tips of the dermal papillae and subepidermal vesicles. Which of the following histopathologic findings would provide the best evidence to support a diagnosis of dermatitis herpetiformis in this patient?
(A) Horn and pseudo-horn cysts
(B) IgA deposits in dermal papillae
(C) Koilocytotic change
(D) Microabscesses in the stratum corneum
(E) Spongiosis

16 A 17-year-old woman is brought to the physician by her parents because "she has been acting strangely" for a couple of days. Over the past 3 months, she has experienced malaise, joint pain, weight loss, and sporadic fever. The patient appears agitated, with a temperature of 38°C (101°F). Other physical findings include malar rash, erythematous-pink plaques with telangiectatic vessels, oral ulcers, and nonblanching purpuric papules on her legs. Laboratory studies show elevated levels of BUN and creatinine. The anti–double-stranded DNA antibody test is positive. Biopsy of sun-damaged lesional skin would most likely show which of the following histopathologic findings in this patient?
(A) Acanthosis, parakeratosis, and neutrophils within the stratum corneum
(B) Early dermal-epidermal separation mediated by eosinophils
(C) Granular distribution of immune complexes in the basement membrane zone
(D) Linear IgA deposits within dermal papillae
(E) Stratum corneum microabscess (Munro)

17 A 14-year-old boy presents with a 6-month history of erythematous papules on his face. Physical examination reveals numerous "blackheads" over the forehead and cheeks. Which of the following bacteria is associated with the development of these lesions?

(A) *Clostridium* sp.
(B) *Lactobacillus* sp.
(C) *Propionibacterium* sp.
(D) *Staphylococcus* sp.
(E) *Streptococcus* sp.

18 A 30-year-old man presents with flat-topped papules that have appeared gradually on the flexor surfaces of his wrists. White streaks and patches are also found on the buccal mucosa of the patient's mouth. Histologically, the lesions showed hyperkeratosis, thickening of the stratum granulosum, and a band-like infiltrate of lymphocytes and macrophages in the upper dermis, disrupting the basal layer of the epidermis. Lymphocytes were mostly of the CD4$^+$ immunophenotype. Which of the following is the appropriate diagnosis?

(A) Dermatitis herpetiformis
(B) Erythema multiforme
(C) Erythema nodosum
(D) Hypersensitivity angiitis
(E) Lichen planus

19 A 66-year-old woman presents with a 5-year history of erythematous, scaly patches on her buttocks. Physical examination reveals plaques with telangiectases, atrophy, and pigmentation. Biopsy of lesional skin shows that the epidermis and papillary dermis are expanded by an extensive infiltrate of atypical lymphocytes. These infiltrating lymphocytes most likely express which of the following "cluster of differentiation" cell surface markers?

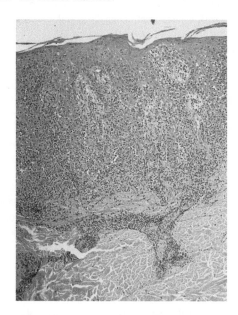

(A) CD4
(B) CD9
(C) CD15
(D) CD20
(E) CD31

20 A 30-year-old woman with chronic hepatitis B presents with numerous red skin lesions that she has had for 5 days. Physical examination reveals multiple, purpuric, 2- to 4-mm papules on the skin (shown in the image). The papules did not blanch under pressure. Biopsy of lesional skin shows necrotizing leukocytoclastic venulitis. Immunofluorescence studies disclose immune complex deposition in vascular walls. Which of the following is the most likely diagnosis?

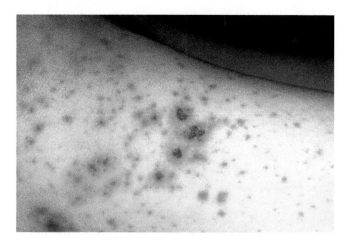

(A) Allergic contact dermatitis
(B) Dermatitis herpetiformis
(C) Erythema multiforme
(D) Erythema nodosum
(E) Hypersensitivity angiitis

21 A 20-year-old man presents to his family physician for treatment of itching after exposure to poison ivy. The patient's hands and arms appeared red and were covered with oozing blisters and crusts (shown in the image). Which of the following represents the most important step in the pathogenesis of the sensitization phase of injury in this patient?

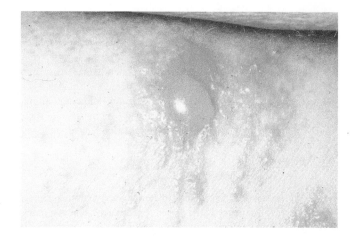

(A) Development of spongiosis
(B) Infiltration of the epidermis by neutrophils
(C) Migration of Langerhans cells into dermal lymphatics
(D) Rapid increase in vascular permeability
(E) Separation of the epidermis from the dermis mediated by eosinophils

22 A 12-year-old girl presents for a routine physical examination. The patient has numerous freckles over her upper trunk and face. Which of the following terms best describes the morphologic appearance of her freckles?

(A) Comedo
(B) Macule
(C) Nodule
(D) Papule
(E) Plaque

23 A 40-year-old woman complains that the skin on her fingers feels stiff. The skin of her face appears tense, and radial furrows are evident around the mouth. A skin biopsy shows loss of dermal appendages and abundant collagen bundles aligned parallel to an atrophic epidermis. Which of the following clinical symptoms is commonly seen in patients with this dermatologic condition?

(A) Facial acne
(B) Dysphagia
(C) Fever and malaise
(D) Polyuria and polydipsia
(E) Urolithiasis

ANSWERS

1 **The answer is E: Internal malignancy.** Seborrheic keratoses are scaly, frequently pigmented, elevated papules or plaques whose scales are easily rubbed off. Microscopically, the lesions are composed of broad anastomosing cords of mature stratified squamous epithelium associated with small cysts of keratin (horn cysts). The sudden appearance of numerous seborrheic keratoses has been associated with internal malignancies (sign of Leser-Trélat), especially gastric adenocarcinoma. Papillomavirus infection (choice D) induces papilloma formation. Choices B and D do not lead to acute plaque eruption.
Diagnosis: Seborrheic keratoses

2 **The answer is B: Cyclin-dependent kinase.** Germline mutations in the *CDKN2A* tumor suppressor gene (also known as *p16*) have been found in some patients who have dysplastic nevus/melanoma and in their family members. This gene encodes an inhibitor of cyclin-dependent kinase that normally functions to suppress cell proliferation. Choices A, D, and E are not related to cell proliferation. Mutations in epidermal growth factor receptor (choice C) are involved in some malignant neoplasms but not dysplastic nevus/melanoma syndrome.
Diagnosis: Dysplastic nevus syndrome

3 **The answer is E: Squamous cell carcinoma.** Actinic keratoses ("from the sun's rays") develop in sun-damaged skin as circumscribed keratotic patches or plaques, commonly on the backs of the hands or the face. Microscopically, the stratum corneum is replaced by a dense parakeratotic scale. The underlying basal keratinocytes display significant atypia. With time, actinic keratoses may evolve into squamous cell carcinoma in situ and, finally, into invasive squamous cell carcinoma. However, most are stable and many regress. Basal cell carcinoma (choice A)

and malignant melanoma (choice D) also arise frequently in sun-exposed skin but are unrelated to actinic keratosis.
Diagnosis: Actinic keratosis

4 **The answer is D: Human herpesvirus type 8.** Kaposi sarcoma is a malignant tumor derived from endothelial cells. This vascular neoplasm is an important cutaneous sign in the AIDS pandemic. Human herpesvirus 8 (HHV-8) is thought to play a role in the pathogenesis of Kaposi sarcoma, however only a small percentage of HHV-8–infected individuals develop Kaposi sarcoma. These malignant tumors most often appear on the hands or feet but may occur anywhere. The histologic appearance of Kaposi sarcoma is highly variable. One form resembles a simple capillary hemangioma. Other forms are highly cellular and vascular spaces are less prominent. Epstein-Barr virus (choice B) is associated with Burkitt lymphoma in sub-Saharan Africa, and human papillomavirus types 16/18 (choice E) are associated with cervical cancer.
Diagnosis: Kaposi sarcoma

5 **The answer is C: Depth of dermal invasion.** Although choices A, B, and D may be factors in melanoma aggressiveness, the evaluation of tumor thickness is recognized as the single strongest prognostic variable for melanoma. Presence of variable melanin pigmentation (choice E) is not a predictor of melanoma growth or spread.
Diagnosis: Melanoma

6 **The answer is D: Ichthyosis vulgaris.** Ichthyosis vulgaris is an autosomal dominant disorder of keratinization characterized by mild hyperkeratosis and reduced or absent keratohyaline granules in the epidermis. Scaly skin results from increased cohesiveness of the stratum corneum. The attenuated stratum granulosum consists of a single layer with small defective keratohyaline granules. Most patients are maintained free of scales with topical treatments. The other choices do not feature autosomal dominant inheritance.
Diagnosis: Ichthyosis vulgaris

7 **The answer is C: Lentigo maligna melanoma.** Lentigo maligna melanoma, also known as Hutchinson melanotic freckle, is a large, pigmented macule that occurs on sun-damaged skin. It develops almost exclusively in fair-skinned, usually elderly, whites. Because it occurs on exposed body surfaces, it is probably related to chronic ultraviolet light exposure, without acute episodes of sunburn, and often occurs in outdoor workers. Acral lentiginous melanoma (choice A) is the most common form of melanoma in dark-skinned people and is generally limited to the palms, soles, and subungual regions. A similar tumor occurs on the mucous membranes and is called mucosal lentiginous melanoma (choice D). Alopecia (choice B) refers to hair loss.
Diagnosis: Melanoma

8 **The answer is D: Neutrophils.** Psoriasis is a disease of the dermis and epidermis that is characterized by persistent epidermal hyperplasia. It is a chronic, frequently familial disorder that features large, erythematous, scaly plaques, commonly on the dorsal extensor cutaneous surfaces. The nucleated layers of the epidermis are thickened several-fold in the rete pegs and are frequently thinner over the dermal papillae. The capillaries of the papillae are dilated and tortuous. Neutrophils emerge at their tips and migrate into the epidermis above the apices of the papillae. Neutrophils may become localized in the epidermal spinous layer or in small Munro microabscesses in the stratum corneum. The dermis below the papillae exhibits a varying number of mononuclear inflammatory cells (choices A and E) around the superficial vascular plexuses.

Diagnosis: Psoriasis

9 **The answer is C: Epidermolysis bullosa (EB).** EB comprises a heterogeneous group of disorders loosely bound by their hereditary nature and by a tendency to form blisters at sites of minor trauma. EB simplex has been attributed to mutations of genes encoding cytokeratin intermediate filaments. The clinical spectrum of the disease ranges from a minor annoyance to a widespread, life-threatening blistering disease. These blisters are almost always noted at birth or shortly thereafter. The classification of these disorders is based on the site of blister formation in the basement membrane zone. Although epidermolytic EB is cosmetically disturbing and sometimes debilitating, it is not life threatening. Blisters seen in bullous pemphigoid (choice A) and pemphigus vulgaris (choice E) are associated with immunoglobulin deposits that are visualized by direct immunofluorescence microscopy. Dermatitis herpetiformis (choice B) occurs at a later age and is associated with gluten hypersensitivity. In ichthyosis vulgaris (choice D), scaly skin results from increased cohesiveness of the stratum corneum.

Diagnosis: Epidermolysis bullosa

10 **The answer is B: Desmoglein-3.** Pemphigus vulgaris is an autoimmune disease caused by autoantibodies to a keratinocyte antigen. The characteristic lesion is a large, easily ruptured blister that leaves extensive denuded or crusted areas. Suprabasal dyshesion results in a blister that has an intact basal layer as a floor and the remaining epidermis as a roof. The blister contains a moderate number of lymphocytes, macrophages, eosinophils, and neutrophils. Distinctive, rounded keratinocytes (termed acantholytic cells) are shed into the vesicle during the process of dyshesion. Circulating IgG antibodies in patients with pemphigus vulgaris react with an epidermal surface antigen called desmoglein-3, a desmosomal protein. Antigen–antibody union results in dyshesion, which is augmented by the release of plasminogen activator and, hence, the activation of plasmin. This proteolytic enzyme acts on the intercellular substance and may be the dominant factor in dyshesion. None of the other choices are related to the pathogenesis of pemphigus vulgaris.

Diagnosis: Pemphigus vulgaris

11 **The answer is A: Basal cell carcinoma (BCC).** BCC is the most common malignant tumor in persons with pale skin. Although it may be locally aggressive, metastases are exceedingly rare. BCC usually develops on the sun-damaged skin of people with fair skin and freckles. The tumor is composed of nests of deeply basophilic epithelial cells with narrow rims of cytoplasm that are attached to the epidermis and protrude into the subjacent papillary dermis. Basaloid keratinocytes are rarely seen in squamous cell carcinoma (choice D) and are not encountered in the other choices.

Diagnosis: Basal cell carcinoma

12 **The answer is E: Human papillomavirus.** Verruca vulgaris, also known as the common wart, is an elevated papule with a verrucous (papillomatous) surface. The warts may be single or multiple and are most frequent on the dorsal surfaces of the hands or on the face. Several human papillomavirus types, including types 2 and 4, have been demonstrated in verruca vulgaris. No malignant potential is recognized. The other choices do not induce papillomas.

Diagnosis: Verruca vulgaris

13 **The answer is D: Erythema nodosum (EN).** EN is a cutaneous disorder that manifests as self-limited, nonsuppurative, tender nodules over the extensor surfaces of the lower extremities. It is triggered by exposure to a variety of agents, including drugs and microorganisms (bacteria, viruses, and fungi), and occurs in association with a number of benign and malignant systemic diseases. The early neutrophilic inflammation suggests that EN may be a response to the activation of complement, with resulting neutrophilic chemotaxis. The subsequent appearance of chronic inflammation, foreign body giant cells, and fibrosis is secondary to necrosis of adipose tissue. The other choices do not feature this distinctive histology.

Diagnosis: Erythema nodosum

14 **The answer is B: Bullous pemphigoid (BP).** BP is a common, autoimmune, blistering disease with clinical similarities to pemphigus vulgaris (thus, the term pemphigoid) but in which acantholysis is absent. Complement-fixing IgG antibodies are directed against two basement membrane proteins, BPAG1 and BPAG2. In contrast to pemphigus vulgaris (choice E), immunofluorescent studies demonstrate linear deposition of C3 and IgG along the epidermal basement membrane zone. The other choices do not feature antibasement membrane antibodies.

Diagnosis: Bullous pemphigoid

15 **The answer is B: IgA deposits in dermal papillae.** Dermatitis herpetiformis is an intensely pruritic cutaneous eruption related to gluten sensitivity, which is characterized by urticaria-like plaques and vesicles over the extensor surfaces of the body. Genetically predisposed patients may develop IgA antibodies to components of gluten in the intestines. The resulting IgA complexes then gain access to the circulation and are deposited in the skin. The release of lysosomal enzymes by inflammatory cells cleaves the epidermis from the dermis. The other choices are not typical histologic findings in dermatitis herpetiformis.

Diagnosis: Dermatitis herpetiformis

16 **The answer is C: Granular distribution of immune complexes in the basement membrane zone.** The patient exhibits signs and symptoms of systemic lupus erythematosus (SLE), a disorder characterized by a variety of autoantibodies and other immune abnormalities indicating B-cell hyperactivity. Epidermal cellular damage initiated by light or other exogenous agents causes the release of a large number of antigens, some of which may return to the skin in the form of immune complexes. Immune complexes are also formed in the skin by a reaction of local DNA with antibody that may also be deposited beneath the epidermal basement membrane zone. The other choices are not features of SLE.

Diagnosis: Systemic lupus erythematosus

17 **The answer is C: *Propionibacterium* sp.** Acne vulgaris is a self-limited, inflammatory disorder of the sebaceous follicles that typically afflicts adolescents, results in the intermittent formation of discrete papular or pustular lesions, and may lead to scarring. The development of acne is related to excessive hormonally induced production of sebum, abnormal cornification of portions of the follicular epithelium, and an inflammatory response to the anaerobic diphtheroid *Propionibacterium acnes*. Choice B (*Lactobacillus* sp.) is not a pathogenic organism and choices A, D, and E usually represent acute bacterial infections.
Diagnosis: Acne vulgaris

18 **The answer is E: Lichen planus.** Lichen planus is a hypersensitivity reaction with lymphocytic infiltrates at the dermal-epidermal junction. The disease is apparently initiated by epidermal injury. This injury causes some epidermal cells to be treated as "foreign." The antigens of such cells are processed by Langerhans cells. The processed antigen induces local macrophage activation and lymphocytic proliferation. Macrophages and T lymphocytes disrupt the stratum basalis resulting in reactive epidermal proliferation (hyperkeratosis). The skin displays multiple, flat-topped, violaceous, polygonal papules. The site of pathologic injury is at the dermal-epidermal junction, where there is a striking infiltrate of lymphocytes, many of which surround apoptotic keratinocytes. These histologic features are not observed in the other choices.
Diagnosis: Lichen planus

19 **The answer is A: CD4.** Mycosis fungoides (MF) is a variant of cutaneous T-cell lymphoma. The most important histologic feature of MF is the presence of lymphocytes in the epidermis (epidermotropism). In late stages, the dermal infiltrate becomes dense to the point of forming tumor nodules. Sézary syndrome refers to the systemic dissemination of MF. Cluster of differentiation (CD) antigens are cell surface molecules that serve as useful markers of cellular identity. Currently some 300 different molecules have been assigned CD numbers. CD4 is a useful marker of helper T lymphocytes. None of the other choices are T-cell markers.
Diagnosis: Mycosis fungoides

20 **The answer is E: Hypersensitivity angiitis.** Cutaneous necrotizing vasculitis (CNV) presents as "palpable purpura" and has also been called allergic cutaneous vasculitis, leukocytoclastic vasculitis, and hypersensitivity angiitis. Circulating immune complexes are deposited in vascular walls. The elaborated C5a complement component attracts neutrophils, which degranulate and release lysosomal enzymes, resulting in endothelial damage and fibrin deposition. CNV may be primary, without a known precipitating event in about half of the cases, or associated with a specific infectious agent (e.g., hepatitis B virus). It may also be a secondary process in a variety of chronic diseases (e.g., ulcerative colitis). Allergic contact dermatitis (choice A) is associated with external contact with an allergen (e.g., poison ivy) and dermatitis herpetiformis (choice B) is secondary to gluten sensitivity. Erythema multiforme (choice C) is an immune complex disease associated with a drug reaction that is histologically different than CNV. Erythema nodosum (choice D) does not feature the deposition of immune complexes.
Diagnosis: Hypersensitivity angiitis, cutaneous necrotizing vasculitis

21 **The answer is C: Migration of Langerhans cells into dermal lymphatics.** Allergic contact dermatitis is a model of spongiotic dermatitis, a reaction pattern in which there is edema in the epidermis. In the initial 24 hours following reexposure to the offending plant (elicitation phase), numerous lymphocytes and macrophages accumulate about the superficial venular bed and extend into the epidermis. The epidermal keratinocytes are partially separated by the edema fluid, creating a sponge-like appearance (spongiosis). During the sensitization phase, low molecular weight haptens combine with carrier proteins at the cell membrane of Langerhans cells. These inflammatory cells carry processed antigen through the lymphatics to regional lymph nodes and present it to CD4+ T lymphocytes. Sensitized T cells then migrate back into the epidermis. Cytokine production leads to the accumulation of more T cells and macrophages and to epidermal cell injury.
Diagnosis: Allergic contact dermatitis

22 **The answer is B: Macule.** Freckles, or ephelides, are small, brown macules that occur on sun-exposed skin, especially in people with fair skin. Freckles usually appear at about age 5 years. The pigmentation of a freckle deepens with exposure to sunlight and fades when light exposure ceases. Freckles show hyperpigmentation of the basal keratinocytes without a concomitant increase in the number of melanocytes. The other choices represent raised lesions of the skin.
Diagnosis: Freckles, ephelides

23 **The answer is B: Dysphagia.** Scleroderma is marked by fibrosis and tightening of the skin. The disease also displays variable structural and functional involvement of internal organs, including the kidneys, lungs, heart, esophagus, and small intestine. Dysphagia due to involvement of the esophagus is common. Patients with early scleroderma usually present with Raynaud phenomenon or nonpitting edema of the hands or fingers. The affected areas become hard and tense. In late stages of the disease, the skin over large parts of the body is thickened, densely fibrotic, and fixed to the underlying tissue. Although scleroderma can affect the kidney, polyuria/polydipsia (choice D) is most commonly a complication of diabetes. The other choices are not related to scleroderma.
Diagnosis: Scleroderma

Chapter 25

The Head and Neck

QUESTIONS

Select the single best answer.

1 A 6-year-old boy presents with painful sores on his upper lip. He was seen for a flu 1 week ago. The lesion appears as 0.2- to 0.4-cm vesicles with focal ulceration. Which of the following is the most likely histologic feature of this skin lesion?
(A) Acute arteritis
(B) Caseating granulomas
(C) Fungal hyphae
(D) Multinucleated epithelial cells
(E) Noncaseating granulomas

2 A 74-year-old man with a 15-year history of diabetes is hospitalized because of end-stage kidney disease. His tongue, inner side of the lips, and buccal mucosa are covered with white, slightly elevated, soft patches (shown in the image). What is the most likely diagnosis?

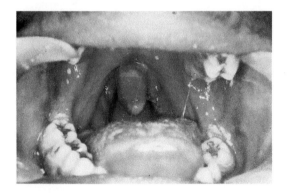

(A) Aphthous stomatitis
(B) Candidiasis
(C) Herpes labialis
(D) Pyogenic granuloma
(E) Xerostomia

3 A 40-year-old woman is hospitalized because of a massive neck infection that developed over a period of 3 days after extraction of an impacted wisdom tooth. She has a high fever, and her lower jaw and entire neck are swollen, red, and painful. Throat culture reveals a mixed bacterial flora, containing both aerobic and anaerobic microorganisms. Which of the following is the most likely diagnosis?
(A) Actinomycosis
(B) Acute necrotizing ulcerative gingivitis
(C) Ludwig angina
(D) Pyogenic granuloma
(E) Scarlet fever

4 A 45-year-old woman presents with a 1-year history of dry mouth and eyes. Physical examination reveals bilateral enlargement of the parotid glands. A biopsy (shown in the image) discloses infiltrates of lymphocytes forming focal germinal centers. Which of the following best describes changes that would be expected in this patient's parotid glands, late in the course of her disease?

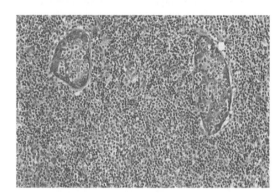

(A) Atrophy
(B) Dysplasia
(C) Hyperplasia
(D) Hypertrophy
(E) Metaplasia

5 A 16-year-old girl presents with a sore throat of 4 months in duration. She describes feeling a lump in her throat. Physical examination reveals a 1-cm cystic lesion at the base of the tongue. This developmental lesion most likely arises as a remnant of which of the following anatomic structures?
(A) Auditory tube
(B) Branchial arches
(C) Facial fusion lines
(D) Rudimentary thymus
(E) Thyroglossal duct

6 A 2-year-old girl was withdrawn from a day care center for excessive irritability. On physical examination, she has multiple, small superficial ulcers of the oral mucosa. The ulcerations heal spontaneously over the next 5 days. Which of the following is the most likely diagnosis?

(A) Aphthous stomatitis
(B) Candidiasis
(C) Gingivitis
(D) Ludwig angina
(E) Pyogenic granuloma

7 A 6-year-old boy presents with a painful sore in his mouth. Physical examination reveals a small, elevated, and focally ulcerated red-purple gingival lesion. A soft red mass measuring 1 cm in diameter is surgically removed. Histologic examination discloses highly vascular granulation tissue, with marked acute and chronic inflammation. What is the most likely diagnosis?

(A) Acute necrotizing gingivitis
(B) Aphthous stomatitis
(C) Herpes labialis
(D) Pyogenic granuloma
(E) Tuberculosis

8 A 60-year-old man, who is a chronic alcoholic, is referred by a homeless shelter for facial ulcers. On physical examination, there are large ulcerations in the mouth and facial tissues with focal exposure of bone. A culture grows *Borrelia vincentii*. Which of the following is the most likely diagnosis?

(A) Acute necrotizing ulcerative gingivitis
(B) Apical granuloma
(C) Ludwig angina
(D) Periodontitis
(E) Pyogenic granuloma

9 A 30-year-old man was told by his dentist that his left upper wisdom tooth showed some decay. Even though the decay was still reparable, tooth extraction was recommended. A whole mount section through the extracted tooth is shown in the image. What is the appropriate diagnosis?

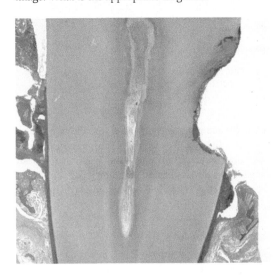

(A) Apical granuloma
(B) Dental caries
(C) Periapical abscess
(D) Periodontitis
(E) Pulpitis

10 A 4-year-old boy from Uganda presents for pre-school physical examination. His parents indicate that hearing loss in his right ear developed 3 years ago following an acute illness. If this child's hearing loss was caused by a viral infection, which of the following was the most likely etiology?

(A) Chickenpox
(B) Epstein-Barr virus
(C) Mumps
(D) Rubella
(E) Yellow fever

11 An 82-year-old man presents with painless swelling below the right ear that has been growing slowly for about a year. Physical examination confirms a cystic lesion. Fine-needle aspiration returns scanty brown fluid, which microscopically consists of a mixture of lymphoid cells and epithelial cells with abundant granular eosinophilic cytoplasm. A biopsy of the mass is shown in the image. Which of the following is the most likely diagnosis?

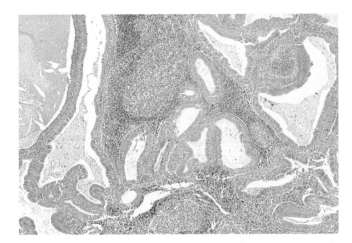

(A) Acinic cell carcinoma
(B) Adenoid cystic carcinoma
(C) Chronic abscess
(D) Pleomorphic adenoma
(E) Warthin tumor

12 A 64-year-old man presents with sores on the gums. Oral examination shows multiple, gingival abscesses adjacent to the teeth and excessive mobility of several teeth. Which of the following is the most likely diagnosis?

(A) Dental caries
(B) Hyperparathyroidism
(C) Osteitis deformans
(D) Periapical granuloma
(E) Periodontal disease

13 A 33-year-old woman presents with a painful gingival lesion. Oral examination shows a 1-cm swelling on the lower right gingiva. A biopsy is taken (shown in the image). Which of the following is the most likely diagnosis?

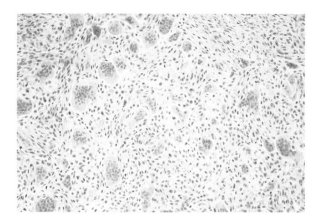

(A) Ameloblastoma
(B) Odontogenic cyst
(C) Peripheral giant-cell granuloma
(D) Radicular cyst
(E) Squamous cell carcinoma

14 A 26-year-old football player complains of persistent nasal blockage, runny nose, and headache. Multiple nasal polyps are identified and resected (shown in the image). Histological examination of the polyps shows that they are benign. Which of the following is the most likely cause of polyps in this patient?

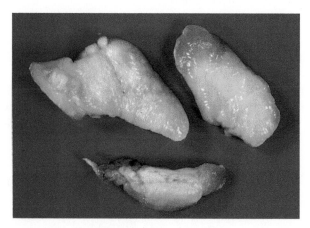

(A) Acute suppurative otitis media
(B) Acute tonsillitis
(C) Acute viral rhinitis
(D) Chronic allergic rhinitis
(E) Chronic otitis media

15 A 55-year-old man presents with recurrent nosebleeds. He complains of persistent runny nose, fever, malaise, and a 20-lb (9-kg) weight loss. Physical examination reveals a "saddle nose" deformity (patient shown in the image). An X-ray film of the chest shows patchy infiltrates. Urinalysis discloses 2+ hematuria. Antibodies directed to which of the following cellular structures would be expected in the serum of this patient?

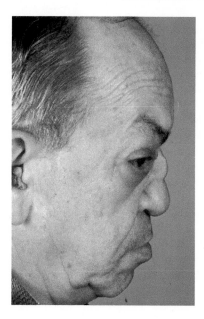

(A) Epithelial nuclei
(B) Mitochondria
(C) Neutrophil cytoplasm
(D) Skeletal muscle
(E) Smooth muscle

16 A 60-year-old woman presents with a 5-month history of "sinus pressure." A 2-cm firm lesion is identified in the right lateral nasal wall. A CT scan reveals involvement of the adjacent paranasal sinus. A biopsy (shown in the image) displays epithelial nests protruding into the submucosa with uniform cellular proliferation and no atypia. Which of the following etiologic agents is most likely associated with the development of this lesion?

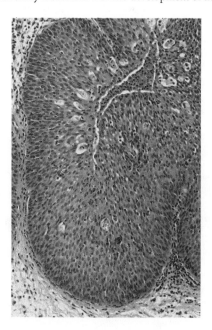

(A) Cytomegalovirus
(B) Epstein-Barr virus
(C) Herpes simplex virus type 1
(D) Human papillomavirus types 6 and 11
(E) *Toxoplasma gondii*

17 An 8-year-old boy presents with a 3-day history of fever and sore throat. His temperature is 38°C (101°F), pulse is 88 per minute, and respirations are 33 per minute. On physical examination, the tonsils are enlarged, boggy, and coated with a purulent exudate. A tonsillar swab is most likely to grow which of the following microorganisms?

(A) *Staphylococcus aureus*
(B) *Staphylococcus epidermidis*
(C) *Streptococcus pneumoniae*
(D) *Streptococcus pyogenes*
(E) *Streptococcus viridans*

18 A 70-year-old woman complains of gradual hearing loss. Which of the following conditions is the most likely cause of conducting hearing loss in this patient?

(A) Acoustic trauma
(B) Chronic otitis media
(C) Labyrinthine toxicity
(D) Mastoiditis
(E) Otosclerosis

19 A 24-year-old man presents with right ear pain that he has had for 3 days. He recently returned from a scuba diving trip to the Caribbean. The patient is afebrile. Otoscopic examination reveals a bulging, right tympanic membrane. What is the most likely diagnosis?

(A) Acute mastoiditis
(B) Acute rhinitis
(C) Acute serous otitis media
(D) Acute sinusitis
(E) Acute suppurative otitis media

20 A 33-year-old man from China presents with a lump in his neck. Physical examination reveals painless, anterior cervical adenopathy. A large necrotizing mass is identified in the posterior nasopharynx, with obstruction of both eustachian tubes. A biopsy of the mass reveals sheets of malignant cells with large nuclei (shown in the image). Which of the following pathogens has been associated with the development of this patient's neoplasm?

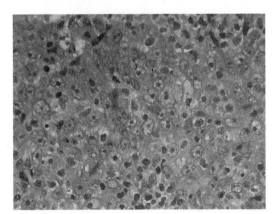

(A) Cytomegalovirus
(B) Epstein-Barr virus
(C) Herpes simplex virus type 2
(D) Human immunodeficiency virus
(E) Human T-cell lymphoma/leukemia virus

21 A 50-year-old woman presents with a slowly enlarging, painful mass at the angle of the right jaw. A biopsy of the mass is shown in the image. Which of the following is the most likely diagnosis?

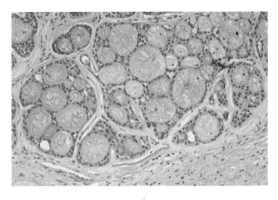

(A) Acinic cell carcinoma
(B) Adenoid cystic carcinoma
(C) Malignant mixed tumor
(D) Malignant oncocytoma
(E) Mucoepidermoid carcinoma

22 A 34-year-old man complains of hearing loss. He has had multiple bouts of ear infections over the last 20 years and was recently diagnosed with chronic suppurative otitis media. Which of the following is the most likely complication of this condition in this patient?

(A) Acoustic neuroma
(B) Cholesteatoma
(C) Chronic rhinitis
(D) Chronic sinusitis
(E) Squamous cell carcinoma

23 A 40-year-old man presents with a 2-month history of a painless lump in his left jaw. A radiograph of the mandible shows a 2-cm multilocular lesion with smooth cyst-like appearance, smooth periphery, expansion of the bone, and thinning of the cortex. A biopsy of the mass is shown in the image. This patient's ameloblastoma is thought to arise from which of the following cells or structures?

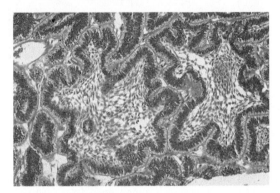

(A) Developmental rests
(B) Odontogenic cyst
(C) Osteoblasts
(D) Osteoclasts
(E) Radicular cyst

24 A 67-year-old woman complains of a white discoloration in her mouth. She has a 60-pack-year history of smoking. Physical examination reveals white plaques on the buccal mucosa, tongue, and floor of the mouth. A biopsy (shown in the image) demonstrates severe epithelial dysplasia. What is the appropriate clinical diagnosis?

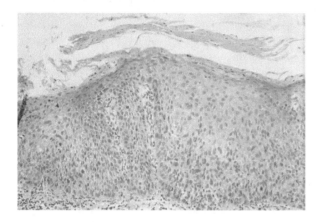

(A) Actinic keratosis
(B) Candidiasis
(C) Leukoplakia
(D) Malakoplakia
(E) Papillomatosis

25 The patient described in Question 24 is at higher risk of developing which of the following neoplasms?
(A) Adenoid cystic carcinoma
(B) Mucoepidermoid carcinoma
(C) Nasopharyngeal carcinoma
(D) Papilloma
(E) Squamous cell carcinoma

26 A 45-year-old man presents with a painless mass in the neck (shown in the image). A 4-cm firm, movable tumor is identified at the angle of the left jaw. A biopsy of the tumor reveals myoepithelial cells intermingled with myxoid, mucoid, and cartilaginous areas. The tumor is removed surgically. Which of the following is the most likely prognosis?

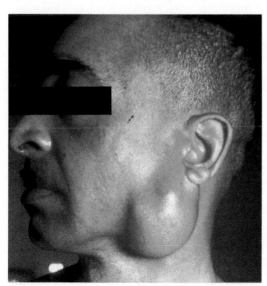

(A) Contralateral spread
(B) Invasion of bone
(C) Local recurrence
(D) Malignant transformation
(E) Pyogenic abscess

ANSWERS

1 **The answer is D: Multinucleated epithelial cells.** Herpes labialis (cold sores, fever blisters) and herpetic stomatitis are caused by herpes virus type 1. They are among the most common viral infections of the lips and oral mucosa in both children and young adults. The disease starts with painful inflammation of the affected mucosa, followed shortly by the formation of vesicles. These vesicles rupture and form shallow, painful ulcers. Microscopically, the herpetic vesicle forms as a result of "ballooning degeneration" of the epithelial cells. Some epithelial cells show intranuclear inclusion bodies. At the edge of the ulcer are large, multinucleated, epithelial cells with "ground glass" homogenized nuclei, often exhibiting nuclear molding. The ulcers heal spontaneously without scar formation. Acute arteritis (choice A) does not cause the described lesions. Choices B, C, and E do not represent acute vesicular lesions.
Diagnosis: Herpes labialis

2 **The answer is B: Candidiasis.** Also termed thrush or moniliasis, candidiasis is caused by a yeast-like fungus, *Candida albicans*, which is a common surface inhabitant of the oral cavity, gastrointestinal tract, and vagina. Oral candidiasis is most common in people with immunocompromised systems or with diabetes, and the incidence in patients with AIDS is 40% to 90%. The oral lesions typically appear as white, slightly elevated, soft patches that consist mainly of fungal hyphae. Choices A, C, and D are generally focal lesions.
Diagnosis: Candidiasis

3 **The answer is C: Ludwig angina.** Ludwig angina is a rapidly spreading cellulitis, or phlegmon, which originates in the submaxillary or sublingual space but extends locally to involve both. The bacteria responsible for this infection originate from the oral flora, but this potentially life-threatening inflammatory process is uncommon in developed countries. After extraction of a tooth, hairline fractures may occur in the lingual cortex of the mandible, providing microorganisms ready access to the submaxillary space. By following the fascial planes, the infection may dissect into the parapharyngeal space and, from there, into the carotid sheath. Actinomycosis (choice A) features branched, filamentous bacteria. Acute necrotizing ulcerative gingivitis (Vincent angina, choice B) does not extend to the neck. Pyogenic granuloma (choice D) is a focal, reactive vascular lesion.
Diagnosis: Ludwig angina

4 **The answer is A: Atrophy.** Sjögren syndrome is a chronic inflammatory disease of the salivary and lacrimal glands; it may be restricted to these sites or may be associated with a systemic collagen vascular disease. Involvement of the salivary glands leads to dry mouth (xerostomia), and disease of the lacrimal glands results in dry eyes (keratoconjunctivitis sicca). Late in the course of the disease, the affected glands become atrophic, with fibrosis and fatty infiltration of the parenchyma. Dysplasia (choice B) is not featured in Sjögren syndrome.

Diagnosis: Sjögren syndrome

5 **The answer is E: Thyroglossal duct.** During its normal development, the thyroid gland descends from the base of the tongue to its final position in the neck. Heterotopic functioning thyroid tissue or a developmental cyst (thyroglossal duct cyst) may occur anywhere along the path of descent. The most common location is at the foramen cecum of the tongue. Symptoms such as dysphonia, sore throat, and awareness of a mass in the throat often become evident during adolescence and pregnancy. The other choices do not present in this anatomic location. In particular, branched cleft cysts that originate from remnants of the branchial arches (choice B) occur in the lateral anterior aspect of the neck or in the parotid gland.

Diagnosis: Thyroglossal duct cyst

6 **The answer is A: Aphthous stomatitis.** Aphthous stomatitis describes a common disease that is characterized by painful, recurrent, solitary or multiple, small ulcers of the oral mucosa. The causative agent is unknown. Microscopically, the lesion consists of a shallow ulcer covered by a fibrinopurulent exudate. Candidiasis (choice B) features white plaques.

Diagnosis: Aphthous stomatitis

7 **The answer is D: Pyogenic granuloma.** Pyogenic granuloma is a reactive vascular lesion that commonly occurs in the oral cavity. Usually some minor trauma to the tissues permits invasion of nonspecific microorganisms. In the oral cavity, pyogenic granulomas, ranging from a few millimeters to a centimeter, are most frequent on the gingiva. The lesion is seen as an elevated, red or purple, soft mass, with a smooth, lobulated, ulcerated surface. Microscopically, the nodule consists of highly vascular granulation tissue that shows varying degrees of acute and chronic inflammation. With time, pyogenic granuloma becomes less vascular and comes to resemble a fibroma. Choices A, B, and C are ulcerating lesions. Tuberculosis (choice E) features granulomatous inflammation.

Diagnosis: Pyogenic granuloma

8 **The answer is A: Acute necrotizing ulcerative gingivitis.** Acute necrotizing ulcerative gingivitis (Vincent angina) represents an infection by two symbiotic organisms; one is a fusiform bacillus, and the other is a spirochete (*B. vincentii*). The fact that these organisms are found in the mouths of many healthy persons suggests that predisposing factors are important in the development of acute necrotizing ulcerative gingivitis. The most important element appears to be decreased resistance to infection as a result of inadequate nutrition, immunodeficiency, or poor oral hygiene. Vincent infection is characterized by punched-out erosions of the interdental papillae. The ulceration tends to spread and eventually to involve all gingival margins, which become covered by a necrotic pseudomembrane. None of the other choices are destructive, ulcerating lesions.

Diagnosis: Necrotizing ulcerative gingivitis

9 **The answer is B: Dental caries.** Caries is the most prevalent chronic disease of the calcified tissues of the teeth. Caries begins with the disintegration of the enamel prisms after decalcification of the interprismatic substance; these events lead to the accumulation of debris and microorganisms. These changes produce a small pit or fissure in the enamel. When the process reaches the dentinoenamel junction, it spreads laterally and also penetrates the dentin along the dentinal tubules. A substantial cavity then forms in the dentin, producing a flask-shaped lesion with a narrow orifice. Only when the vascular pulp of the tooth is invaded does an inflammatory reaction (pulpitis) appear (choice E). Apical granuloma (choice A), the most common sequel of pulpitis, is the formation of chronically inflamed periapical granulation tissue. Periapical abscess (choice C) is also a result of pulpitis. Periodontitis (choice D) is an inflammatory condition of the marginal gingiva.

Diagnosis: Dental caries

10 **The answer is C: Mumps.** Mumps is the most common cause of deafness among the postnatal viral infections. The infection can cause rapid hearing loss, which is unilateral in 80% of cases. By contrast, prenatal infection of the labyrinth with rubella (choice D) is usually bilateral, with permanent loss of cochlear and vestibular function. A number of other viruses are suspected to cause labyrinthitis, including influenza and parainfluenza viruses, Epstein-Barr virus (choice B), herpesviruses, and adenoviruses. Temporal bone specimens of such cases reveal severe damage to the organ of Corti, with almost total loss of both inner and outer hair cells.

Diagnosis: Mumps

11 **The answer is E: Warthin tumor.** Warthin tumor is a benign neoplasm of the parotid gland, composed of cystic glandular spaces embedded in dense lymphoid tissue. This tumor is the most common monomorphic adenoma. Although the neoplasm is clearly benign, it can be bilateral (15% of cases) or multifocal within the same gland. Warthin tumor is the only tumor of the salivary glands that is more common in men than in women. These lesions generally occur after the age of 30, with most arising after age 50 years. Pleomorphic adenoma (choice D) has a biphasic appearance, which represents an admixture of epithelial and stromal elements. Acinic cell carcinoma (choice A) is an uncommon malignancy. Adenoid cystic carcinoma (choice B) is a slow-growing malignant neoplasm of the salivary gland, which invades locally and tends to recur after surgery.

Diagnosis: Warthin tumor, adenolymphoma

12 **The answer is E: Periodontal disease.** Periodontal disease refers to acute and chronic disorders of the soft tissues surrounding the teeth, which eventually lead to the loss of supporting bone. Chronic periodontal disease typically occurs in adults, particularly in persons with poor oral hygiene. However, many persons with apparently impeccable habits, but a strong family history of periodontal disease, manifest the disorder. Chronic periodontitis causes loss of more teeth in adults than does any other disease, including caries. Periapical granuloma (choice D) is the most common sequel to pulpitis and represents chronically inflamed periapical granulation tissue.

Diagnosis: Periodontal disease

13 **The answer is C: Peripheral giant-cell granuloma.** Peripheral giant-cell granuloma is an unusual proliferative reaction to local injury that is seen as a mass on the gingiva or the alveolar process. The adjective "peripheral" denotes the superficial, extraosseous location of the lesion, as opposed to the "central" giant-cell granulomas that occur within the jawbones. Peripheral giant-cell granuloma is seen as a mass covered by mucous membrane, which can be ulcerated. Histological examination reveals a nonencapsulated lesion with numerous multinucleated giant cells embedded in a fibrous stroma that also contains ovoid or spindle-shaped mesenchymal cells. The other choices do not typically feature multinucleated giant cells.

Diagnosis: Peripheral giant-cell granuloma

14 The answer is D: Chronic allergic rhinitis. Sinonasal inflammatory polyps are nonneoplastic lesions of the mucosa. Most polyps arise from the lateral nasal wall or the ethmoid recess. They may be unilateral or bilateral and single or multiple. Symptoms include nasal obstruction, rhinorrhea, and headaches. The etiology involves multiple factors, including allergy, cystic fibrosis, infections, diabetes mellitus, and aspirin intolerance. Microscopically, sinonasal allergic polyps are lined externally by respiratory epithelium and contain mucous glands within a loose mucoid stroma, which is infiltrated by plasma cells, lymphocytes, and numerous eosinophils. Neither acute tonsillitis (choice B) nor acute viral rhinitis (choice C) leads to nasal polyps.

Diagnosis: Nasal polyps

15 The answer is C: Neutrophil cytoplasm. Wegener granulomatosis is a disease of unknown origin that shares some features with lethal midline granuloma. Both diseases are characterized by necrotizing, ulcerated, mucosal lesions. Lethal midline granuloma is a sign of an underlying lymphoid malignancy, whereas Wegener granulomatosis is an inflammatory disease. Evidence points to an autoimmune etiology for Wegener granulomatosis. In most instances the lesions are not limited to the upper respiratory tract; they also involve the lungs and the kidneys. More than 90% of patients with Wegener granulomatosis exhibit antineutrophil cytoplasmic antibody (ANCA); of these patients, 75% have C-ANCA. Antibodies directed against the other choices are not associated with the clinical syndrome described.

Diagnosis: Wegener granulomatosis

16 The answer is D: Human papillomavirus types 6 and 11. Papillomas are the most common tumors of the nasal cavity. Human papillomavirus types 6 and 11 cause papillomas, which may be histologically diagnosed as either squamous or inverted. Epstein-Barr virus infection (choice B) is related to nasopharyngeal carcinoma.

Diagnosis: Sinonasal inverted papilloma

17 The answer is D: *Streptococcus pyogenes*. Acute tonsillitis may be caused by bacterial or viral infections. *Streptococcus pyogenes* (group A β-hemolytic streptococci, choice D) is the most common etiologic agent in acute suppurative tonsillitis.

Diagnosis: Tonsillitis, acute

18 The answer is E: Otosclerosis. Otosclerosis refers to the formation of new spongy bone about the stapes and the oval window, which results in progressive deafness. This condition is an autosomal dominant hereditary defect and is the most common cause of conductive hearing loss in young and middle-aged adults in the United States. Ten percent of white and 1% of black adult Americans have some otosclerosis, although 90% of cases are asymptomatic. The other choices are much less common causes of hearing loss.

Diagnosis: Otosclerosis

19 The answer is C: Acute serous otitis media. Obstruction of the eustachian tube may result from sudden changes in atmospheric pressure (e.g., during flying in an aircraft or deep-sea diving). This effect is particularly severe in the presence of an upper respiratory tract infection, an acute allergic reaction, or viral or bacterial infection at the orifice of the eustachian tube. Inflammation may also occur without bacterial invasion of the middle ear. More than half of children in the United States have had at least one episode of serous otitis media before their third birthday. It has become increasingly evident that repeated bouts of otitis media in early childhood often contribute to unsuspected hearing loss, which is due to residual (usually sterile) fluid in the middle ear. Acute suppurative otitis media (choice E) is unlikely without fever.

Diagnosis: Serous otitis media, acute

20 The answer is B: Epstein-Barr virus. Nasopharyngeal carcinoma is an epithelial cancer of the nasopharynx that is classified into keratinizing and nonkeratinizing subtypes. Nonkeratinizing nasopharyngeal carcinoma is associated with EBV infection. Most patients have anti-EBV IgA in their serum. Both differentiated and undifferentiated nonkeratinizing nasopharyngeal carcinomas are immunoreactive with antibodies to cytokeratins. Choices A, C, and D are noncarcinogenic viruses. Choice E does not cause malignant transformation of epithelial cells.

Diagnosis: Nasopharyngeal carcinoma

21 The answer is B: Adenoid cystic carcinoma. Adenoid cystic carcinoma is a slowly growing malignant neoplasm of the salivary gland that is notorious for its tendency to invade locally and to recur after surgical resection. The tumor cells are small, have scant cytoplasm, and grow in solid sheets or as small groups, strands, or columns. Within these structures, the tumor cells interconnect to enclose cystic spaces, resulting in a solid, tubular or cribriform (sieve-like) arrangement. The other choices do not exhibit the typical cribriform pattern.

Diagnosis: Adenoid cystic carcinoma

22 The answer is B: Cholesteatoma. Cholesteatoma is a complication of chronic suppurative otitis and a rupture of the eardrum. Cholesteatoma is a mass of accumulated keratin and squamous mucosa that results from the growth of squamous epithelium from the external ear canal through the perforated eardrum into the middle ear. Microscopically, cholesteatomas are identical to epidermal inclusion cysts and are surrounded by granulation tissue and fibrosis. The keratin mass frequently becomes infected and shields the bacteria from antibiotics. Squamous cell carcinoma (choice E) rarely occurs in the ear.

Diagnosis: Cholesteatoma

23 **The answer is A: Developmental rests.** Ameloblastomas (adamantinomas) are tumors of epithelial odontogenic origin and represent the most common clinically significant odontogenic tumor. They are slow-growing, locally invasive tumors that generally follow a benign clinical course. Microscopically, ameloblastoma resembles the enamel organ in its various stages of differentiation, and a single tumor may show various histologic patterns. The centers of these cell nests consist of loosely arranged, large polyhedral cells that resemble the stellate reticulum of the developing tooth. Choices B and E are acquired nonneoplastic lesions of the oral cavity. Cells of normal bone (choices C and D) do not give rise to this characteristic odontogenic tumor.

Diagnosis: Ameloblastoma

24 **The answer is C: Leukoplakia.** Leukoplakia is a descriptive term for many reactive, preneoplastic, and neoplastic lesions of the oral mucosa. Leukoplakic lesions are not necessarily premalignant and demonstrate a spectrum of histopathologic changes, ranging from increased surface keratinization without dysplasia to invasive keratinizing squamous carcinoma. Candidiasis (choice B) also presents with whitish plaques but does not induce dysplasia. Actinic keratosis (choice A) involves sun-exposed skin and malakoplakia (choice D) occurs in the bladder. Papillomatosis (choice E) does not present as a flat white lesion.

Diagnosis: Leukoplakia

25 **The answer is E: Squamous cell carcinoma.** Although the probability of squamous cell carcinoma developing in a patient with oral leukoplakia is low, there is still a risk (10% to 12%) of malignant transformation. Carcinogenic factors that lead to the induction of cancer usually affect more than one site in the oral mucosa, and the tumors may therefore be multiple. Choices A, B, and C do not arise from the oral epithelium and choice D is not a complication of epithelial dysplasia.

Diagnosis: Squamous cell carcinoma

26 **The answer is C: Local recurrence.** Pleomorphic adenoma, the most common tumor of the salivary glands, is a benign neoplasm characterized by a biphasic appearance which represents an admixture of epithelial and stromal elements. At surgery, tumor projections can be missed if the tumor is not carefully dissected. Tumor implanted during surgery or tumor nodules left behind continue to grow as recurrences in the scar tissue of the previous operation. Recurrence of pleomorphic adenoma represents local growth and does not reflect malignancy. Malignant transformation (choice D) is exceedingly rare.

Diagnosis: Pleomorphic adenoma

Chapter 26

Bones, Joints, and Soft Tissues

QUESTIONS

Select the single best answer.

1 A 30-year-old man with dwarfism is admitted to the hospital for hip replacement due to severe osteoarthritis. He has short arms and legs and a relatively large head. His parents do not show signs of this congenital disease. This patient most likely has a spontaneous mutation in the gene encoding which of the following proteins?
(A) Collagen type I
(B) Dystrophin
(C) Fibroblast growth factor receptor
(D) Growth hormone receptor
(E) Insulin-like growth factor

2 A 2-year-old boy is treated for recurrent fractures of his long bones. Physical examination reveals blue sclerae, loose joints, abnormal teeth, and poor hearing. Molecular diagnostic studies will most likely demonstrate a mutation in the gene encoding which of the following proteins?
(A) Collagen
(B) Dystrophin
(C) Lysyl hydroxylase
(D) Fibrillin
(E) Fibroblast growth factor receptor

3 A 9-year-old boy is evaluated for signs of precocious puberty. Laboratory tests demonstrate a 21-hydroxylase deficiency and increased serum levels of androgens. A CT scan reveals enlargement of the adrenal glands bilaterally. If this patient is untreated, short stature will result as a consequence of which of the following mechanisms of disease?
(A) Decreased growth hormone production
(B) End-organ resistance to androgens
(C) Impaired osteoblast activity
(D) Premature epiphyseal plate closure
(E) Unresponsiveness to bone morphogenetic protein

4 A 17-year-old girl suffers a spiral fracture of her right tibia, and the leg is casted. Unfortunately, the fracture does not heal correctly due to excessive motion and interposition of soft tissue at the fracture site. Which of the following represents the most likely complication of nonunion in this patient?

(A) Codman triangle formation
(B) Cup-shaped epiphysis
(C) Involucrum formation
(D) Osteomyelitis
(E) Pseudoarthrosis

5 A 50-year-old woman presents with lower back pain of 3 weeks in duration. Radiologic studies reveal several discrete lytic lesions in the lumbar back and pelvis. Laboratory studies show elevated serum levels of alkaline phosphatase. Serum calcium, serum protein, and peripheral blood smears are normal. Aspiration biopsy of a pelvic lesion shows keratin-positive cells. Which of the following is the most likely diagnosis?
(A) Chondrosarcoma
(B) Metastatic carcinoma
(C) Osteochondroma
(D) Osteosarcoma
(E) Plasmacytoma

6 A 6-year-old child with mild hydrocephalus suffers chronic infections and dies of intractable chronic anemia. At autopsy, his bones are dense and misshapen. The femur, in particular, shows obliteration of the marrow space. Histologically, the bones demonstrate disorganization of bony trabeculae by retention of primary spongiosa and further obliteration of the marrow spaces by secondary spongiosa (shown in the image). Hematopoietic bone marrow cells are sparse. The disorder is caused by mutations in genes that regulate which of the following cell types?

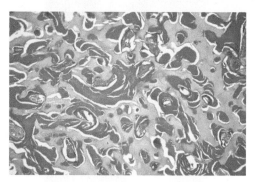

(A) Fibroblasts
(B) Myofibroblasts
(C) Normoblasts
(D) Osteoblasts
(E) Osteoclasts

291

7 A 33-year-old woman presents with a spontaneous fracture of her femoral head. She has suffered from Crohn disease for 20 years. Multiple surgical procedures have resulted in the removal of much of her small bowel. She has had profound weight loss over the last 10 years. The bone is pinned. Histologically, the resected femoral head shows bony trabeculae that are covered by a thicker-than-normal layer of osteoid (shown in the image). In this section, the osteoid is stained red, and mineralized bone is stained black. Which of the following best describes the pathogenesis of this lesion?

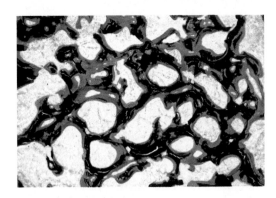

(A) Degenerative changes in the subchondral bone
(B) Enhanced osteoblast activity
(C) Impaired mineralization of osteoid
(D) Inflammatory synovium with pannus formation
(E) Subperiosteal bone resorption

8 An 18-year-old man presents with bone pain about his knee that he has had for 6 weeks. Radiologic studies reveal a lytic lesion of the distal end of the femur, which arises in the metaphysis, extends into the proximal diaphysis, and elevates the periosteum. Serum levels of alkaline phosphatase are markedly elevated. The lesion is removed, and the cut surface of the surgical specimen is shown in the image. Molecular studies of this tumor would most likely reveal a mutation in the gene encoding which of the following proteins?

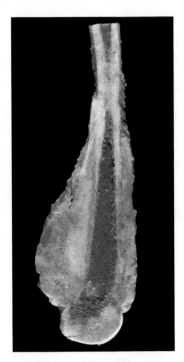

(A) Cyclin A
(B) Cyclin D
(C) Fibroblast growth factor receptor
(D) Rb tumor suppressor protein
(E) Stimulatory guanine nucleotide–binding protein

9 A 10-year-old boy complains of increasing pain in his left hip. He began limping shortly after playing a baseball game at school. He is afebrile. An X-ray of the femoral head shows a fracture and irregular densities of the cancellous bone. You make a diagnosis of Legg-Calvé-Perthes disease. Which of the following best describes the pathologic findings in this patient?

(A) Avascular osteonecrosis
(B) Chondroma
(C) Fibrous dysplasia
(D) Osteitis fibrosa cystica
(E) Osteopetrosis

10 A 50-year-old man presents with a 2-day history of left leg pain. His temperature is 38.7°C (103°F). He has a harsh systolic murmur and echocardiographic evidence of bacterial endocarditis. If this patient has developed hematogenous osteomyelitis, his bone infection would most likely be found in which of the following anatomic locations?

(A) Body of a flat bone
(B) Diaphysis of a long bone
(C) Epiphysis of a long bone
(D) Metaphysis of a long bone
(E) Periosteum of a long bone

11 A 74-year-old, obese woman (BMI = 33 kg/m²) complains of chronic pain in her back, knees, and fingers. The pain typically subsides at rest. On physical examination, the distal interphalangeal joints are enlarged and tender. Which of the following best describes the pathogenesis of joint pain in this patient?

(A) Acute inflammation of the ligaments
(B) Degeneration of articular cartilage
(C) Degenerative changes of cortical bone
(D) Inflammatory synovium with pannus formation
(E) Reduction of the volume of synovial fluid

12 A 60-year-old woman with arthritis suffers a massive stroke and expires. At autopsy, the proximal phalangeal joint tissue shows pannus, synovial cell hyperplasia, and lymphoid follicles. Which of the following best describes the pathogenesis of pannus formation in this patient?

(A) Calcification of the synovium
(B) Chronic inflammation of synovium
(C) Degeneration of cartilage
(D) Dislocation of a portion of bone
(E) Necrosis of fibroadipose tissue

13 A 9-year-old boy complains of 2 weeks of pain in the hip. His temperature is 38°C (101°F). Laboratory studies show an elevated erythrocyte sedimentation rate. An X-ray reveals a mottled radiolucent defect in the upper femur, with abundant periosteal new bone formation. Fine-needle aspiration returns numerous neutrophils and cocci. *Staphylococcus aureus* is cultured from the bone lesion. A biopsy shows a fragment of necrotic bone embedded in fibrinopurulent exudate. Which of the following terms best describes the necrotic bone?

(A) Brodie abscess
(B) Cloaca
(C) Involucrum
(D) Osteophyte
(E) Sequestrum

14 A 40-year-old woman complains of morning stiffness in her hands. On physical examination, her finger joints are painful, swollen, and warm. X-ray examination of the hands shows narrowing of the joint spaces and erosion of joint surfaces of the metacarpal/phalangeal joints. The adjacent bones show osteoporosis. A synovial biopsy reveals prominent lymphoid follicles, synovial hyperplasia, and villous folds (shown in the image). Laboratory studies conducted on a blood sample from this patient will most likely show polyclonal antibodies directed against which of the following proteins?

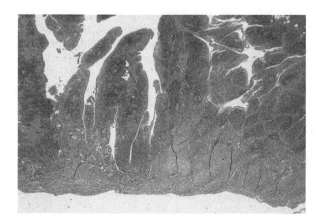

(A) Double-stranded DNA
(B) Fab2 portion of IgM
(C) Fc portion of IgG
(D) Ribonucleoprotein
(E) Topoisomerase I

15 A 55-year-old man presents with pain in the left arm. Laboratory studies show elevated serum levels of calcium and parathyroid hormone. An X-ray of the left arm reveals multiple small bone cysts and pathologic fractures. Biopsy of the affected bone discloses numerous giant cells in a cellular and fibrous stroma. The patient undergoes removal of a parathyroid adenoma. Which of the following best describes the pathogenesis of bone pain and pathologic fractures in this patient?

(A) Enhanced osteoblast activity
(B) Impaired mineralization of osteoid
(C) Increased bone resorption
(D) Increased mineralization of bone
(E) Osteoporosis

16 A 67-year-old man from England develops bow-legs and leg pain over a period of 5 years. He also complains of progressive hearing loss over the last 2 years. A bone biopsy shows a mosaic pattern with prominent cement lines and increased osteoblastic and osteoclastic activity. Serum electrolyte levels are normal. This patient is at increased risk for developing which of the following diseases?

(A) Amyloidosis
(B) Multiple myeloma
(C) Osteogenic sarcoma
(D) Pulmonary embolism
(E) Renal failure

17 A 60-year-old man with a history of gout presents with multiple rubbery nodules on his hands (shown in the image). Which of the following best explains the pathogenesis of this patient's underlying condition?

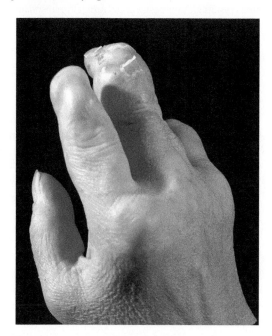

(A) Autoimmune relapsing polychondritis
(B) High dietary intake of purine-rich foods
(C) Hypercalcemia and chondrocalcinosis
(D) Impaired renal excretion of uric acid
(E) Increased calcium hydroxyapatite deposition

18 A 23-year-old man complains of stiffness and pain in his lower back that causes him to awaken at night. He first noticed morning stiffness in his lower back during his college years. He also describes occasional pain in his right eye and sensitivity to light. An X-ray of the sacroiliac region shows fusion of the small joint spaces in the posterior spine and ossification of the intervertebral discs. Serologic tests for rheumatoid factor and antinuclear antibodies are negative. This patient most likely expresses which of the following human leukocyte antigen (HLA) haplotypes?

(A) B15
(B) B19
(C) B27
(D) B31
(E) B9

19 A 28-year-old man complains of burning pain on urination, as well as pain in his fingers and left eye. He also relates a recent episode of bacillary diarrhea contracted during a visit to Mexico. Physical examination confirms arthritis and conjunctivitis. The patient responds well to treatment with NSAIDs. Which of the following is the most likely diagnosis?
(A) Ankylosing spondylitis
(B) Infectious arthritis
(C) Osteomyelitis
(D) Reiter syndrome
(E) Rheumatoid arthritis

20 An 85-year-old man presents with a 3-week history of painful swelling of his right knee. Aspiration of joint fluid returns numerous neutrophils and crystals, which are described as rhomboid and "coffin-like." Chemical analysis shows that these crystals are composed of calcium pyrophosphate. Which of the following is the most likely diagnosis?
(A) Ankylosing spondylitis
(B) Gout
(C) Infectious arthritis
(D) Pseudogout
(E) Rheumatoid arthritis

21 A 10-year-old boy complains of pain in his hands and feet. His temperature is 38°C (101°F). Physical examination reveals a faint pericardial friction rub. His spleen, liver, and axillary lymph nodes are enlarged. Which of the following is the most likely diagnosis?
(A) Gaucher disease
(B) Gout
(C) Juvenile arthritis
(D) Psoriatic arthritis
(E) Reiter syndrome

22 A 58-year-old woman fractures her hip after slipping on an icy sidewalk. An X-ray shows generalized osteopenia. A bone biopsy reveals attenuated bony trabeculae and a normal ratio of mineral-to-matrix. Serum calcium and phosphorus levels are normal. Which of the following best explains the pathogenesis of osteopenia in this postmenopausal woman?
(A) Impaired mineralization of osteoid
(B) Increased osteoblast activity
(C) Increased mineralization of bone
(D) Increased osteoclast activity
(E) Mosaic bone formation

23 A 16-year-old boy presents with a swelling on his left tibia. An X-ray of the leg shows a destructive process, with indistinct borders and an "onion-skin" pattern of periosteal bone. Histologic examination of a biopsy reveals uniform small cells with round, dark blue nuclei (shown in the image). A PAS stain demonstrates abundant intracellular glycogen.

Immunohistochemistry for leukocyte common antigen is negative. Which of the following is the most likely chromosomal abnormality in this tumor?

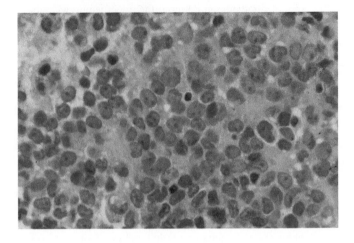

(A) t(11;22)
(B) t(14;18)
(C) t(8;14)
(D) t(9;22)
(E) t(3;16)

24 A 2-year-old boy presents with a rash. On physical examination, he has a crusty, red skin lesion at the hairline and on the extensor surfaces of his extremities and abdomen. Exophthalmos is noted. An X-ray film of the head shows multiple, radiolucent lesions in the skull. A biopsy of one of the skull lesions shows large, plump cells with pale, eosinophilic, foamy cytoplasm and convoluted nuclei (shown in the image). What is the most likely diagnosis?

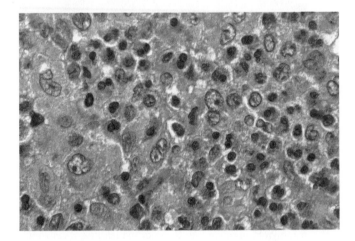

(A) Ewing sarcoma
(B) Giant cell tumor of bone
(C) Hand-Schüller-Christian disease
(D) Large B-cell lymphoma
(E) Multiple myeloma

25 A 17-year-old boy fractures his left tibia in a skiing accident. One year later, an X-ray of the leg discloses reactive bone formation in the calf muscle at the site of injury. Which of the following is the most likely diagnosis?

(A) Myositis ossificans
(B) Fibrous dysplasia
(C) Malignant fibrous histiocytoma
(D) Nodular fasciitis
(E) Synovial sarcoma

26 A 16-year-old boy presents with a 2-week history of pain in his right leg. He says that he has been taking aspirin to relieve the pain. An X-ray of the leg shows a 1-cm sharply demarcated, radiolucent lesion in the diaphysis of the tibia surrounded by dense, sclerotic bone. The lesion is surgically removed, and the gross specimen is shown in the image. Microscopically, the tumor shows irregular trabeculae of woven bone surrounded by osteoblasts, osteoclasts, and fibrovascular marrow. What is the appropriate diagnosis?

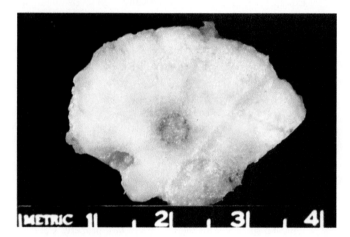

(A) Chondroblastoma
(B) Giant cell tumor of bone
(C) Osteoblastoma
(D) Osteoid osteoma
(E) Solitary chondroma

27 A 68-year-old woman presents with a lump in the soft tissue of her neck. Physical examination reveals a 0.5-cm subcutaneous tumor. Biopsy of the mass shows a benign neoplasm. The patient is told that she has the most common soft tissue tumor. What is the appropriate diagnosis?

(A) Fibroma
(B) Leiomyoma
(C) Lipoma
(D) Pleomorphic adenoma
(E) Rhabdomyosarcoma

28 A 56-year-old woman receives high-dose radiation therapy for thyroid carcinoma. One year later, the patient presents with a subcutaneous mass at the site of irradiation. A photomicrograph of the biopsy is shown in the image. Which of the following is the most likely diagnosis?

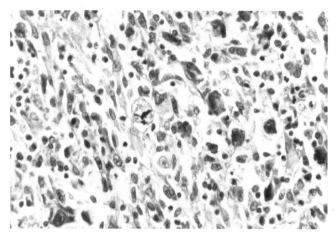

(A) Hodgkin lymphoma
(B) Leiomyosarcoma
(C) Malignant fibrous histiocytoma
(D) Rhabdomyosarcoma
(E) Synovial sarcoma

29 A 40-year-old woman presents with pain and swelling in her left elbow that has lasted 6 months. Physical examination reveals a 0.5-cm soft tissue mass. Biopsy of the mass discloses a biphasic histologic pattern consisting of cuboidal epithelial and spindle-shaped mesenchymal cells. Which of the following is the most likely diagnosis?

(A) Liposarcoma
(B) Malignant fibrous histiocytoma
(C) Nodular fasciitis
(D) Rhabdomyosarcoma
(E) Synovial sarcoma

30 A 50-year-old man complains of fever and severe pain in his great toe of 24 hours in duration. The pain developed in the morning and became so severe that he could not walk. Laboratory findings include leukocytosis, hyperuricemia, and hyperlipidemia. An X-ray of the affected joint reveals punched-out lesions in the juxta-articular bone. An aspirate of joint fluid returns urate crystals and neutrophils. Which of the following would be the most likely pathologic finding within the periarticular soft tissue of this patient?

(A) Osteophyte
(B) Pannus
(C) Reactive bone
(D) Rheumatoid nodule
(E) Tophus

31 A 35-year-old woman has multiple cartilaginous lesions in her long and short bones. A radiograph of the hand (shown in the image) reveals bulbous swellings. A biopsy shows abnormally arranged hyaline cartilage, with scattered zones of proliferation. This patient is at risk for which of the following bone diseases?

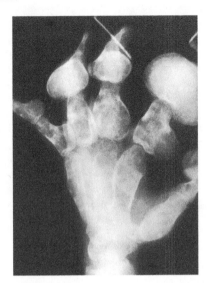

(A) Chondrosarcoma
(B) Giant cell tumor of bone
(C) Osteosarcoma
(D) Histocytic lymphoma
(E) Synovial sarcoma

32 A 24-year-old man on chronic corticosteroid therapy for severe asthma presents with a 6-month history of increasing hip pain. This patient most likely exhibits symptoms of which of the following metabolic bone diseases?
(A) Gaucher disease
(B) Osteomalacia
(C) Osteopetrosis
(D) Osteoporosis
(E) Paget disease

ANSWERS

1 **The answer is C: Fibroblast growth factor receptor.** Achondroplasia refers to a syndrome of short-limbed dwarfism and macrocephaly and represents a failure of normal epiphyseal cartilage formation. It is the most common genetic form of dwarfism and is inherited as an autosomal dominant trait. However, most cases represent new mutations. Achondroplasia is caused by an activating mutation in the fibroblast growth factor-3 receptor. This mutation negatively regulates chondrocyte proliferation and differentiation and arrests the development of the growth plate. A defective growth hormone receptor (choice D) is responsible for rare cases of dwarfism (Laron dwarfism). Mutations in dystrophin (choice B) are encountered in cases of Duchenne muscular dystrophy. Congenital deficiency of insulin-like growth factor (choice E) has not been reported as a cause of achondroplasia.
Diagnosis: Achondroplasia

2 **The answer is A: Collagen.** Osteogenesis imperfecta (OI) refers to a group of mainly autosomal dominant, heritable disorders of connective tissue, caused by mutations in the gene for type I collagen; this affects the skeleton, joints, ears, ligaments, teeth, sclerae, and skin. The pathogenesis of OI involves mutations of *COL1A1* and *COL1A2* genes, which encode the α1 and α2 chains of type I procollagen, the major structural protein of bone. Mutations in lysyl hydroxylase gene (choice C) are seen in patients with Ehlers-Danlos syndrome, and mutations in the fibrillin gene (choice D) account for Marfan syndrome. Mutations in the dystrophin gene (choice B) cause Duchenne muscular dystrophy. Mutations in the fibroblast growth factor receptor gene (choice E) may result in achondroplasia.
Diagnosis: Osteogenesis imperfecta

3 **The answer is D: Premature epiphyseal plate closure.** Congenital deficiency of 21-hydroxylase results in adrenogenital syndrome, which is associated with virilization of external genitalia in female infants (pseudohermaphroditism). Males exhibit precocious puberty. Eventually, high levels of adrenal androgens lead to premature closure of the epiphyses and stunted growth. The other choices are not related to the adrenogenital syndrome.
Diagnosis: Adrenogenital syndrome, adrenal cortical hyperplasia

4 **The answer is E: Pseudoarthrosis.** If a fracture site does not heal, the condition is termed nonunion. Causes of nonunion include interposition of soft tissues at the fracture site, excessive motion, infection, poor blood supply, and other factors mentioned in the question. Continued movement at the unhealed fracture site may also lead to pseudoarthrosis, a condition in which joint-like tissue is formed. In such cases, the fracture never heals, and the joint-like material must be removed surgically for the fracture to heal properly. Codman triangle (choice A) is an X-ray finding of a bone involved in osteosarcoma, where, an incomplete rim of reactive bone adjacent to tumor is lifted from the cortical surface. Involucrum (choice C) is the viable bone that surrounds necrotic bone (sequestrum) in osteomyelitis. Osteomyelitis (choice D) is an uncommon complication of a closed fracture.
Diagnosis: Nonunion of healing fracture

5 **The answer is B: Metastatic carcinoma.** Multiple lytic lesions associated with keratin-positive cells strongly suggest metastatic bone cancer. Metastatic carcinoma is the most common tumor of bone, and skeletal metastases are found in at least 85% of cancer cases that have run their full clinical course. The vertebral column is the most commonly affected bony structure. Tumor cells usually arrive in the bone by way of the bloodstream. Some tumors (thyroid, gastrointestinal tract, kidney, neuroblastoma) produce mostly lytic lesions. A few neoplasms (prostate, breast, lung, stomach) stimulate osteoblastic components to make bone. The other choices are not keratin positive.
Diagnosis: Metastatic bone cancer

6 **The answer is E: Osteoclasts.** Osteopetrosis, also known as "marble bone" disease or Albers-Schönberg disease, is a group of rare, inherited disorders. The most common autosomal recessive form is a severe, sometimes fatal disease affecting infants and children. The sclerotic skeleton of osteopetrosis is the result of failed osteoclastic bone resorption. The disease is caused by mutations in genes that govern osteoclast formation or function. Because osteoclast function is arrested, osteopetrosis is characterized by (1) the retention of the primary spongiosum with its cartilage cores, (2) lack of funnelization of the metaphysis, and (3) a thickened cortex. The result is short, block-like, radiodense bones, and hence the term marble bone disease. Choices A, B, and C do not regulate bone organization. Increased osteoblast activity (choice D) has not been demonstrated in patients with osteopetrosis.

Diagnosis: Osteopetrosis, Albers-Schönberg disease

7   The answer is C: Impaired mineralization of osteoid. Osteomalacia (soft bones) is a disorder of adults characterized by inadequate mineralization of newly formed bone matrix. Diverse conditions associated with osteomalacia and rickets include abnormalities in vitamin D metabolism, phosphate deficiency states, and defects in the mineralization process itself. In osteomalacia, the bony trabeculae are rimmed by broad layers of osteoid, whereas the bone spicules in osteoporosis are thin but normally mineralized. Intrinsic diseases of the small intestine, cholestatic disorders of the liver, biliary obstruction, and chronic pancreatic insufficiency are the most frequent causes of osteomalacia in the United States. Malabsorption of vitamin D and calcium complicates a number of small intestinal diseases, including celiac disease, Crohn disease, and scleroderma. Enhanced osteoblast activity (choice B) is encountered in new bone formation. Inflammatory synovium with pannus formation (choice D) is a feature of rheumatoid arthritis.

Diagnosis: Osteomalacia

8   The answer is D: Rb tumor suppressor protein. Osteosarcoma is a highly malignant bone tumor characterized by formation of bone tissue by tumor cells. It is most frequent in adolescents between the ages of 10 and 20 years. Almost two thirds of cases of osteosarcoma exhibit mutations in the retinoblastoma (*Rb*) gene, and many tumors also contain mutations in *p53*. Often, the periosteum produces an incomplete rim of reactive bone adjacent to the site where it is lifted from the cortical surface by the tumor. When this appears on an X-ray as a shell of bone intersecting the cortex at one end and open at the other end, it is referred to as Codman triangle. A "sunburst" periosteal reaction is often superimposed. Mutations in the fibroblast growth factor receptor gene (choice C) are a cause of achondroplasia. Deregulation of cyclins (choices A and B) and cyclin-dependent kinases are associated with several neoplasms.

Diagnosis: Osteosarcoma

9   The answer is A: Avascular osteonecrosis. Osteonecrosis, also known as avascular necrosis, refers to the death of bone and marrow in the absence of infection. Such bone infarcts may be caused by a variety of conditions, such as trauma, thrombi, emboli, and corticosteroids. Growing bones of children and adolescents are often affected, and in most instances, the cause of such infarctions is not evident. Legg-Calvé-Perthes disease refers to osteonecrosis in the femoral head in children. Collapse of the femoral head may lead to joint incongruity

and severe osteoarthritis. Chondroma (choice B) is a benign, intraosseous tumor composed of well-differentiated hyaline cartilage. Fibrous dysplasia (choice C) is a developmental abnormality of the skeleton, characterized by a disorganized mixture of fibrous and osseous elements in the interior of the affected bones. Osteitis fibrosa cystica (choice D) occurs in primary hyperparathyroidism.

Diagnosis: Avascular osteonecrosis

10   The answer is D: Metaphysis of a long bone. Hematogenous osteomyelitis primarily affects the metaphyseal area of the long bones (knee, ankle, hip) because of the unique vascular supply in this region. Normally, arterioles enter the calcified portion of the growth plate, form a loop, and then drain into the medullary cavity without establishing a capillary bed. This vascular loop permits slowing and sludging of blood flow, allowing bacteria time to penetrate the walls of the blood vessels and establish an infective focus within the bone marrow. Osteomyelitis may break into the periosteum (choice E) but does not originate there. Vascular loops do not reach the epiphysis (choice C). Choices A and B would be distinctly uncommon.

Diagnosis: Osteomyelitis

11   The answer is B: Degeneration of articular cartilage. Osteoarthritis is a slowly progressive destruction of the articular cartilage that is manifested in the weight-bearing joints and fingers of older persons or in the joints of younger persons subjected to trauma. Osteoarthritis is the single most common form of joint disease. The disorder is not a single nosologic entity but rather a group of conditions that have in common the mechanical destruction of a joint. Inflammation of synovium with pannus formation (choice D) occurs in patients with rheumatoid arthritis.

Diagnosis: Osteoarthritis

12   The answer is B: Chronic inflammation of synovium. Rheumatoid arthritis (RA) is a systemic, chronic inflammatory disease in which chronic polyarthritis involves diarthrodial joints symmetrically and bilaterally. Synovial lining cells undergo hyperplasia. The result is a synovial lining thrown into numerous villi and frond-like folds that fill the peripheral recesses of the joint. As the synovium undergoes hyperplasia and hypertrophy, it creeps over the surface of the articular cartilage and adjacent structures. This inflammatory synovium is termed a pannus (cloak). The pannus covers the articular cartilage and isolates it from the synovial fluid. Synovial calcification (choice A) does not occur in RA. Pannus may destroy cartilage (choice C) by depriving it of nourishment.

Diagnosis: Rheumatoid arthritis

13   The answer is E: Sequestrum. Infectious organisms may reach the bone through the bloodstream. If the infection is not contained, pus and bacteria extend into the endosteal vascular channels that supply the cortex and spread throughout the Volkmann and Haversian canals of the cortex. Eventually, pus forms underneath the periosteum, shearing off the perforating arteries of the periosteum and further devitalizing the cortex. This expansion may shear off the perforating arteries that supply the cortex with blood, leading to necrosis of the cortex. The necrotic bone is called a sequestrum. Brodie abscess (choice A) consists of reactive bone from the periosteum and the endosteum that surrounds and contains the infection. Cloaca (choice B) is the hole found in the bone during formation of a draining sinus. Involucrum (choice C) refers to a lesion in which periosteal new bone formation forms a sheath around the necrotic sequestrum. Osteophytes (choice D) are bone nodules appearing on the peripheral portion of the joint surface that are complications of osteoarthritis.

Diagnosis: Osteomyelitis

14 The answer is C: Fc portion of IgG. Immunologic mechanisms play an important role in the pathogenesis of rheumatoid arthritis (RA). Lymphocytes and plasma cells accumulate in the synovium, where they produce immunoglobulins, mainly of the IgG class. Some 80% of patients with classic RA are positive for rheumatoid factor (RF). This factor actually represents multiple antibodies, principally IgM, but sometimes IgG or IgA, directed against the Fc fragment of IgG. Significant titers of RF are also found in patients with related collagen vascular diseases, such as systemic lupus erythematosus, scleroderma, and dermatomyositis. The presence of RF in high titer is associated with severe and unremitting disease, many systemic complications, and a serious prognosis. Antibodies against choices A, D, and E are seen in patients with other collagen vascular/systemic autoimmune diseases.

Diagnosis: Rheumatoid arthritis

15 The answer is C: Increased bone resorption. In patients with primary hyperparathyroidism, osteoclasts are stimulated to resorb bone. From the subperiosteal and endosteal surfaces, osteoclasts bore their way into the cortex as cutting cones. This process is termed dissecting osteitis. As the disease progresses, the trabecular bone is resorbed, and the marrow is replaced by loose fibrosis. Cystic degeneration ultimately occurs, leading to areas of fibrosis that contain reactive woven bone, and hemosiderin-laden macrophages often display many giant cells, which are actually osteoclasts. Because of its macroscopic appearance, this lesion has been termed a brown tumor. This is not a true tumor, but rather a repair reaction. Impaired mineralization of osteoid (choice B) is a feature of osteomalacia. Osteoporosis (choice E) is characterized by decreased but otherwise normally mineralized bone.

Diagnosis: Hyperparathyroidism, osteitis fibrosa cystica

16 The answer is C: Osteogenic sarcoma. Paget disease is a chronic condition characterized by lesions of bone resulting from disordered remodeling, in which excessive bone resorption initially results in lytic lesions, followed by disorganized and excessive bone formation. The diagnostic hallmark in late disease is an abnormal arrangement of lamellar bone, in which islands of irregular bone formation, resembling pieces of a jigsaw puzzle, are separated by prominent cement lines. Persons of English descent have a high incidence of this disease. Neoplastic transformation may occur in a focus of Paget disease, usually in the femur, humerus, or pelvis. This complication occurs in less than 1% of all cases; however, the incidence of osteogenic sarcoma is still 1,000 times higher than that in the general population. The other choices are not associated with disorganized bone.

Diagnosis: Paget disease, osteogenic sarcoma

17 The answer is D: Impaired renal excretion of uric acid. Gout is a heterogeneous group of diseases in which the common denominator is an increased serum uric acid level and deposition of urate crystals in the joints and kidneys. A tophus (shown in the photograph) is an extracellular soft tissue deposit of urate crystals surrounded by foreign-body giant cells and mononuclear cells. Most cases (85%) of idiopathic gout result from an as yet unexplained impairment of uric acid excretion by the kidneys. When sodium urate crystals precipitate from supersaturated body fluids, they absorb fibronectin, complement, and a number of other proteins on their surfaces. Neutrophils that have ingested urate crystals release activated oxygen species and lysosomal enzymes, which mediate tissue injury and promote an inflammatory response. A high dietary intake of purine-rich foods (choice B) does not lead to gout, although endogenous overproduction of purines is associated with this condition.

Diagnosis: Gout

18 The answer is C: B27. Ankylosing spondylitis is an inflammatory arthropathy of the vertebral column and sacroiliac joints. It may be accompanied by asymmetric, peripheral arthritis (30% of patients) and systemic manifestations. Ankylosing spondylitis is most common in young men, and the peak incidence is at age 20 years. More than 90% of patients are positive for human leukocyte antigen-B27 (HLA-B27), although the disorder affects only 1% of persons with this haplotype. None of the other haplotypes are related to the pathogenesis of ankylosing spondylitis.

Diagnosis: Ankylosing spondylitis

19 The answer is D: Reiter syndrome. Reiter syndrome is a triad that includes (1) seronegative polyarthritis, (2) conjunctivitis, and (3) nonspecific urethritis. The disorder is almost exclusively encountered in men and usually follows venereal exposure or an episode of bacillary dysentery. As in ankylosing spondylitis, Reiter syndrome is associated with HLA-B27 antigen in up to 90% of patients. In fact, after an attack of dysentery, 20% of HLA-B27–positive men develop Reiter syndrome. The pathologic features of Reiter arthritis are comparable to those of rheumatoid arthritis. The other choices do not typically affect the eye.

Diagnosis: Reiter syndrome

20 The answer is D: Pseudogout. Calcium pyrophosphate dihydrate (CPPD)–deposition disease refers to the accumulation of this compound in synovial membranes (pseudogout), joint cartilage (chondrocalcinosis), ligaments, and tendons. CPPD-deposition disease is principally a condition of old age, with half of the population older than 85 years being afflicted. Pseudogout refers to self-limited attacks of acute arthritis lasting from 1 day to 4 weeks and involving one or two joints. Some 25% of patients with CPPD-deposition disease have an acute onset of gout-like symptoms, manifesting as inflammation and swelling of the knees, ankles, wrists, elbows, hips, or shoulders. The synovial fluid exhibits abundant leukocytes containing CPPD crystals. Gout (choice B) features deposition of urate crystals. Crystal deposition does not occur in rheumatoid arthritis (choice E).

Diagnosis: Chondrocalcinosis, pseudogout

21 The answer is C: Juvenile arthritis. Juvenile arthritis (Still disease) refers to a number of different chronic arthritic conditions in children. Twenty percent of children with polyarticular juvenile arthritis have prominent systemic symptoms that include fever, rash, hepatosplenomegaly, lymphadenopathy, pleuritis, and anemia. Many children with juvenile arthritis develop rheumatoid arthritis, ankylosing spondylitis, psoriatic arthritis, and other connective tissue diseases. Gout (choice B) is a disease mainly of adult men and does not cause organomegaly. Reiter syndrome (choice E) occurs almost exclusively in men and usually follows venereal exposure. Psoriatic arthritis (choice D) is excluded by lack of psoriasis.

Diagnosis: Juvenile arthritis

22 The answer is D: Increased osteoclast activity. Osteoporosis is a metabolic bone disease characterized by diffuse skeletal lesions in which normally mineralized bone is decreased in mass to the point that it no longer provides adequate mechanical support. The remaining bone exhibits a normal ratio of mineralized to nonmineralized (osteoid) matrix (therefore, not choices A and C). Bone loss and eventually fractures are the hallmarks of osteoporosis. Primary osteoporosis occurs principally in postmenopausal women (type 1) and elderly persons of both sexes (type 2). Type 1 primary osteoporosis is due to an absolute increase in osteoclast activity. The increased number of osteoclasts that appear in the early postmenopausal skeleton is the direct result of estrogen withdrawal. Type 2 osteoporosis reflects decreased osteoblast activity (therefore, not choice B). Mosaic bone formation (choice E) is a feature of Paget disease.

Diagnosis: Osteoporosis, osteopenia

23 The answer is A: t(11;22). Ewing sarcoma (EWS) is an uncommon malignant bone tumor composed of small, uniform, round cells. It represents only 5% of all bone tumors and is found in children and adolescents. EWS is thought to arise from primitive marrow elements or immature mesenchymal cells. Virtually all of these tumors have a reciprocal translocation between chromosomes 11 and 22, which results in the fusion of the amino terminus of the *EWS1* gene to the *FLI-1* gene, which encodes a nuclear transcription factor. Chromosomal translocation t(14;18) (choice B) is found in follicular lymphomas; t(8;14) (choice C) is present in Burkitt lymphoma; and t(9;22) (choice D) occurs in chronic myelogenous leukemia.

Diagnosis: Ewing sarcoma

24 The answer is C: Hand-Schüller-Christian disease. Langerhans cell histiocytosis is a generic term for three entities characterized by the proliferation of Langerhans cells in various tissues: (1) eosinophilic granuloma, a localized form; (2) Hand-Schüller-Christian disease, a disseminated variant; and (3) Letterer-Siwe disease, a fulminant and often fatal generalized disease. Hand-Schüller-Christian disease occurs in younger children (age 2 to 5 years). Radiolucent bony lesions characterize the disorder and occur most frequently in the calvaria, ribs, pelvis, and scapulae. A lesion may infiltrate the retro-orbital space, producing exophthalmos. Infiltration of the stalk of the hypothalamus by the proliferated Langerhans cells leads to diabetes insipidus. Crusty, red, weepy skin lesions occur at the hairline and on the extensor surfaces of the extremities, abdomen, and occasionally soles of the feet.

Ewing sarcoma (choice A) is composed of small, uniform, round cells.

Diagnosis: Langerhans cell histiocytosis, Hand-Schüller-Christian disease

25 The answer is A: Myositis ossificans. Myositis ossificans affects young persons and, although it is entirely benign, often mimics a malignant neoplasm. The lesion typically results from blunt trauma to the muscle and soft tissues, usually of the lower limb. Peripheral neovascularization of the resulting hematoma leads in a short time to the formation of bone spicules in the soft tissue because the local environment is similar to that of an initial hematoma in a healing fracture. Because myositis ossificans often occurs near a bone, on radiography, it may be misdiagnosed as a malignant bone-forming tumor. The other choices are unrelated to prior trauma.

Diagnosis: Myositis ossificans

26 The answer is D: Osteoid osteoma. Osteoid osteoma is a small, painful, benign lesion of bone composed of osseous tissue (the nidus) and surrounded by a halo of reactive bone formation. The tumor typically occurs in young persons ranging in age from 5 to 25 years. Osteoid osteoma frequently arises in the cortex of the diaphysis of the tubular bones of the lower extremity. Osteoid osteoma is a spherical, hyperemic tumor of about 1 cm in diameter that is considerably softer than the surrounding bone and easily enucleated at surgery. Reactive, sclerotic bone surrounds the nidus. Chondroblastoma (choice A) features primitive chondroblasts and cartilage matrix. Giant cell tumor (choice B) of bone is a locally aggressive neoplasm composed of multinucleated, osteoclastic giant cells. Osteoblastoma (choice C) is a benign neoplasm that is histologically similar to osteoid osteoma but larger and not accompanied by nocturnal pain relieved by aspirin. Solitary chondroma (choice E) is a benign, intraosseous tumor composed of well-differentiated hyaline cartilage.

Diagnosis: Osteoid osteoma

27 The answer is C: Lipoma. Lipoma is composed of well-differentiated adipocytes and is the most common soft tissue mass. This benign, circumscribed tumor can originate at any site in the body that contains adipose tissue, but most appear in the subcutaneous tissues of the upper half of the body, especially on the trunk and neck. Lipomas are encountered mainly in adults. Histologically, a lipoma is often indistinguishable from normal adipose tissue. Fibroma (choice A) and leiomyoma (choice B) are benign neoplasms of fibroblasts and smooth muscle cells, respectively. Pleomorphic adenoma (choice D) is a mixed neoplasm of the salivary gland.

Diagnosis: Lipoma

28 The answer is C: Malignant fibrous histiocytoma. Malignant fibrous histiocytoma (MFH) is a soft tissue tumor that contains foci of histiocytic (macrophage) differentiation and is the most frequent sarcoma encountered after radiation therapy. Histologically, MFH displays a highly variable morphologic pattern, with areas of spindle-shaped tumor cells arrayed in an irregularly whorled (storiform) pattern adjacent to pleomorphic fields. The spindle cells tend to be well differentiated and resemble fibroblasts. The other choices do not typically arise as a consequence of radiation treatment.

Diagnosis: Malignant fibrous histiocytoma

29   **The answer is E: Synovial sarcoma.** Synovial sarcoma is a highly malignant soft tissue tumor that arises in the region of a joint. Synovial sarcoma occurs principally in adolescents and young adults as a painful or tender mass in the vicinity of a large joint, particularly the knee. The neoplasm consists of spindle-shaped mesenchymal cells and cuboidal epithelial-like cells. The latter stain with antibodies to keratin, form glands and clefts, and are presumably epithelial. The other tumors listed exhibit some histologic polymorphism, but their cells do not show any epithelial features or markers of differentiation.

Diagnosis: Synovial sarcoma

30   **The answer is E: Tophus.** Chronic accumulation of uric acid crystals leads to the formation of nodules (tophi) that contain granuloma-like aggregates of macrophages. These granuloma-like areas are found in cartilage, in any of the soft tissues around joints, and even in the subchondral bone marrow adjacent to joints. Osteophytes (choice A) are a complication of osteoarthritis. Pannus (choice B) is featured in rheumatoid arthritis. Rheumatoid nodules (choice D) are found in extra-articular locations.

Diagnosis: Gout

31   **The answer is A: Chondrosarcoma.** Enchondromatosis, also termed Ollier disease, is a bone disorder characterized by the development of numerous cartilaginous masses that lead to bony deformities. The condition is not strictly a disease of delayed maturation of bone, but one in which residual hyaline cartilage, anlage cartilage, or cartilage from the growth plate does not undergo endochondral ossification and remains in the bones. As a consequence, the bones show multiple, tumor-like masses of abnormally arranged hyaline cartilage (enchondromas), with zones of proliferative and hypertrophied cartilage. Enchondromas exhibit a strong tendency to undergo malignant change into chondrosarcomas in adult life. None of the other choices are related to cartilaginous tumors.

Diagnosis: Enchondromatosis, Ollier disease

32   **The answer is D: Osteoporosis.** Risk factors for osteoporosis include smoking, vitamin D deficiency, low body mass index, hypogonadism, a sedentary lifestyle, and glucocorticoid therapy (seen in this patient). Bone loss and fractures are the hallmarks of osteoporosis, regardless of the underlying cause. Choices A and C are congenital disorders that are not related to corticosteroid therapy. Choices B and E are acquired conditions but they are not related to corticosteroid therapy.

Diagnosis: Osteoporosis

Chapter 27

Skeletal Muscle

QUESTIONS

Select the single best answer.

1 A 4-year-old boy is brought to the physician by his parents because he falls a lot, cannot jump, and tires easily. Physical examination reveals weakness in the pelvic and shoulder girdles and enlargement of the child's calf muscles. The serum level of creatine kinase is elevated. A biopsy of calf muscle reveals marked variation in size and shape of muscle fibers. There are foci of muscle fiber necrosis, myophagocytosis, regenerating fibers, and fibrosis. Which of the following is the most likely cause of death expected in this patient?

(A) Dissecting aortic aneurysm
(B) Disseminated intravascular coagulation
(C) Pulmonary embolism
(D) Respiratory insufficiency
(E) Rhabdomyosarcoma

2 Molecular diagnostic assays performed on muscle biopsy from the patient described in Question 1 would show alterations in the length of the primary transcript for which of the following muscle-associated proteins?

(A) Creatine kinase
(B) Desmin
(C) Dystrophin
(D) Glycogen phosphorylase
(E) Myosin

3 A 10-year-old girl complains of persistent redness of the skin over her knuckles and around the nail beds. She describes easy fatigability and can rise only with difficulty from a squatting position. Physical examination reveals erythema over the knuckles and a heliotropic rash. A muscle biopsy shows infiltrates of B and T lymphocytes around blood vessels and in connective tissue of the perimysium. Elevated serum levels of which of the following would be expected in this patient?

(A) Alkaline phosphatase
(B) Alpha-fetoprotein
(C) Carcinoembryonic antigen
(D) Creatine kinase
(E) Urea-nitrogen

4 A 25-year-old woman complains of weakness and easy fatigability, which is most pronounced in the late afternoon. She describes difficulty reading and tiredness while watching television. She has problems chewing and swallowing and loses her voice while talking. Physical examination reveals ptosis and diplopia. Laboratory studies would most likely demonstrate serum autoantibodies directed against which of the following proteins?

(A) Acetylcholine receptor
(B) Phosphodiesterase
(C) Desmin
(D) Dystrophin
(E) Troponin

5 Which of the following may be of therapeutic benefit to the patient described in Question 4?

(A) Adrenalectomy
(B) Parathyroidectomy
(C) Thymectomy
(D) Thyroidectomy
(E) Vagotomy

6 A 60-year-old man recovering from a "flu" complains of marked fatigability. He reports that he cannot climb stairs two at a time as he used to. He also describes pain in his thighs. A muscle biopsy (shown in the image) demonstrates a mononuclear inflammatory cell infiltrate chiefly in the endomysium. Immunostaining shows that most of these inflammatory cells are CD8⁺ T lymphocytes. What is the appropriate diagnosis?

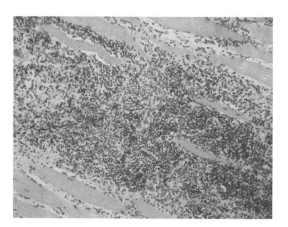

(A) Dermatomyositis
(B) Myasthenia gravis
(C) Myotonic dystrophy
(D) Polymyositis
(E) Werdnig-Hoffman disease

7 A 60-year-old man who had been treated for lung cancer complains of a rash on his chest and pain in his upper arms and calves. He cannot raise his arms and climbs the stairs only with difficulty. A muscle biopsy shows perivascular infiltrates of lymphocytes and plasma cells extending in between the muscle fibers. Immunofluorescence reveals immune complexes in the walls of intramuscular blood vessels. Which of the following is the most likely diagnosis?
(A) Becker muscular dystrophy
(B) Dermatomyositis
(C) Lambert-Eaton myasthenic syndrome
(D) Myasthenia gravis
(E) Toxic myopathy

8 A 70-year-old man who had been treated for small cell carcinoma of the lung develops marked weakness of his legs and arms. He also complained of mouth dryness, double vision, and drooping upper eyelids. On physical examination there is diffuse muscle weakness and wasting. A muscle biopsy is normal. Laboratory studies demonstrate serum IgG autoantibodies that recognize voltage-sensitive calcium channels in motor nerve terminals. Which of the following is the most likely diagnosis?
(A) Becker muscular dystrophy
(B) Dermatomyositis
(C) Lambert-Eaton myasthenic syndrome
(D) Myasthenia gravis
(E) Toxic myopathy

9 A 40-year-old man presents with muscle weakness. He cannot open his hand for a handshake and cannot extend his arm after flexing it. On physical examination, he has marked atrophy of leg and arm muscles, ptosis, and a fixed facial expression. There is testicular atrophy. Laboratory studies demonstrate mild diabetes. A muscle biopsy reveals atrophy of type I fibers, hypertrophy of type II fibers, and numerous fibers with centrally located nuclei. Which of the following is the most likely diagnosis?
(A) Dermatomyositis
(B) Duchenne muscular dystrophy
(C) Limb-girdle muscular dystrophy
(D) Myasthenia gravis
(E) Myotonic dystrophy

10 A 20-year-old man reports muscle cramping after vigorous exercise. He noted darkening of his urine after recently running a half-marathon. A urinalysis at that time showed myoglobinuria. A muscle biopsy displays no morphologic abnormalities. Which of the following is the most likely diagnosis?
(A) Carnitine palmityl transferase deficiency
(B) Lambert-Eaton myasthenic syndrome
(C) Mitochondrial encephalomyopathy
(D) Pompe disease
(E) Toxic myopathy

11 A 3-month-old boy presents with severe hypotonia and areflexia. His tongue and heart are enlarged. A muscle biopsy displays massive accumulation of membrane-bound glycogen and disappearance of the myofilaments and other sarcoplasmic organelles. The patient dies after 1 year. Which of the following is the most likely diagnosis?
(A) Carnitine deficiency
(B) Duchenne muscular dystrophy
(C) Hurler syndrome
(D) Niemann-Pick disease
(E) Pompe disease

12 A 42-year-old woman presents with muscle weakness. She has difficulty climbing stairs and lately tires while combing her hair. A muscle biopsy demonstrates lymphocytic infiltration with single-fiber necrosis. In addition, muscle fibers exhibit basophilic granular material. An electron micrograph of the cytoplasmic material is shown. Which of the following is the most likely diagnosis?

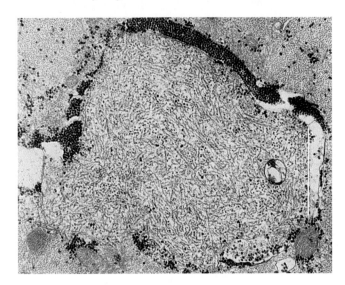

(A) Amyotrophic lateral sclerosis
(B) Becker muscular dystrophy
(C) Inclusion body myositis
(D) Myasthenia gravis
(E) Myotonic dystrophy

13 A healthy 28-year-old woman collapses near the end of a summer marathon. In the emergency room, the patient is noted to have hot dry skin with little sweating. Her temperature is 40.4°C (104.8°F). Laboratory findings reveal high levels of creatine kinase. The urine is dark red and contains myoglobin. Which of the following would be most expected in the muscle tissue of this patient?
(A) Amyloid deposition
(B) Gangrene
(C) Lymphocytic infiltration
(D) Microabscesses
(E) Rhabdomyolysis

14 A 22-year-old woman injured her leg in a motor vehicle accident and subsequently suffers from weakness of her left lower leg. A biopsy of the gastrocnemius muscle is obtained after 4 months (shown in the image). Which of the following best characterizes this pathology?

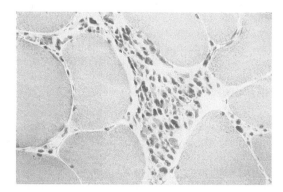

(A) Autoimmune myopathy
(B) Compensatory hypertrophy
(C) Denervation
(D) Mitochondrial depletion
(E) Target fibers

15 A 28-year-old man begins a program of vigorous body building. After 6 months, his biceps would be expected to exhibit which of the following adaptive cellular changes?
(A) Hyperplasia of type I fibers
(B) Hyperplasia of type II fibers
(C) Hypertrophy of type I fibers
(D) Hypertrophy of type II fibers
(E) Hypoplasia of type I and II fibers with hyperplasia of myoblasts

ANSWERS

1 **The answer is D: Respiratory insufficiency.** Duchenne muscular dystrophy is a severe, progressive, X-linked, inherited condition characterized by progressive degeneration of muscles, particularly those of the pelvic and shoulder girdles. The weakness is noted mainly around the pelvic and shoulder girdles (proximal muscle weakness) and is relentlessly progressive. "Pseudohypertrophy" (enlargement of a muscle due to abundant replacement of muscle fibers by fibroadipose tissue) of the calf muscles eventually develops. Patients are usually wheelchair bound by the age of 10 years and bedridden by age 15 years. The most common causes of death are complications of respiratory insufficiency caused by muscular weakness or cardiac arrhythmia due to myocardial involvement. The other choices are not complications of Duchenne muscular dystrophy.
Diagnosis: Duchenne muscular dystrophy

2 **The answer is C: Dystrophin.** Duchenne muscular dystrophy is caused by mutations of a large gene on the short arm of the X chromosome (Xp21). This gene codes for dystrophin, a protein localized to the inner surface of the sarcolemma. Dystrophin links the subsarcolemmal cytoskeleton to the exterior of the cell through a transmembrane complex of proteins and glycoproteins that binds to laminin. Dystrophin-deficient muscle fibers thus lack the normal interaction between the sarcolemma and the extracellular matrix. This disruption may be responsible for the observed increased osmotic fragility of dystrophic muscle, the excessive influx of calcium ions, and the release of soluble muscle enzymes such as creatine kinase into the serum. The other proteins are not altered in patients with Duchenne muscular dystrophy.
Diagnosis: Duchenne muscular dystrophy

3 **The answer is D: Creatine kinase.** The inflammatory myopathies represent a heterogeneous group of acquired disorders, all of which feature symmetric proximal muscle weakness, increased serum levels of muscle-derived enzymes, and nonsuppurative inflammation of skeletal muscle. They are thought to have an autoimmune origin. The most common morphologic characteristics in the inflammatory myopathies are (1) inflammatory cells, (2) necrosis and phagocytosis of muscle fibers, (3) a mixture of regenerating and atrophic fibers, and (4) fibrosis. Dermatomyositis is distinguished from the other myopathies (i.e., polymyositis and inclusion body myositis) by the presence of a characteristic heliotropic rash on the upper eyelids, face, and trunk. Patients with inflammatory myopathies have increased serum levels of creatine kinase and other muscle enzymes. Elevated serum alkaline phosphatase (choice A) is associated with liver and bone disease. Alphafetoprotein and carcinoembryonic antigen (choices B and C) are markers of neoplasia. Elevated blood urea-nitrogen (choice E) is associated with renal disease.
Diagnosis: Dermatomyositis

4 **The answer is A: Acetylcholine receptor.** Myasthenia gravis is an acquired autoimmune disease characterized by abnormal muscular fatigability. It is caused by circulating antibodies to the acetylcholine receptor at the myoneural junction (motor endplate). Antibodies to the acetylcholine receptor can be demonstrated in the serum of most patients with myasthenia gravis and localized in muscle biopsies by immunohistochemistry. The clinical severity of the condition is variable, and symptoms tend to wax and wane. The other choices are not related to myasthenia gravis.
Diagnosis: Myasthenia gravis

5 **The answer is C: Thymectomy.** The thymus clearly plays an important role in the pathogenesis of myasthenia gravis. Up to 40% of patients with thymoma develop myasthenia gravis, and surgical removal of the tumor is often curative. Other patients with myasthenia gravis have thymic hyperplasia, and in such cases, thymectomy is often an effective treatment. Acetylcholine receptors have been demonstrated on the surface of some thymic cells in both thymoma and thymic hyperplasia. None of the other choices are curative for myasthenia gravis. Abnormalities of the other organs are not associated with myasthenia gravis.
Diagnosis: Myasthenia gravis

6 **The answer is D: Polymyositis.** Polymyositis is related to direct muscle cell damage produced by cytotoxic T cells. Healthy muscle fibers are initially surrounded by CD8+ T lymphocytes and macrophages (see photomicrograph), after which muscle fibers degenerate. There is a frequent association between polymyositis and anti-Jo-1, an antibody against histidyl-tRNA synthetase, with the concomitant presence of interstitial lung disease, Raynaud phenomenon, and nonerosive arthritis. Although viral infections (e.g., influenza) may trigger polymyositis, muscle tissue has not yielded a virus on culture. An inflammatory myopathy indistinguishable from polymyositis occurs in many cases of HIV infection, but the role of the lentivirus is unclear. None of the other choices are associated with an infiltrate of cytotoxic T lymphocytes.

Diagnosis: Polymyositis

7   The answer is B: Dermatomyositis.   Dermatomyositis is an immune-mediated microangiopathy that leads to obliteration of capillaries, ischemic injury, and muscle damage. Immunofluorescence demonstrates that the walls of many capillaries contain C5b-9 proteins (i.e., membrane attack complex). When dermatomyositis occurs in a middle-aged man, it is associated with an increased risk of epithelial cancer, most commonly carcinoma of the lung. By contrast, polymyositis and inclusion body myositis have only a chance association with malignancy. Lambert-Eaton myasthenic syndrome (choice C) is also seen in patients with lung cancer, but as with the other incorrect choices, it is not associated with a skin rash or muscle inflammation.

Diagnosis: Dermatomyositis

8   The answer is C: Lambert-Eaton myasthenic syndrome.   Lambert-Eaton syndrome is a paraneoplastic disorder that manifests as muscular weakness, wasting, and fatigability of the proximal limbs and trunk. Also termed myasthenic–myopathic syndrome, the disease is usually associated with small cell carcinoma of the lung, although it may also occur in patients with other malignant diseases. Like myasthenia gravis, the disease seems to have an autoimmune basis because it can be transferred to mice by IgG from patients and it responds to treatment with corticosteroids. The pathogenic IgG autoantibodies recognize voltage-sensitive calcium channels that are expressed both in motor nerve terminals and in the cells of the lung cancer. The calcium channels, which are necessary for release of acetylcholine, are greatly reduced in the presynaptic membrane in these patients, thereby interfering with neuromuscular transmission. Antichannel antibodies are not encountered in the other choices.

Diagnosis: Lambert-Eaton myasthenic syndrome

9   The answer is E: Myotonic dystrophy.   Myotonic dystrophy, the most common form of adult muscular dystrophy, is an autosomal dominant disorder characterized by slowing muscle relaxation (myotonia) and progressive muscle weakness and wasting. In addition to skeletal muscle, myotonic dystrophy affects many systems, including the heart, smooth muscle, central nervous system, endocrine glands, and eye. Myotonic dystrophy can be separated into two clinical groups: adult onset and congenital. Most adult patients display atrophy of type I fibers and hypertrophy of type II fibers. Unlike the other choices, internally situated nuclei are a constant feature. Necrosis and regeneration, although occasionally present, are not as prominent as they are in Duchenne muscular dystrophy (choice B).

Diagnosis: Myotonic dystrophy

10   The answer is A: Carnitine palmityl transferase deficiency.   Patients with carnitine palmityl transferase deficiency cannot metabolize long-chain fatty acids because of an inability to transport these lipids into the mitochondria, where they undergo β-oxidation. After prolonged exercise, these patients have muscular pain, which may progress to myoglobinuria. After such an episode, fibers regenerate and restore muscle structure. Biopsy specimens show no microscopic abnormalities, and the diagnosis depends on the biochemical assay for carnitine palmityl transferase activity. The other choices do not feature exercise-induced myoglobinuria.

Diagnosis: Carnitine palmityl transferase deficiency

11   The answer is E: Pompe disease.   Glycogen-storage diseases are autosomal recessive, inherited, metabolic disorders characterized by an inability to degrade glycogen. The first acid maltase deficiency to be recognized, described by Pompe, is the most severe form and occurs in the neonatal or early infantile stage. These patients have severe hypotonia and areflexia. Sometimes, the patients have an enlarged tongue and cardiomegaly and die of cardiac failure, usually within the first 2 years of life. Many tissues are affected, but the most significant involvement is in skeletal and cardiac muscle, the central nervous system, and the liver. The serum creatine kinase level is only slightly to moderately increased. Hurler syndrome (choice C) is an inherited defect in mucopolysaccharide metabolism. Glycogen accumulation is not a feature of the other choices.

Diagnosis: Pompe disease

12   The answer is C: Inclusion body myositis.   The pathologic features of inclusion body myositis resemble those of polymyositis and consist of single-fiber necrosis and regeneration with predominantly endomysial cytotoxic T cells. The inclusions are stained by Congo red and represent a form of intracellular amyloid that can be demonstrated by electron microscopy. The fibers in the electron micrograph shown here represent amyloid filaments. These filaments are immunoreactive for β-amyloid protein—same type of amyloid present in the senile plaques of Alzheimer disease. The pathogenic significance of these inclusions is not understood. None of the other disorders feature amyloid deposition or inclusions.

Diagnosis: Inclusion body myositis

13   The answer is E: Rhabdomyolysis.   Rhabdomyolysis refers to the dissolution of skeletal muscle fibers and the release of myoglobin into the circulation, an event that may result in myoglobinuria and acute renal failure. The disorder may be acute, subacute, or chronic. During acute rhabdomyolysis, the muscles are swollen, tender, and profoundly weak. Rhabdomyolysis may complicate heat stroke or malignant hyperthermia after administration of an anesthetic such as halothane. Pathologic changes in rhabdomyolysis correspond to an active, noninflammatory myopathy, with scattered necrosis of muscle fibers and varying degrees of degeneration and regeneration. None of the other choices are seen in acute rhabdomyolysis.

Diagnosis: Heat stroke, rhabdomyolysis

14 **The answer is C: Denervation.** A muscle biopsy is a highly sensitive test for detecting a lesion of the lower motor neuron, but the pattern of denervation does not identify the cause of the lesion. When a skeletal muscle fiber becomes separated from contact with its lower motor neuron, it invariably atrophies due to the progressive loss of myofibrils. On cross section, the atrophic fiber has a characteristic angular configuration, seemingly compressed by surrounding normal muscle fibers. If the fiber is not reinnervated, the atrophy proceeds to complete loss of myofibrils, and the nuclei condense into aggregates. The photomicrograph in this case shows small groups of angular atrophic fibers reflecting advanced denervation. In the end stage, the muscle fibers disappear and are replaced chiefly by adipose tissue. The other choices are not related to denervation.

Diagnosis: Skeletal muscle atrophy, denervation

15 **The answer is D: Hypertrophy of type II fibers.** Stimulation of type II fibers elicits a faster, shorter, and more powerful contraction than occurs in type I fibers. Type II muscle fibers are suitable for rapid contractions of brief duration and react to strength training with hypertrophy. Androgenic steroids also induce hypertrophy of type II fibers, and disuse of the muscle results in their selective atrophy. Skeletal muscle does not respond to an increased workload by increasing the number of fibers (hyperplasia).

Diagnosis: Skeletal muscle hypertrophy

Chapter 28

The Nervous System

QUESTIONS

Select the single best answer.

1 A female neonate is noted at birth to have a gross deformity of her lower back. Examination of the subcutaneous lesion reveals disorganized neural tissue with entrapment of nerve roots. What is the appropriate diagnosis?
(A) Meningocele
(B) Meningomyelocele
(C) Rachischisis
(D) Spina bifida occulta
(E) Syringomyelia

2 The parents of the neonate described in Question 1 ask about the risks for similar birth defects in their future offspring. You mention that supplementation of the maternal diet can reduce the incidence of neural tube defects. What is this important dietary supplement?
(A) Folic acid
(B) Niacin
(C) Thiamine
(D) Vitamin B_6
(E) Vitamin B_{12}

3 A male neonate is noted at birth to have paralysis of the lower limbs. The infant fails to thrive and expires. The brainstem and cerebellum are examined at autopsy (shown in the image). What is the diagnosis?

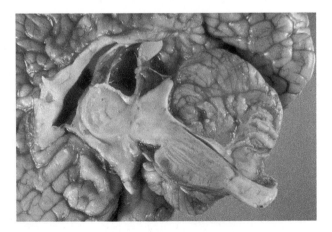

(A) Anencephaly
(B) Arnold-Chiari malformation
(C) Holoprosencephaly
(D) Hydromyelia
(E) Lissencephaly

4 A female neonate is noted to have a pronounced enlargement of her head (shown in the image). She develops convulsions. MRI reveals excessive accumulation of cerebrospinal fluid, ventricular enlargement, and atrophy of the cerebral cortex. This developmental birth defect was most likely caused by which of the following mechanisms of disease?

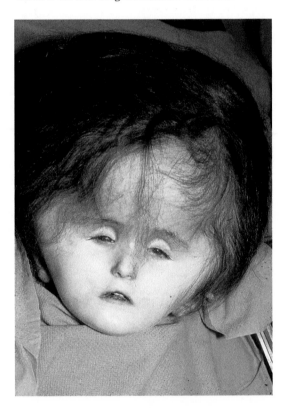

(A) Atresia of the aqueduct of Sylvius
(B) Birth trauma
(C) Congenital brain tumor
(D) Maternal folate deficiency
(E) Oligohydramnios

306

5 Which anatomic structure/region produced the CSF that accumulated in the brain of the neonate described in Question 4?

(A) Arachnoid
(B) Choroid plexus
(C) Corpus callosum
(D) Pia mater
(E) Subependymal areas of the cerebral hemispheres

6 A 3-year-old girl who has been mentally retarded since birth is killed in a drowning accident. The superior surface of the brain at autopsy is shown in the image. What is the diagnosis for this gross deformity of the brain?

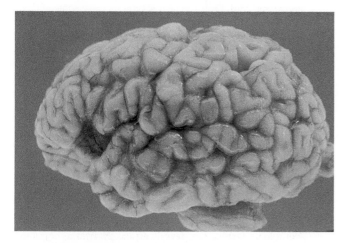

(A) Arrhinencephaly
(B) Holoprosencephaly
(C) Lissencephaly
(D) Pachygyria
(E) Polymicrogyria

7 A 2-week-old male neonate has frequent generalized seizures and fails to thrive. Physical examination reveals facial dysmorphology, including cleft palate and low-set ears. A coronal section of the brain at autopsy is shown in the image. Which of the following is the most likely cause of this congenital birth defect?

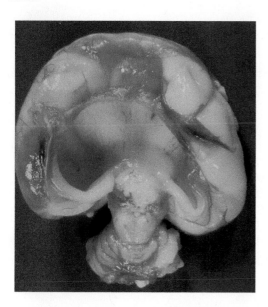

(A) Bacterial meningitis
(B) Birth trauma
(C) Chromosomal abnormality
(D) Fetal alcohol syndrome
(E) TORCH syndrome

8 A 50-year-old man presents with a "staggering" gait and "lightning pain" in his hands and legs. His past medical history is significant for an aortic aneurysm and aortic insufficiency. Neurologic examination reveals impaired senses of vibration, as well as touch and pain in the lower extremities. The patient subsequently dies of pneumonia. Autopsy discloses obliterative endarteritis of meningeal blood vessels and atrophy of the posterior columns of the spinal cord. What is the appropriate diagnosis?

(A) Amyotrophic lateral sclerosis
(B) Friedreich ataxia
(C) Huntington disease
(D) Tabes dorsalis
(E) Vitamin B_{12} deficiency (subacute combined degeneration)

9 A 76-year-old man is admitted to the hospital for evaluation of progressive memory loss and disorientation. The pupils are small but react normally to light. Muscle tone is normal. A lumbar puncture returns clear, colorless CSF under normal pressure. An electroencephalogram shows diffuse slowing. A CT scan of the brain reveals moderate atrophy. Which of the following is the most likely diagnosis?

(A) Alzheimer disease
(B) Creutzfeldt-Jakob disease
(C) Glioblastoma multiforme
(D) Huntington disease
(E) Pick disease

10 A 66-year-old woman vocalist complains of difficulty remembering her favorite songs. This problem continues to worsen over the next several months, and the patient becomes increasingly withdrawn from her family. When examined, she evidences dementia and gait disturbance. MRI demonstrates mild cerebral atrophy. Analysis of CSF shows no inflammatory cells and normal levels of glucose and protein. An electroencephalogram reveals periodic spike-wave complexes. One month later, the patient is bedridden and nonresponsive, and subsequently dies. A section of brain tissue obtained at autopsy is shown in the image. This patient most likely has which of the following categories of organ-specific amyloidosis?

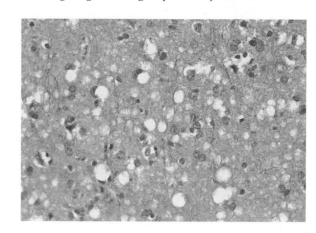

(A) Aβ
(B) AA
(C) AE
(D) AL
(E) APrP

11 What key feature distinguishes normal proteins from their pathologic forms in the brain of the patient described in Question 10?
(A) ATPase activity
(B) Glycolipid anchor
(C) Three-dimensional conformation
(D) Tyrosine kinase activity
(E) Zinc finger domain

12 An 88-year-old woman with Alzheimer disease dies of congestive heart failure. Examination of the brain at autopsy shows bilateral atrophy of the gyri, particularly in the frontal and hippocampal cortex. What additional finding might be expected in the brain of this patient?
(A) Cerebritis
(B) Hydrocephalus ex vacuo
(C) Lissencephaly
(D) Pachygyria
(E) Periventricular patches of demyelination

13 A 35-year-old man presents with a history of behavioral and personality changes and unusual involuntary movements. Physical examination reveals chorea and dystonia. The patient's mother and maternal grandfather had similar clinical symptoms. His mother died in a psychiatric institute, and his maternal grandfather committed suicide. MRI shows bilateral cerebral atrophy and enlargement of the lateral ventricles. Marked atrophy would also be expected in which of the following regions of this patient's brain?
(A) Anterior horn of the spinal cord
(B) Caudate nuclei
(C) Cerebellum
(D) Hypothalamus
(E) Substantia nigra

14 Which of the following gene abnormalities would be expected in the patient described in Question 13?
(A) Deletion of an exon in the gene for presenilin
(B) Expansion of a trinucleotide repeat
(C) Frame shift mutation in the gene for superoxide dismutase
(D) Nondisjunction during meiosis of chromosome 21
(E) Point mutation in the gene for the prion protein

15 A 20-year-old woman with mild scoliosis complains of a 3-month history of difficulty walking. Physical and neurologic examinations reveal dysarthria, lower-limb areflexia, extensor plantar reflexes, and sensory loss. Genetic studies show evidence of a trinucleotide repeat expansion syndrome. The family asks for information regarding their daughter's prognosis. You are cognizant of the fact that the length of this child's trinucleotide repeat is directly related

to the rate of clinical progression, as well as the probability that she will develop which of the following life-threatening complications?
(A) Aplastic anemia
(B) Astrocytoma
(C) Cardiomyopathy
(D) Cerebral amyloidosis
(E) Tuberous sclerosis

16 A 35-year-old woman complains of urinary incontinence and blurred vision for 2 months. A funduscopic examination shows no abnormalities. Two months later, the patient develops double vision and numbness in the fingers of her left hand. MRI shows scattered plaques in the patient's brain and spinal cord. Over the next several months, some of these plaques diminish in size, while others appear in new locations. These plaques would most likely show selective loss of which of the following proteins?
(A) β-Amyloid
(B) Glial fibrillary acidic protein
(C) Myelin
(D) Synaptophysin
(E) α-Synuclein

17 A 30-year-old woman presents with an 8-day history of mild tremor in her arms and impaired balance when walking. Vital signs are normal. Her symptoms disappear the following week. About 18 months later, the patient experiences another episode of weakness and requires assistance when walking. Neurologic examination reveals ataxia, dysarthria, decreased vibratory sensation in her legs, absent abdominal reflexes, increased deep tendon reflexes, and a Babinski sign on the left. Fifteen years after the onset of symptoms, the patient becomes bedridden and dies. A coronal section of the patient's brain at autopsy is stained for myelin with luxol fast blue (shown in the image). Which of the following histopathologic findings would be expected in these plaques?

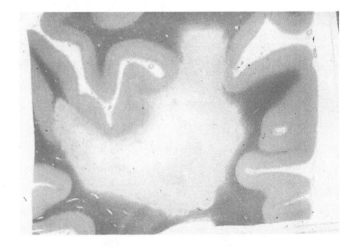

(A) Astrogliosis
(B) Lewy bodies
(C) Negri bodies
(D) Neurofibrillary tangles
(E) Myelin figures

18 A 45-year-old woman is rushed to the emergency room following an automobile accident. Ten hours after admission, the patient complains of a severe headache and blurred vision. An X-ray film of the cranium shows a fracture of the temporal-parietal bone. Despite emergency craniotomy, the patient dies. Which of the following pathologic findings would be expected at autopsy?

(A) Epidural hematoma
(B) Intracerebral hemorrhage
(C) Intraventricular hemorrhage
(D) Subarachnoid hemorrhage
(E) Subdural hematoma

19 A 68-year-old woman complains of difficulty getting out of a chair. On examination, the patient shows reduced facial expression, a resting tremor, cogwheel rigidity, and bradykinesia (slowness of voluntary movements). The patient dies of congestive heart failure 10 years later. Microscopic examination of brain tissue at autopsy is shown in the image. The spherical, eosinophilic inclusions in the cytoplasm of this pigmented neuron are composed of which of the following proteins?

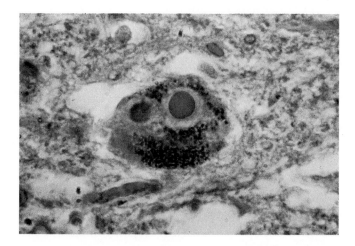

(A) β-Amyloid
(B) Polyglutamine
(C) PrP^{sc}
(D) α-Synuclein
(E) Tau

20 A 50-year-old woman presents with a 3-month history of easy fatigability, a smooth sore tongue, numbness and tingling of the feet, and weakness of the legs. The hemoglobin is 5.6 g/dL, WBC count is 5,100/μL, and platelets are 240,000/μL. A hematologic evaluation reveals a megaloblastic anemia that is not reversed by folate therapy. Peripheral neuropathy in this patient is most likely associated with which of the following pathologic findings?

(A) Atrophy of frontal cortex
(B) Atrophy of mammillary bodies
(C) Degeneration of anterior horn cells in the spinal column
(D) Degeneration of the posterior columns of the spinal cord
(E) Spongiform degeneration of the cerebellum

21 A 60-year-old man with a history of smoking and chronic bronchitis complains of difficulty walking. On examination, the patient appears stiff and stooped, shows an expressionless face, and speaks in a monotonous voice. A tremor of his fingers is apparent but ceases when he tries to reach for something. The patient dies 3 years later of metastatic lung cancer. At autopsy, the substantia nigra of the patient (right) differs from that of a normal brain (left). This pathologic finding is associated with which of the following biochemical changes?

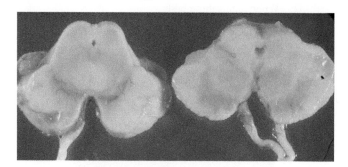

(A) Increased β-amyloid biosynthesis
(B) Increased release of NMDA
(C) Increased synthesis of GABA
(D) Reduced levels of dopamine
(E) Reduced tau protein self-assembly

22 A 60-year-old chronic alcoholic was found in a state of mental confusion. Physical and neurologic examinations reveal horizontal diplopia, strabismus, amblyopia, nystagmus, ataxia, and peripheral neuropathy. The patient subsequently develops lobar pneumonia and expires. Examination of the brain at autopsy shows calcification and brownish discoloration of atrophic mammillary bodies. Petechiae in the quadrigeminal plate and periaqueductal regions of the midbrain are also observed. Which of the following best explains the pathogenesis of these clinical and pathologic findings?

(A) AIDS-related encephalopathy
(B) Amyotrophic lateral sclerosis
(C) Hepatic encephalopathy
(D) Hepatorenal syndrome
(E) Thiamine deficiency

23 A 15-year-old boy is rushed to the emergency room after suffering a tonic-clonic seizure 4 weeks after a spelunking expedition. The boy appears irritable and agitated, and his parents state that he has difficulty swallowing fluids. Lumbar puncture shows numerous lymphocytes. The patient becomes delirious, slips into a coma, and expires. At autopsy, the brain stem shows infiltrates of lymphocytes around small blood vessels and evidence of neuronophagia. Some neurons contain eosinophilic inclusions. What is the proper name for these neuronal inclusions?

(A) Councilman bodies
(B) Hirano bodies
(C) Lewy bodies
(D) Negri bodies
(E) Psammoma bodies

24 A 10-month-old girl is brought to the emergency room with severe, unremitting watery diarrhea. Her blood pressure is 80 mm Hg systolic, and the pulse is 120 per minute. Which of the following is a potentially lethal complication of systemic dehydration in this patient?

(A) Diffuse axonal shearing
(B) Intraventricular hemorrhage
(C) Midbrain hemorrhage
(D) Pontine hemorrhage
(E) Venous sinus thrombosis

25 A 54-year-old woman dies 48 hours after suffering severe head injuries in an automobile accident. Just before her death, her left pupil becomes fixed and dilated. An inferior view of the patient's brain at autopsy is shown in the image. Which of the following was the most likely cause of death?

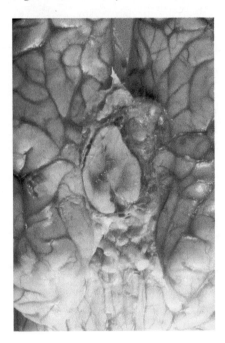

(A) Diffuse axonal shearing
(B) Laminar necrosis
(C) Thrombosis of sagittal sinus
(D) Transtentorial herniation
(E) Watershed infarct

26 Further examination of the brainstem at autopsy of the patient described in Question 25 would most likely reveal which of the following pathologic findings?

(A) Cervical contusion
(B) Duret hemorrhages
(C) Encephalomalacia
(D) Pontine myelinolysis
(E) Ruptured saccular aneurysm

27 An 18-year-old man suffers massive trauma in a motorcycle accident. A CT scan shows multiple intracerebral hemorrhages. The patient expires after 6 months in a coma. At autopsy, there are cystic cavities within the frontal and temporal lobes, corresponding to the areas of prior hemorrhage. These cavities were formed in large measure due to the phagocytic activity of which of the following cell types?

(A) Astrocytes
(B) Endothelial cells
(C) Microglial cells
(D) Neutrophils
(E) Oligodendrocytes

28 A 22-year-old boxer suffers a concussion during a boxing match and is rushed to the emergency room. According to his trainer, the blow deflected his head upward and posteriorly. Loss of consciousness in this patient presumably occurred because of a functional paralysis of neurons in which of the following anatomic regions of his brain?

(A) Brainstem reticular formation
(B) Cerebellum
(C) Hypothalamus
(D) Periventricular white matter
(E) Temporoparietal area

29 The patient described in Question 28 persists in a vegetative coma for several months and then expires. A section of the temporal lobe shows massive proliferation of cells with a star-shaped appearance (shown in the image). Which of the following best accounts for this cellular response to injury?

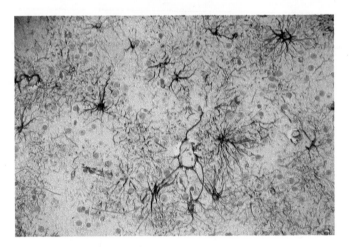

(A) Axonal regeneration
(B) Chromatolysis
(C) Gliosis
(D) Leukodystrophy
(E) Neuronophagia

30 A 68-year-old obese woman (BMI = 34 kg/m²) suffers a stroke and expires. Histologic examination of the brain at autopsy reveals extensive arteriolar lipohyalinosis and numerous Charcot-Bouchard aneurysms. Which of the following best accounts for the pathogenesis of these autopsy findings?

(A) Atherosclerosis
(B) Autoimmunity
(C) Diabetes
(D) Hypertension
(E) Vasculitis

31 A 12-year-old boy is rushed to the emergency room in a coma after falling from an upper story window of his home. MRI shows a subdural hematoma over the left hemisphere. What is the most likely source of intracranial bleeding in this patient?

(A) Bridging veins
(B) Charcot-Bouchard aneurysm
(C) Internal carotid artery
(D) Middle meningeal artery
(E) Sagittal sinus

32 Two months later, the patient described in Question 31 experiences increasing headaches and muscle weakness and suffers a tonic-clonic seizure. What is the most likely explanation for this patient's new clinical presentation?

(A) Rebleeding from previous hematoma
(B) Ruptured saccular aneurysm
(C) Sagittal sinus thrombosis
(D) Thromboembolism to middle meningeal artery
(E) Watershed infarcts

33 A 5-year-old boy is brought to the emergency room with fever, vomiting, and convulsions. The patient is febrile to 39.5°C (104°F). Physical examination reveals cervical rigidity and pain in the neck and knees. Acute inflammation most likely involves which anatomic region of the patient's brain?

(A) Choroid plexus
(B) Ependyma
(C) Hypothalamus
(D) Lateral ventricles
(E) Leptomeninges

34 A 32-year-old woman presents with a 2-day history of headache, vomiting, and fever. Physical examination reveals cervical rigidity and knee pain with hip flexion. Lumbar puncture demonstrates an abundance of neutrophils and decreased levels of glucose. Which of the following diseases is most likely associated with these clinical laboratory findings?

(A) Meningococcal meningitis
(B) Neurosarcoidosis
(C) Staphylococcal meningitis
(D) Tuberculous meningitis
(E) Viral meningitis

35 A 3-day-old infant presents with a fever of 38.7°C (103°F) and convulsions. The infant is started on broad-spectrum antibiotics and antiviral medications but slips into a coma and expires. At autopsy, the brain shows a purulent exudate in the subarachnoid space at the base of the brain (shown in the image). What was the most likely cause of suppurative meningitis in this neonate?

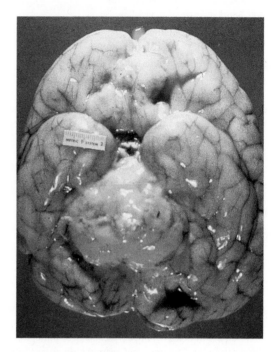

(A) *Candida albicans*
(B) *Cryptococcus neoformans*
(C) *Escherichia coli*
(D) *Haemophilus influenzae*
(E) *Neisseria meningitidis*

36 A 1-year-old boy presents with a delay in motor development. Progressive muscle weakness and blindness ensue, and the patient dies within a year. The brain at autopsy shows swollen neurons that contain numerous lysosomes filled with lipid. Which of the following is the most likely diagnosis?

(A) AL amyloidosis
(B) Hurler syndrome
(C) Phenylketonuria
(D) Tay-Sachs disease
(E) Tuberous sclerosis

37 A 59-year-old woman presents with headache and mild fever of 3 days in duration. On physical examination, the patient appears confused and inattentive. On the following day, she is rushed to the emergency room after suffering a generalized seizure. Lumbar puncture shows increased levels of CSF protein, but cultures are negative, and the white cell count is not elevated. PCR analysis of the CSF fluid shows evidence of herpes simplex type 1. This infection most likely involves which of the following anatomic regions of the patient's brain?

(A) Basal ganglia
(B) Brainstem nuclei
(C) Cerebral hemispheres
(D) Subependymal areas of the cerebral hemispheres
(E) Temporal lobes

38 The patient described in Question 37 is started on antiviral medication but becomes increasingly unresponsive and expires. Examination of affected brain tissue at autopsy would most likely reveal which of the following pathologic findings?
(A) Charcot-Bouchard aneurysms
(B) Focal plaques of demyelination
(C) Neurofibrillary tangles
(D) Perivascular cuffs of lymphocytes
(E) Spongiform degeneration

39 A 2-day-old neonate exhibits convulsions. Imaging studies disclose mild hydrocephaly, as well as areas of calcification in periventricular areas and in the brain stem. The neonate is started on broad-spectrum antibiotics but dies within 2 days. Examination of the brain at autopsy reveals pink intranuclear inclusions in Purkinje cells. Which of the following is the most likely etiology of cerebral calcification and convulsions in this neonate?
(A) *Cryptococcus neoformans*
(B) Cytomegalovirus
(C) Human immunodeficiency virus
(D) Poliovirus
(E) *Toxoplasma gondii*

40 A 48-year-old man with AIDS is admitted to the hospital with a headache, fever of 38.7°C (103°F), and persistent cough. His CD4 cell count is less than 500/μL. Lumbar puncture returns cloudy fluid, and microscopic examination shows numerous encapsulated microorganisms (shown in the image). Which of the following pathogens is the most likely cause of meningitis in this patient?

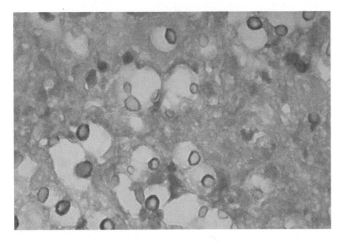

(A) *Aspergillus flavus*
(B) *Cryptococcus neoformans*
(C) *Mycobacterium tuberculosis*
(D) *Neisseria meningitidis*
(E) *Toxoplasma gondii*

41 A 30-year-old woman presents to the emergency room complaining that she has the "worst headache" of her life. Her temperature is 37°C (98.6°F), blood pressure 135/85 mm Hg, and

pulse 90 per minute. The patient shows no evidence of muscle weakness or ataxia. Imaging studies reveal subarachnoid hemorrhage, and an angiogram shows a saccular aneurysm. Which of the following best describes the pathogenesis of aneurysm formation in this patient?
(A) Atherosclerosis
(B) Bacterial infection
(C) Congenital weakness
(D) Diabetes mellitus
(E) Systemic hypertension

42 Which of the following is the most likely anatomic location of the ruptured aneurysm in the patient described in Question 41?
(A) Circle of Willis
(B) Internal carotid artery
(C) Middle meningeal artery
(D) Striate artery
(E) Vertebral artery

43 A 62-year-old man with a history of poorly controlled hypertension and diabetes presents with sudden onset of weakness. His blood pressure is 200/115 mm Hg, and his pulse is 80 per minute. An X-ray film of the chest demonstrates cardiomegaly and pulmonary edema. A CT scan of the brain reveals intra-parenchymal hemorrhage. The patient becomes unresponsive and eventually expires. Which of the following was the most likely site for cerebral hemorrhage in this patient?
(A) Basal ganglia/thalamic area
(B) Frontal lobe cortex (cortical layers IV through VI)
(C) Medulla
(D) Midbrain
(E) Sommer's sector of the hippocampus

44 A 42-year-old man with AIDS dementia complex dies of respiratory insufficiency secondary to *Pneumocystis carinii* pneumonia. Examination of the brain at autopsy reveals mild cerebral atrophy, with dilation of the lateral ventricles. Which of the following best explains the pathogenesis of neuronal injury in this patient?
(A) Accumulation of lysosomal storage material
(B) Apoptosis of oligodendrocytes
(C) Lytic infection of neurons by HIV
(D) Necrotizing vasculitis that results in multiple cerebral infarcts
(E) Release of neurotoxic cytokines from macrophages

45 A 27-year-old man presents with dementia, weakness, visual loss, and ataxia 1 year after receiving a cadaveric kidney transplant. Which of the following is the most likely cause of this patient's CNS disorder?
(A) Adrenoleukodystrophy
(B) Gaucher disease
(C) Metachromatic leukodystrophy
(D) Progressive multifocal leukoencephalopathy
(E) Subacute sclerosing panencephalitis

46 A 45-year-old man with AIDS is admitted to the hospital with a productive cough, fever, and night sweats. An X-ray film of the chest shows an ill-defined area of consolidation at the periphery of the right middle lobe and mediastinal lymphadenopathy. A sputum culture grows acid-fast bacilli. The patient develops severe headache and neck rigidity. Which of the following brain areas is most likely affected by this patient's infection?

(A) Base of the brain
(B) Cerebellum
(C) Hippocampus
(D) Periventricular white matter
(E) Temporal-occipital sulcus

47 A 65-year-old homeless man is found in the street and is brought to the emergency room with severe lethargy. He is treated with intravenous fluids but lapses into a coma and expires. Examination of the brainstem at autopsy shows a soft lesion in the tegmentum of the pons. A section stained for myelin with luxol fast blue is shown in the image. Which of the following is associated with this disorder?

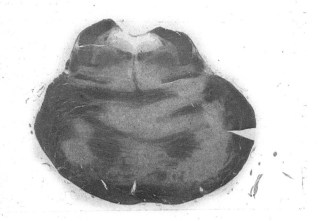

(A) AIDS
(B) Alcoholism
(C) Hypertension
(D) Multiple sclerosis
(E) Viral infection

48 A 79-year-old man presents to the emergency room with severe right-sided weakness. He has noticed increasing difficulty using his right hand over the past several months and now walks with great difficulty. His past medical history is significant for colon cancer that was resected 5 years ago. He has poorly controlled hypertension and admits to smoking two packs of cigarettes a day for the past 50 years. A CT scan of the brain reveals a discrete globoid lesion in the frontal lobe with a prominent halo of edema. A CT-guided biopsy reveals neoplastic cells. Which of the following is the most likely diagnosis?

(A) Craniopharyngioma
(B) Glioblastoma multiforme
(C) Medulloblastoma
(D) Meningioma
(E) Metastatic cancer

49 A 34-year-old intravenous drug abuser presents to the emergency room with a 24-hour history of fever and shaking chills. His temperature is 38.7°C (103°F), pulse 92 per minute, and blood pressure 140/80 mm Hg. Cardiac auscultation reveals a harsh systolic murmur. Blood cultures are positive for *Staphylococcus aureus*. The patient suddenly develops left-sided paralysis. Imaging studies would most likely reveal occlusion of which of the following arteries?

(A) Anterior meningeal
(B) Basilar
(C) Cerebellar
(D) Common carotid
(E) Middle cerebral

50 A 56-year-old man is rushed to the emergency room after collapsing while shoveling snow. The patient has no pulse on admission but is resuscitated. Laboratory studies show elevated serum levels of cardiac-specific proteins, and ECG confirms a transmural infarct of the left ventricle. The patient expires 2 weeks later of cardiac tamponade. Examination of the patient's brain at autopsy would most likely reveal necrosis of Purkinje cells and selective loss of neurons in which of the following regions?

(A) Frontal lobes
(B) Hippocampus
(C) Hypothalamus
(D) Occipital lobes
(E) Thalamus

51 A 30-year-old woman suffers massive trauma in an automobile accident and expires 4 days later of respiratory insufficiency. A horizontal section of the patient's brain at autopsy reveals numerous petechiae scattered throughout the white matter. Which of the following is the most likely explanation for this pathologic finding?

(A) Fat embolism
(B) Global ischemia
(C) Occlusion of middle cerebral artery
(D) Sepsis
(E) Uremia

52 A 67-year-old man with a history of ischemic heart disease is rushed to the emergency room after collapsing in his garden. A CT scan demonstrates a large infarct of the left frontal lobe. The patient dies, and the brain is examined at autopsy (shown in the image). This lesion was caused by thrombosis of which of the following blood vessels?

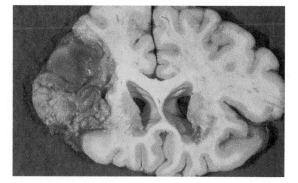

(A) External carotid artery
(B) Internal carotid artery
(C) Middle cerebral artery
(D) Sagittal venous sinus
(E) Vertebral artery

53 A 70-year-old man with a history of senile dementia and a recent myocardial infarct dies of multiple organ system failure following occlusion of the superior mesenteric artery. Examination of the patient's brain at autopsy reveals aneurysmal dilation of the basilar artery (shown in the image). Which of the following is the most common complication of this pathologic finding?

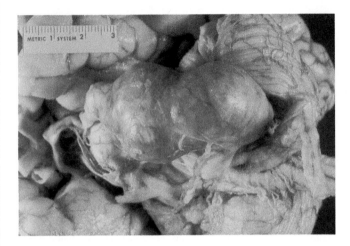

(A) Dissection
(B) Hemorrhage
(C) Infection
(D) Thrombosis
(E) Transformation

54 A 55-year-old man is brought to the emergency room after a near-drowning accident while boating. The patient has no pulse when the paramedics arrive, but he is resuscitated. The patient never regains consciousness and expires 3 days later. Examination of the brain at autopsy reveals a watershed zone of infarction in the left cerebral hemisphere. Which of the following best describes the pathogenesis of this infarct?

(A) Disseminated intravascular coagulation
(B) Prolonged hypotension
(C) Sagittal sinus thrombosis
(D) Spontaneous cerebral hemorrhage
(E) Thromboembolism

55 A 52-year-old man is brought to the emergency room 2 hours after being involved in an automobile accident. The patient denies striking his head, although his head was thrust forward and backward. His vital signs are normal, and he returns home. The following day, the patient's wife notices that he is lethargic. By the time the ambulance arrives at the emergency room, the patient is comatose. Which of the following is the most likely cause of the decline in mental status in this patient?

(A) Diffuse axonal injury
(B) Duret hemorrhages
(C) Ruptured saccular aneurysm
(D) Spinal cord contusions
(E) Watershed infarcts

56 A 45-year-old man presents with weakness and wasting of the muscles of his right hand for 8 months. Physical examination shows fasciculations of the hand. The patient's speech is impaired, and 6 years later, he dies of respiratory insufficiency. Autopsy shows atrophy of ventral roots in the spinal cord. Which of the following is the most likely diagnosis?

(A) Amyotrophic lateral sclerosis
(B) Gerstman Straussler-Scheinker disease
(C) Huntington disease
(D) Multiple infarct dementia
(E) Pick disease

57 A 6-month-old girl with metachromatic leukodystrophy (MLD) fails to thrive and dies of respiratory insufficiency. Histologic examination of the child's brain at autopsy shows marked accumulation of metachromatic material in the white matter and prominent astrogliosis. Laboratory studies confirm an accumulation of cerebroside. This patient most likely suffered from an inborn error of metabolism, characterized by a deficiency of which of the following enzymes?

(A) Arylsulfatase
(B) Galactosidase
(C) Mannosidase
(D) N-acetyl-hexosaminidase
(E) Phenylalanine hydroxylase

58 A 5-year-old girl exhibits a progressive decline in motor and sensory functions and is quickly reduced to a vegetative state. MRI reveals confluent, bilaterally symmetric, demyelination. At autopsy, the brain shows gliosis and perivascular infiltrates of lymphocytes. Laboratory studies disclose high levels of saturated very long–chain fatty acids in tissues and body fluids. This patient's leukodystrophy is most likely caused by an inborn error in the function of what cell component?

(A) Golgi apparatus
(B) Mitochondria
(C) Nuclear envelope
(D) Peroxisome
(E) Plasma membrane

59 An 8-month-old boy exhibits severe motor, sensory, and cognitive impairments. Brain biopsy shows a disease of white matter characterized by the accumulation of "globoid cells." Biochemical studies reveal an absence of galactocerebroside β-galactosidase activity. What is the appropriate diagnosis?

(A) Alexander disease
(B) Hurler disease
(C) Krabbe disease
(D) Metachromatic leukodystrophy
(E) Glycogen storage disease

60 An 8-year-old girl is brought to the physician by her parents, who express concerns about their daughters' academic performance and recent changes in behavior. Her vital signs are normal. Neurologic examination reveals motor and sensory impairments. Lumbar puncture shows no biochemical abnormalities. At autopsy, the brain shows prominent intranuclear inclusions in neurons and oligodendroglia, marked gliosis in gray and white matter, and demyelination. PCR analysis of the brain tissue shows the presence of a defective form of the measles virus. Which of the following is the appropriate diagnosis?

(A) Fatal familial insomnia
(B) Granulomatous vasculitis of the central nervous system
(C) Progressive multifocal leukoencephalopathy
(D) Spongiform encephalopathy
(E) Subacute sclerosing panencephalitis

61 A 36-year-old woman with inoperable brain cancer lapses into a coma and dies of cardiorespiratory failure. A horizontal section of the patient's brain at autopsy is shown in the image. Dilation of the ventricular system in this patient was most likely caused by obstruction at which of the following anatomic locations?

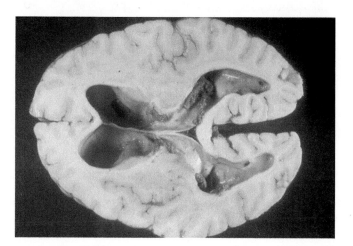

(A) Aqueduct of Sylvius
(B) Central spinal canal
(C) Foramen of Luschka
(D) Foramen of Magendie
(E) Virchow-Robin spaces

62 A 60-year-old man is brought to the emergency room in a coma. Physical examination reveals an emaciated man with a distended abdomen, jaundice, ascites, and a slightly enlarged liver and spleen. Laboratory studies show elevated levels of blood ammonia. A liver biopsy demonstrates cirrhosis. Histologic examination of brain tissue from this patient would most likely show prominent changes in the nuclei of which of the following cell types?

(A) Astrocytes
(B) Ependymal lining cells
(C) Microglia
(D) Neurons
(E) Oligodendroglia

63 A 2-year-old boy is brought to the physician by his parents, who complain that their son continually loses his balance. They also report that his speech seems more slurred. Physical examination confirms the truncal ataxia and wide-based gait. The child appears lethargic, and there is bobbing of the head while he is sitting. Muscle tone is normal. This patient may have a midline tumor in which anatomic portion of the brain?

(A) Cerebellum
(B) Corpus callosum
(C) Frontal lobes
(D) Hypothalamus
(E) Meninges

64 A lumbar puncture is performed in the patient described in Question 63, and neoplastic cells are found. A suboccipital craniotomy is performed, and a tumor is resected. Microscopic examination of the surgical specimen would most likely reveal which of the following histologic patterns?

(A) Malignant epithelial cells with prominent tonofilaments
(B) Perivascular collections of neoplastic lymphocytes
(C) Small, hyperchromatic cells and rare neuroblastic rosettes
(D) Vacuolated tumor cells and an abundant capillary network
(E) Whorled pattern of meningothelial cells and psammoma bodies

65 A 24-year-old woman presents with a 4-month history of headaches and unsteadiness in walking. She reports a tendency to fall to the right and a loss of coordinated movements in her right hand and leg. Her father and paternal aunt died of renal cell carcinoma. A paternal grandfather had a history of spinal cord tumors, and her sister is seeing an ophthalmologist for "retinal angiomas." On examination, the woman has a wide-based gait. She is unable to stand on her right leg and has intentional tremor and dysdiadokinesia of the right upper extremity. MRI reveals a right-sided parasagittal tumor of the cerebellum. A biopsy of the lesion demonstrates a hemangioblastoma. Which of the following is the most likely diagnosis?

(A) Down syndrome
(B) Multiple endocrine neoplasia type 2A (Sipple syndrome)
(C) Neurofibromatosis type 1
(D) Sturge-Weber syndrome
(E) Von Hippel-Lindau syndrome

66 A 65-year-old woman with a history of breast cancer and a recent melanoma presents to the emergency room following a tonic-clonic seizure. Blood chemistry values are within normal limits. There is no history of drug or alcohol use. MRI of the brain shows bilateral cerebral edema and a cystic, frontal lobe lesion. Frozen section obtained from a CT-guided biopsy reveals a hemorrhagic nodule of neoplastic cells. Immunohistochemical stains for which of the following antigens would be most helpful in making your diagnosis definitive for melanoma?

(A) Alpha-fetoprotein
(B) HMB-45
(C) Human chorionic gonadotropin
(D) Neuron-specific enolase
(E) Synaptophysin

67 A 68-year-old man presents with a 2-week history of tonic-clonic seizures that initially involve his left arm but have more recently progressed to involve his left leg. The seizures are accompanied by muscle weakness but no other neurologic signs. The cranial nerves are intact; and the Babinski sign is present. A CT scan reveals a mass in the left cerebral hemisphere. A left frontoparietal craniotomy is performed. Histologic examination of the brain biopsy is shown in the image. Which of the following is the appropriate diagnosis?

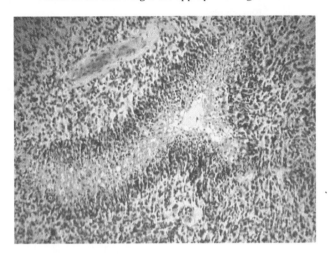

(A) Craniopharyngioma
(B) Ependymoma
(C) Ganglioglioma
(D) Glioblastoma multiforme
(E) Meningioma

68 A 65-year-old woman presents with a 3-week history of intractable headaches. Her vital signs and CBC are normal. Two weeks later, the patient develops left-sided hemiparesis. MRI reveals a large, necrotic tumor in the right hemisphere of the cerebrum, extending across the corpus callosum into the left hemisphere. A coronal section of the patient's brain at autopsy is shown in the image. This tumor is most likely derived from which of the following cell types?

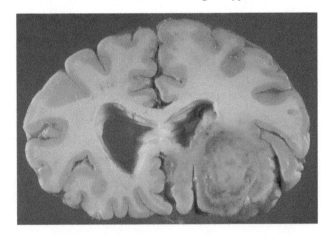

(A) Astrocytes
(B) Ependymal lining cells
(C) Microglia
(D) Neurons
(E) Oligodendroglia

69 A 50-year-old man presents with a 5-month history of severe headaches. Vital signs and CBC are normal. Imaging studies demonstrate a mass in the fourth ventricle and hydrocephalus. The results of a CT-guided biopsy are shown in the image. What is the appropriate diagnosis for this patient's malignant neoplasm?

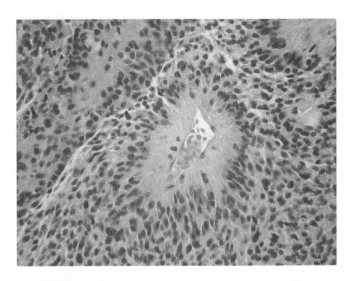

(A) Craniopharyngioma
(B) Ependymoma
(C) Glioblastoma multiforme
(D) Oligodendroglioma
(E) Schwannoma

70 A 45-year-old woman is brought to the emergency room after experiencing a generalized seizure. An X-ray film of the skull reveals a lytic bone mass. A CBC is normal. A portion of the skull and the adherent mass are removed. Microscopic examination of the surgical specimen is shown in the image. What is the appropriate diagnosis?

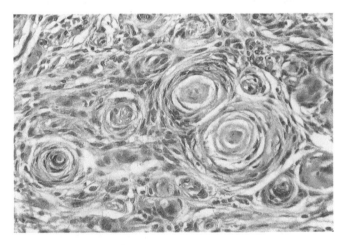

(A) Glioblastoma multiforme
(B) Hemangioblastoma
(C) Medulloblastoma
(D) Meningioma
(E) Oligodendroglioma

71 A 26-year-old woman with a history of bitemporal hemianopsia and diabetes insipidus develops meningococcal infection and dies of septic shock. Examination of the brain at autopsy reveals a large cystic tumor mass replacing the midline structures in the region of the hypothalamus (shown in the image). This tumor is derived from epithelial cells originating in which of the following embryonic structures?

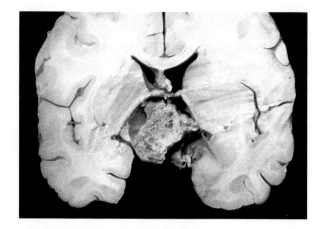

(A) Diencephalon
(B) Mesencephalon
(C) Nasopharynx
(D) Prosencephalon
(E) Third pharyngeal arch

72 A 48-year-old man with AIDS is admitted to the hospital with a fever of 38.7°C (103°F), persistent cough, and diarrhea. His CD4 cell count is less than 500/μL. The patient is started on broad-spectrum antibiotics. He has also experienced a recent decline in cognitive function. He is at increased risk of developing which of the following CNS neoplasms?
(A) Ependymoma
(B) Glioblastoma
(C) Lymphoma
(D) Medulloblastoma
(E) Oligodendroglioma

73 A 14-year-old boy complains of a 4-month history of fatigue, abdominal pain, and yellowing of his eyes and skin. Physical examination shows tremor of both hands, lack of coordination, and mild jaundice. An ophthalmic examination reveals Kayser-Fleischer rings. Degenerative changes are present in which of the following anatomic regions of the CNS in this patient?
(A) Cerebellum
(B) Corpus striatum
(C) Paraventricular white matter
(D) Pons
(E) Temporal-occipital sulcus

74 A 50-year-old man presents to the emergency room after suffering an epileptic seizure. Vital signs are normal. An X-ray of the patient's head shows a mass in the left cerebral hemisphere with scattered foci of calcification. Histologic examination of a brain biopsy is shown in the image. Which of the following is the appropriate diagnosis?

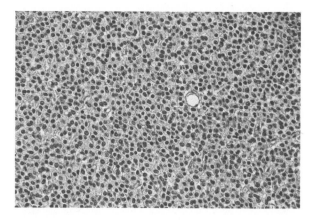

(A) Ependymoma
(B) Glioblastoma
(C) Hemangioblastoma
(D) Meningioma
(E) Oligodendroglioma

75 A 20-year-old man complains of increasing difficulty in hearing over the past several years. Physical examination confirms bilateral sensorineural hearing deficits. MRI discloses bilateral cerebellopontine angle tumors, consistent with schwannomas. This patient has a strong family history for benign tumors, including low-grade gliomas and meningiomas on his mother's side of the family. Which of the following is the probable diagnosis?
(A) Neurofibromatosis type 1
(B) Neurofibromatosis type 2
(C) Sturge-Weber syndrome
(D) Tuberous sclerosis
(E) Von Hippel-Lindau syndrome

76 An 80-year-old woman wanders away from a nursing home and dies in a pedestrian-motor vehicle accident. A silver-stained section of her brain at autopsy reveals numerous lesions in the cerebral cortex (shown in the image). Which of the following terms best describes these pathologic findings?

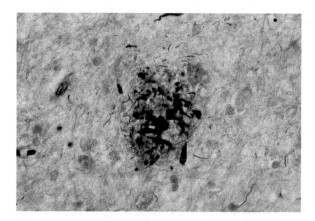

(A) Granulovacuolar degeneration
(B) Lewy bodies
(C) Neuritic plaques
(D) Neurofibrillary tangles
(E) Spongiform encephalopathy

77 A 14-year-old girl is rushed to the emergency room after receiving a gunshot wound to the head and is pronounced dead on arrival. If this child died due to an immediate "blast effect" of the penetrating wound, the autopsy would likely show herniation of the tonsils of the cerebellum into which anatomic space?
(A) Aqueduct of Sylvius
(B) Central spinal canal
(C) Foramen magnum
(D) Foramen of Magendie
(E) Posterior fossa

78 A 60-year-old man with a 15-year history of diabetes mellitus type 2 complains of deep burning pain and sensitivity to touch over his hands and fingers. Nerve conduction studies show slow transmission of impulses and diminished muscle stretch reflexes in both ankles and knees. Sensations to vibrations and light touch are also markedly diminished. Laboratory analysis of CSF shows no biochemical abnormalities. Which of the following is the most likely type of peripheral nerve disease in this patient?
(A) Autonomic neuropathy
(B) Distal polyneuropathy
(C) Inflammatory neuropathy
(D) Mononeuropathy
(E) Paraproteinemic neuropathy

79 A 35-year-old man with Down syndrome dies of acute lymphoblastic leukemia. Gross examination of the patient's brain at autopsy shows mild microcephaly and underdevelopment of the superior temporal gyri. Histologic examination would most likely show which of the following neuropathologic changes?
(A) AA amyloidosis
(B) Lewy bodies
(C) Negri bodies
(D) Neurofibrillary tangles
(E) Spongiform encephalopathy

ANSWERS

1 **The answer is B: Meningomyelocele.** Neural tube defects (dysraphic anomalies) reflect impaired closure of the dorsal aspect of the vertebral column. These abnormalities are classified according the extent of the defect, ranging in severity from spina bifida occulta to meningocele, meningomyelocele, and rachischisis. Spina bifida (choice D) is restricted to the vertebral arches and is usually asymptomatic. Meningocele (choice A) permits protrusion of the meninges as a fluid-filled sac. Meningomyelocele (choice B) exposes the spinal canal and causes the nerve roots to be entrapped. Rachischisis (choice C) is an extreme defect, often without a recognizable spinal cord. Syringomyelia (choice E) is a congenital malformation, in which a tubular cavitation (syrinx) extends for variable distances along the entire length of the spinal cord.
Diagnosis: Neural tube defect, meningomyelocele

2 **The answer is A: Folic acid.** Maternal folic acid deficiency has been associated with an increased incidence of neural tube defects, and folic acid has, therefore, been approved for inclu-

sion as a food supplement in commercial flour. Deficiencies of vitamins in the other choices are not associated with congenital dysraphic anomalies. Niacin deficiency results in pellagra. Thiamine deficiency (choice C) causes Wernicke syndrome and beriberi. Vitamin B_{12} deficiency (choice E) leads to pernicious anemia.
Diagnosis: Neural tube defect

3 **The answer is B: Arnold-Chiari malformation.** Arnold-Chiari malformation is a condition in which the brainstem and cerebellum are compacted into a shallow, bowl-shaped posterior fossa with a low-positioned tentorium. The cerebellar vermis is herniated below the level of the foramen magnum in the photograph shown. Anencephaly (choice A) refers to the congenital absence of all or part of the brain. Holoprosencephaly (choice C) is a microcephalic brain in which the interhemispheric fissure is absent. Hydromyelia (choice D) is the term for dilation of the central canal of the spinal cord.
Diagnosis: Arnold-Chiari malformation

4 **The answer is A: Atresia of the aqueduct of Sylvius.** Congenital hydrocephalus refers to an excessive amount of CSF and ventricular enlargement. Congenital atresia of the aqueduct of Sylvius is the most common cause of congenital hydrocephalus, occurring in 1 in 1,000 live births. Histologic examination of the midbrain may disclose multiple atretic channels or an aqueduct narrowed by gliosis. Congenital brain tumors (choice C) are rare. The other choices are not associated with congenital hydrocephalus. Because the infantile cranium expands easily, symptoms of increased intracranial pressure are generally absent. However, convulsions are common, and optic atrophy with blindness can occur.
Diagnosis: Hydrocephalus

5 **The answer is B: Choroid plexus.** Cerebrospinal fluid (CSF) constitutes an accessory circulatory system adapted to the needs of the CNS. CSF is formed principally by the choroid plexus at a rate of approximately 500 mL per day. The choroid plexus stretches along the roof of the third ventricle and then angles posteriorly to span the lateral ventricles. It flows from its intraventricular origin to sites of reabsorption, principally through the arachnoid villi, into the dural sinuses. The fluid transports metabolites, serves as a medium for clearing metabolic waste, and protects or "cushions" the structures contained within it. CSF is not produced in any of the other structures.
Diagnosis: Hydrocephalus

6 **The answer is E: Polymicrogyria.** Abnormalities of the cerebral gyri are frequently associated with mental retardation. Polymicrogyria is a congenital disorder in which the surface of the brain exhibits an excessive number of small, irregularly sized, randomly distributed gyral folds. Arrhinencephaly (choice A) refers to absence of the olfactory tracts. Lissencephaly (choice C) is a congenital disorder in which the cortical surface of the cerebral hemispheres is smooth or has imperfectly formed gyri. Pachygyria (choice D) is a condition in which the gyri are reduced in number and usually broad.
Diagnosis: Polymicrogyria

7 **The answer is C: Chromosomal abnormality.** Congenital defects of the CNS are often associated with chromosomal abnormalities, which are best exemplified by trisomies of chromosomes 13 to 15 (holoprosencephaly) and chromosome 21 (Down syndrome). Holoprosencephaly refers to a microcephalic brain in which the interhemispheric fissure is absent. The horseshoe-shaped cerebral hemispheres have fused frontal poles, across which the gyri show an irregular horizontal orientation. Holoprosencephaly is rarely compatible with life beyond a few weeks or months. All of the other choices are acquired disorders that do not affect gross brain morphology.
Diagnosis: Holoprosencephaly

8 **The answer is D: Tabes dorsalis.** Tabes dorsalis is a feature of tertiary syphilis and is characterized by chronic fibrosing meningitis, which constricts the posterior root of the spinal cord. The posterior roots contain sensory nerves that originate in the spinal ganglia and form the posterior columns of the spinal cord. Compression of sensory nerves that originate in the posterior roots causes lancinating pain in extremities. It also damages the transmission of proprioceptive impulses, causing gait disturbances (ataxia). Amyotrophic lateral sclerosis (choice A) is a motor neuron disease that does not affect the posterior columns. Friedreich ataxia (choice B) is an autosomal dominant trait that involves the spinal cord in a complex way. It affects not only the centripetal pathways (spinocerebellar and posterior columns), but also the efferent corticospinal tracts. Subacute combined degeneration (choice E) is due to vitamin B_{12} deficiency and involves not only the posterior columns, but also the anterior horn cells and the spinocerebellar and corticospinal tracts.
Diagnosis: Syphilis

9 **The answer is A: Alzheimer disease.** Alzheimer disease is the most common cause of dementia in the elderly, accounting for more than half of all cases. Alzheimer's original patients were younger than 65 years of age, but the disease now refers to dementias that display characteristic pathologic findings. Alzheimer disease is an insidious and progressive neurologic disorder, characterized clinically by loss of memory, cognitive impairment, difficulty with language, and eventual dementia. It features atrophy of the brain, which can be recognized by CT scan as widening of the sulci and bilateral atrophy of the gyri, particularly the frontal and hippocampal cortex. These clinical and morphologic features are not typically observed in the other choices. Bronchopneumonia is the usual lethal outcome of Alzheimer disease.
Diagnosis: Alzheimer disease

10 **The answer is E: APrP.** The brain biopsy shows spongiform degeneration of the gray matter, characterized by individual and clustered vacuoles, with no evidence of inflammation. Prion diseases are recognized clinically by slowly progressive ataxia and dementia and pathologically by the accumulation of fibrillar or insoluble prion proteins, degeneration of neurons, and vacuolization (spongiform degeneration). Spongiform encephalopathies are transmissible, and inadvertent human transmission of Creutzfeldt-Jakob disease (CJD) has followed the administration of contaminated human pituitary growth hormone, corneal transplantation from a diseased donor, insufficiently sterilized neurosurgical instruments, and surgi-

cal implantation of contaminated dura. APrP amyloid is found in patients with spongiform encephalopathies. Prion proteins (PrPs) are natural plasma membrane constituents found in a variety of cells, including the central nervous system. The residual PrP, now in an altered conformation, may serve as a template for the association of additional PrP molecules. In so doing, they confer the new PrP conformation (PrP^{sc}). Such altered PrP and its aggregates form fibrils with the characteristic of amyloid and are believed to play a role in a group of human and animal degenerative diseases of the central nervous system, such as kuru, CJD, Gerstmann-Straussler-Sheinker disease, scrapie, and bovine spongiform encephalopathy (mad cow disease). The other forms of amyloid are not associated with spongiform encephalopathies.
Diagnosis: Creutzfeldt-Jakob disease, spongiform encephalopathy

11 **The answer is C: Three-dimensional conformation.** The normal prion gene product (PrP) is a constitutively expressed, cell-surface glycoprotein that is bound to the plasma membrane by a glycolipid anchor. The highest levels of PrP mRNA are found in CNS neurons. Remarkably, the normal cellular prion protein (PrP^C) and the pathogenic (infectious) prion protein (scrapie PrP or PrP^{SC}) do not differ in amino acid sequence. However, they represent different three-dimensional conformations. Specifically, PrP^C is rich in α-helix configuration, whereas the β-pleated sheet configuration is predominant in PrP^{SC}. This is an epigenetic phenomenon. Newly converted proteins then change other PrP^C proteins into pathogenic PrP^{SC}. The result is an autocatalytic, exponentially expanding accrual of abnormal PrP^{SC}. About 15% of prion diseases are familial and reflect mutations that predispose to abnormal protein folding.
Diagnosis: Creutzfeldt-Jakob disease, spongiform encephalopathy

12 **The answer is B: Hydrocephalus ex vacuo.** The brain of patients with Alzheimer disease loses approximately 200 g in an interval of 3 to 8 years. The gyri narrow, the sulci widen, and cortical atrophy becomes apparent. In turn, these changes lead to widening of the lateral ventricles (hydrocephalus ex vacuo). Hydrocephalus ex vacuo refers to enlargement of the ventricular system as a compensatory response to severe brain atrophy and is unrelated to obstructive lesions. The atrophy is bilateral and symmetric, and targets the frontal and hippocampal cortex. Choices C and D are congenital disorders. Choice E is common in patients with multiple sclerosis.
Diagnosis: Alzheimer disease, hydrocephalus ex vacuo

13 **The answer is B: Caudate nuclei.** Huntington disease (HD) is an autosomal dominant genetic disorder characterized by involuntary movements of all parts of the body, deterioration of cognitive function, and often severe emotional disturbance. The huntingtin gene product is widely expressed in tissues throughout the body and in all regions of the CNS by neurons and glia. On gross examination of brains from patients who died of HD, the frontal cortex is symmetrically and moderately atrophic, whereas the lateral ventricles appear disproportionately enlarged, owing to the loss of the normal convex curvature of the caudate nuclei. There is symmetric atrophy of the caudate nuclei, with lesser involvement of the putamen.

Biochemical assays at the termination of the disease show a marked decreased in γ-aminobutyric acid and glutamic acid decarboxylase. Choices A, C, and D are not involved in Huntington disease. Pathology of the substantia nigra (choice E) characterizes Parkinson disease.

Diagnosis: Huntington disease

14   The answer is B: Expansion of a trinucleotide repeat. A large group of hereditary neurodegenerative diseases are classified on a genetic basis as trinucleotide repeat expansion syndromes. The triplet repeat mutation disorders include Huntington disease (HD), fragile X syndrome, and Friedreich ataxia. Trinucleotide repeats are a normal feature of many genes, but expansion of the number of repeats confers pathogenicity. In HD, the expansion lies within the coding region of a gene segment and results in the production of a toxic protein, namely huntingtin. The other choices reflect genetic abnormalities that are not related to Huntington disease.

Diagnosis: Huntington disease

15   The answer is C: Cardiomyopathy. Friedreich ataxia is the most common inherited ataxia. Although the inheritance pattern is autosomal recessive, many cases arise sporadically as new mutations without a family history. The onset of symptoms is usually before age 25 years, followed by an unremitting and progressive course of about 30 years before death. The hallmark of Friedreich ataxia is a combined ataxia of both the upper and lower limbs. Dysarthria, lower-limb areflexia, extensor plantar reflexes, and sensory loss also occur in most patients. Frequently associated systemic abnormalities are deformities of the skeleton system (scoliosis), diabetes mellitus, and hypertrophic cardiomyopathy (which commonly causes death). The candidate gene encodes a mitochondrial protein (frataxin) involved in iron transport. Friedreich ataxia is associated with an unstable expansion of a trinucleotide repeat that presumably interferes with transcription or RNA processing. The highest levels of frataxin gene expression are found in the heart and spinal cord. The other choices are not associated with trinucleotide repeat expansion syndromes.

Diagnosis: Friedreich ataxia

16   The answer is C: Myelin. Multiple sclerosis (MS) is a chronic demyelinating disease that is the most common chronic CNS disease of young adults in the United States. The disorder affects sensory and motor functions and is characterized by exacerbations and remissions over many years. MS may present with a variety of symptoms, such as sensory deficits, sphincter weakness, and tremors. Forty percent of cases are marked by eye problems, such as loss of visual fields, blindness in one eye, or diplopia. The demyelinated plaque is the hallmark of MS. Evolving plaques are marked by: selective loss of myelin in a region of axonal preservation; a few lymphocytes that cluster about small veins and arteries; an influx of macrophages; and considerable edema. Intracellular deposits of α-synuclein (choice E) are seen in patients with Parkinson disease.

Diagnosis: Multiple sclerosis

17   The answer is A: Astrogliosis. Multiple sclerosis is punctuated by abrupt and brief episodes of clinical progression,

interspersed with periods of relative stability. Each exacerbation reflects the formation of additional demyelinated plaques. Plaques of demyelinated white matter are typically found around the lateral ventricles of the cerebrum, in the cerebellum, and in the spinal cord. End-stage lesions feature astrogliosis, thick-walled blood vessels, moderate perivascular inflammation, and a secondary loss of axons. Lewy bodies (choice B) are features of Parkinson disease. Negri bodies (choice C) are encountered in rabies. Neurofibrillary tangles (choice D) are features of Alzheimer disease. Whorled "myelin figures" (choice E) represent lysosomal storage of unmetabolized gangliosides in the neurons of patients with Tay-Sachs disease.

Diagnosis: Multiple sclerosis

18   The answer is A: Epidural hematoma. Epidural hematoma is the accumulation of blood between the calvaria and the dura. It usually results from a blow to the head, and unless treated promptly, it is generally fatal. The temporal bone is one of the thinnest bones of the skull and is particularly vulnerable to fracture, so that seemingly minor trauma may fracture it. An epidural hematoma usually results from a traumatic bone fracture that severs the middle meningeal artery. The other choices are not characteristic complications of temporal bone fracture.

Diagnosis: Epidural hematoma

19   The answer is D: α-Synuclein. Parkinson disease (PD) is a common movement disorder characterized pathologically by the loss of neurons, primarily in the substantia nigra, and the accumulation of eosinophilic inclusions termed Lewy bodies, formed by filamentous aggregates of α-synuclein. Accumulating evidence suggests that oxidative stress produced by the auto-oxidation of catecholamines during melanin formation injures pigmented neurons in the substantia nigra by promoting the misfolding of α-synuclein. Clinically, PD features tremors at rest, muscular rigidity, expressionless countenance, emotional liability, and, less commonly, cognitive impairments, including dementia late in the disease course. The other choices are not characterized by demarcated inclusions within neurons of the substantia nigra.

Diagnosis: Parkinson disease

20   The answer is D: Degeneration of the posterior columns of the spinal cord. Subacute combined degeneration results from a lack of vitamin B_{12} (pernicious anemia) and leads to lesions in the posterolateral portions of the spinal cord. Vitamin B_{12} is required for DNA synthesis, and its deficiency results in large (megaloblastic) nuclei in all bone marrow lineages. A burning sensation in the soles of the feet and other paresthesias herald the onset of this rapidly progressive and poorly reversible neurologic disorder. Initially, there is symmetric myelin and axonal loss at the thoracic level of the spinal cord. With time, the affected spinal cord exhibits gliosis and atrophy, especially in the posterolateral areas of the cord. The other anatomic locations are not adversely affected by vitamin B_{12} deficiency.

Diagnosis: Subacute combined degeneration, pernicious anemia

21   The answer is D: Reduced levels of dopamine. The substantia nigra is a component of the extrapyramidal system that relays information to the basal ganglia through dopaminergic synapses. Normal aging is associated with a loss of neurons in the substantia nigra and reduced levels of dopamine, but these features are more exaggerated in patients with Parkinson disease (PD). Degeneration in the pars compacta of the substantia nigra is characterized by macroscopic nigral pallor, microscopic loss of pigmented neurons, pigment granules found extracellularly or within macrophages, gliosis, and, in some surviving neurons, cytoplasmic inclusions that have an eosinophilic core surrounded by a clear halo (Lewy bodies). The vast majority of cases of Parkinson disease are idiopathic, but the disease has been recorded after viral encephalitis (von Economo encephalitis) and after intake of the toxic chemical methyl-phenyl-tetrahydropyridine. None of the other choices reflects damage to the substantia nigra.

Diagnosis: Parkinson disease

22 The answer is E: Thiamine deficiency. Wernicke syndrome is secondary to thiamine (vitamin B₁) deficiency. It is characterized clinically by the rapid onset of a disturbance in thermal regulation, altered consciousness, ophthalmoplegia, nystagmus, and ataxia and pathologically by lesions in the hypothalamus and mamillary bodies, the periaqueductal regions of the midbrain, and the tegmentum of the pons. Atrophy of the superior portion of cerebellar vermis also occurs. The syndrome arises most commonly in association with chronic alcoholism. Wernicke syndrome may progress rapidly to death but is reversed by the administration of thiamine. Wernicke-Korsakoff syndrome refers to a state of disordered recent memory often compensated for by confabulation. Choices C and D are consequences of hepatic failure that are not related to thiamine deficiency. Choice B (amyotrophic lateral sclerosis) is a chronic neurological disorder unrelated to vitamins.

Diagnosis: Wernicke encephalopathy

23 The answer is D: Negri bodies. Rabies is an encephalitis caused by the rabies virus, which is transmitted to humans through contaminated saliva introduced by a bite. Dogs, wolves, foxes, and skunks are the principal reservoirs, but the infection is also acquired from the bite of rabid bats, which often inhabit caves. Viral replication initiates at the site of the bite, and transport to the CNS is mediated by viral entry into peripheral nerves. Destruction of the brainstem neurons by rabies virus initiates painful spasms of the throat, difficulty swallowing, and a tendency to aspirate fluids, which has prompted the designation "hydrophobia." Encephalopathy progresses to death within 1 to several weeks. Pathologic features of rabies encephalitis include perivascular cuffing by lymphocytes, neuronophagia, microglial nodules, and "Negri bodies," which are distinctive eosinophilic, cytoplasmic inclusions in infected nerve cells. Councilman bodies (choice A) are remnants of apoptotic hepatocytes seen in acute viral hepatitis. Lewy bodies (choice C) are features of Parkinson disease.

Diagnosis: Rabies

24 The answer is E: Venous sinus thrombosis. The cerebral veins empty into large venous sinuses, the most prominent of which is the sagittal sinus, because it accommodates the venous drainage from the superior portions of the cerebral hemispheres. Venous sinus thrombosis in the brain is a potentially lethal complication of systemic dehydration, as occurs in infants with severe

gastrointestinal fluid loss. Because venous obstruction causes stagnation upstream, abrupt thrombosis of the sagittal sinus results in bilateral hemorrhagic infarctions of the frontal lobe regions. Dehydration is not a cause of hemorrhage (choices B, C, and D). Choice A (diffuse axonal shearing) reflects trauma.

Diagnosis: Sagittal sinus thrombosis

25 The answer is D: Transtentorial herniation. Head trauma can cause extensive intracranial hemorrhage and cerebral edema. After compensatory mechanisms have been exhausted, the brain is shifted laterally away from the side of the lesion. The medial temporal lobe on the side of the hematoma is compressed against the midbrain to displace it downward through the opening created by the tentorium, a fatal event known as transtentorial herniation. Thus, the oculomotor nerve may be compressed against the edge of the tentorium, causing third-nerve palsy. The pupil, generally on the side of the lesion, becomes fixed and dilated. The herniated uncus also compresses the vasculature of the midbrain, especially the mesencephalic veins. Venous stagnation in the midbrain causes further hypoxia and impairs neuronal function. Choices B and E are related to global anoxia. Diffuse axonal shearing (choice A) is a microscopic diagnosis.

Diagnosis: Transtentorial herniation

26 The answer is B: Duret hemorrhages. In patients with transtentorial herniation, the uncus of the hippocampus is herniated downward to displace the midbrain, which is the site of secondary (Duret) hemorrhages. Duret hemorrhages in a case of transtentorial herniation tend to be midline and occupy the brainstem from the upper midbrain to the midpons. Pontine myelinolysis (choice D) is seen in chronic alcoholics. Encephalomalacia (choice C) occurs after brain infarcts.

Diagnosis: Transtentorial herniation

27 The answer is C: Microglial cells. Microglia are phagocytic macrophage-derived cells of the CNS, accounting for 5% of all glial cells. In response to necrosis, macroglia become phagocytic, accumulate lipids and other cellular debris, and are designated gitter cells. Some reactive microglia exhibit a prominent elongated nucleus, in which case they are referred to as rod cells. After microglial phagocytosis, astrocytosis (choice A) then leads to local scar formation, which persists as telltale evidence of a prior injury.

Diagnosis: Cerebral contusion

28 The answer is A: Brainstem reticular formation. Concussion is defined as the transient loss of consciousness due to trauma. Consciousness is a positive neurologic activity that depends on the function of specific neurons, especially in the brainstem reticular formation. In the current case, a blow that deflects the head upward and posteriorly, often with a rotary component, imparts quick torque on the brainstem and causes functional paralysis of the neurons of the reticular formation. By contrast, a blow to the temporoparietal area (choice E) may lead to a skull fracture but does not generally cause a concussion because lateral movement of the cerebral hemispheres is prevented by the falx. Contusion of the cerebellum (choice B) is unlikely to cause loss of consciousness.

Diagnosis: Subdural hematoma, concussion

29 The answer is C: Gliosis. Astrocytes are star-shaped glial cells that far outnumber neurons throughout the CNS. Astrocytes proliferate locally in response to injuries (e.g., trauma, abscess, tumors, infarcts, and hemorrhages). This process, referred to as astrocytosis or gliosis, is readily demonstrated by immunostaining for glial fibrillary acidic protein (shown in photomicrograph). Astrocytosis evolves in hours to days and persists to an extent that is usually commensurate with the severity of the initiating injury. The result is a "glial scar" composed of reactive astrocytes and their processes. Neuronophagia (choice E) is a function of microglia.

Diagnosis: Astrogliosis

30 The answer is D: Hypertension. Hypertension compromises the integrity of cerebral arterioles by causing the deposition of lipid in, and hyalinization of, the arterial walls, an alteration referred to as lipohyalinosis. Further weakening of the wall leads to the formation of Charcot-Bouchard aneurysms, which are located mainly along the trunk of a vessel rather than at its bifurcation. Although the other choices affect blood vessels, they do not typically cause cerebral microaneurysms.

Diagnosis: Hypertensive stroke, cerebral hemorrhage

31 The answer is A: Bridging veins. Subdural hematoma reflects torn bridging veins in the subdural space. Unlike the epidural space, the subdural space can expand. Because bleeding in this situation is from veins, it usually stops spontaneously after an accumulation of 25 to 50 mL because of a local tamponade effect. However, this effect also can compress severed bridging veins and cause thrombosis. Because the brain is symmetric and a force applied in the sagittal plane similarly affects both cerebral hemispheres, it is not surprising that subdural hematomas are frequently bilateral. Tearing of the middle meningeal artery (choice D) causes epidural hemorrhage.

Diagnosis: Subdural hematoma

32 The answer is A: Rebleeding from previous hematoma. Subdural hemorrhages tend to stop spontaneously, owing to low pressure within the torn veins and external compression by the hematoma. The blood eventually coagulates, and granulation tissue grows into the wound. The organizing subdural hematoma may enlarge because of repeated trauma. Even minor trauma, such as shaking the head, may cause rebleeding. The other choices do not represent complications of subdural hemorrhage.

Diagnosis: Subdural hematoma

33 The answer is E: Leptomeninges. Meningitis is a dangerous infection caused by a variety of microorganisms. Leptomeningitis denotes an inflammatory process localized to the pia/arachnoid. This compartment houses the CSF, an excellent culture medium for most microorganisms. With few exceptions, all forms of meningitis are initiated by microorganisms, suppurative bacteria being the principal offenders. In untreated cases, delirium gives way to coma and death. The other choices are rarely affected by bacteria.

Diagnosis: Bacterial meningitis

34 The answer is A: Meningococcal meningitis. The presence of neutrophils in the CSF is the most definitive index of bacterial meningitis. By contrast, lymphocytes are the hallmark of tuberculosis and the viral meningitides (choice E), as well as some chronic infections. The classic signs of meningitis include cervical rigidity, knee pain with hip flexion (Kernig sign), and knee/hip flexion when the neck is flexed (Brudzinski sign). *Staphylococcus* (choice C) is rarely a cause of meningitis. CSF neutrophils are not predominant in tuberculous meningitis (choice D).

Diagnosis: Meningococcal meningitis

35 The answer is C: *Escherichia coli*. *E. coli* is the prime cause of meningitis in the newborn, whose resistance to Gram-negative bacteria has not fully developed. The transplacental transfer of maternal IgG imparts protection to the newborn against many bacteria, but *E. coli* requires IgM for neutralization. At autopsy, the brain shows a creamy exudate in the leptomeninges (see photograph). Choices A and B do not lead to meningitis. *Haemophilus influenzae* (choice D) and *Neisseria meningitides* (choice E) cause meningitis at a later age.

Diagnosis: Bacterial meningitis

36 The answer is D: Tay-Sachs disease. Tay-Sachs disease is a lethal, autosomal recessive disorder caused by an inborn deficiency of hexosaminidase A, which permits the accumulation of ganglioside GM1 in CNS neurons. The disease is fatal in infancy and early childhood. Retinal involvement increases macular transparency and is responsible for a cherry-red spot in the macula. On histologic examination, lipid droplets are seen in the cytoplasm of distended nerve cells of the CNS and peripheral nervous system. Electron microscopy reveals the lipid within lysosomes in the form of whorled "myelin figures." Swollen neurons that exhibit marked vacuolization of the perikaryon and contain lysosomes filled with lipid can also occur in other lipid-storage diseases (e.g., Gaucher disease, Niemann-Pick disease). The other diseases do not produce such neuronal changes.

Diagnosis: Tay-Sachs disease

37 The answer is E: Temporal lobes. The manifestations of viral infections of CNS parenchyma are heterogeneous, owing to viral tropism to specific regions of the brain. Herpes simplex targets the temporal lobes. The mechanisms of viral tropism in general are unknown but may reflect specific binding of viruses to sites on the plasma membranes of CNS cells, the ability of viruses to remain latent, or selective replication in distinct intracellular microenvironments. Brainstem nuclei (choice B) are affected by poliovirus.

Diagnosis: Herpes encephalitis

38 The answer is D: Perivascular cuffs of lymphocytes. The classic hallmark of most CNS viral infections is the presence of perivascular lymphocytes around arteries and arterioles. The other choices are not features of acute viral infection.

Diagnosis: Herpes encephalitis

39 The answer is B: Cytomegalovirus (CMV). CMV is one of the agents of the so-called TORCH syndrome. CMV crosses the placenta to induce encephalitis in utero. CMV particles are demonstrated as intranuclear and intracytoplasmic inclusions in neurons and astrocytes. The lesions in the embryonic CNS predominate in the periventricular areas and are

characterized by necrosis and calcification. Because of the proximity of these lesions to the third ventricle and the aqueduct, they are prone to induce hydrocephalus. Toxoplamosis (choice E) does not feature intranuclear inclusions.
Diagnosis: Viral encephalitis

40 **The answer is B: *Cryptococcus neoformans.*** Cryptococcal meningitis is an indolent infection in which the virulence of the causative agent marginally exceeds the resistance of the host. In most cases, it acts opportunistically in immunocompromised persons (e.g., patients who have AIDS). The organisms vary in size from 5 to 15 μm in diameter and reproduce by budding. When a drop of contaminated CSF is mixed with India ink, microscopic examination shows a clear halo about the encapsulated organism. The tissue response to *C. neoformans* in the meninges is typically sparse. The other choices are not typical CNS infections in patients with AIDS.
Diagnosis: Cryptococcal meningitis

41 **The answer is C: Congenital weakness.** Rupture of a berry (saccular) aneurysm results in life-threatening subarachnoid hemorrhage, with a 35% mortality during the initial hemorrhage. A sudden severe headache characteristically heralds the onset of subarachnoid hemorrhage and may be followed by coma. Berry aneurysms are the consequence of arterial defects that are presumed to arise during embryogenesis. The muscular layer of a blood vessel that bifurcates into two branches may fail to interdigitate adequately across the branch point, thereby creating a point of congenital muscular weakness that is bridged only by endothelium, the internal elastic membrane, and a thin adventitia. Over time, the blood flow from the parent vessel exerts pressure at the point of bifurcation and expands the congenital defect. Atherosclerosis (choice A) results in aneurysms that produce a mass effect. Hypertension (choice E) is associated with arteriolar lipohyalinosis and induces Charcot-Bouchard aneurysms. Bacterial infection (choice B) leads to mycotic aneurysms.
Diagnosis: Berry aneurysm

42 **The answer is A: Circle of Willis.** More than 90% of saccular aneurysms occur in the circle of Willis at branch points in the carotid system. They are equally distributed at the junction of (1) the anterior cerebral and anterior communicating arteries, (2) the internal carotid-posterior communicating-anterior cerebral-anterior choroidal arteries, and (3) the trifurcation of the middle cerebral artery. Lesions of the other arteries do not cause subarachnoid hemorrhage.
Diagnosis: Berry aneurysm

43 **The answer is A: Basal ganglia/thalamic area.** Cerebral hemorrhage causes stroke (apoplexy). Cerebral hemorrhages that occur without trauma are referred to as "spontaneous," although most are related to preexisting vascular lesions (Charcot-Bouchard aneurysms) or are the consequence of long-standing hypertension. Hypertensive intracerebral hemorrhage occurs at preferential sites, which in order of frequency are the basal ganglia-thalamus (65%), pons (15%), and cerebellum (8%). Necrosis of pyramidal neurons of Sommer's sector in the hippocampus (choice E) occurs as a consequence of global anoxia.
Diagnosis: Cerebral hemorrhage

44 **The answer is E: Release of neurotoxic cytokines from macrophages.** In most patients with AIDS encephalopathy, the disease is attributable to an active infection of the CNS by the virus itself. Macrophages and microglial cells in the CNS are productively infected by HIV-1. Although neurons and astrocytes may interact with the virus, they do not seem to be infected but are injured indirectly by cytokines or other neurotoxic factors released by macrophages. Dementia is the most common clinical manifestation of AIDS encephalopathy, which ranges from mild to severe cognitive impairment, with paralysis and loss of sensory functions. The other choices are not typical complications of AIDS.
Diagnosis: AIDS dementia complex

45 **The answer is D: Progressive multifocal leukoencephalopathy (PML).** PML is a relentlessly destructive disease caused by JC virus, which principally affects the white matter in brain. Typical lesions appear as widely disseminated discrete foci of demyelination near the gray-white junction in the cerebral hemispheres and the brainstem. Most commonly, PML is a terminal complication in immunosuppressed patients, such as those treated for cancer or lupus erythematosus, organ transplant patients, and persons with AIDS. Adrenoleukodystrophy (choice A), Gaucher disease (choice B), and metachromatic leukodystrophy (choice C) are caused by inborn errors of metabolism. Subacute sclerosing panencephalitis (choice E) is a chronic, lethal, viral infection of the brain caused by measles virus.
Diagnosis: Progressive multifocal leukoencephalopathy

46 **The answer is A: Base of the brain.** Tuberculous meningitis has a predilection for the base of the brain, and infarcts are often found in the distribution of the striate arteries. Inadequately treated tuberculous meningitis results in meningeal fibrosis, communicating hydrocephalus, and arteritis, with the last leading to infarcts. Less often, parenchymal tuberculosis produces tuberculomas (i.e., solitary masses with central caseous necrosis surrounded by granulomatous tissue; choices B, C, D, and E).
Diagnosis: Tuberculosis

47 **The answer is B: Alcoholism.** Central pontine myelinolysis is a rare demyelinating disorder that features selective demyelination in the pons. The lesions are often too small to have clinical manifestations and are discovered only at autopsy. However, some patients develop quadriparesis, pseudobulbar palsy, or severe depression of consciousness (pseudocoma). Central pontine myelinolysis is thought to arise from overly rapid correction of hyponatremia in alcoholics or malnourished persons. Demyelination in patients with multiple sclerosis (choice D) is preferentially located in other parts of the brain.
Diagnosis: Central pontine myelinosis

48 **The answer is E: Metastatic cancer.** Metastatic tumors reach the intracranial compartment through the bloodstream, generally in patients with advanced cancer. Tumors of different organs vary in their incidence of intracranial metastases (e.g., melanoma-high, liver-low). Most metastatic lesions seed to the gray-white junction, reflecting the rich capillary bed in this area. A metastasis contrasts with a primary glioma (choice B) or medulloblastoma (choice C) in its discrete appearance, globoid shape, and prominent halo of edema.

Diagnosis: Metastatic cancer

49 **The answer is E: Middle cerebral.** Septicemia and cardiac murmurs in an intravenous drug abuser suggest bacterial endocarditis. Infected thromboemboli from the heart valves cause infarcts and abscesses in various organs, including brain, kidneys, spleen, intestines, and upper and lower extremities. Because the trifurcation of the middle cerebral artery is a site of a major stepdown in vascular caliber, it is the predominant site occluded by emboli, most of which emanate from the heart. The other choices are much less common sites of occlusion.

Diagnosis: Bacterial endocarditis, cerebral infarction

50 **The answer is B: Hippocampus.** Inadequate perfusion of the brain results from generalized low blood flow due to extracranial events that lead to global ischemia (cardiac arrest, external hemorrhage) or from occlusive cerebrovascular disease (cerebral artery thrombosis), which produces regional ischemia and often a localized infarct. Global ischemia also results from hypoxia (near-drowning, carbon monoxide poisoning, suffocation). The pattern of injury produced by global ischemia or hypoxia reflects the anatomy of the cerebral vasculature and the selective vulnerability of individual neurons to oxygen deprivation. Although the other choices may be affected, selective neuronal sensitivity to a lack of oxygen is expressed most dramatically in the Purkinje cells of the cerebellum and the pyramidal neurons of Sommer's sector in the hippocampus.

Diagnosis: Global ischemia

51 **The answer is A: Fat embolism.** Small emboli, notably those composed of fat or air, occlude capillaries. Fat emboli originating from bone fractures are carried downstream through the cerebral vessels until the caliber of the emboli exceeds that of the blood vessels, at which point they lodge and block blood flow. The distal capillary endothelium becomes hypoxic and permeable, and petechiae develop, most commonly in the white matter. Although sepsis (choice D) sometimes leads to brain petechiae, the patient's condition does not support this conclusion. None of the other choices are characterized by petechiae in the brain.

Diagnosis: Fat embolism

52 **The answer is C: Middle cerebral artery.** The diversity of the neurologic deficits caused by stroke directly reflects the consequences of occluding different cerebral vessels. For example, the lengthy and slender striate arteries, which take origin from the proximal middle cerebral artery, are commonly occluded by atherosclerosis and thrombosis. The resultant infarct often transects the internal capsule and produces hemiparesis or hemiplegia. The trifurcation of the middle cerebral artery is a favored site for lodgment of emboli and for thrombosis secondary to atherosclerotic damage. Occlusion of the middle cerebral artery at this site deprives the parietal cortex of circulation and produces motor and sensory deficits. When the dominant hemisphere is involved, these lesions are commonly accompanied by aphasia. Occlusion of the vertebral artery (choice E) results in infarcts of the cerebellum.

Diagnosis: Cerebral infarction

53 **The answer is D: Thrombosis.** Aneurysms caused by atherosclerosis are localized mainly in major cerebral arteries (vertebral, basilar, and internal carotid), which are favored sites of atherosclerosis. Fibrous replacement of the media and destruction of the internal elastic membrane weakens the arterial wall and causes aneurysmal dilation. Although hemorrhage (choice B) and dissection (choice A) may occur, the major complication of an atherosclerotic aneurysm is thrombosis.

Diagnosis: Atherosclerotic aneurysm

54 **The answer is B: Prolonged hypotension.** The anterior, middle, and posterior cerebral arteries perfuse partially overlapping territories, but there are no anastomoses between their terminal branches. Because this overlap zone is not as richly perfused as the primary territories of the anterior and the middle cerebral arteries, reduced blood flow in these arteries will diminish perfusion more severely in the partial overlap zone (watershed area), thereby causing a parasagittal watershed infarct. None of the other choices are associated with watershed infarcts.

Diagnosis: Watershed infarct

55 **The answer is A: Diffuse axonal injury.** The consequences of traumatic brain injury may be internal and subtle. The parasagittal cortex is anchored to arachnoid villi, whereas the lateral aspects of the cerebrum move more freely. This anatomical feature, together with the differential density of gray and white matter, permits generation of shearing forces between different brain regions, leading to diffuse axonal shearing injuries, particularly in vehicular accidents. Shearing injuries can distort or disrupt axons, causing them to retract into "spheroids," as well as lose myelin. This type of injury typically occurs in parasagittal white matter and may be accompanied by multiple small hemorrhages. Duret hemorrhage (choice B) occurs in the uncus during transtentorial herniation.

Diagnosis: Traumatic brain injury

56 **The answer is A: Amyotrophic lateral sclerosis (ALS).** ALS is a degenerative disease of motor neurons of the brain and spinal cord that results in progressive weakness and wasting of the extremities and eventually impairment of respiratory muscles. The disease affects motor neurons in three locations: (1) the anterior horn cells of the spinal cord; (2) the motor nuclei of the brainstem, particularly the hypoglossal nuclei; and (3) the upper motor neurons of the cerebral cortex. The injury to the motor neurons leads to the degeneration of their axons, visualized in striking alterations of the lateral pyramidal pathways in the spinal cord. The defining histologic change in ALS is a loss of large motor neurons accompanied by mild gliosis. ALS begins as weakness and wasting of the muscles of the hand, often accompanied by painful cramps of the muscles of the arm. The other choices do not affect the motor neurons of the spinal cord.

Diagnosis: Amyotrophic lateral sclerosis

57 **The answer is A: Arylsulfatase.** MLD, the most common leukodystrophy, is an autosomal recessive disorder of myelin metabolism that is characterized by the accumulation of a cerebroside (galactosyl sulfatide) in the white matter of the brain and peripheral nerves. MLD is caused by a deficiency in the activity of arylsulfatase, a lysosomal enzyme involved in the degradation of myelin sulfatides. Accordingly, there is progressive accumulation of sulfatides within the lysosomes of myelin-forming Schwann cells and oligodendrocytes. Although the other choices are involved in congenital metabolic disorders, their deficiencies do not cause metachromatic leukodystrophy.

Diagnosis: Metachromatic leukodystrophy

58 The answer is D: Peroxisome. Adrenoleukodystrophy (ALD) refers to an X-linked disorder in which dysfunction of the adrenal cortex and demyelination of the nervous system are associated with high levels of saturated very long–chain fatty acids in tissues and body fluids. ALD occurs in children between the ages of 3 and 10 years. The disease progresses rapidly, and the body is quickly reduced to a vegetative state. A defect in the peroxisomal membrane prevents the normal activation of free fatty acids by the addition of coenzyme A. As a result, these fatty acids accumulate in gangliosides and myelin. Defects in the other organelles are not related to the accumulation of very long-chain fatty acids.

Diagnosis: Adrenoleukodystrophy

59 The answer is C: Krabbe disease. Krabbe disease is a rapidly progressive, invariably fatal, autosomal recessive neurologic disorder caused by a deficiency of galactocerebroside β-galactosidases. The condition appears in young infants and is defined by the presence of perivascular aggregates of mononuclear and multinucleated cells (globoid cells) in the white matter. The globoid cells are macrophages that contain undigested galactosylceramide. Alexander disease (choice A) is a rare neurologic disorder, also of infants, characterized by mutations in the gene encoding glial fibrillary acidic protein, which leads to aggregates of fibrous structures, known as Rosenthal fibers. Hurler disease (choice B) features the accumulation of mucopolysaccharides.

Diagnosis: Krabbe disease

60 The answer is E: Subacute sclerosing panencephalitis (SSPE). SSPE is a chronic, lethal, viral infection of the brain caused by a reactivation of a latent measles virus. In children, the course is protracted, and inflammation occurs primarily in cerebral gray matter. In adults, SSPE may follow a more rapid course. The infection is highlighted by prominent intranuclear inclusions in neurons and oligodendroglia, marked gliosis in affected gray and white matter (hence sclerosing), patchy loss of myelin, and ubiquitous perivascular lymphocytes and macrophages. Choices A and D are prion diseases. Choice C is caused by activation of a latent JC virus.

Diagnosis: Subacute sclerosing panencephalitis

61 The answer is A: Aqueduct of Sylvius. Hydrocephalus refers to dilation of the ventricles by accumulated CSF. When obstruction to the flow of CSF in the brain is within the ventricles, hydrocephalus is designated "noncommunicating." In noncommunicating hydrocephalus, the flow of CSF through the ventricular system may be obstructed at the aqueduct of Sylvius by congenital malformations, neoplasms (as in this case), inflammation, or hemorrhage. The mass of an intracranial neoplasm, combined with edema or hydrocephalus, causes increased intracranial pressure, which leads to headaches and

vomiting. Choices C and D connect the 4th ventricle with the subarachnoid space and are the primary routes for escape of CSF into the posterior cerebellomedullary cistern (cisterna magna). Virchow-Robin spaces (choice E) surround blood vessels as they enter the brain.

Diagnosis: Hydrocephalus

62 The answer is A: Astrocytes. Hepatic encephalopathy is a common clinical expression of liver failure, manifested as delirium, seizures, and coma. In general, the clinical symptoms greatly exceed their morphologic correlates, which are restricted to the appearance of altered astroglia (termed Alzheimer type II astrocytes), which show enlarged nuclei and marginated chromatin, especially in the thalamus. The development of hepatic encephalopathy is caused by increased serum concentrations of neurotoxic substances, including ammonia. None of the other choices include cells that are altered by hepatic encephalopathy.

Diagnosis: Hepatic encephalopathy

63 The answer is A: Cerebellum. The neuroectoderm may (albeit infrequently) give rise to a neoplasm of neuronal heritage. These tumors occur most often in childhood, and their cellular composition is usually primitive. An example is medulloblastoma, which arises in the cerebellum, generally in the first decade of life. This entity is usually situated in the vermis. Its growth is rapid and regional infiltration is extensive. Children with medulloblastoma are first seen with cerebellar dysfunction or hydrocephalus. Tumors in the other areas do not ordinarily produce the symptoms described.

Diagnosis: Medulloblastoma

64 The answer is C: Small, hyperchromatic cells and rare neuroblastic rosettes. Medulloblastomas and, less commonly ependymomas and pineal parenchymal tumors, have a propensity to disseminate by way of the CSF throughout the CNS. Since medulloblastomas are close to the fourth ventricle, they may disseminate downstream into the spinal cord. The detection of neuronal and progenitor cell markers (e.g., synaptophysin or nestin) may be diagnostically informative in distinguishing these tumors from metastatic epithelial tumors, lymphomas, or other neuroectodermal malignancies. Medulloblastomas are characterized by cells with hyperchromatic, round-to-oval nuclei and scant cytoplasm, which often crowd together with no structural pattern. The neuroblastic character of the cells is occasionally expressed in rosette formation, a histologic feature of neuroblasts. The other choices do not describe midline, cerebellar tumors arising in children.

Diagnosis: Medulloblastoma

65 The answer is E: Von Hippel-Lindau syndrome. Von Hippel-Lindau syndrome is a hereditary disorder in which cerebellar hemangioblastomas are associated with retinal angiomas and other tumors (e.g., renal cell carcinoma) due to mutations in the *VHL* tumor suppressor gene. Hemangioblastoma is a highly vascularized tumor that originates predominantly in the cerebellum. It features endothelium-lined canals interspersed with plump cells. In 20% of cases, these cells secrete erythropoietin and induce polycythemia. Sturge-Weber syndrome (choice D) is a nonfamilial congenital disorder that features a facial port-wine stain (*nevus flammeus*) and angiomas of the leptomeninges. The other choices do not feature vascular tumors.

Diagnosis: Von Hippel-Lindau syndrome, hemangioblastoma

66 **The answer is B: HMB-45.** Metastatic tumors are the most common intracranial neoplasms. They reach the intracranial compartment through the bloodstream, generally in patients with advanced cancer. Tumors of different organs vary in their incidence of intracranial metastases. For example, a patient with disseminated melanoma has a greater than 50% likelihood of acquiring intracranial metastases, whereas the incidence of such metastases in carcinoma of the breast and lung is 35%, and the incidence for cancer of the kidney or colon is only 5%. HMB-45 is a useful tumor marker for melanoma. Neuron-specific enolase (choice D) and synaptophysin (choice E) are markers for neurons.

Diagnosis: Melanoma, metastatic cancer

67 **The answer is D: Glioblastoma multiforme.** Glioblastoma multiforme is a brain tumor composed of malignant astroglial cells, which show marked pleomorphism and are often multinucleated. Because of their invasive properties and vascular changes ("arteritic obliteration"), the tumors feature patchy yellow areas of necrosis and red zones of hemorrhage. The term multiforme derives from the variegated gross appearance of these tumors and the histologic pleomorphism of the tumor cells. The other choices do not display the characteristic palisading of tumor cells around necrotic areas (see photomicrograph).

Diagnosis: Glioblastoma multiforme

68 **The answer is A: Astrocytes.** Unlike the other choices, glioblastoma multiforme can invade the contralateral hemisphere across the corpus callosum and present as a bilateral "butterfly-like" lesion. None of the other cells contribute to glioblastoma multiforme.

Diagnosis: Glioblastoma multiforme

69 **The answer is B: Ependymoma.** Ependymoma originates in the lining of the cavities that contain cerebrospinal fluid. The tumor is most common in the fourth ventricle, where it produces obstruction and results in hydrocephalus. The cells of an ependymoma characteristically have an "epithelial" appearance, similar to that of normal ependymal cells. They may arrange around blood vessels forming perivascular pseudorosettes. Ependymomas may also originate from the lining of the central canal of the spinal cord and the filum terminale. Together with astrocytomas (choice A), ependymomas are the most common neoplasms of the spinal cord. Because of their central location, they cannot be easily resected.

Diagnosis: Ependymoma

70 **The answer is D: Meningioma.** Meningiomas are benign intracranial tumors that arise from the arachnoid villi and produce symptoms by compressing adjacent brain tissue. They account for almost 20% of all primary intracranial neoplasms. Meningiomas occur at almost any intracranial site but are most common in parasagittal regions of the cerebral hemispheres, the olfactory groove, and the lateral sphenoid

wing. On gross examination, most meningiomas appear as well-circumscribed, firm, bosselated masses of variable size. The histologic hallmark of meningiomas is a whorled pattern of "meningothelial" cells (see photomicrograph). The indolent growth of meningiomas enables them to enlarge slowly for years before becoming symptomatic, during which time they displace the brain but do not infiltrate it. Although benign, meningiomas have a propensity to erode contiguous bone. Choices A, C, and E are malignant bone tumors. Choice B (hemangioblastoma) is characterized by vascular proliferation.

Diagnosis: Meningioma

71 **The answer is C: Nasopharynx.** Craniopharyngiomas are solid and cystic lesions located above the sella turcica that arise from the epithelium of Rathke pouch. This structure is a part of the embryonic nasopharynx that migrates cephalad and gives origin to the anterior lobe of the hypophysis. Some cystic lesions are lined by squamous epithelium, whereas others, referred to as adamantinomas, are solid and resemble tumors of dentigerous origin. Neoplasms derived from ectopic tissues compress adjacent structures. Craniopharyngiomas generally become symptomatic in the first two decades of life, creating visual deficits and headaches. They may cause pituitary failure, including diabetes insipidus. Choices A, B, and D represent neural structures. The third pharyngeal arch (choice E) is distal to the nasopharynx and gives rise to the thymus and parathyroid glands.

Diagnosis: Craniopharyngioma

72 **The answer is C: Lymphoma.** Lymphomas may arise as a primary B-cell lesion in the brain in a manner analogous to its occurrence in the stomach, small bowel, or testis, but the overwhelming majority of lymphomas are metastatic to the brain from other sites. Primary lymphoma of the brain often originates deep in the cerebral hemispheres, commonly in bilateral periventricular positions. A mixture of small and large lymphocytes is angiocentric. Lymphomas often arise in the context of immunosuppression and in patients with AIDS. In some instances, they have been linked etiologically to infection with EBV. AIDS does not give rise to tumors of neural origin (choices A, B, D, and E).

Diagnosis: Lymphoma

73 **The answer is B: Corpus striatum.** Wilson disease is an autosomal recessive condition in which excess copper may deposit in the liver and brain. Chronic hepatitis leads to cirrhosis in young people. Ocular lesions, so-called Kayser-Fleischer rings, represent deposition of copper in Descemet membrane in the iris. Lack of coordination and tremor (extrapyramidal neurologic symptoms) are related to degenerative changes in the corpus striatum. Deposition of copper is not observed in the other anatomic regions of the brain.

Diagnosis: Wilson disease

74 **The answer is E: Oligodendroglioma.** Oligodendrogliomas arise in the white matter and grow slowly. They occur predominantly in the white matter of the cerebral hemispheres of adults. Histologically, the tumors have small rounded nuclei similar to normal oligodendrocytes, but they also exhibit increased cell density and cellular pleomorphism. Calcospher-ites, which may be visualized radiographically, are occasionally scattered randomly throughout the lesion. The other choices do not feature uniform monomorphic cells.

Diagnosis: Oligodendroglioma

75 **The answer is B: Neurofibromatosis type 2.** Neurofibromato-sis type 2 refers to a syndrome defined by bilateral tumors of the eighth cranial nerve (acoustic neuromas), and commonly, by meningiomas and gliomas. Acoustic neuromas are intrac-ranial schwannomas that are restricted to the eighth cranial nerve. Some schwannomas exhibit deletions or mutations of the *NF2* gene. Neurofibromatosis type 1 (choice A) exhibits neurofibromas but not acoustic neuromas. None of the other choices lead to acoustic Schwannomas.

Diagnosis: Neurofibromatosis type 2

76 **The answer is C: Neuritic plaques.** Microscopic changes in Alzheimer disease are dominated by the presence of senile (neuritic) plaques, neurofibrillary tangles, and neuron loss. In end-stage disease, neuritic plaques converge to occupy large volumes of the cerebral gray matter. The plaques are positive for Congo red and exhibit immunoreactivity for Aβ at the core and periphery. Neurofibrillary tangles are formed by large intra-cytoplasmic masses of tau filaments. Remarkably, most cases of Alzheimer disease are also associated with Lewy bodies. Thus, Alzheimer disease features a "triple" brain amyloidosis, owing to accumulations of filamentous tau, Aβ, and α-synuclein. Granu-lovacuolar degeneration (choice A), Lewy bodies (choice B), and neurofibrillary tangles (choice D) are all seen in the brains of patients with Alzheimer disease, however, these lesions are not evident in the slide that accompanies this case (see photo-micrograph). Spongiform encephalopathy (clustered vacuoles within the gray matter, choice E) is featured in prion disease.

Diagnosis: Alzheimer disease

77 **The answer is C: Foramen magnum.** Penetrating wounds produce hemorrhage and blast effects. The "blast effect" of a high-velocity projectile causes an immediate increase in supratentorial pressure and results in death because of impac-tion of the cerebellum and medulla into the foramen magnum. A low-velocity projectile increases the pressure at a more grad-ual rate through hemorrhage and edema. The other choices do not represent areas of herniation.

Diagnosis: Bullet wound

78 **The answer is B: Distal polyneuropathy.** Peripheral neuropathy is a process that affects the function of one or more peripheral nerves. Diabetic neuropathy is the most common neuropathy in the United States. Other common causes include alcohol-ism, renal failure, neurotoxic drugs, autoimmune diseases, monoclonal gammopathy, and HIV infection. The pathologic findings are limited to axonal degeneration or segmental demy-elination, or a combination of both. Diabetes affects both the sensory and the motor portions of the peripheral nervous system and most often presents as distal polyneuropathy. Auto-nomic neuropathy (choice A) and mononeuropathy (choice D) are less common. The pathogenesis of these disorders is not fully understood, but they may be related to metabolic dis-turbances or to disease of small blood vessels. Vasculitis and paraproteinemia (choices C and E) are not features of diabetes. Peripheral sensory or sensorimotor neuropathy typically pres-ents with cramps or deep burning pain, cutaneous hyperesthe-sia, or insensitivity to changes of temperature.

Diagnosis: Diabetes mellitus

79 **The answer is D: Neurofibrillary tangles.** One of the most intriguing neurologic features of Down syndrome (trisomy 21) is its association with Alzheimer disease. The morpho-logic lesions characteristic of Alzheimer disease progress in all patients with Down syndrome and are universally demonstrable by age 35 years. These changes include gran-ulovacuolar degeneration, neurofibrillary tangles, senile (neuritic) plaques, and loss of neurons. The gene for amy-loid precursor protein (APP) is located on chromosome 21, and the additional dose of the gene product in patients with trisomy 21 may predispose to precocious accumulation of Aβ. Some patients with the familial form of Alzheimer dis-ease harbor mutations in APP or presenilin genes. These mutations lead to increased production of Aβ—the amy-loidogenic fragment of APP. None of the other choices are associated with the pathogenesis of Down syndrome or Alzheimer disease.

Diagnosis: Down syndrome, amyloidosis

Chapter 29

The Eye

QUESTIONS

Select the single best answer.

1 A 15-year-old boy who emigrated to the United States from Sudan presents with bilateral eye irritation and itching. Physical examination reveals photophobia, conjunctivitis, and fibrovascular opacity in the superior cornea (shown in the image). Giemsa staining of a conjunctival scrape demonstrates cytoplasmic inclusion bodies. What term describes the corneal lesion?

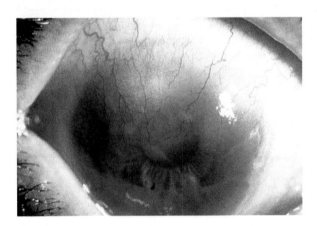

(A) Glaucoma
(B) Keratitis
(C) Pannus
(D) Pinguecula
(E) Pterygium

2 A 29-year-old woman complains of nervousness and weakness of 6 months in duration. She says that she is increasingly intolerant of heat and frequently sweats. She has experienced a 9-kg (20-lb) weight loss over the past 2 months despite normal caloric intake and says that she frequently finds her heart racing. Physical examination reveals a symmetrically enlarged thyroid and exophthalmos. Which of the following best explains the pathogenesis of bilateral exophthalmos in this patient?

(A) Acute orbital inflammation
(B) Enlargement of the eyeball
(C) Orbital deposits of thyroid hormone
(D) Orbital hemorrhage
(E) Swelling of the extraocular muscles

3 A 56-year-old obese, diabetic woman (BMI = 32 kg/m²) complains of declining visual acuity. Funduscopic examination shows peripheral retinal capillary microaneurysms, deep and superficial retinal hemorrhages, "waxy" hard exudates, areas of capillary closure, and vitreoretinal neovascularization. Urinalysis reveals 3+ proteinuria and 3+ glucosuria. Which of the following is the most important pathogenetic factor underlying this patient's retinopathy?

(A) Hyperlipidemia
(B) Hypoalbuminemia
(C) Hypoglycemia
(D) Retinal ischemia
(E) Systemic hypertension

4 A 65-year-old man complains of gradual loss of peripheral vision over the past 2 years. Ophthalmic examination shows elevated intraocular pressure. Funduscopic examination reveals "optic cupping." Which of the following best explains the loss of visual field sensitivity in this patient?

(A) Corneal abrasion
(B) Degeneration of the choroid
(C) Fixed dilation of the pupil
(D) Retinal degeneration
(E) Retinal ischemia

5 The patient described in Question 4 has no underlying ocular disease. Which of the following types of glaucoma is most likely present?

(A) Closed-angle
(B) Congenital
(C) Low tension
(D) Open-angle
(E) Secondary

6 A 28-year-old man consults his physician regarding his vision. He describes a 6-month history of increasing night blindness. Two of his maternal uncles have the same condition. Visual examination reveals a marked constriction of the patient's peripheral visual field. Funduscopic examination would likely show which of the following pathologic findings?

(A) Cherry-red spot
(B) Cotton-wool spots
(C) Microaneurysms
(D) Optic cupping
(E) Pigment accumulation

328

7 A 3-year-old child presents with a red and painful left eye. Ophthalmic examination reveals swelling of the eyelid and a purulent exudate. What is the proper name for this condition?

(A) Conjunctivitis
(B) Glaucoma
(C) Keratitis
(D) Pinguecula
(E) Retinitis

8 A 54-year-old woman with rheumatoid arthritis presents with a 2-year history of dry eyes and dry mouth. Physical examination confirms xerostomia (dry mouth) and xerophthalmia (dry eyes) and reveals enlarged lacrimal glands bilaterally. Histologic examination of the lacrimal glands would likely show an infiltrate of which of the following inflammatory cell types?

(A) Fibroblasts
(B) Lymphocytes
(C) Macrophages
(D) Mast cells
(E) Neutrophils

9 A 55-year-old obese woman (BMI = 34 kg/m²) with a history of hypertension and hypercholesterolemia complains of nodular lesions on the nasal aspect of both of her eyelids. The lesions are yellow and nonpainful. Biopsy of a lesion would likely show an accumulation of which of the following cells?

(A) Fibroblasts
(B) Lymphocytes
(C) Macrophages
(D) Mast cells
(E) Neutrophils

10 A 67-year-old man complains of a lesion in his left eye. Physical examination reveals a triangular fold of vascularized conjunctiva growing horizontally into the cornea in the shape of an insect wing. Which of the following terms best describes this patient's lesion?

(A) Loiasis
(B) Onchocerciasis
(C) Pinguecula
(D) Pterygium
(E) Siderosis bulbi

11 A 70-year-old man who was born prematurely and has been blind since birth suffers a stroke and expires. The eye at autopsy is shown in the image. Which of the following was the most likely cause of this man's blindness?

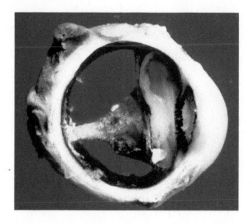

(A) Autoimmune hemolytic disease
(B) Birth trauma
(C) Congenital hypothyroidism
(D) Diabetes
(E) Oxygen toxicity

12 A 65-year-old man complains of decreased visual acuity in one eye of 5 years in duration. Physical examination reveals a white discoloration in one pupil (shown in the image). Which of the following best explains the pathogenesis of this patient's loss of vision?

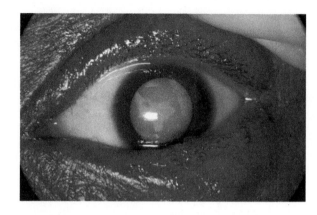

(A) Chronic conjunctivitis
(B) Degeneration of the lens
(C) Fibrovascular occlusion of the cornea
(D) Increased intraocular pressure
(E) Retinal ischemia

13 A 58-year-old obese woman (BMI = 32 kg/m²) complains of declining visual acuity of 6 months in duration. Physical examination reveals a pulse of 82 per minute, respirations 20 per minute, and blood pressure 195/110 mm Hg. Funduscopic examination shows "cotton-wool spots," retinal hemorrhage, "macular star," edema of the optic nerve, and arteriovenious nicking of retinal arterioles. A photograph of the ocular fundus is shown. These findings are best explained by which of the following mechanisms?

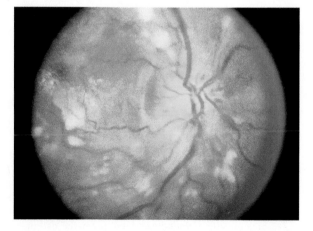

(A) Central retinal artery occlusion
(B) Central retinal vein occlusion
(C) Gangliosidosis
(D) Hypertensive retinopathy
(E) Pigmentary retinopathy

14 A 67-year-old man with a history of ischemic heart disease presents with 4 days of blurred vision in his left eye. Which of the following findings on funduscopic examination would characterize the pathologic consequences of central *retinal vein* occlusion in this patient?
(A) Cherry-red macula
(B) Cotton-wool patches
(C) Flame-shaped hemorrhages
(D) Macular star
(E) Microaneurysms

15 If the patient described in Question 14 suffered from central *retinal artery* occlusion, which of the following pathologic findings would be expected on funduscopic examination?
(A) Cherry-red macula
(B) Cotton-wool patches
(C) Macular star
(D) Microaneurysms
(E) Neovascularization

16 A 60-year-old woman with a history of adult-onset (type 2) diabetes suffers a massive stroke and expires. A flat preparation of the retina at autopsy is shown in the image. Which of the following pathologic features of diabetic retinopathy is evident in this specimen?

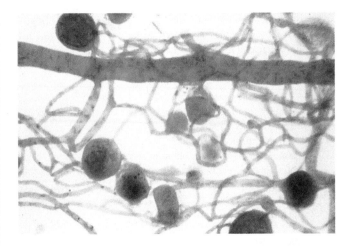

(A) Cotton-wool patches
(B) Flame-shaped hemorrhages
(C) Inflammatory exudate
(D) Lacy vacuolization
(E) Microaneurysms

17 A 13-year-old girl presents because of increased thirst, hunger, and frequent urination over the past few months. Urinalysis discloses 3+ glucosuria. The blood sugar is 275 mg/dL. The patient receives counseling on the self-administration of insulin. Six years later, she complains of blurred vision. Ophthalmic examination reveals "snow-flake" cataracts. An accumulation of which of the following biologic compounds best accounts for the pathogenesis of cataracts in this patient?

(A) Glycogen in the iris
(B) Hemoglobin in the lens
(C) Lipid in the lens
(D) Lipid in the retina
(E) Sorbitol in the lens

18 A 50-year-old man presents with loss of vision in his left eye after a motorcycle accident. Funduscopy reveals separation of the sensory retina from the retinal pigmentary epithelium. Which of the following is the likely cause of retinal detachment?
(A) Autoimmune uveitis
(B) Increased intraocular pressure
(C) Intraocular hemorrhage
(D) Macular degeneration
(E) Retinitis pigmentosa

19 A 15-year-old boy sees an optometrist to obtain his first pair of eye glasses. An eye examination reveals 20/80 vision in both eyes. Which of the following best explains the pathogenesis of myopia in this patient?
(A) Decreased anteroposterior diameter of the eye
(B) Increased anteroposterior diameter of the eye
(C) Increased thickness of the lens
(D) Sensory retinal degeneration
(E) Water retention in the aqueous humor

20 A 4-year-old boy presents with a white pupil that his parents first noticed about 4 months ago. A history of an eye tumor in a first cousin is provided. Ophthalmic examination shows a tumor in the left eye (patient shown in the image), after which the eye is enucleated. A mutation in which of the following genes was most likely associated with the development of this tumor?

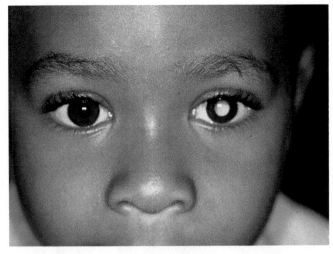

(A) *p53*
(B) *C-myc*
(C) *N-myc*
(D) *Rb*
(E) *RET*

21 A 55-year-old woman presents with a 3-month history of reduced visual acuity of her right eye. Funduscopic examination reveals a dark mass located beneath the choroid vessels. Biopsy of the mass shows spindle-shaped cells and epithelioid cells, many of which contain pigment. The enucleated eye is shown in the image. This mushroom-shaped tumor most likely originated from which of the following anatomic locations?

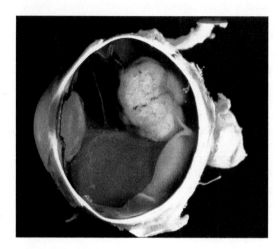

(A) Cornea
(B) Lens
(C) Retina
(D) Sclera
(E) Uvea

22 A 67-year-old woman complains that she has had poor vision for 4 years. Ophthalmic examination shows a selective loss of central vision. Which of the following is the most likely diagnosis?

(A) Cataract
(B) Corneal dystrophy
(C) Gaucher disease
(D) Macular degeneration
(E) Retinitis pigmentosa

ANSWERS

1 **The answer is C: Pannus.** Trachoma is a chronic, contagious conjunctivitis caused by *Chlamydia trachomatis*. When inoculated into the eye, the organism reproduces within the conjunctival epithelium, inciting a mixed acute and chronic inflammatory infiltrate. As the disease progresses, lymphoid aggregates enlarge, and the conjunctiva becomes focally hypertrophic and scarred. The cornea is invaded by blood vessels, and fibroblasts form a trachomatous pannus. In children, the disease usually heals spontaneously. In adults, it may cause blindness, especially if combined with bacterial superinfection. Pinguecula (choice D) is a yellowish conjunctival lump usually located nasal to the corneoscleral limbus. Pterygium (choice E) is a fold of vascularized cornea not related to infectious agents, which grows horizontally onto the cornea in the shape of an insect wing.
Diagnosis: Trachoma

2 **The answer is E: Swelling of the extraocular muscles.** The most common cause of proptosis (forward protrusion of the eye) is thyroid disease, followed by orbital dermoid cysts and hemangiomas. Exophthalmos may precede or follow other manifestations of thyroid dysfunction. This condition is caused by enlargement of the extraocular muscles within the orbit. The muscles themselves are normal, but they are swollen by mucinous edema, the accumulation of fibroblasts, and infiltration by lymphocytes. Complications of severe exophthalmos include corneal exposure with subsequent ulceration and optic nerve compression. The other choices are not complications of hyperthyroidism.
Diagnosis: Graves disease, exophthalmos

3 **The answer is D: Retinal ischemia.** The eye is frequently involved in diabetes mellitus, and ocular symptoms occur in 20% to 40% of diabetics, even at the clinical onset of the disease. Virtually all patients with type 1 (insulin-dependent) diabetes and many of those with type 2 (non–insulin-dependent) diabetes develop some background retinopathy within 5 to 15 years of the onset of diabetes. Retinal ischemia can account for most features of diabetic retinopathy, including cotton-wool spots, capillary closure, microaneurysms, and retinal neovascularization. Ischemia results from narrowing or occlusion of retinal arterioles (as from arteriolosclerosis or platelet and lipid thrombi) or from atherosclerosis of the central retinal or ophthalmic arteries. The frequency of proliferative retinopathy correlates with the degree of glycemic control (i.e., hyperglycemia, not hypoglycemia, see choice C); the better the control, the lower is the rate of retinopathy. Systemic hypertension (choice E) may also be a contributing factor in diabetics.
Diagnosis: Diabetic retinopathy

4 **The answer is D: Retinal degeneration.** Glaucoma refers to a collection of disorders that feature an optic neuropathy accompanied by a characteristic excavation of the optic nerve head and a progressive loss of visual field sensitivity. In most cases, glaucoma is produced by increased intraocular pressure (ocular hypertension). Increased intraocular pressure, however, does not necessarily cause glaucoma. In certain pathologic states, aqueous humor accumulates within the eye, and the intraocular pressure increases. Temporary or permanent impairment of vision results from pressure-induced degenerative changes in the retina and optic nerve head and from corneal edema and opacification. The other choices are not complications of glaucoma.
Diagnosis: Glaucoma

5 **The answer is D: Open-angle.** Primary glaucoma develops in a person with no apparent underlying eye disease. The disorder is subdivided into open-angle glaucoma, in which the anterior chamber angle is open and appears normal, and closed-angle glaucoma, in which the anterior chamber is shallower than normal and the angle is abnormally narrow. Primary open-angle glaucoma is the most frequent type of glaucoma and is a major cause of blindness in the United States. The angle of the anterior chamber is open and appears normal, but increased resistance to the outflow of the aqueous humor is present within the vicinity of Schlemm canal. Primary closed-angle glaucoma (choice A) afflicts persons whose iris is displaced anteriorly. When the pupil dilates, the iris obstructs the anterior chamber angle, thereby impairing fluid drainage and raising intraocular pressure. Acute primary closed-angle glaucoma, low tension glaucoma (choice C), is an ocular emergency, and it is essential to start ocular hypotensive treatment within the first 24 to 48 hours if vision is to be maintained. Primary closed-angle glaucoma affects both eyes, but it may become apparent in one eye 2 to 5 years before it is noted in the other. Congenital glaucoma (choice B) refers to glaucoma caused by obstruction to the aqueous drainage by developmental anomalies. Causes of secondary glaucoma (choice E) include inflammation, hemorrhage, neovascularization of the iris, and adhesions.

Diagnosis: Glaucoma

6 The answer is E: Pigment accumulation. Retinitis pigmentosa (pigmentary retinopathy) is a generic term that refers to a variety of bilateral, progressive, degenerative retinopathies. They are characterized clinically by night blindness and constriction of peripheral visual fields and pathologically by the loss of retinal photoreceptors (rods and cones) and pigment accumulation within the retina. In retinitis pigmentosa, the destruction of rods and later cones is followed by migration of retinal pigment epithelial cells into the sensory retina. Melanin appears within slender processes of spidery cells and accumulates mainly around small branching retinal blood vessels, like spicules of bone. The retinal blood vessels then gradually attenuate, and the optic nerve head acquires a characteristic waxy pallor. Half of all patients with retinitis pigmentosa have a family history of the disease. Cherry-red spot (choice A) describes a bright central foveola that occurs in the setting of lysosomal storage diseases and central retinal artery occlusion. Cotton-wool spots (choice B) are observed in diabetics and patients with hypertension. Microaneurysms (choice C) are encountered in patients with hypertension.

Diagnosis: Retinitis pigmentosa

7 The answer is A: Conjunctivitis. Microorganisms lodging on the surface of the eye frequently cause conjunctivitis, although keratitis or corneal ulcer may also occur. At some stage in life, virtually everyone has viral or bacterial conjunctivitis. This most common of eye diseases is characterized by hyperemic conjunctival blood vessels (pink eye). The inflammatory exudates that accumulate in the conjunctival sac commonly crust, causing the eyelids to stick together in the morning. Choices B, C, and E affect other anatomic structures in the eye. Choice D (pinguecula) is a yellow lump in the conjunctiva that is not infected.

Diagnosis: Conjunctivitis

8 The answer is B: Lymphocytes. This patient has Sjögren (sicca) syndrome, an autoimmune disease characterized by an intense lymphocytic infiltration of the salivary and lacrimal glands. Patients develop xerostomia and xerophthalmia. The other choices are not characteristic of autoimmune disease.

Diagnosis: Sjögren syndrome

9 The answer is C: Macrophages. Xanthelasmas are yellow plaques of lipid-containing macrophages that usually are located on the eyelids. They are frequently seen in patients with familial hypercholesterolemia but may occur in persons without lipid disorders. The other cells do not store lipid material.

Diagnosis: Familial hypercholesterolemia, xanthelasma

10 The answer is D: Pterygium. Pterygium is a fold of vascularized conjunctiva that grows horizontally onto the cornea in the shape of an insect wing (hence the name). It is often associated with a pinguecula (conjunctival lump, choice C) and frequently recurs after excision.

Diagnosis: Pterygium

11 The answer is E: Oxygen toxicity. Retinopathy of prematurity, also termed retrolental fibroplasia, is a bilateral, iatrogenic, retinal disorder that occurs predominantly in premature infants who have been treated after birth with oxygen. The entity was originally called retrolental fibroplasia because of a mass of scarred tissue behind the lens in advanced cases. In premature infants exposed to excessive amounts of oxygen (e.g., in an incubator), the developing retinal blood vessels become obliterated, and the peripheral retina, which is normally avascular until the end of fetal life, does not vascularize. The condition is unrelated to birth trauma (choice B).

Diagnosis: Retinopathy of prematurity, retrolental fibroplasia

12 The answer is B: Degeneration of the lens. Cataracts represent opacifications in the crystalline lens. They are a major cause of visual impairment and blindness throughout the world and are the outcome of numerous conditions. Clefts appear between the lens fibers, and degenerated lens material accumulates in these open spaces. The most common cataract in the United States is associated with aging (age-related cataract), although the risk is increased with diabetes, heavy exposure to ultraviolet light, certain genetic disorders, and many other conditions. The degenerated lens material exerts osmotic pressure, causing the damaged lens to increase in volume by imbibing water. Such a swollen lens may obstruct the pupil and cause glaucoma (phacomorphic glaucoma). In a mature cataract, the entire lens degenerates, and its volume diminishes because lenticular debris escapes into the aqueous humor through a degenerated lens capsule (hypermature cataract). The other choices do not affect the ocular lens.

Diagnosis: Cataract

13 The answer is D: Hypertensive retinopathy. Characteristic features of hypertensive retinopathy include arteriolar narrowing, hemorrhages in the retinal nerve fiber layer (flame-shaped hemorrhages), exudates, including some that radiate from the center of the macula (macular star). Arteriolosclerosis accompanies longstanding hypertension and commonly affects the retinal and choroidal vessels. The lumina of the thickened retinal arterioles become narrowed, increasingly tortuous, and of irregular caliber. At sites where the arterioles cross veins, the latter appear kinked (arteriovenous nicking). Small superficial or deep retinal hemorrhages often accompany retinal arteriolosclerosis. Impaired axoplasmic flow within the nerve fiber layer, caused by ischemia, results in swollen axons with cytoplasmic bodies. Such structures resemble cotton on funduscopy (cotton-wool spots). None of the other choices are associated with the ophthalmologic features shown in the photomicrograph.

Diagnosis: Hypertensive retinopathy

14 The answer is C: Flame-shaped hemorrhages. Central retinal vein occlusion is more common than occlusion of the retinal artery. It typically evolves gradually and has a better prognosis. Funduscopic examination typically reveals flame-shaped hemorrhages. The intraocular pressure tends to be elevated. Retinal hemorrhages are also a feature of other disorders, including hypertension and diabetes mellitus, as well as central retinal vein occlusion. The appearance varies with the location. Hemorrhages in the nerve fiber layer spread between axons and cause a flame-shaped appearance on funduscopy, whereas deep retinal hemorrhages tend to be round. When located between the retinal pigment epithelium and Bruch membrane, blood appears as a dark mass and clinically may resemble a melanoma. The other choices are not characteristic of central retinal vein occlusion.
Diagnosis: Retinal occlusive vascular disease

15 The answer is A: Cherry-red macula. Central retinal artery occlusion may follow thrombosis of the retinal artery, as in atherosclerosis, giant cell arteritis, or embolization to that vessel. Intracellular edema, manifested by retinal pallor, is prominent, especially in the macula, where the ganglion cells are most numerous. The foveola stands out in sharp contrast as a prominent cherry-red spot. The lack of retinal circulation reduces the retinal arterioles to delicate threads. Permanent blindness follows central retinal artery obstruction unless ischemia is of short duration. Cherry-red macula is also seen in patients with lysosomal storage diseases. In these patients, intracytoplasmic lysosomal inclusions within the multilayered ganglion cell layer of the macula impart a striking pallor to the affected retina. As a result, the central foveola appears bright red because of the underlying choroidal vasculature. Cotton-wool patches (choice B) and neovascularization (choice E) are noted in patients with diabetic retinopathy. Macular star (choice C) and microaneurysms (choice D) occur in patients with hypertensive retinopathy.
Diagnosis: Retinal occlusive vascular disease

16 The answer is E: Microaneurysms. This autopsy specimen shows capillary microaneurysms. Background diabetic retinopathy exhibits capillary microaneurysms, small hemorrhages (dot and blot hemorrhages), and exudates. These lesions usually do not impair vision unless associated with macular edema. After many years, diabetic retinopathy becomes proliferative. Delicate new blood vessels grow along with fibrous and glial tissue toward the vitreous body. Neovascularization of the retina is a prominent feature of diabetic retinopathy and of other conditions caused by retinal ischemia. Tortuous new vessels first appear on the surface of the retina and optic nerve head and then grow into the vitreous cavity. None of the other choices are shown in the photomicrograph.
Diagnosis: Diabetic retinopathy

17 The answer is E: Sorbitol in the lens. Patients with type 1 diabetes often develop bilateral "snowflake" cataracts. These consist of a blanket of white needle-shaped opacities in the lens immediately beneath the anterior and posterior lens capsule. The opacities coalesce within a few weeks in adolescents and within days in children, until the whole lens become opaque. Snowflake cataracts can be produced experimentally in young animals and result from an osmotic effect caused by the accumulation of sorbitol, the alcohol derived from glucose. The increased sorbitol content of the lens causes imbibition of water and enlargement of the lens. The accumulation of glycogen (choice A) in the iris causes lacy vacuolization. Lipemia retinalis (choice D) accounts for the waxy streaks seen by funduscopy. Bleeding (choice B) occurs in the cornea and vitreous body and can cause glaucoma.
Diagnosis: Cataract, diabetic retinopathy

18 The answer is C: Intraocular hemorrhage. Traumatic hemorrhages separate the sensory retina from the retinal pigment epithelium. Factors predisposing to retinal detachment also include retinal defects (e.g., certain retinal degenerations), vitreous traction, and diminished pressure on the retina (e.g., after vitreous loss). After accidental or surgical perforation of the globe, choroidal hemorrhages may detach the choroid and displace the retina, vitreous body, and lens through the wound. The other choices are not associated with retinal detachment.
Diagnosis: Retinal detachment

19 The answer is B: Increased anteroposterior diameter of the eye. Myopia (near-sightedness) is a refractive ocular abnormality in which light from the visualized object focuses at a point in front of the retina because of a longer than usual anteroposterior diameter of the eye. Myopia affects more than 70 million persons in the United States, requiring correction with glasses, contact lenses, or laser treatment. Choice A causes the focal point to be behind the retina causing hyperopia (far-sightedness). The other choices do not involve the point of focus.
Diagnosis: Myopia

20 The answer is D: *Rb*. Retinoblastoma is the most common intraocular malignant neoplasm of childhood, affecting 1:25,000 children. Most frequently the tumor is seen within the first 2 years of life and sometimes even at birth. The presenting signs include a white pupil (leukocoria), squint (strabismus), poor vision, spontaneous hyphema, and a red, painful eye. Secondary glaucoma is a frequent complication. Although most retinoblastomas occur sporadically, about 7% are inherited and are related to a germline mutation in the retinoblastoma gene, which functions as a tumor suppressor. The Rb protein functions to regulate the cell cycle at a checkpoint before S phase. *RET* protooncogene mutations (choice E) are seen in patients with multiple endocrine neoplasia type 2.
Diagnosis: Retinoblastoma

21 The answer is E: Uvea. The eye and adjacent structures contain a variety of cell types, and malignant neoplasms arise from them. Malignant melanoma is the most common primary intraocular malignancy. The tumor arises within the eye from uveal melanocytes or nevi. Microscopically, uveal melanomas are generally composed of variable numbers of spindle-shaped cells and polygonal cells with distinct cell borders and prominent nucleoli (epithelioid cells). Melanocytes are found in both the uvea and the retina, but the retinal melanocytes do not undergo malignant transformation as readily as those in the uvea. The choroid is the most common site of origin of ocular melanomas. Retinoblastoma arises from immature retinal neurons (choice C).
Diagnosis: Melanoma

22 **The answer is D: Macular degeneration.** The most common cause of amblyopia (impaired visual acuity) in the United States is age-related macular degeneration. The center of the macula (foveola) is the point of greatest visual acuity. In this area, a high concentration of cones rests on the retinal pigment epithelium. Surrounding the macula, the retina has a multilay- ered concentration of ganglion cells. With aging, the macula may degenerate, in which case central vision is impaired. Retinitis pigmentosa (choice E) begins in the periphery of the retina, leading to night blindness. The other choices are not associated with central vision.

Diagnosis: Macular degeneration

Chapter 30

Cytopathology

QUESTIONS

Select the single best answer.

1. A 31-year-old woman complains of increased vaginal discharge of 3 months in duration. A cervical Pap smear is obtained. Two superficial squamous cells (shown in the image) display enlarged nuclei and perinuclear vacuoles (koilocytotic atypia). What is the appropriate diagnosis?

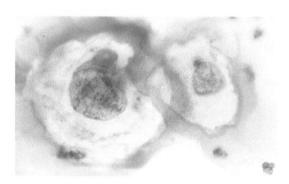

(A) Chlamydia infection
(B) Endometrial adenocarcinoma
(C) Herpes simplex virus infection
(D) Human papillomavirus (HPV) infection
(E) Invasive squamous cell carcinoma

2. A 33-year-old woman complains of vaginal spotting after intercourse. A cervical Pap smear is taken, and the results are shown in the image. A normal squamous epithelial cell is in the right upper corner. Which of the following is the most likely diagnosis?

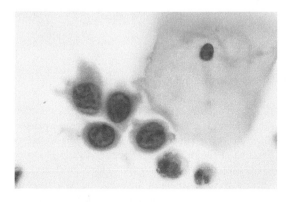

(A) Herpes simplex virus infection
(B) High-grade cervical dysplasia
(C) Human papillomavirus infection
(D) Low-grade cervical dysplasia
(E) Vaginal clear cell adenocarcinoma

3. For the patient described in Question 2, which of the following cytologic features observed in the Pap smear would provide the best evidence to substantiate a diagnosis of invasive squamous cell carcinoma?

(A) Atrophy
(B) Dysplasia
(C) Metaplasia
(D) Nuclear inclusion bodies
(E) Pleomorphism

4. A 30-year-old woman presents for a routine physical examination. A cervical Pap smear is taken. A cluster of multinucleated squamous cells is shown in the image. A normal superficial squamous cell is present at the top of the field. This patient most likely has which of the following gynecologic diseases?

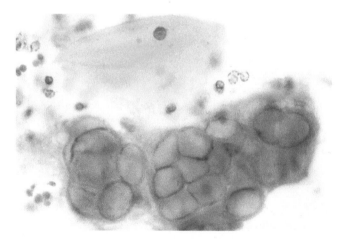

(A) Endometrial adenocarcinoma
(B) Herpes simplex virus infection
(C) High-grade cervical dysplasia
(D) Human papillomavirus infection
(E) Invasive squamous cell carcinoma

335

5 An 85-year-old woman presents with increasing fatigue and weight loss over the past 3 months. A CT scan of the abdomen reveals a 4-cm retroperitoneal mass. Fine-needle aspiration reveals numerous, large, noncleaved dissociated cells. By flow cytometry, the cells are positive for CD10, CD19, CD20, IgM, and lambda light chain. Which of the following is the appropriate diagnosis?
(A) Acute myelogenous leukemia
(B) Adult T-cell lymphoma/leukemia
(C) B-cell lymphoma
(D) Hodgkin disease
(E) T-cell lymphoma

6 A 59-year-old man presents with a 3-week history of painless hematuria. Physical examination is unremarkable. Urinalysis shows 2+ hematuria. A CT scan of the abdomen reveals an exophytic mass in the renal pelvis. Cytologic examination of a fine-needle aspiration of the renal pelvis is shown in the image. These cells show which of the following patterns of arrangement?

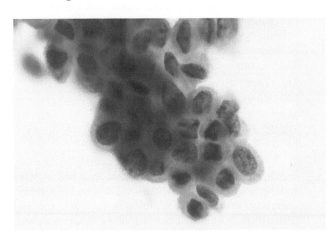

(A) Follicular configuration
(B) Glandular structures
(C) Papillary configuration
(D) Pearls
(E) Rosettes

7 A 2-month-old girl is brought to the physician because her parents noticed an enlargement in her abdomen. Physical examination reveals a flank mass over the left kidney. Twenty-four–hour urinalysis shows elevated levels of metanephrines. A CT scan of the abdomen reveals an 8-cm suprarenal mass. Fine-needle aspiration of the mass is performed. Cytologic examination of the aspirate would most likely show neoplastic cells with which of the following patterns of arrangement?
(A) Glandular structures
(B) Papillae
(C) Pearls
(D) Rosettes
(E) Syncytia

8 A 60-year-old man presents with a 4-month history of increasing weight loss and shortness of breath. He has smoked two packs of cigarettes a day for 20 years. His past medical history is significant for emphysema and chronic bronchitis. A chest X-ray shows a mass in the left main stem bronchus. Cytologic examination of a bronchial brushing shows pleomorphic keratinized cells with large irregular and pyknotic nuclei. These cells would most likely show which of the following patterns of arrangement on cytologic examination?
(A) Follicular configuration
(B) Glandular structures
(C) Papillary configuration
(D) Pearls
(E) Rosettes

9 A 36-year-old HIV-positive man presents with persistent dry cough, fatigue, and low-grade fever. Physical examination shows marked pallor and respiratory distress. An X-ray film of the chest reveals diffuse, bilateral, interstitial infiltrates. Bronchoalveolar lavage demonstrates a foamy alveolar cast composed of small cysts (shown in the image). What is the most likely diagnosis?

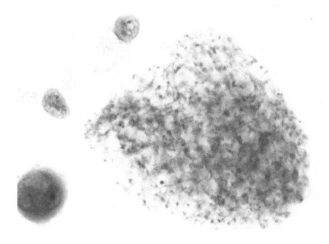

(A) Adenocarcinoma
(B) Herpesvirus infection
(C) Human papillomavirus infection
(D) *Pneumocystis carinii* pneumonia
(E) Small cell carcinoma

10 A 45-year-old woman complains of gradual swelling in her neck of 6 months in duration. Physical examination reveals an enlarged and nodular thyroid gland. A fine-needle aspiration of a nodule in the left lobe of the thyroid is performed. Cytologic examination of the aspirate shows follicular cells, macrophages, and abundant colloid. What is the appropriate diagnosis?
(A) Chronic lymphocytic thyroiditis
(B) Follicular adenoma
(C) Hürthle cell carcinoma
(D) Multinodular goiter
(E) Papillary carcinoma of thyroid

11 A 35-year-old woman comes to the physician after noticing a lump in her neck. Physical examination reveals a palpable nodule in an enlarged thyroid gland. A fine-needle aspiration of the left lobe of the thyroid is performed. Cytologic examination of the aspirate reveals malignant cells (shown in the image). These cells show which of the following patterns of arrangement, appropriate for tumor cells arising in this location?

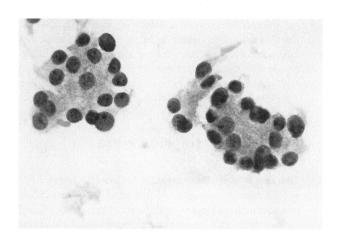

(A) Apocrine glands
(B) Follicular configuration
(C) Keratin pearls
(D) Mucin-secreting glands
(E) Multinucleated giant cells

12 A 35-year-old woman presents after noticing a gradual enlargement of her neck over the past 6 months. Physical examination reveals a diffusely enlarged thyroid gland. Cytologic examination of a fine-needle aspirate of the thyroid shows follicular cells and abundant lymphoid cells. Which of the following is the appropriate diagnosis?
(A) Follicular adenoma
(B) Goiter
(C) Graves disease
(D) Hashimoto thyroiditis
(E) Hürthle cell carcinoma

13 A 67-year-old man presents with chest wall pain and chronic nonproductive cough. A chest X-ray reveals a pleural-based mass and a large pleural effusion. A sputum sample is shown in the image. Fluid obtained from the left pleural cavity shows numerous single and clustered neoplastic cells. Which of the following is the most likely diagnosis?

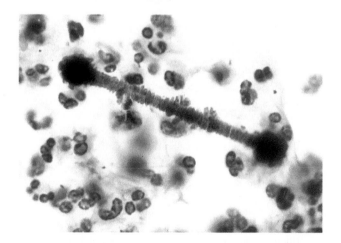

(A) Malignant lymphoma
(B) Malignant melanoma
(C) Mesothelioma
(D) Squamous cell carcinoma
(E) Transitional cell carcinoma

14 A 54-year-old man presents with a 4-month history of progressive weight loss. He has smoked three packs of cigarettes a day for 30 years. An X-ray film of the chest shows a mass in the right upper lobe. The bronchial brush specimen is shown in the image. Special stains are positive for mucin. Which of the following is the most likely diagnosis?

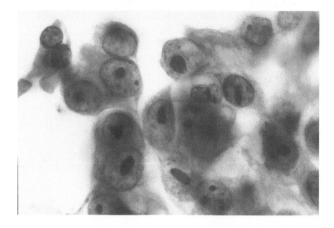

(A) Adenocarcinoma
(B) Malignant lymphoma
(C) Small cell carcinoma
(D) Squamous cell carcinoma
(E) Transitional cell carcinoma

15 A 55-year-old woman presents with a 4-month history of increasing abdominal girth and pelvic discomfort. Physical examination reveals ascites, and pelvic examination demonstrates an adnexal mass. A blood test for CA-125 is positive. A tap of the ascites returns numerous epithelial cells with papillary fronds. A small cluster of cells is shown in the image. Which of the following is the most likely diagnosis?

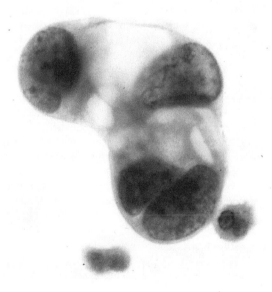

(A) Adenocarcinoma of the ovary
(B) Malignant melanoma
(C) Mesothelioma
(D) Neuroblastoma
(E) Transitional cell carcinoma of bladder

16 A 64-year-old man presents with a history of weight loss and progressive yellowing of the skin and sclera. Ultrasound examination of the liver shows multiple lesions. A fine-needle aspiration is performed under ultrasound guidance. The smear discloses numerous round cells, with poorly defined cytoplasm, eccentric nuclei, and prominent nucleoli. The cytoplasm of these cells contains pigmented granules (shown in the image). Immunohistochemical stains are positive for the HMB-45 antigen. What is the appropriate diagnosis?

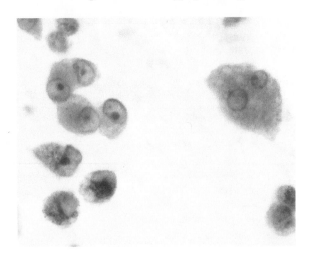

(A) Hepatic adenoma
(B) Hepatocellular carcinoma
(C) Metastatic adenocarcinoma
(D) Metastatic melanoma
(E) Metastatic squamous cell carcinoma

ANSWERS

1 **The answer is D: Human papillomavirus (HPV) infection.** HPV is a DNA virus that infects a variety of skin and mucosal surfaces to produce wart-like lesions (verrucae and condylomata). In the female reproductive tract, HPV infections are linked to the pathogenesis of cervical cancer. The morphologic hallmark of HPV infection is koilocytotic atypia, a term that denotes the presence of sharply demarcated, large perinuclear vacuoles, combined with alterations in the chromatin pattern of squamous epithelial cells. These perinuclear vacuoles are filled with replicating virus particles. Endometrial adenocarcinoma (choice B) demonstrates eccentric nuclei with irregular nuclear membranes and abnormally distributed chromatin. Herpes simplex virus infection (choice C) demonstrates multinucleation and "ground glass" nuclei. Invasive squamous cell carcinoma (choice E) is characterized by pleomorphic elongate squamous cells, with enlarged, irregular, and hyperchromatic nuclei.
Diagnosis: Human papillomavirus

2 **The answer is B: High-grade cervical dysplasia.** Cervical squamous intraepithelial lesions (SILs) show a spectrum of changes from low-grade SIL with mild dysplasia (cervical intraepithelial neoplasia, CIN1) to high-grade SIL with severe dysplasia (CIN3, carcinoma in situ). In low-grade CIN1, the dysplastic cells have abundant cytoplasm, and the nuclei

are enlarged and hyperchromatic. In high-grade dysplasia, the dysplastic cells have a higher nuclear-cytoplasmic ratio. Low-grade dysplasia (choice D) is incorrect because the dysplastic cells shown here have minimal cytoplasm and a very high nucleus to cytoplasm ratio. Herpes simplex virus infection (choice A) shows multinucleation and "ground glass" nuclei. Human papillomavirus infection (choice C) features perinuclear vacuoles.
Diagnosis: Cervical intraepithelial neoplasia

3 **The answer is E: Pleomorphism.** Squamous intraepithelial lesions must be distinguished from invasive lesions. In invasive squamous cell carcinoma, the neoplastic cells are usually pleomorphic, with caudate and elongate forms, and coarsely granular or pyknotic chromatin. Choices A, B, and C represent morphologic characteristics of cellular adaptation to chronic persistent stress. Nuclear inclusion bodies (choice D) likely represent viral infection.
Diagnosis: Squamous cell carcinoma of the cervix

4 **The answer is B: Herpes simplex virus infection.** Herpes simplex virus type 2 is a DNA virus that is a common cause of sexually transmitted genital infections. Multinucleated giant cells with "ground glass" appearance of the nuclei are typical. The other choices do not present with multinucleated giant cells.
Diagnosis: Genital herpes

5 **The answer is C: B-cell lymphoma.** Lymphomas are malignant proliferations of lymphocytes or lymphoblasts. The World Health Organization classification distinguishes between Hodgkin lymphoma and B-cell and T-cell lymphomas (non-Hodgkin lymphomas). B-cell lymphomas are characterized by their expression of cell surface immunoglobulin heavy and light chains and other cell surface CD antigens (e.g., CD20). The other choices do not express cell surface immunoglobulin heavy or light chains.
Diagnosis: B-cell lymphoma

6 **The answer is C: Papillary configuration.** The relation between cells is a helpful criterion for cytologic diagnosis. Cells may appear singly, in small groups, in monolayer sheets, in syncytia, or in three-dimensional clusters. Cell clusters may form papillary configurations (e.g., papillary transitional cell carcinoma), glandular structures (e.g., adenocarcinoma), follicles (e.g., follicular adenoma of thyroid), rosettes (e.g., neuroblastoma), or pearls (e.g., squamous cell carcinoma). Transitional cell carcinomas (this case) typically form papillary structures with a fibrovascular core. The nuclei are crowded and hyperchromatic.
Diagnosis: Transitional cell carcinoma of the urothelium

7 **The answer is D: Rosettes.** The clinical features of this case are most consistent with neuroblastoma. This malignant neural crest tumor is composed of neuroblasts and originates in the adrenal medulla or sympathetic ganglia. Microscopically, the tumor is composed of dense sheets of small, round to fusiform cells with hyperchromatic nuclei and scanty cytoplasm. Characteristic rosettes are defined by a rim of dark tumor cells in a circumferential arrangement around a central pale fibrillar core.
Diagnosis: Neuroblastoma

8 **The answer is D: Pearls.** Squamous cell carcinoma accounts for 30% of all invasive lung cancers in the United States. Following chronic injury (e.g., cigarette smoking), the metaplastic bronchial epithelium follows a sequence of dysplasia, carcinoma in situ, and invasive carcinoma, similar to that in the cervix. Well-differentiated tumors display keratin "pearls," which appear as small, rounded nests of brightly eosinophilic aggregates of keratin surrounded by concentric layers of squamous epithelial cells. Glandular structures (choice B) would be indicative of adenocarcinoma. The other choices are unlikely to exhibit keratinization.
Diagnosis: Squamous cell carcinoma of the lung

9 **The answer is D: *Pneumocystis carinii* pneumonia.** *P. carinii* (now correctly termed *P. jiroveci*) causes progressive, often fatal pneumonia in persons with severely impaired cell-mediated immunity and is one of the most common opportunistic pathogens in persons with AIDS. About 80% of all untreated patients with AIDS develop *P. carinii* pneumonia in the course of their illness. The morphologic hallmark of *P. carinii* pneumonia is foamy alveolar casts composed of small cysts. None of the other choices display a foamy appearance shown in the photomicrograph.
Diagnosis: *Pneumocystis* pneumonia

10 **The answer is D: Multinodular goiter.** Multinodular (nontoxic) goiter refers to an enlargement of the thyroid that is not associated with functional, inflammatory, or neoplastic alterations. Microscopically, thyroid nodules are lined by hyperplastic follicular epithelial cells and are distended with colloid. The other choices would show neoplastic cells (choices B, C, and E) or chronic inflammatory cells (choice A).
Diagnosis: Goiter

11 **The answer is B: Follicular configuration.** Follicular thyroid carcinoma does not contain papillae or other architectural elements. On cytologic examination, the tumor cells form small follicles, with scant colloid and mild nuclear atypia. Keratin pearls (choice C) or mucin secretion (choice D) are not observed.
Diagnosis: Follicular carcinoma of the thyroid

12 **The answer is D: Hashimoto thyroiditis.** Chronic, autoimmune thyroiditis displays a conspicuous infiltrate of lymphocytes and plasma cells. The inflammatory infiltrates are focally arranged in lymphoid follicles, often with germinal centers. Lymphoid infiltrates are not features of the other choices.
Diagnosis: Hashimoto thyroiditis, chronic lymphocytic thyroiditis

13 **The answer is C: Mesothelioma.** The sputum sample shows a ferruginous body, which appears as a yellow, beaded structures with clubbed ends. Also termed asbestos bodies, they are formed by the precipitation of iron and protein complexes on asbestos fibers. Asbestos exposure is a well-known risk factor for the development of mesothelioma. The other choices are not associated with asbestos exposure.
Diagnosis: Mesothelioma, ferruginous bodies

14 **The answer is A: Adenocarcinoma.** Adenocarcinoma accounts for a third of all invasive lung cancers. Cytologic examination of bronchial brush specimens shows clustered epithelial cells with highly atypical nuclei, prominent nucleoli, and cytoplasmic vacuoles. Mucin secretion is rarely, if ever, encountered in the other choices.
Diagnosis: Adenocarcinoma of the lung

15 **The answer is A: Adenocarcinoma of the ovary.** Ovarian cancer is most common in women between the ages of 40 and 60 years. By the time an ovarian cancer has attained a size of 10 to 15 cm, it has often spread beyond the ovary and seeded the peritoneum ("peritoneal carcinomatosis"). Monoclonal antibody to a tumor antigen (CA-125) detects about 90% of tumors that have already spread. The neoplastic cells shown here exhibit nuclear atypia, and their cytoplasm contains prominent secretory vacuoles. Although the other choices may metastasize to the ovary, they are unlikely to express CA-125 or demonstrate secretory vacuoles.
Diagnosis: Adenocarcinoma of the ovary

16 **The answer is D: Metastatic melanoma.** The brown pigment in the cytoplasm is composed of fine melanin granules, which is characteristic of malignant melanoma. HMB-45 antigen is commonly expressed in melanoma cells. Intracellular pigment is not encountered in the other choices.
Diagnosis: Melanoma

Appendix A
NORMAL REFERENCE RANGE*

Laboratory Test	Reference Range
CLINICAL CHEMISTRY TESTS (SERUM)	
Alanine aminotransferase (ALT)	
Male	1–45 IU/L @ 37°C
Female	1–30 IU/L @ 37°C
Albumin	3.0–5.0 g/dL
Alkaline phosphatase	
0–17 years	40–400 IU/L @ 37°C
18–99 years	30–160 IU/L @ 37°C
Alpha-1-antitrypsin, total	96–199 mg/dL
Ammonia	11–35 µmol/L
Amylase	<132 U/L
Aspartate aminotransferase (AST)	
Male	7–42 IU/L @ 37°C
Female	7–35 IU/L @ 37°C
Bilirubin, direct	0.0–0.4 mg/dL
Bilirubin, total	0.2–1.2 mg/dL
Calcium	8.5–10.5 mg/dL
Cardio C-reactive protein (low-risk)	<1.2 mg/dL
Chloride	98–109 mmol/L
Cholesterol, HDL (desirable)	>60 mg/dL
Cholesterol, LDL (desirable)	<100 mg/dL
Cholesterol, total	<200 mg/dL
CO_2	24–32 mmol/L
Complement C-3	88–201 mg/dL
Complement C-4	16–47 mg/dL
Creatine kinase (CK)	
Male	25–215 IU/L @ 37°C
Female	25–185 IU/L @ 37°C
Creatinine	0.5–1.4 mg/dL
Ferritin	
Male	15–300 ng/mL
Female	10–160 ng/mL
Folate (folic acid)	3–18 ng/mL
Folate, red cell	145–540 ng/mL
Glucose, fasting	50–100 mg/dL
Hemoglobin A_2	1.7%–3.4%
Hemoglobin, plasma, free	0–10 mg/dL
Immunoglobulins	
IgA	69–382 mg/dL
IgG	723–1,685 mg/dL
IgM	63–277 mg/dL
Insulin	10–26 mIU/mL
Iron	
Male	55–160 µg/dL
Female	40–155µg/dL
Iron-binding capacity	250–400 µg/dL
Lactate dehydrogenase (LD)	100–200 U/L
Lead	
Child	0–9.9 µg/dL
Adult	0–25 µg/dL
Lipase	<52 U/L
Magnesium	1.3–2.1 mEq/L
Mercury	0–13 mg/L
Phosphate	2.5–4.5 mg/dL
Potassium	3.5–5.0 mmol/L
Protein, total	6.0–8.5 g/dL
Sodium	135–146 mmol/L
Triglycerides (desirable)	<150 mg/dL
Troponin I	<0.5 ng/mL
Urate (uric acid)	
Male	3.5–8.0 mg/dL
Female	2.2–7.0 mg/dL
Urea-N (blood urea nitrogen)	10–30 mg/dL
Vitamin B_{12} (cobalamin)	200–1100 pg/dL

Laboratory Test	Reference Range	
ARTERIAL BLOOD GASES (HEPARINIZED WHOLE BLOOD)		
pH	7.35–7.45	
pO_2	83–108 mm Hg	
pCO_2	31–45 mm Hg	
HEMATOLOGY TESTS		
Complete Blood Count Adult Male		
Leukocytes	$4–11 \times 10^9$/L	
Erythrocytes	$4.5–6.0 \times 10^{12}$/L	
Hemoglobin	14–17 g/dL	
Hematocrit	42%–52%	
MCV	80–99 fL	
MCH	26–34 pg	
MCHC	32–36.5 g/dL	
RDW	11.0%–15.8%	
Platelets	$140–400 \times 10^9$/L	
MPV	9–13 fL	
Erythrocyte sedimentation rate	0–10 mm/hr	
Complete Blood Count Adult Female		
Leukocytes	$4–11 \times 10^9$/L	
Erythrocytes	$3.7–5.2 \times 10^{12}$/L	
Hemoglobin	12.5–15 g/dL	
Hematocrit	36%–46%	
MCV	80–99 fL	
MCH	26–34 pg	
MCHC	32–36.5 g/dL	
RDW	11.0%–15.8%	
Platelets	$140–400 \times 10^9$/L	
MPV	9–13 fL	
Erythrocyte sedimentation rate	0–20 mm/hr	
Automated Differential (Adult)	**Relative %**	**Absolute** $(\times 10^9$/L$)$
Neutrophils	40–73	1.7–7.0
Lymphocytes	20–44	1–4.0
Monocytes	3–13	0.2–0.9
Eosinophils	0–6	0.1–0.5
Basophils	0–3	0.0–0.2
Reticulocytes	0.5–1.5	20–76
COAGULATION TESTS (CITRATED PLASMA)		
d-Dimer	<0.45 µg/mL	
Partial thromboplastin time (PTT), activated	22–38 seconds	
Prothrombin time (PT)	12.0–15.4 seconds	
Fibrinogen	226–454 mg/dL	
ENDOCRINE TESTS AND TUMOR MARKERS (SERUM)		
Alpha-fetoprotein (AFP), nonmaternal	<7.7 ng/mL	
Angiotensin converting enzyme (ACE)	35–140 nmol/mL/min	
Carcinoembryonic antigen (CEA)		
Nonsmoker	3.5 ng/mL	
Smoker	0–5.0 ng/mL	
Corticotropin (ACTH)	9–52 pg/mL	
Cortisol, serum		
8–10 AM	4–24 µg/dL	
4–6 PM	2–12 µg/dL	
Growth hormone		
0–1 year	15–40 ng/mL (fasting)	
1 year–adult	0–5 (fasting)	
Human chorionic gonadotropin (hCG)		
Time after conception		
1st week	0–50 mIU/mL	
1 month	1,000–20,000 mIU/mL	
3 months	20,000–200,000 mIU/mL	
Insulin	10–26 mIU/mL	
17-Ketosteroids, total	5–20 mg/24 hours	

Laboratory Test	Reference Range	Laboratory Test	Reference Range
Parathyroid hormone, intact		Glucose, quantitative	<500 mg/24 hours
Child	1–43 pg/mL	17-Hydroxycorticosteroids	3–11 mg/24 hours
Adult	10–55 pg/mL	Magnesium	1.0–24.0 mEq/24 hours
Prolactin	0–19 ng/mL	Mercury	0–20 µg/L
Prostate-specific antigen, male >40 years	0–4 ng/mL	Osmolality (10 mL random	
Triiodothyronine (T-3), total	90–200 ng/dL	specimen)	300–900 mOsmol/kg
Thyroxine (T-4), free	0.7–1.6 ng/dL	Oxalate	3.6–38 mg/24 hours
Testosterone, total		pH	5.0–8.0
Male	270–1,070 ng/dL	Phosphate	400–1,400 mg/24 hours
Female	10–70 ng/dL	Protein, total	<150 mg/24 hours
Thyroid-stimulating hormone (TSH)	0.4–4.8 µIU/mL	Urate (uric acid)	250–750 mg/24 hours
URINE TESTS		CEREBROSPINAL FLUID	
Calcium, quantitative	0–150 mg/24 hours	Glucose	40–70 mg/dL
Cortisol, free	<50 µg/24 hours	Protein	
Creatinine		*Neonate*	15–130 mg/dL
Male	1,000–2,000 mg/24 hours	*Adult*	15–55 mg/dL
Female	800–1,800 mg/24 hours		
Electrolytes (24-hour collection or 10 mL)		BODY MASS INDEX	
Potassium	25–120 mmol/24 hours	BMI (adult)	19–25 kg/m^2
Sodium	40–220 mmol/24 hours		
Chloride	110–250 mmol/24 hours		

*Normal Reference Range data provided by Clinical Laboratories, Department of Pathology, Thomas Jefferson University Hospital, Philadelphia. Normal reference range data vary considerably between institutions.

Appendix B
COMMON ABBREVIATIONS

Abbreviation	Expanded Form
ACTH	Corticotropin
ADH	Antidiuretic hormone
AFP	Alpha-fetoprotein
AIDS	Acquired immunodeficiency syndrome
ALL	Acute lymphoblastic leukemia
ALT	Alanine aminotransferase
AML	Acute myeloblastic leukemia
ANA	Antinuclear antibody
ANCA	Antineutrophil cytoplasmic antibody
AST	Aspartate aminotransferase
ATP	Adenosine triphosphate
ATPase	Adenosine triphosphatase
BMI	Body mass index
BPH	Benign prostatic hyperplasia
BUN	Blood urea nitrogen
C	Complement
cAMP	Cyclic adenosine monophosphate
CBC	Complete blood cell count
CD	Clusters of differentiation
CEA	Carcinoembryonic antigen
CFU	Colony-forming unit
cGMP	Cyclic guanosine monophosphate
CK	Creatine kinase
CMV	Cytomegalovirus
CNS	Central nervous system
CT	Computed tomography
DIC	Disseminated intravascular coagulation
DNA	Deoxyribonucleic acid
DNase	Deoxyribonuclease
EBV	Epstein-Barr virus
ECG	Electrocardiogram
FISH	Fluorescence in situ hybridization
FSH	Follicle-stimulating hormone
GI	Gastrointestinal
HbS	Sickle cell hemoglobin
HBsAg	Hepatitis B surface antigen
HBV	Hepatitis B virus
hCG	Human chorionic gonadotropin
HCV	Hepatitis C virus
HDL	High-density lipoprotein
hGH	Human growth hormone
HIV	Human immunodeficiency virus
HLA	Human leukocyte antigen
HMG-CoA	3-hydroxy-3-methylglutaryl coenzyme A

Abbreviation	Expanded Form
HPF	High-power field
HPV	Human papillomavirus
HSV	Herpes simplex virus
HTLV	Human T-lymphotrophic virus
Ig	Immunoglobulin (IgM, IgG, IgA, IgE)
IL	Interleukin
ITP	Idiopathic thrombocytopenic purpura
IV	Intravenous
Kb	Kilobase (DNA)
LDH	Lactate dehydrogenase
LDL	Low-density lipoprotein
LH	Luteinizing hormone
MCH	Mean corpuscular hemoglobin
MCHC	Mean corpuscular hemoglobin concentration
MCV	Mean corpuscular volume
MEN	Multiple endocrine neoplasia
MRI	Magnetic resonance imaging
mRNA	Messenger RNA
NK	Natural killer
NSAID	Nonsteroidal anti-inflammatory drug
$PaCO_2$	Partial pressure of carbon dioxide, arterial
PaO_2	Partial pressure of oxygen, arterial
PAS	Periodic acid-Schiff
PCR	Polymerase chain reaction
pH	Hydrogen ion concentration
PID	Pelvic inflammatory disease
PSA	Prostate-specific antigen
PT	Prothrombin time
PTH	Parathyroid hormone
PTT	Partial thromboplastin time
RBC	Red blood cell
RNA	Ribonucleic acid
RSV	Respiratory syncytial virus
SIDS	Sudden infant death syndrome
STD	Sexually transmitted disease
SLE	Systemic lupus erythematosus
T3	Triiodothyronine
T4	Thyroxine
TB	Tuberculosis
TNF-α	Tumor necrosis factor-α
TSH	Thyrotropin
TTP	Thrombotic thrombocytopenic purpura
UV	Ultraviolet
WBC	White blood cell

Appendix C
FIGURE CREDITS

Chapter 1

Q1-1: Image from Rubin E, Gorstein F, Rubin R, et al., eds. Rubin's Pathology: Clinicopathologic Foundations of Medicine. 4th Ed. Philadelphia: Lippincott Williams & Wilkins, 2005.

Q1-3: Image from Rubin R, Strayer D, eds. Rubin's Pathology: Clinicopathologic Foundations of Medicine. 5th Ed. Baltimore: Lippincott Williams & Wilkins, 2008.

Q1-5: Image from Okazaki H, Scheithauer BW. Atlas of Neuropathology. New York: Gower Medical Publishing, 1988.

Q1-7: Image from Rubin E, Gorstein F, Rubin R, et al., eds. Rubin's Pathology: Clinicopathologic Foundations of Medicine. 4th Ed. Philadelphia: Lippincott Williams & Wilkins, 2005.

Q1-11: Image from Rubin E, Gorstein F, Rubin R, et al., eds. Rubin's Pathology: Clinicopathologic Foundations of Medicine. 4th Ed. Philadelphia: Lippincott Williams & Wilkins, 2005.

Q1-13: Image from Rubin E, Gorstein F, Rubin R, et al., eds. Rubin's Pathology: Clinicopathologic Foundations of Medicine. 4th Ed. Philadelphia: Lippincott Williams & Wilkins, 2005.

Q1-15: Image from Rubin E, Gorstein F, Rubin R, et al., eds. Rubin's Pathology: Clinicopathologic Foundations of Medicine. 4th Ed. Philadelphia: Lippincott Williams & Wilkins, 2005.

Q1-20: Image from Rubin E, Gorstein F, Rubin R, et al., eds. Rubin's Pathology: Clinicopathologic Foundations of Medicine. 4th Ed. Philadelphia: Lippincott Williams & Wilkins, 2005.

Q1-22: Image from Rubin E, Gorstein F, Rubin R, et al., eds. Rubin's Pathology: Clinicopathologic Foundations of Medicine. 4th Ed. Philadelphia: Lippincott Williams & Wilkins, 2005.

Q1-24: Image from Rubin E, Gorstein F, Rubin R, et al., eds. Rubin's Pathology: Clinicopathologic Foundations of Medicine. 4th Ed Philadelphia: Lippincott Williams & Wilkins, 2005.

Q1-29: Image from Rubin R, Strayer D, eds. Rubin's Pathology: Clinicopathologic Foundations of Medicine. 5th Ed. Baltimore: Lippincott Williams & Wilkins, 2008.

Q1-33: Image from Rubin R, Strayer D, eds. Rubin's Pathology: Clinicopathologic Foundations of Medicine. 5th Ed. Baltimore: Lippincott Williams & Wilkins, 2008.

Q1-34: Image from Rubin E, Gorstein F, Rubin R, et al., eds. Rubin's Pathology: Clinicopathologic Foundations of Medicine. 4th Ed. Philadelphia: Lippincott Williams & Wilkins, 2005.

Q1-37: Image from Rubin E, Gorstein F, Rubin R, et al., eds. Rubin's Pathology: Clinicopathologic Foundations of Medicine. 4th Ed. Philadelphia: Lippincott Williams & Wilkins, 2005.

Q1-42: Image from Rubin R, Strayer D, eds. Rubin's Pathology: Clinicopathologic Foundations of Medicine. 5th Ed. Baltimore: Lippincott Williams & Wilkins, 2008.

Q1-44: Image from Rubin R, Strayer D, eds. Rubin's Pathology: Clinicopathologic Foundations of Medicine. 5th Ed. Baltimore: Lippincott Williams & Wilkins, 2008.

Chapter 2

Q2-8: Image from Okazaki H, Scheithauer BW. Atlas of Neuropathology. New York: Gower Medical Publishing, 1988.

Q2-14: Image from Rubin R, Strayer D, eds. Rubin's Pathology: Clinicopathologic Foundations of Medicine. 5th Ed. Baltimore: Lippincott Williams & Wilkins, 2008.

Q2-16: Image from Rubin R, Strayer D, eds. Rubin's Pathology: Clinicopathologic Foundations of Medicine. 5th Ed. Baltimore: Lippincott Williams & Wilkins, 2008.

Q2-31: Image from Rubin E, Gorstein F, Rubin R, et al., eds. Rubin's Pathology: Clinicopathologic Foundations of Medicine. 4th Ed. Philadelphia: Lippincott Williams & Wilkins, 2005.

Q2-33: Image from Rubin R, Strayer D, eds. Rubin's Pathology: Clinicopathologic Foundations of Medicine. 5th Ed. Baltimore: Lippincott Williams & Wilkins, 2008.

Q2-38: Image from Rubin R, Strayer D, eds. Rubin's Pathology: Clinicopathologic Foundations of Medicine. 5th Ed. Baltimore: Lippincott Williams & Wilkins, 2008.

Chapter 3

Q3-3: Image from Rubin E, Gorstein F, Rubin R, et al., eds. Rubin's Pathology: Clinicopathologic Foundations of Medicine. 4th Ed. Philadelphia: Lippincott Williams & Wilkins, 2005.

Q3-6: Image from Rubin E, Gorstein F, Rubin R, et al., eds. Rubin's Pathology: Clinicopathologic Foundations of Medicine. 4th Ed. Philadelphia: Lippincott Williams & Wilkins, 2005.

Q3-9: Image from Rubin E, Gorstein F, Rubin R, et al., eds. Rubin's Pathology: Clinicopathologic Foundations of Medicine. 4th Ed. Philadelphia: Lippincott Williams & Wilkins, 2005.

Q3-11: Image from Rubin E, Gorstein F, Rubin R, et al., eds. Rubin's Pathology: Clinicopathologic Foundations of Medicine. 4th Ed. Philadelphia: Lippincott Williams & Wilkins, 2005.

Q3-22: Image from Okazaki H, Scheithauer BW. Atlas of Neuropathology. New York, Gower Medical Publishing, 1988.

Q3-24: Image from Rubin R, Strayer D, eds. Rubin's Pathology: Clinicopathologic Foundations of Medicine. 5th Ed. Baltimore: Lippincott Williams & Wilkins, 2008.

Chapter 4

Q4-18: Image from Sandoz Pharmaceutical Corporation.

Q4-23: Image from Rubin R, Strayer D, eds. Rubin's Pathology: Clinicopathologic Foundations of Medicine. 5th Ed. Baltimore: Lippincott Williams & Wilkins, 2008.

Chapter 5

Q5-2: Image from Rubin E, Gorstein F, Rubin R, et al., eds. Rubin's Pathology: Clinicopathologic Foundations of Medicine. 4th Ed. Philadelphia: Lippincott Williams & Wilkins, 2005.

Q5-6: Image from Rubin E, Gorstein F, Rubin R, et al., eds. Rubin's Pathology: Clinicopathologic Foundations of Medicine. 4th Ed. Philadelphia: Lippincott Williams & Wilkins, 2005.

Q5-8: Image from Rubin E, Gorstein F, Rubin R, et al., eds. Rubin's Pathology: Clinicopathologic Foundations of Medicine. 4th Ed. Philadelphia: Lippincott Williams & Wilkins, 2005.

Q5-12: Image from Rubin R, Strayer D, eds. Rubin's Pathology: Clinicopathologic Foundations of Medicine. 5th Ed. Baltimore: Lippincott Williams & Wilkins, 2008.

Q5-15: Image from Rubin E, Gorstein F, Rubin R, et al., eds. Rubin's Pathology: Clinicopathologic Foundations of Medicine. 4th Ed. Philadelphia: Lippincott Williams & Wilkins, 2005.

Q5-31: Image from Rubin E, Gorstein F, Rubin R, et al., eds. Rubin's Pathology: Clinicopathologic Foundations of Medicine. 4th Ed. Philadelphia: Lippincott Williams & Wilkins, 2005.

Q5-33: Image from Bullough PG, Vigorita VJ. Atlas of Orthopaedic Pathology. New York: Gower Medical Publishing, 1984.

Q5-38: Image from Rubin R, Strayer D, eds. Rubin's Pathology: Clinicopathologic Foundations of Medicine. 5th Ed. Baltimore: Lippincott Williams & Wilkins, 2008.

Q5-41: Image from Rubin R, Strayer D, eds. Rubin's Pathology: Clinicopathologic Foundations of Medicine. 5th Ed. Baltimore: Lippincott Williams & Wilkins, 2008.

Q5-42: Image from Rubin R, Strayer D, eds. Rubin's Pathology: Clinicopathologic Foundations of Medicine. 5th Ed. Baltimore: Lippincott Williams & Wilkins, 2008.

Q5-43: Image from Elder D. Synopsis and Atlas of Lever's Histopathology of the Skin. Philadelphia: Lippincott Williams & Wilkins, 1999.

Q5-44: Image from Rubin R, Strayer D, eds. Rubin's Pathology: Clinicopathologic Foundations of Medicine. 5th Ed. Baltimore: Lippincott Williams & Wilkins, 2008.

Chapter 6

Q6-3: Image from Rubin R, Strayer D, eds. Rubin's Pathology: Clinicopathologic Foundations of Medicine. 5th Ed. Baltimore: Lippincott Williams & Wilkins, 2008.

Q6-7: Image from Rubin E, Gorstein F, Rubin R, et al., eds. Rubin's Pathology: Clinicopathologic Foundations of Medicine. 4th Ed. Philadelphia: Lippincott Williams & Wilkins, 2005.

Q6-17: Image from Rubin R, Strayer D, eds. Rubin's Pathology: Clinicopathologic Foundations of Medicine. 5th Ed. Baltimore: Lippincott Williams & Wilkins, 2008.

Q6-20: Image from Rubin R, Strayer D, eds. Rubin's Pathology: Clinicopathologic Foundations of Medicine. 5th Ed. Baltimore: Lippincott Williams & Wilkins, 2008.

Q6-24: Image from Rubin R, Strayer D, eds. Rubin's Pathology: Clinicopathologic Foundations of Medicine. 5th Ed. Baltimore: Lippincott Williams & Wilkins, 2008.

Q6-39: Image from Rubin R, Strayer D, eds. Rubin's Pathology: Clinicopathologic Foundations of Medicine. 5th Ed. Baltimore: Lippincott Williams & Wilkins, 2008.

Chapter 7

Q7-10: Image from UBC Pulmonary Registry, St Paul's Hospital.

Q7-11: Image from Rubin E, Gorstein F, Rubin R, et al., eds. Rubin's Pathology: Clinicopathologic Foundations of Medicine. 4th Ed. Philadelphia: Lippincott Williams & Wilkins, 2005.

Q7-24: Image from Dr. Greg J. Davis, Department of Pathology, University of Kentucky College of Medicine.

Q7-26: Image from Rubin E, Gorstein F, Rubin R, et al., eds. Rubin's Pathology: Clinicopathologic Foundations of Medicine. 4th Ed. Philadelphia: Lippincott Williams & Wilkins, 2005.

Q7-27: Image from Dr. Greg J. Davis, Department of Pathology, University of Kentucky College of Medicine.

Q7-29: Image from Rubin E, Gorstein F, Rubin R, et al., eds. Rubin's Pathology: Clinicopathologic Foundations of Medicine. 4th Ed. Philadelphia: Lippincott Williams & Wilkins, 2005.

Q7-31: Image from Rubin E, Gorstein F, Rubin R, et al., eds. Rubin's Pathology: Clinicopathologic Foundations of Medicine. 4th Ed. Philadelphia: Lippincott Williams & Wilkins, 2005.

Q7-35: Image from Rubin R, Strayer D, eds. Rubin's Pathology: Clinicopathologic Foundations of Medicine. 5th Ed. Baltimore: Lippincott Williams & Wilkins, 2008.

Q7-36: Image from UBC Pulmonary Registry, St Paul's Hospital.

Q7-37: Image from Rubin R, Strayer D, eds. Rubin's Pathology: Clinicopathologic Foundations of Medicine. 5th Ed. Baltimore: Lippincott Williams & Wilkins, 2008.

Q7-39: Image from Rubin R, Strayer D, eds. Rubin's Pathology: Clinicopathologic Foundations of Medicine. 5th Ed. Baltimore: Lippincott Williams & Wilkins, 2008.

Q7-40: Image from Rubin R, Strayer D, eds. Rubin's Pathology: Clinicopathologic Foundations of Medicine. 5th Ed. Baltimore: Lippincott Williams & Wilkins, 2008.

Chapter 8

Q8-1: Image from Rubin R, Strayer D, eds. Rubin's Pathology: Clinicopathologic Foundations of Medicine. 5th Ed. Baltimore: Lippincott Williams & Wilkins, 2008.

Q8-2: Image from Courtesy of the Armed Forces Institute of Pathology.

Q8-23: Image from Rubin R, Strayer D, eds. Rubin's Pathology: Clinicopathologic Foundations of Medicine. 5th Ed. Baltimore: Lippincott Williams & Wilkins, 2008.

Chapter 9

Q9-4: Image from Rubin E, Gorstein F, Rubin R, et al., eds. Rubin's Pathology: Clinicopathologic Foundations of Medicine. 4th Ed. Philadelphia: Lippincott Williams & Wilkins, 2005.

Q9-10: Image from Rubin E, Gorstein F, Rubin R, et al., eds. Rubin's Pathology: Clinicopathologic Foundations of Medicine. 4th Ed. Philadelphia: Lippincott Williams & Wilkins, 2005.

Q9-12: Image from Rubin E, Gorstein F, Rubin R, et al., eds. Rubin's Pathology: Clinicopathologic Foundations of Medicine. 4th Ed. Philadelphia: Lippincott Williams & Wilkins, 2005.

Q9-13: Image from Rubin E, Gorstein F, Rubin R, et al., eds. Rubin's Pathology: Clinicopathologic Foundations of Medicine. 4th Ed. Philadelphia: Lippincott Williams & Wilkins, 2005.

Q9-16: Image from Rubin E, Gorstein F, Rubin R, et al., eds. Rubin's Pathology: Clinicopathologic Foundations of Medicine. 4th Ed. Philadelphia: Lippincott Williams & Wilkins, 2005.

Q9-21: Image from Rubin E, Gorstein F, Rubin R, et al., eds. Rubin's Pathology: Clinicopathologic Foundations of Medicine. 4th Ed. Philadelphia: Lippincott Williams & Wilkins, 2005.

Q9-24: Image from Rubin E, Gorstein F, Rubin R, et al., eds. Rubin's Pathology: Clinicopathologic Foundations of Medicine. 4th Ed. Philadelphia: Lippincott Williams & Wilkins, 2005.

Q9-26: Image from Rubin E, Gorstein F, Rubin R, et al., eds. Rubin's Pathology: Clinicopathologic Foundations of Medicine. 4th Ed. Philadelphia: Lippincott Williams & Wilkins, 2005.

Q9-30: Image from Farrar Wek, Wood MJ, Innes JA, et al. Infectious Diseases Text and Color Atlas. 2nd Ed. New York: Gower Medical Publishing, 1992.

Q9-33: Image from Rubin E, Gorstein F, Rubin R, et al., eds. Rubin's Pathology: Clinicopathologic Foundations of Medicine. 4th Ed. Philadelphia: Lippincott Williams & Wilkins, 2005.

Q9-35: Image from Rubin E, Gorstein F, Rubin R, et al., eds. Rubin's Pathology: Clinicopathologic Foundations of Medicine. 4th Ed. Philadelphia: Lippincott Williams & Wilkins, 2005.

Q9-38: Image from Rubin E, Gorstein F, Rubin R, et al., eds. Rubin's Pathology: Clinicopathologic Foundations of Medicine. 4th Ed. Philadelphia: Lippincott Williams & Wilkins, 2005.

Q9-41: Image from Rubin E, Gorstein F, Rubin R, et al., eds. Rubin's Pathology: Clinicopathologic Foundations of Medicine. 4th Ed. Philadelphia: Lippincott Williams & Wilkins, 2005.

Q9-44: Image from Rubin E, Gorstein F, Rubin R, et al., eds. Rubin's Pathology: Clinicopathologic Foundations of Medicine. 4th Ed. Philadelphia: Lippincott Williams & Wilkins, 2005.

Q9-46: Image from Rubin E, Gorstein F, Rubin R, et al., eds. Rubin's Pathology: Clinicopathologic Foundations of Medicine. 4th Ed. Philadelphia: Lippincott Williams & Wilkins, 2005.

Q9-51: Image from Rubin R, Strayer D, eds. Rubin's Pathology: Clinicopathologic Foundations of Medicine. 5th Ed. Baltimore: Lippincott Williams & Wilkins, 2008.

Q9-55: Image from Rubin E, Gorstein F, Rubin R, et al., eds. Rubin's Pathology: Clinicopathologic Foundations of Medicine. 4th Ed. Philadelphia: Lippincott Williams & Wilkins, 2005.

Q9-61: Image from Rubin E, Gorstein F, Rubin R, et al., eds. Rubin's Pathology: Clinicopathologic Foundations of Medicine. 4th Ed. Philadelphia: Lippincott Williams & Wilkins, 2005.

Chapter 10

Q10-1: Image from Rubin E, Gorstein F, Rubin R, et al., eds. Rubin's Pathology: Clinicopathologic Foundations of Medicine. 4th Ed. Philadelphia: Lippincott Williams & Wilkins, 2005.

Q10-3: Image from Rubin E, Gorstein F, Rubin R, et al., eds. Rubin's Pathology: Clinicopathologic Foundations of Medicine. 4th Ed. Philadelphia: Lippincott Williams & Wilkins, 2005.

Q10-5: Image from Rubin E, Gorstein F, Rubin R, et al., eds. Rubin's Pathology: Clinicopathologic Foundations of Medicine. 4th Ed. Philadelphia: Lippincott Williams & Wilkins, 2005.

Q10-7: Image from Rubin R, Strayer D, eds. Rubin's Pathology: Clinicopathologic Foundations of Medicine. 5th Ed. Baltimore: Lippincott Williams & Wilkins, 2008.

Q10-8: Image from Rubin E, Gorstein F, Rubin R, et al., eds. Rubin's Pathology: Clinicopathologic Foundations of Medicine. 4th Ed. Philadelphia: Lippincott Williams & Wilkins, 2005.

Q10-9: Image from Rubin E, Gorstein F, Rubin R, et al., eds. Rubin's Pathology: Clinicopathologic Foundations of Medicine. 4th Ed. Philadelphia: Lippincott Williams & Wilkins, 2005.

Q10-10: Image from Rubin E, Gorstein F, Rubin R, et al., eds. Rubin's Pathology: Clinicopathologic Foundations of Medicine. 4th Ed. Philadelphia: Lippincott Williams & Wilkins, 2005.

Q10-13: Image from Dr. Kevin C. Kain, Centre for Travel and Tropical Medicine, Toronto General Hospital.

Q10-16: Image from Rubin E, Gorstein F, Rubin R, et al., eds. Rubin's Pathology: Clinicopathologic Foundations of Medicine. 4th Ed. Philadelphia: Lippincott Williams & Wilkins, 2005.

Q10-17: Image from Rubin E, Gorstein F, Rubin R, et al., eds. Rubin's Pathology: Clinicopathologic Foundations of Medicine. 4th Ed. Philadelphia: Lippincott Williams & Wilkins, 2005.

Q10-19: Image from Rubin E, Gorstein F, Rubin R, et al., eds. Rubin's Pathology: Clinicopathologic Foundations of Medicine. 4th Ed. Philadelphia: Lippincott Williams & Wilkins, 2005.

Q10-25: Image from Rubin E, Gorstein F, Rubin R, et al., eds. Rubin's Pathology: Clinicopathologic Foundations of Medicine. 4th Ed. Philadelphia: Lippincott Williams & Wilkins, 2005.

Q10-28: Image from Rubin E, Gorstein F, Rubin R, et al., eds. Rubin's Pathology: Clinicopathologic Foundations of Medicine. 4th Ed. Philadelphia: Lippincott Williams & Wilkins, 2005.

Q10-29: Image from Rubin R, Strayer D, eds. Rubin's Pathology: Clinicopathologic Foundations of Medicine. 5th Ed. Baltimore: Lippincott Williams & Wilkins, 2008.

Q10-30: Image from Rubin E, Gorstein F, Rubin R, et al., eds. Rubin's Pathology: Clinicopathologic Foundations of Medicine. 4th Ed. Philadelphia: Lippincott Williams & Wilkins, 2005.

Q10-33: Image from Rubin E, Gorstein F, Rubin R, et al., eds. Rubin's Pathology: Clinicopathologic Foundations of Medicine. 4th Ed. Philadelphia: Lippincott Williams & Wilkins, 2005.

Q10-34: Image from Rubin R, Strayer D, eds. Rubin's Pathology: Clinicopathologic Foundations of Medicine. 5th Ed. Baltimore: Lippincott Williams & Wilkins, 2008.

Q10-36: Image from Rubin E, Gorstein F, Rubin R, et al., eds. Rubin's Pathology: Clinicopathologic Foundations of Medicine. 4th Ed. Philadelphia: Lippincott Williams & Wilkins, 2005.

Q10-37: Image from Rubin E, Gorstein F, Rubin R, et al., eds. Rubin's Pathology: Clinicopathologic Foundations of Medicine. 4th Ed. Philadelphia: Lippincott Williams & Wilkins, 2005.

Q10-40: Image from Rubin R, Strayer D, eds. Rubin's Pathology: Clinicopathologic Foundations of Medicine. 5th Ed. Baltimore: Lippincott Williams & Wilkins, 2008.

Chapter 11

Q11-7: Image from Rubin E, Gorstein F, Rubin R, et al., eds. Rubin's Pathology: Clinicopathologic Foundations of Medicine. 4th Ed. Philadelphia: Lippincott Williams & Wilkins, 2005.

Q11-9: Image from Rubin E, Gorstein F, Rubin R, et al., eds. Rubin's Pathology: Clinicopathologic Foundations of Medicine. 4th Ed. Philadelphia: Lippincott Williams & Wilkins, 2005.

Q11-11: Image from Rubin E, Gorstein F, Rubin R, et al., eds. Rubin's Pathology: Clinicopathologic Foundations of Medicine. 4th Ed. Philadelphia: Lippincott Williams & Wilkins, 2005.

Q11-17: Image from Rubin E, Gorstein F, Rubin R, et al., eds. Rubin's Pathology: Clinicopathologic Foundations of Medicine. 4th Ed. Philadelphia: Lippincott Williams & Wilkins, 2005.

Q11-19: Image from Rubin E, Gorstein F, Rubin R, et al., eds. Rubin's Pathology: Clinicopathologic Foundations of Medicine. 4th Ed. Philadelphia: Lippincott Williams & Wilkins, 2005.

Q11-20: Image from Rubin E, Gorstein F, Rubin R, et al., eds. Rubin's Pathology: Clinicopathologic Foundations of Medicine. 4th Ed. Philadelphia: Lippincott Williams & Wilkins, 2005.

Q11-22: Image from Rubin E, Gorstein F, Rubin R, et al., eds. Rubin's Pathology: Clinicopathologic Foundations of Medicine. 4th Ed. Philadelphia: Lippincott Williams & Wilkins, 2005.

Q11-23: Image from Rubin E, Gorstein F, Rubin R, et al., eds. Rubin's Pathology: Clinicopathologic Foundations of Medicine. 4th Ed. Philadelphia: Lippincott Williams & Wilkins, 2005.

Q11-27: Image from Rubin E, Gorstein F, Rubin R, et al., eds. Rubin's Pathology: Clinicopathologic Foundations of Medicine. 4th Ed. Philadelphia: Lippincott Williams & Wilkins, 2005.

Q11-28: Image from Rubin E, Gorstein F, Rubin R, et al., eds. Rubin's Pathology: Clinicopathologic Foundations of Medicine. 4th Ed. Philadelphia: Lippincott Williams & Wilkins, 2005.

Q11-33: Image from Rubin R, Strayer D, eds. Rubin's Pathology: Clinicopathologic Foundations of Medicine. 5th Ed. Baltimore: Lippincott Williams & Wilkins, 2008.

Q11-37: Image from Rubin E, Gorstein F, Rubin R, et al., eds. Rubin's Pathology: Clinicopathologic Foundations of Medicine. 4th Ed. Philadelphia: Lippincott Williams & Wilkins, 2005.

Q11-40: Image from Rubin E, Gorstein F, Rubin R, et al., eds. Rubin's Pathology: Clinicopathologic Foundations of Medicine. 4th Ed. Philadelphia: Lippincott Williams & Wilkins, 2005.

Q11-41: Image from Rubin E, Gorstein F, Rubin R, et al., eds. Rubin's Pathology: Clinicopathologic Foundations of Medicine. 4th Ed. Philadelphia: Lippincott Williams & Wilkins, 2005.

Q11-42: Image from Rubin E, Gorstein F, Rubin R, et al., eds. Rubin's Pathology: Clinicopathologic Foundations of Medicine. 4th Ed. Philadelphia: Lippincott Williams & Wilkins, 2005.

Q11-43: Image from Rubin E, Gorstein F, Rubin R, et al., eds. Rubin's Pathology: Clinicopathologic Foundations of Medicine. 4th Ed. Philadelphia: Lippincott Williams & Wilkins, 2005.

Q11-44: Image from Rubin E, Gorstein F, Rubin R, et al., eds. Rubin's Pathology: Clinicopathologic Foundations of Medicine. 4th Ed. Philadelphia: Lippincott Williams & Wilkins, 2005.

Q11-46: Image from Rubin R, Strayer D, eds. Rubin's Pathology: Clinicopathologic Foundations of Medicine. 5th Ed. Baltimore: Lippincott Williams & Wilkins, 2008.

Q11-47: Image from Rubin R, Strayer D, eds. Rubin's Pathology: Clinicopathologic Foundations of Medicine. 5th Ed. Baltimore: Lippincott Williams & Wilkins, 2008.

Chapter 12

Q12-4: Image from Rubin E, Gorstein F, Rubin R, et al., eds. Rubin's Pathology: Clinicopathologic Foundations of Medicine. 4th Ed. Philadelphia: Lippincott Williams & Wilkins, 2005.

Q12-10: Image from Rubin E, Gorstein F, Rubin R, et al., eds. Rubin's Pathology: Clinicopathologic Foundations of Medicine. 4th Ed. Philadelphia: Lippincott Williams & Wilkins, 2005.

Q12-11: Image from Rubin E, Gorstein F, Rubin R, et al., eds. Rubin's Pathology: Clinicopathologic Foundations of Medicine. 4th Ed. Philadelphia: Lippincott Williams & Wilkins, 2005.

Q12-13: Image from Rubin E, Gorstein F, Rubin R, et al., eds. Rubin's Pathology: Clinicopathologic Foundations of Medicine. 4th Ed. Philadelphia: Lippincott Williams & Wilkins, 2005.

Q12-14: Image from Rubin E, Gorstein F, Rubin R, et al., eds. Rubin's Pathology: Clinicopathologic Foundations of Medicine. 4th Ed. Philadelphia: Lippincott Williams & Wilkins, 2005.

Q12-19: Image from Rubin E, Gorstein F, Rubin R, et al., eds. Rubin's Pathology: Clinicopathologic Foundations of Medicine. 4th Ed. Philadelphia: Lippincott Williams & Wilkins, 2005.

Q12-20: Image from Rubin E, Gorstein F, Rubin R, et al., eds. Rubin's Pathology: Clinicopathologic Foundations of Medicine. 4th Ed. Philadelphia: Lippincott Williams & Wilkins, 2005.

Q12-24: Image from Rubin E, Gorstein F, Rubin R, et al., eds. Rubin's Pathology: Clinicopathologic Foundations of Medicine. 4th Ed. Philadelphia: Lippincott Williams & Wilkins, 2005.

Q12-28: Image from Rubin E, Gorstein F, Rubin R, et al., eds. Rubin's Pathology: Clinicopathologic Foundations of Medicine. 4th Ed. Philadelphia: Lippincott Williams & Wilkins, 2005.

Q12-29: Image from Rubin E, Gorstein F, Rubin R, et al., eds. Rubin's Pathology: Clinicopathologic Foundations of Medicine. 4th Ed. Philadelphia: Lippincott Williams & Wilkins, 2005.

Q12-31: Image from Rubin E, Gorstein F, Rubin R, et al., eds. Rubin's Pathology: Clinicopathologic Foundations of Medicine. 4th Ed. Philadelphia: Lippincott Williams & Wilkins, 2005.

Q12-33: Image from Rubin E, Gorstein F, Rubin R, et al., eds. Rubin's Pathology: Clinicopathologic Foundations of Medicine. 4th Ed. Philadelphia: Lippincott Williams & Wilkins, 2005.

Q12-34: Image from Rubin E, Gorstein F, Rubin R, et al., eds. Rubin's Pathology: Clinicopathologic Foundations of Medicine. 4th Ed. Philadelphia: Lippincott Williams & Wilkins, 2005.

Q12-35: Image from Rubin E, Gorstein F, Rubin R, et al., eds. Rubin's Pathology: Clinicopathologic Foundations of Medicine. 4th Ed. Philadelphia: Lippincott Williams & Wilkins, 2005.

Q12-36: Image from Rubin E, Gorstein F, Rubin R, et al., eds. Rubin's Pathology: Clinicopathologic Foundations of Medicine. 4th Ed. Philadelphia: Lippincott Williams & Wilkins, 2005.

Q12-37: Image from Rubin E, Gorstein F, Rubin R, et al., eds. Rubin's Pathology: Clinicopathologic Foundations of Medicine. 4th Ed. Philadelphia: Lippincott Williams & Wilkins, 2005.

Q12-38: Image from Rubin E, Gorstein F, Rubin R, et al., eds. Rubin's Pathology: Clinicopathologic Foundations of Medicine. 4th Ed. Philadelphia: Lippincott Williams & Wilkins, 2005.

Q12-39: Image from Rubin E, Gorstein F, Rubin R, et al., eds. Rubin's Pathology: Clinicopathologic Foundations of Medicine. 4th Ed. Philadelphia: Lippincott Williams & Wilkins, 2005.

Q12-40: Image from Rubin E, Gorstein F, Rubin R, et al., eds. Rubin's Pathology: Clinicopathologic Foundations of Medicine. 4th Ed. Philadelphia: Lippincott Williams & Wilkins, 2005.

Q12-41: Image from Rubin E, Gorstein F, Rubin R, et al., eds. Rubin's Pathology: Clinicopathologic Foundations of Medicine. 4th Ed. Philadelphia: Lippincott Williams & Wilkins, 2005.

Q12-42: Image from Rubin E, Gorstein F, Rubin R, et al., eds. Rubin's Pathology: Clinicopathologic Foundations of Medicine. 4th Ed. Philadelphia: Lippincott Williams & Wilkins, 2005.

Q12-44: Image from Rubin E, Gorstein F, Rubin R, et al., eds. Rubin's Pathology: Clinicopathologic Foundations of Medicine. 4th Ed. Philadelphia: Lippincott Williams & Wilkins, 2005.

Q12-45: Image from Rubin E, Gorstein F, Rubin R, et al., eds. Rubin's Pathology: Clinicopathologic Foundations of Medicine. 4th Ed. Philadelphia: Lippincott Williams & Wilkins, 2005.

Q12-46: Image from Rubin E, Gorstein F, Rubin R, et al., eds. Rubin's Pathology: Clinicopathologic Foundations of Medicine. 4th Ed. Philadelphia: Lippincott Williams & Wilkins, 2005.

Q12-47: Image from Rubin E, Gorstein F, Rubin R, et al., eds. Rubin's Pathology: Clinicopathologic Foundations of Medicine. 4th Ed. Philadelphia: Lippincott Williams & Wilkins, 2005.

Q12-48: Image from Rubin E, Gorstein F, Rubin R, et al., eds. Rubin's Pathology: Clinicopathologic Foundations of Medicine. 4th Ed. Philadelphia: Lippincott Williams & Wilkins, 2005.

Q12-49: Image from Rubin E, Gorstein F, Rubin R, et al., eds. Rubin's Pathology: Clinicopathologic Foundations of Medicine. 4th Ed. Philadelphia: Lippincott Williams & Wilkins, 2005.

Q12-50: Image from Rubin E, Gorstein F, Rubin R, et al., eds. Rubin's Pathology: Clinicopathologic Foundations of Medicine. 4th Ed. Philadelphia: Lippincott Williams & Wilkins, 2005.

Chapter 13

Q13-4: Image from Rubin E, Gorstein F, Rubin R, et al., eds. Rubin's Pathology: Clinicopathologic Foundations of Medicine. 4th Ed. Philadelphia: Lippincott Williams & Wilkins, 2005.

Q13-10: Image from Rubin E, Gorstein F, Rubin R, et al., eds. Rubin's Pathology: Clinicopathologic Foundations of Medicine. 4th Ed. Philadelphia: Lippincott Williams & Wilkins, 2005.

Q13-14: Image from Rubin E, Gorstein F, Rubin R, et al., eds. Rubin's Pathology: Clinicopathologic Foundations of Medicine. 4th Ed. Philadelphia: Lippincott Williams & Wilkins, 2005.

Q13-19: Image from Rubin E, Gorstein F, Rubin R, et al., eds. Rubin's Pathology: Clinicopathologic Foundations of Medicine. 4th Ed. Philadelphia: Lippincott Williams & Wilkins, 2005.

Q13-22: Image from Rubin E, Gorstein F, Rubin R, et al., eds. Rubin's Pathology: Clinicopathologic Foundations of Medicine. 4th Ed. Philadelphia: Lippincott Williams & Wilkins, 2005.

Q13-25: Image from Rubin E, Gorstein F, Rubin R, et al., eds. Rubin's Pathology: Clinicopathologic Foundations of Medicine. 4th Ed. Philadelphia: Lippincott Williams & Wilkins, 2005.

Q13-26: Image from Rubin E, Gorstein F, Rubin R, et al., eds. Rubin's Pathology: Clinicopathologic Foundations of Medicine. 4th Ed. Philadelphia: Lippincott Williams & Wilkins, 2005.

Q13-27: Image from Mitros FA. Atlas of Gastrointestinal Pathology. New York: Gower Medical Publishing, 1988.

Q13-29: Image from Rubin R, Strayer D, eds. Rubin's Pathology: Clinicopathologic Foundations of Medicine. 5th Ed. Baltimore: Lippincott Williams & Wilkins, 2008.

Q13-31: Image from Rubin R, Strayer D, eds. Rubin's Pathology: Clinicopathologic Foundations of Medicine. 5th Ed. Baltimore: Lippincott Williams & Wilkins, 2008.

Q13-32: Image from Rubin E, Gorstein F, Rubin R, et al., eds. Rubin's Pathology: Clinicopathologic Foundations of Medicine. 4th Ed. Philadelphia: Lippincott Williams & Wilkins, 2005.

Q13-33: Image from Rubin E, Gorstein F, Rubin R, et al., eds. Rubin's Pathology: Clinicopathologic Foundations of Medicine. 4th Ed. Philadelphia: Lippincott Williams & Wilkins, 2005.

Q13-34: Image from Rubin E, Gorstein F, Rubin R, et al., eds. Rubin's Pathology: Clinicopathologic Foundations of Medicine. 4th Ed. Philadelphia: Lippincott Williams & Wilkins, 2005.

Q13-35: Image from Rubin E, Gorstein F, Rubin R, et al., eds. Rubin's Pathology: Clinicopathologic Foundations of Medicine. 4th Ed. Philadelphia: Lippincott Williams & Wilkins, 2005.

Q13-36: Image from Rubin R, Strayer D, eds. Rubin's Pathology: Clinicopathologic Foundations of Medicine. 5th Ed. Baltimore: Lippincott Williams & Wilkins, 2008.

Q13-39: Image from Rubin E, Gorstein F, Rubin R, et al., eds. Rubin's Pathology: Clinicopathologic Foundations of Medicine. 4th Ed. Philadelphia: Lippincott Williams & Wilkins, 2005.

Q13-43: Image from Rubin E, Gorstein F, Rubin R, et al., eds. Rubin's Pathology: Clinicopathologic Foundations of Medicine. 4th Ed. Philadelphia: Lippincott Williams & Wilkins, 2005.

Q13-54: Image from Rubin E, Gorstein F, Rubin R, et al., eds. Rubin's Pathology: Clinicopathologic Foundations of Medicine. 4th Ed. Philadelphia: Lippincott Williams & Wilkins, 2005.

Q13-57: Image from Rubin E, Gorstein F, Rubin R, et al., eds. Rubin's Pathology: Clinicopathologic Foundations of Medicine. 4th Ed. Philadelphia: Lippincott Williams & Wilkins, 2005.

Q13-60: Image from Mitros FA. Atlas of Gastrointestinal Pathology. New York: Gower Medical Publishing, 1988.

Chapter 14

Q14-7: Image from Rubin E, Gorstein F, Rubin R, et al., eds. Rubin's Pathology: Clinicopathologic Foundations of Medicine. 4th Ed. Philadelphia: Lippincott Williams & Wilkins, 2005.

Q14-8: Image from Rubin E, Gorstein F, Rubin R, et al., eds. Rubin's Pathology: Clinicopathologic Foundations of Medicine. 4th Ed. Philadelphia: Lippincott Williams & Wilkins, 2005.

Q14-11: Image from Rubin E, Gorstein F, Rubin R, et al., eds. Rubin's Pathology: Clinicopathologic Foundations of Medicine. 4th Ed. Philadelphia: Lippincott Williams & Wilkins, 2005.

Q14-16: Image from Rubin E, Gorstein F, Rubin R, et al., eds. Rubin's Pathology: Clinicopathologic Foundations of Medicine. 4th Ed. Philadelphia: Lippincott Williams & Wilkins, 2005.

Q14-17: Image from Rubin E, Gorstein F, Rubin R, et al., eds. Rubin's Pathology: Clinicopathologic Foundations of Medicine. 4th Ed. Philadelphia: Lippincott Williams & Wilkins, 2005.

Q14-18: Image from Rubin E, Gorstein F, Rubin R, et al., eds. Rubin's Pathology: Clinicopathologic Foundations of Medicine. 4th Ed. Philadelphia: Lippincott Williams & Wilkins, 2005.

Q14-19: Image from Yanoff M. Ocular Pathology: A Color Atlas. New York: Gower Medical Publishing, 1988.

Q14-20: Image from Rubin E, Gorstein F, Rubin R, et al., eds. Rubin's Pathology: Clinicopathologic Foundations of Medicine. 4th Ed. Philadelphia: Lippincott Williams & Wilkins, 2005.

Q14-23: Image from Rubin E, Gorstein F, Rubin R, et al., eds. Rubin's Pathology: Clinicopathologic Foundations of Medicine. 4th Ed. Philadelphia: Lippincott Williams & Wilkins, 2005.

Q14-24: Image from Rubin R, Strayer D, eds. Rubin's Pathology: Clinicopathologic Foundations of Medicine. 5th Ed. Baltimore: Lippincott Williams & Wilkins, 2008.

Q14-25: Image from Rubin E, Gorstein F, Rubin R, et al., eds. Rubin's Pathology: Clinicopathologic Foundations of Medicine. 4th Ed. Philadelphia: Lippincott Williams & Wilkins, 2005.

Q14-26: Image from Rubin E, Gorstein F, Rubin R, et al., eds. Rubin's Pathology: Clinicopathologic Foundations of Medicine. 4th Ed. Philadelphia: Lippincott Williams & Wilkins, 2005.

Q14-28: Image from Rubin E, Gorstein F, Rubin R, et al., eds. Rubin's Pathology: Clinicopathologic Foundations of Medicine. 4th Ed. Philadelphia: Lippincott Williams & Wilkins, 2005.

Q14-31: Image from Rubin E, Gorstein F, Rubin R, et al., eds. Rubin's Pathology: Clinicopathologic Foundations of Medicine. 4th Ed. Philadelphia: Lippincott Williams & Wilkins, 2005.

Q14-34: Image from Rubin E, Gorstein F, Rubin R, et al., eds. Rubin's Pathology: Clinicopathologic Foundations of Medicine. 4th Ed. Philadelphia: Lippincott Williams & Wilkins, 2005.

Q14-38: Image from Rubin E, Gorstein F, Rubin R, et al., eds. Rubin's Pathology: Clinicopathologic Foundations of Medicine. 4th Ed. Philadelphia: Lippincott Williams & Wilkins, 2005.

Q14-39: Image from Rubin E, Gorstein F, Rubin R, et al., eds. Rubin's Pathology: Clinicopathologic Foundations of Medicine. 4th Ed. Philadelphia: Lippincott Williams & Wilkins, 2005.

Q14-40: Image from Rubin E, Gorstein F, Rubin R, et al., eds. Rubin's Pathology: Clinicopathologic Foundations of Medicine. 4th Ed. Philadelphia: Lippincott Williams & Wilkins, 2005.

Q14-45: Image from Rubin E, Gorstein F, Rubin R, et al., eds. Rubin's Pathology: Clinicopathologic Foundations of Medicine. 4th Ed. Philadelphia: Lippincott Williams & Wilkins, 2005.

Q14-49: Image from Rubin R, Strayer D, eds. Rubin's Pathology: Clinicopathologic Foundations of Medicine. 5th Ed. Baltimore: Lippincott Williams & Wilkins, 2008.

Chapter 15

Q15-7: Image from Rubin E, Gorstein F, Rubin R, et al., eds. Rubin's Pathology: Clinicopathologic Foundations of Medicine. 4th Ed. Philadelphia: Lippincott Williams & Wilkins, 2005.

Q15-9: Image from Rubin E, Gorstein F, Rubin R, et al., eds. Rubin's Pathology: Clinicopathologic Foundations of Medicine. 4th Ed. Philadelphia: Lippincott Williams & Wilkins, 2005.

Q15-14: Image from Rubin E, Gorstein F, Rubin R, et al., eds. Rubin's Pathology: Clinicopathologic Foundations of Medicine. 4th Ed. Philadelphia: Lippincott Williams & Wilkins, 2005.

Q15-17: Image from Rubin R, Strayer D, eds. Rubin's Pathology: Clinicopathologic Foundations of Medicine. 5th Ed. Baltimore: Lippincott Williams & Wilkins, 2008.

Chapter 16

Q16-1: Image from Rubin E, Gorstein F, Rubin R, et al., eds. Rubin's Pathology: Clinicopathologic Foundations of Medicine. 4th Ed. Philadelphia: Lippincott Williams & Wilkins, 2005.

Q16-2: Image from Rubin E, Gorstein F, Rubin R, et al., eds. Rubin's Pathology: Clinicopathologic Foundations of Medicine. 4th Ed. Philadelphia: Lippincott Williams & Wilkins, 2005.

Q16-8: Image from Rubin E, Gorstein F, Rubin R, et al., eds. Rubin's Pathology: Clinicopathologic Foundations of Medicine. 4th Ed. Philadelphia: Lippincott Williams & Wilkins, 2005.

Q16-13: Image from Rubin E, Gorstein F, Rubin R, et al., eds. Rubin's Pathology: Clinicopathologic Foundations of Medicine. 4th Ed. Philadelphia: Lippincott Williams & Wilkins, 2005.

Q16-19: Image from Rubin E, Gorstein F, Rubin R, et al., eds. Rubin's Pathology: Clinicopathologic Foundations of Medicine. 4th Ed. Philadelphia: Lippincott Williams & Wilkins, 2005.

Q16-23: Image from Rubin E, Gorstein F, Rubin R, et al., eds. Rubin's Pathology: Clinicopathologic Foundations of Medicine. 4th Ed. Philadelphia: Lippincott Williams & Wilkins, 2005.

Q16-24: Image from Rubin E, Gorstein F, Rubin R, et al., eds. Rubin's Pathology: Clinicopathologic Foundations of Medicine. 4th Ed. Philadelphia: Lippincott Williams & Wilkins, 2005.

Q16-27: Image from Rubin E, Gorstein F, Rubin R, et al., eds. Rubin's Pathology: Clinicopathologic Foundations of Medicine. 4th Ed. Philadelphia: Lippincott Williams & Wilkins, 2005.

Q16-28: Image from Rubin E, Gorstein F, Rubin R, et al., eds. Rubin's Pathology: Clinicopathologic Foundations of Medicine. 4th Ed. Philadelphia: Lippincott Williams & Wilkins, 2005.

Q16-30: Image from Rubin E, Gorstein F, Rubin R, et al., eds. Rubin's Pathology: Clinicopathologic Foundations of Medicine. 4th Ed. Philadelphia: Lippincott Williams & Wilkins, 2005.

Q16-34: Image from Rubin E, Gorstein F, Rubin R, et al., eds. Rubin's Pathology: Clinicopathologic Foundations of Medicine. 4th Ed. Philadelphia: Lippincott Williams & Wilkins, 2005.

Q16-36: Image from Rubin E, Gorstein F, Rubin R, et al., eds. Rubin's Pathology: Clinicopathologic Foundations of Medicine. 4th Ed. Philadelphia: Lippincott Williams & Wilkins, 2005.

Q16-40: Image from Rubin E, Gorstein F, Rubin R, et al., eds. Rubin's Pathology: Clinicopathologic Foundations of Medicine. 4th Ed. Philadelphia: Lippincott Williams & Wilkins, 2005.

Q16-41: Image from Rubin E, Gorstein F, Rubin R, et al., eds. Rubin's Pathology: Clinicopathologic Foundations of Medicine. 4th Ed. Philadelphia: Lippincott Williams & Wilkins, 2005.

Q16-42: Image from Rubin E, Gorstein F, Rubin R, et al., eds. Rubin's Pathology: Clinicopathologic Foundations of Medicine. 4th Ed. Philadelphia: Lippincott Williams & Wilkins, 2005.

Q16-44: Image from Rubin E, Gorstein F, Rubin R, et al., eds. Rubin's Pathology: Clinicopathologic Foundations of Medicine. 4th Ed. Philadelphia: Lippincott Williams & Wilkins, 2005.

Q16-45: Image from Rubin E, Gorstein F, Rubin R, et al., eds. Rubin's Pathology: Clinicopathologic Foundations of Medicine. 4th Ed. Philadelphia: Lippincott Williams & Wilkins, 2005.

Q16-46: Image from Rubin E, Gorstein F, Rubin R, et al., eds. Rubin's Pathology: Clinicopathologic Foundations of Medicine. 4th Ed. Philadelphia: Lippincott Williams & Wilkins, 2005.

Q16-53: Image from Rubin E, Gorstein F, Rubin R, et al., eds. Rubin's Pathology: Clinicopathologic Foundations of Medicine. 4th Ed. Philadelphia: Lippincott Williams & Wilkins, 2005.

Q16-55: Image from Rubin E, Gorstein F, Rubin R, et al., eds. Rubin's Pathology: Clinicopathologic Foundations of Medicine. 4th Ed. Philadelphia: Lippincott Williams & Wilkins, 2005.

Q16-56: Image from Rubin E, Gorstein F, Rubin R, et al., eds. Rubin's Pathology: Clinicopathologic Foundations of Medicine. 4th Ed. Philadelphia: Lippincott Williams & Wilkins, 2005.

Q16-58: Image from Rubin E, Gorstein F, Rubin R, et al., eds. Rubin's Pathology: Clinicopathologic Foundations of Medicine. 4th Ed. Philadelphia: Lippincott Williams & Wilkins, 2005.

Q16-59: Image from Rubin E, Gorstein F, Rubin R, et al., eds. Rubin's Pathology: Clinicopathologic Foundations of Medicine. 4th Ed. Philadelphia: Lippincott Williams & Wilkins, 2005.

Chapter 17

Q17-1: Image from Wiss MA, Mills SE. Atlas of Genitourinary Tract Disorders. New York: Gower Medical Publishers, 1988.

Q17-7: Image from Rubin E, Gorstein F, Rubin R, et al., eds. Rubin's Pathology: Clinicopathologic Foundations of Medicine. 4th Ed. Philadelphia: Lippincott Williams & Wilkins, 2005.

Q17-8: Image from Rubin E, Gorstein F, Rubin R, et al., eds. Rubin's Pathology: Clinicopathologic Foundations of Medicine. 4th Ed. Philadelphia: Lippincott Williams & Wilkins, 2005.

Q17-9: Image from Rubin E, Gorstein F, Rubin R, et al., eds. Rubin's Pathology: Clinicopathologic Foundations of Medicine. 4th Ed. Philadelphia: Lippincott Williams & Wilkins, 2005.

Q17-10: Image from Rubin E, Gorstein F, Rubin R, et al., eds. Rubin's Pathology: Clinicopathologic Foundations of Medicine. 4th Ed. Philadelphia: Lippincott Williams & Wilkins, 2005.

Q17-16: Image from Rubin E, Gorstein F, Rubin R, et al., eds. Rubin's Pathology: Clinicopathologic Foundations of Medicine. 4th Ed. Philadelphia: Lippincott Williams & Wilkins, 2005.

Q17-20: Image from Rubin R, Strayer D, eds. Rubin's Pathology: Clinicopathologic Foundations of Medicine. 5th Ed. Baltimore: Lippincott Williams & Wilkins, 2008.

Q17-26: Image from Rubin E, Gorstein F, Rubin R, et al., eds. Rubin's Pathology: Clinicopathologic Foundations of Medicine. 4th Ed. Philadelphia: Lippincott Williams & Wilkins, 2005.

Q17-27: Image from Rubin R, Strayer D, eds. Rubin's Pathology: Clinicopathologic Foundations of Medicine. 5th Ed. Baltimore: Lippincott Williams & Wilkins, 2008.

Q17-39: Image from Rubin R, Strayer D, eds. Rubin's Pathology: Clinicopathologic Foundations of Medicine. 5th Ed. Baltimore: Lippincott Williams & Wilkins, 2008.

Q17-41: Image from Rubin E, Gorstein F, Rubin R, et al., eds. Rubin's Pathology: Clinicopathologic Foundations of Medicine. 4th Ed. Philadelphia: Lippincott Williams & Wilkins, 2005.

Q17-46: Image from Rubin E, Gorstein F, Rubin R, et al., eds. Rubin's Pathology: Clinicopathologic Foundations of Medicine. 4th Ed. Philadelphia: Lippincott Williams & Wilkins, 2005.

Chapter 18

Q18-4: Image from Rubin E, Gorstein F, Rubin R, et al., eds. Rubin's Pathology: Clinicopathologic Foundations of Medicine. 4th Ed. Philadelphia: Lippincott Williams & Wilkins, 2005.

Q18-8: Image from Rubin E, Gorstein F, Rubin R, et al., eds. Rubin's Pathology: Clinicopathologic Foundations of Medicine. 4th Ed. Philadelphia: Lippincott Williams & Wilkins, 2005.

Q18-9: Image from Rubin E, Gorstein F, Rubin R, et al., eds. Rubin's Pathology: Clinicopathologic Foundations of Medicine. 4th Ed. Philadelphia: Lippincott Williams & Wilkins, 2005.

Q18-12: Image from Rubin E, Gorstein F, Rubin R, et al., eds. Rubin's Pathology: Clinicopathologic Foundations of Medicine. 4th Ed. Philadelphia: Lippincott Williams & Wilkins, 2005.

Q18-13: Image from Rubin E, Gorstein F, Rubin R, et al., eds. Rubin's Pathology: Clinicopathologic Foundations of Medicine. 4th Ed. Philadelphia: Lippincott Williams & Wilkins, 2005.

Q18-15: Image from Rubin E, Gorstein F, Rubin R, et al., eds. Rubin's Pathology: Clinicopathologic Foundations of Medicine. 4th Ed. Philadelphia: Lippincott Williams & Wilkins, 2005.

Q18-17: Image from Stanley J. Robboy, MD, and Gynecologic Pathology Associates, Durham and Chapel Hill, North Carolina.

Q18-19: Image from Rubin E, Gorstein F, Rubin R, et al., eds. Rubin's Pathology: Clinicopathologic Foundations of Medicine. 4th Ed. Philadelphia: Lippincott Williams & Wilkins, 2005.

Q18-20: Image from Rubin E, Gorstein F, Rubin R, et al., eds. Rubin's Pathology: Clinicopathologic Foundations of Medicine. 4th Ed. Philadelphia: Lippincott Williams & Wilkins, 2005.

Q18-22: Image from Stanley J. Robboy, MD, and Gynecologic Pathology Associates, Durham and Chapel Hill, North Carolina.

Q18-28: Image from Rubin E, Gorstein F, Rubin R, et al., eds. Rubin's Pathology: Clinicopathologic Foundations of Medicine. 4th Ed. Philadelphia: Lippincott Williams & Wilkins, 2005.

Q18-30: Image from Rubin E, Gorstein F, Rubin R, et al., eds. Rubin's Pathology: Clinicopathologic Foundations of Medicine. 4th Ed. Philadelphia: Lippincott Williams & Wilkins, 2005.

Q18-31: Image from Woodruff JD, Parmley TH. Atlas of Gynecologic Pathology. New York: Gower Medical Publishing, 1988.

Q18-33: Image from Rubin E, Gorstein F, Rubin R, et al., eds. Rubin's Pathology: Clinicopathologic Foundations of Medicine. 4th Ed. Philadelphia: Lippincott Williams & Wilkins, 2005.

Q18-34: Image from Rubin R, Strayer D, eds. Rubin's Pathology: Clinicopathologic Foundations of Medicine. 5th Ed. Baltimore: Lippincott Williams & Wilkins, 2008.

Q18-37: Image from Rubin E, Gorstein F, Rubin R, et al., eds. Rubin's Pathology: Clinicopathologic Foundations of Medicine. 4th Ed. Philadelphia: Lippincott Williams & Wilkins, 2005.

Q18-38: Image from Rubin E, Gorstein F, Rubin R, et al., eds. Rubin's Pathology: Clinicopathologic Foundations of Medicine. 4th Ed. Philadelphia: Lippincott Williams & Wilkins, 2005.

Q18-41: Image from Rubin E, Gorstein F, Rubin R, et al., eds. Rubin's Pathology: Clinicopathologic Foundations of Medicine. 4th Ed. Philadelphia: Lippincott Williams & Wilkins, 2005.

Q18-45: Image from Rubin E, Gorstein F, Rubin R, et al., eds. Rubin's Pathology: Clinicopathologic Foundations of Medicine. 4th Ed. Philadelphia: Lippincott Williams & Wilkins, 2005.

Chapter 19

Q19-3: Image from Rubin E, Gorstein F, Rubin R, et al., eds. Rubin's Pathology: Clinicopathologic Foundations of Medicine. 4th Ed. Philadelphia: Lippincott Williams & Wilkins, 2005.

Q19-4: Image from Rubin R, Strayer D, eds. Rubin's Pathology: Clinicopathologic Foundations of Medicine. 5th Ed. Baltimore: Lippincott Williams & Wilkins, 2008.

Q19-11: Image from Rubin R, Strayer D, eds. Rubin's Pathology: Clinicopathologic Foundations of Medicine. 5th Ed. Baltimore: Lippincott Williams & Wilkins, 2008.

Q19-13: Image from Rubin E, Gorstein F, Rubin R, et al., eds. Rubin's Pathology: Clinicopathologic Foundations of Medicine. 4th Ed. Philadelphia: Lippincott Williams & Wilkins, 2005.

Q19-15: Image from Rubin E, Gorstein F, Rubin R, et al., eds. Rubin's Pathology: Clinicopathologic Foundations of Medicine. 4th Ed. Philadelphia: Lippincott Williams & Wilkins, 2005.

Q19-16: Image from Rubin E, Gorstein F, Rubin R, et al., eds. Rubin's Pathology: Clinicopathologic Foundations of Medicine. 4th Ed. Philadelphia: Lippincott Williams & Wilkins, 2005.

Q19-17: Image from Rubin E, Gorstein F, Rubin R, et al., eds. Rubin's Pathology: Clinicopathologic Foundations of Medicine. 4th Ed. Philadelphia: Lippincott Williams & Wilkins, 2005.

Q19-18: Image from Rubin E, Gorstein F, Rubin R, et al., eds. Rubin's Pathology: Clinicopathologic Foundations of Medicine. 4th Ed. Philadelphia: Lippincott Williams & Wilkins, 2005.

Q19-19: Image from Rubin E, Gorstein F, Rubin R, et al., eds. Rubin's Pathology: Clinicopathologic Foundations of Medicine. 4th Ed. Philadelphia: Lippincott Williams & Wilkins, 2005.

Q19-21: Image from Rubin E, Gorstein F, Rubin R, et al., eds. Rubin's Pathology: Clinicopathologic Foundations of Medicine. 4th Ed. Philadelphia: Lippincott Williams & Wilkins, 2005.

Q19-23: Image from Rubin E, Gorstein F, Rubin R, et al., eds. Rubin's Pathology: Clinicopathologic Foundations of Medicine. 4th Ed. Philadelphia: Lippincott Williams & Wilkins, 2005.

Q19-25: Image from Rubin E, Gorstein F, Rubin R, et al., eds. Rubin's Pathology: Clinicopathologic Foundations of Medicine. 4th Ed. Philadelphia: Lippincott Williams & Wilkins, 2005.

Chapter 20

Q20-7: Image from Rubin E, Gorstein F, Rubin R, et al., eds. Rubin's Pathology: Clinicopathologic Foundations of Medicine. 4th Ed. Philadelphia: Lippincott Williams & Wilkins, 2005.

Q20-9: Image from Rubin E, Gorstein F, Rubin R, et al., eds. Rubin's Pathology: Clinicopathologic Foundations of Medicine. 4th Ed. Philadelphia: Lippincott Williams & Wilkins, 2005.

Q20-11: Image from Rubin E, Gorstein F, Rubin R, et al., eds. Rubin's Pathology: Clinicopathologic Foundations of Medicine. 4th Ed. Philadelphia: Lippincott Williams & Wilkins, 2005.

Q20-12: Image from Rubin E, Gorstein F, Rubin R, et al., eds. Rubin's Pathology: Clinicopathologic Foundations of Medicine. 4th Ed. Philadelphia: Lippincott Williams & Wilkins, 2005.

Q20-15: Image from Rubin E, Gorstein F, Rubin R, et al., eds. Rubin's Pathology: Clinicopathologic Foundations of Medicine. 4th Ed. Philadelphia: Lippincott Williams & Wilkins, 2005.

Q20-18: Image from Rubin E, Gorstein F, Rubin R, et al., eds. Rubin's Pathology: Clinicopathologic Foundations of Medicine. 4th Ed. Philadelphia: Lippincott Williams & Wilkins, 2005.

Q20-22: Image from Rubin E, Gorstein F, Rubin R, et al., eds. Rubin's Pathology: Clinicopathologic Foundations of Medicine. 4th Ed. Philadelphia: Lippincott Williams & Wilkins, 2005.

Q20-23: Image from Rubin E, Gorstein F, Rubin R, et al., eds. Rubin's Pathology: Clinicopathologic Foundations of Medicine. 4th Ed. Philadelphia: Lippincott Williams & Wilkins, 2005.

Q20-25: Image from Rubin E, Gorstein F, Rubin R, et al., eds. Rubin's Pathology: Clinicopathologic Foundations of Medicine. 4th Ed. Philadelphia: Lippincott Williams & Wilkins, 2005.

Q20-26: Image from Rubin E, Gorstein F, Rubin R, et al., eds. Rubin's Pathology: Clinicopathologic Foundations of Medicine. 4th Ed. Philadelphia: Lippincott Williams & Wilkins, 2005.

Q20-28: Image from Rubin E, Gorstein F, Rubin R, et al., eds. Rubin's Pathology: Clinicopathologic Foundations of Medicine. 4th Ed. Philadelphia: Lippincott Williams & Wilkins, 2005.

Q20-30: Image from Rubin E, Gorstein F, Rubin R, et al., eds. Rubin's Pathology: Clinicopathologic Foundations of Medicine. 4th Ed. Philadelphia: Lippincott Williams & Wilkins, 2005.

Q20-32: Image from Rubin E, Gorstein F, Rubin R, et al., eds. Rubin's Pathology: Clinicopathologic Foundations of Medicine. 4th Ed. Philadelphia: Lippincott Williams & Wilkins, 2005.

Q20-33: Image from Rubin E, Gorstein F, Rubin R, et al., eds. Rubin's Pathology: Clinicopathologic Foundations of Medicine. 4th Ed. Philadelphia: Lippincott Williams & Wilkins, 2005.

Q20-34: Image from Rubin E, Gorstein F, Rubin R, et al., eds. Rubin's Pathology: Clinicopathologic Foundations of Medicine. 4th Ed. Philadelphia: Lippincott Williams & Wilkins, 2005.

Q20-38: Image from Rubin E, Gorstein F, Rubin R, et al., eds. Rubin's Pathology: Clinicopathologic Foundations of Medicine. 4th Ed. Philadelphia: Lippincott Williams & Wilkins, 2005.

Q20-39: Image from Rubin E, Gorstein F, Rubin R, et al., eds. Rubin's Pathology: Clinicopathologic Foundations of Medicine. 4th Ed. Philadelphia: Lippincott Williams & Wilkins, 2005.

Q20-41: Image from Rubin E, Gorstein F, Rubin R, et al., eds. Rubin's Pathology: Clinicopathologic Foundations of Medicine. 4th Ed. Philadelphia: Lippincott Williams & Wilkins, 2005.

Q20-42: Image from Rubin E, Gorstein F, Rubin R, et al., eds. Rubin's Pathology: Clinicopathologic Foundations of Medicine. 4th Ed. Philadelphia: Lippincott Williams & Wilkins, 2005.

Q20-44: Image from Rubin E, Gorstein F, Rubin R, et al., eds. Rubin's Pathology: Clinicopathologic Foundations of Medicine. 4th Ed. Philadelphia: Lippincott Williams & Wilkins, 2005.

Q20-52: Image from Rubin E, Gorstein F, Rubin R, et al., eds. Rubin's Pathology: Clinicopathologic Foundations of Medicine. 4th Ed. Philadelphia: Lippincott Williams & Wilkins, 2005.

Q20-53: Image from Rubin E, Gorstein F, Rubin R, et al., eds. Rubin's Pathology: Clinicopathologic Foundations of Medicine. 4th Ed. Philadelphia: Lippincott Williams & Wilkins, 2005.

Q20-54: Image from Rubin E, Gorstein F, Rubin R, et al., eds. Rubin's Pathology: Clinicopathologic Foundations of Medicine. 4th Ed. Philadelphia: Lippincott Williams & Wilkins, 2005.

Q20-59: Image from Rubin E, Gorstein F, Rubin R, et al., eds. Rubin's Pathology: Clinicopathologic Foundations of Medicine. 4th Ed. Philadelphia: Lippincott Williams & Wilkins, 2005.

Q20-62: Image from Rubin E, Gorstein F, Rubin R, et al., eds. Rubin's Pathology: Clinicopathologic Foundations of Medicine. 4th Ed. Philadelphia: Lippincott Williams & Wilkins, 2005.

Q20-66: Image from Rubin E, Gorstein F, Rubin R, et al., eds. Rubin's Pathology: Clinicopathologic Foundations of Medicine. 4th Ed. Philadelphia: Lippincott Williams & Wilkins, 2005.

Chapter 21

Q21-1: Image from Rubin E, Gorstein F, Rubin R, et al., eds. Rubin's Pathology: Clinicopathologic Foundations of Medicine. 4th Ed. Philadelphia: Lippincott Williams & Wilkins, 2005.

Q21-7: Image from Rubin E, Gorstein F, Rubin R, et al., eds. Rubin's Pathology: Clinicopathologic Foundations of Medicine. 4th Ed. Philadelphia: Lippincott Williams & Wilkins, 2005.

Q21-10: Image from Rubin R, Strayer D, eds. Rubin's Pathology: Clinicopathologic Foundations of Medicine. 5th Ed. Baltimore: Lippincott Williams & Wilkins, 2008.

Q21-13: Image from Rubin E, Gorstein F, Rubin R, et al., eds. Rubin's Pathology: Clinicopathologic Foundations of Medicine. 4th Ed. Philadelphia: Lippincott Williams & Wilkins, 2005.

Q21-15: Image from Rubin E, Gorstein F, Rubin R, et al., eds. Rubin's Pathology: Clinicopathologic Foundations of Medicine. 4th Ed. Philadelphia: Lippincott Williams & Wilkins, 2005.

Q21-21: Image from Rubin R, Strayer D, eds. Rubin's Pathology: Clinicopathologic Foundations of Medicine. 5th Ed. Baltimore: Lippincott Williams & Wilkins, 2008.

Q21-29: Image from Rubin E, Gorstein F, Rubin R, et al., eds. Rubin's Pathology: Clinicopathologic Foundations of Medicine. 4th Ed. Philadelphia: Lippincott Williams & Wilkins, 2005.

Q21-30: Image from Rubin E, Gorstein F, Rubin R, et al., eds. Rubin's Pathology: Clinicopathologic Foundations of Medicine. 4th Ed. Philadelphia: Lippincott Williams & Wilkins, 2005.

Q21-32: Image from Rubin E, Gorstein F, Rubin R, et al., eds. Rubin's Pathology: Clinicopathologic Foundations of Medicine. 4th Ed. Philadelphia: Lippincott Williams & Wilkins, 2005.

Q21-33: Image from Rubin E, Gorstein F, Rubin R, et al., eds. Rubin's Pathology: Clinicopathologic Foundations of Medicine. 4th Ed. Philadelphia: Lippincott Williams & Wilkins, 2005.

Q21-34: Image from Rubin E, Gorstein F, Rubin R, et al., eds. Rubin's Pathology: Clinicopathologic Foundations of Medicine. 4th Ed. Philadelphia: Lippincott Williams & Wilkins, 2005.

Q21-36: Image from Rubin E, Gorstein F, Rubin R, et al., eds. Rubin's Pathology: Clinicopathologic Foundations of Medicine. 4th Ed. Philadelphia: Lippincott Williams & Wilkins, 2005.

Q21-37: Image from Rubin E, Gorstein F, Rubin R, et al., eds. Rubin's Pathology: Clinicopathologic Foundations of Medicine. 4th Ed. Philadelphia: Lippincott Williams & Wilkins, 2005.

Q21-38: Image from Rubin E, Gorstein F, Rubin R, et al., eds. Rubin's Pathology: Clinicopathologic Foundations of Medicine. 4th Ed. Philadelphia: Lippincott Williams & Wilkins, 2005.

Q21-40: Image from Rubin E, Gorstein F, Rubin R, et al., eds. Rubin's Pathology: Clinicopathologic Foundations of Medicine. 4th Ed. Philadelphia: Lippincott Williams & Wilkins, 2005.

Q21-41: Image from Rubin E, Gorstein F, Rubin R, et al., eds. Rubin's Pathology: Clinicopathologic Foundations of Medicine. 4th Ed. Philadelphia: Lippincott Williams & Wilkins, 2005.

Q21-45: Image from Rubin E, Gorstein F, Rubin R, et al., eds. Rubin's Pathology: Clinicopathologic Foundations of Medicine. 4th Ed. Philadelphia: Lippincott Williams & Wilkins, 2005.

Chapter 22

Q22-1: Image from Rubin E, Gorstein F, Rubin R, et al., eds. Rubin's Pathology: Clinicopathologic Foundations of Medicine. 4th Ed. Philadelphia: Lippincott Williams & Wilkins, 2005.

Q22-10: Image from Rubin E, Gorstein F, Rubin R, et al., eds. Rubin's Pathology: Clinicopathologic Foundations of Medicine. 4th Ed. Philadelphia: Lippincott Williams & Wilkins, 2005.

Chapter 23

Q23-3: Image from Rubin E, Gorstein F, Rubin R, et al., eds. Rubin's Pathology: Clinicopathologic Foundations of Medicine. 4th Ed. Philadelphia: Lippincott Williams & Wilkins, 2005.

Q23-4: Image from Rubin E, Gorstein F, Rubin R, et al., eds. Rubin's Pathology: Clinicopathologic Foundations of Medicine. 4th Ed. Philadelphia: Lippincott Williams & Wilkins, 2005.

Q23-8: Image from Rubin E, Gorstein F, Rubin R, et al., eds. Rubin's Pathology: Clinicopathologic Foundations of Medicine. 4th Ed. Philadelphia: Lippincott Williams & Wilkins, 2005.

Chapter 24

Q24-4: Image from Rubin E, Gorstein F, Rubin R, et al., eds. Rubin's Pathology: Clinicopathologic Foundations of Medicine. 4th Ed. Philadelphia: Lippincott Williams & Wilkins, 2005.

Q24-5: Image from Rubin E, Gorstein F, Rubin R, et al., eds. Rubin's Pathology: Clinicopathologic Foundations of Medicine. 4th Ed. Philadelphia: Lippincott Williams & Wilkins, 2005.

Q24-6: Image from Elder D. Synopsis and Atlas of Lever's Histopathology of the Skin. Philadelphia: Lippincott Williams & Wilkins, 1999.

Q24-7: Image from Rubin E, Gorstein F, Rubin R, et al., eds. Rubin's Pathology: Clinicopathologic Foundations of Medicine. 4th Ed. Philadelphia: Lippincott Williams & Wilkins, 2005.

Q24-10: Image from Rubin E, Gorstein F, Rubin R, et al., eds. Rubin's Pathology: Clinicopathologic Foundations of Medicine. 4th Ed. Philadelphia: Lippincott Williams & Wilkins, 2005.

Q24-11: Image from Rubin E, Gorstein F, Rubin R, et al., eds. Rubin's Pathology: Clinicopathologic Foundations of Medicine. 4th Ed. Philadelphia: Lippincott Williams & Wilkins, 2005.

Q24-12: Image from Rubin E, Gorstein F, Rubin R, et al., eds. Rubin's Pathology: Clinicopathologic Foundations of Medicine. 4th Ed. Philadelphia: Lippincott Williams & Wilkins, 2005.

Q24-14: Image from Elder D. Synopsis and Atlas of Lever's Histopathology of the Skin. Philadelphia: Lippincott Williams & Wilkins, 1999.

Q24-19: Image from Rubin E, Gorstein F, Rubin R, et al., eds. Rubin's Pathology: Clinicopathologic Foundations of Medicine. 4th Ed. Philadelphia: Lippincott Williams & Wilkins, 2005.

Q24-20: Image from Elder D. Synopsis and Atlas of Lever's Histopathology of the Skin. Philadelphia: Lippincott Williams & Wilkins, 1999.

Q24-21: Image from Elder D. Synopsis and Atlas of Lever's Histopathology of the Skin. Philadelphia: Lippincott Williams & Wilkins, 1999.

Chapter 25

Q25-2: Image from Rubin E, Gorstein F, Rubin R, et al., eds. Rubin's Pathology: Clinicopathologic Foundations of Medicine. 4th Ed. Philadelphia: Lippincott Williams & Wilkins, 2005.

Q25-4: Image from Rubin E, Gorstein F, Rubin R, et al., eds. Rubin's Pathology: Clinicopathologic Foundations of Medicine. 4th Ed. Philadelphia: Lippincott Williams & Wilkins, 2005.

Q25-9: Image from Rubin E, Gorstein F, Rubin R, et al., eds. Rubin's Pathology: Clinicopathologic Foundations of Medicine. 4th Ed. Philadelphia: Lippincott Williams & Wilkins, 2005.

Q25-11: Image from Rubin E, Gorstein F, Rubin R, et al., eds. Rubin's Pathology: Clinicopathologic Foundations of Medicine. 4th Ed. Philadelphia: Lippincott Williams & Wilkins, 2005.

Q25-13: Image from Rubin E, Gorstein F, Rubin R, et al., eds. Rubin's Pathology: Clinicopathologic Foundations of Medicine. 4th Ed. Philadelphia: Lippincott Williams & Wilkins, 2005.

Q25-14: Image from Rubin E, Gorstein F, Rubin R, et al., eds. Rubin's Pathology: Clinicopathologic Foundations of Medicine. 4th Ed. Philadelphia: Lippincott Williams & Wilkins, 2005.

Q25-15: Image from Rubin E, Gorstein F, Rubin R, et al., eds. Rubin's Pathology: Clinicopathologic Foundations of Medicine. 4th Ed. Philadelphia: Lippincott Williams & Wilkins, 2005.

Q25-16: Image from Rubin E, Gorstein F, Rubin R, et al., eds. Rubin's Pathology: Clinicopathologic Foundations of Medicine. 4th Ed. Philadelphia: Lippincott Williams & Wilkins, 2005.

Q25-20: Image from Rubin E, Gorstein F, Rubin R, et al., eds. Rubin's Pathology: Clinicopathologic Foundations of Medicine. 4th Ed. Philadelphia: Lippincott Williams & Wilkins, 2005.

Q25-21: Image from Rubin E, Gorstein F, Rubin R, et al., eds. Rubin's Pathology: Clinicopathologic Foundations of Medicine. 4th Ed. Philadelphia: Lippincott Williams & Wilkins, 2005.

Q25-23: Image from Rubin E, Gorstein F, Rubin R, et al., eds. Rubin's Pathology: Clinicopathologic Foundations of Medicine. 4th Ed. Philadelphia: Lippincott Williams & Wilkins, 2005.

Q25-24: Image from Rubin E, Gorstein F, Rubin R, et al., eds. Rubin's Pathology: Clinicopathologic Foundations of Medicine. 4th Ed. Philadelphia: Lippincott Williams & Wilkins, 2005.

Q25-26: Image from Rubin E, Gorstein F, Rubin R, et al., eds. Rubin's Pathology: Clinicopathologic Foundations of Medicine. 4th Ed. Philadelphia: Lippincott Williams & Wilkins, 2005.

Chapter 26

Q26-6: Image from Rubin E, Gorstein F, Rubin R, et al., eds. Rubin's Pathology: Clinicopathologic Foundations of Medicine. 4th Ed. Philadelphia: Lippincott Williams & Wilkins, 2005.

Q26-7: Image from Rubin E, Gorstein F, Rubin R, et al., eds. Rubin's Pathology: Clinicopathologic Foundations of Medicine. 4th Ed. Philadelphia: Lippincott Williams & Wilkins, 2005.

Q26-8: Image from Rubin E, Gorstein F, Rubin R, et al., eds. Rubin's Pathology: Clinicopathologic Foundations of Medicine. 4th Ed. Philadelphia: Lippincott Williams & Wilkins, 2005.

Q26-14: Image from Rubin E, Gorstein F, Rubin R, et al., eds. Rubin's Pathology: Clinicopathologic Foundations of Medicine. 4th Ed. Philadelphia: Lippincott Williams & Wilkins, 2005.

Q26-17: Image from Rubin E, Gorstein F, Rubin R, et al., eds. Rubin's Pathology: Clinicopathologic Foundations of Medicine. 4th Ed. Philadelphia: Lippincott Williams & Wilkins, 2005.

Q26-23: Image from Rubin E, Gorstein F, Rubin R, et al., eds. Rubin's Pathology: Clinicopathologic Foundations of Medicine. 4th Ed. Philadelphia: Lippincott Williams & Wilkins, 2005.

Q26-24: Image from Rubin E, Gorstein F, Rubin R, et al., eds. Rubin's Pathology: Clinicopathologic Foundations of Medicine. 4th Ed. Philadelphia: Lippincott Williams & Wilkins, 2005.

Q26-26: Image from Rubin E, Gorstein F, Rubin R, et al., eds. Rubin's Pathology: Clinicopathologic Foundations of Medicine. 4th Ed. Philadelphia: Lippincott Williams & Wilkins, 2005.

Q26-28: Image from Rubin E, Gorstein F, Rubin R, et al., eds. Rubin's Pathology: Clinicopathologic Foundations of Medicine. 4th Ed. Philadelphia: Lippincott Williams & Wilkins, 2005.

Q26-31: Image from Rubin E, Gorstein F, Rubin R, et al., eds. Rubin's Pathology: Clinicopathologic Foundations of Medicine. 4th Ed. Philadelphia: Lippincott Williams & Wilkins, 2005.

Chapter 27

Q27-6: Image from Rubin R, Strayer D, eds. Rubin's Pathology: Clinicopathologic Foundations of Medicine. 5th Ed. Baltimore: Lippincott Williams & Wilkins, 2008.

Q27-12: Image from Rubin E, Gorstein F, Rubin R, et al., eds. Rubin's Pathology: Clinicopathologic Foundations of Medicine. 4th Ed. Philadelphia: Lippincott Williams & Wilkins, 2005.

Q27-14: Image from Rubin E, Gorstein F, Rubin R, et al., eds. Rubin's Pathology: Clinicopathologic Foundations of Medicine. 4th Ed. Philadelphia: Lippincott Williams & Wilkins, 2005.

Chapter 28

Q28-3: Image from Rubin E, Gorstein F, Rubin R, et al., eds. Rubin's Pathology: Clinicopathologic Foundations of Medicine. 4th Ed. Philadelphia: Lippincott Williams & Wilkins, 2005.

Q28-4: Image from Rubin E, Gorstein F, Rubin R, et al., eds. Rubin's Pathology: Clinicopathologic Foundations of Medicine. 4th Ed. Philadelphia: Lippincott Williams & Wilkins, 2005.

Q28-6: Image from Rubin E, Gorstein F, Rubin R, et al., eds. Rubin's Pathology: Clinicopathologic Foundations of Medicine. 4th Ed. Philadelphia: Lippincott Williams & Wilkins, 2005.

Q28-7: Image from Rubin E, Gorstein F, Rubin R, et al., eds. Rubin's Pathology: Clinicopathologic Foundations of Medicine. 4th Ed. Philadelphia: Lippincott Williams & Wilkins, 2005.

Q28-10: Image from Rubin E, Gorstein F, Rubin R, et al., eds. Rubin's Pathology: Clinicopathologic Foundations of Medicine. 4th Ed. Philadelphia: Lippincott Williams & Wilkins, 2005.

Q28-17: Image from Rubin E, Gorstein F, Rubin R, et al., eds. Rubin's Pathology: Clinicopathologic Foundations of Medicine. 4th Ed. Philadelphia: Lippincott Williams & Wilkins, 2005.

Q28-19: Image from Rubin E, Gorstein F, Rubin R, et al., eds. Rubin's Pathology: Clinicopathologic Foundations of Medicine. 4th Ed. Philadelphia: Lippincott Williams & Wilkins, 2005.

Q28-21: Image from Rubin R, Strayer D, eds. Rubin's Pathology: Clinicopathologic Foundations of Medicine. 5th Ed. Baltimore: Lippincott Williams & Wilkins, 2008.

Q28-25: Image from Rubin E, Gorstein F, Rubin R, et al., eds. Rubin's Pathology: Clinicopathologic Foundations of Medicine. 4th Ed. Philadelphia: Lippincott Williams & Wilkins, 2005.

Q28-29: Image from Rubin E, Gorstein F, Rubin R, et al., eds. Rubin's Pathology: Clinicopathologic Foundations of Medicine. 4th Ed. Philadelphia: Lippincott Williams & Wilkins, 2005.

Q28-35: Image from Rubin E, Gorstein F, Rubin R, et al., eds. Rubin's Pathology: Clinicopathologic Foundations of Medicine. 4th Ed. Philadelphia: Lippincott Williams & Wilkins, 2005.

Q28-40: Image from Rubin E, Gorstein F, Rubin R, et al., eds. Rubin's Pathology: Clinicopathologic Foundations of Medicine. 4th Ed. Philadelphia: Lippincott Williams & Wilkins, 2005.

Q28-47: Image from Rubin E, Gorstein F, Rubin R, et al., eds. Rubin's Pathology: Clinicopathologic Foundations of Medicine. 4th Ed. Philadelphia: Lippincott Williams & Wilkins, 2005.

Q28-52: Image from Rubin E, Gorstein F, Rubin R, et al., eds. Rubin's Pathology: Clinicopathologic Foundations of Medicine. 4th Ed. Philadelphia: Lippincott Williams & Wilkins, 2005.

Q28-53: Image from Rubin E, Gorstein F, Rubin R, et al., eds. Rubin's Pathology: Clinicopathologic Foundations of Medicine. 4th Ed. Philadelphia: Lippincott Williams & Wilkins, 2005.

Q28-61: Image from Rubin E, Gorstein F, Rubin R, et al., eds. Rubin's Pathology: Clinicopathologic Foundations of Medicine. 4th Ed. Philadelphia: Lippincott Williams & Wilkins, 2005.

Q28-67: Image from Rubin E, Gorstein F, Rubin R, et al., eds. Rubin's Pathology: Clinicopathologic Foundations of Medicine. 4th Ed. Philadelphia: Lippincott Williams & Wilkins, 2005.

Q28-68: Image from Rubin E, Gorstein F, Rubin R, et al., eds. Rubin's Pathology: Clinicopathologic Foundations of Medicine. 4th Ed. Philadelphia: Lippincott Williams & Wilkins, 2005.

Q28-69: Image from Rubin E, Gorstein F, Rubin R, et al., eds. Rubin's Pathology: Clinicopathologic Foundations of Medicine. 4th Ed. Philadelphia: Lippincott Williams & Wilkins, 2005.

Q28-70: Image from Rubin E, Gorstein F, Rubin R, et al., eds. Rubin's Pathology: Clinicopathologic Foundations of Medicine. 4th Ed. Philadelphia: Lippincott Williams & Wilkins, 2005.

Q28-71: Image from Rubin E, Gorstein F, Rubin R, et al., eds. Rubin's Pathology: Clinicopathologic Foundations of Medicine. 4th Ed. Philadelphia: Lippincott Williams & Wilkins, 2005.

Q28-74: Image from Rubin E, Gorstein F, Rubin R, et al., eds. Rubin's Pathology: Clinicopathologic Foundations of Medicine. 4th Ed. Philadelphia: Lippincott Williams & Wilkins, 2005.

Chapter 29

Q29-1: Image from Rubin E, Gorstein F, Rubin R, et al., eds. Rubin's Pathology: Clinicopathologic Foundations of Medicine. 4th Ed. Philadelphia: Lippincott Williams & Wilkins, 2005.

Q29-11: Image from Rubin E, Gorstein F, Rubin R, et al., eds. Rubin's Pathology: Clinicopathologic Foundations of Medicine. 4th Ed. Philadelphia: Lippincott Williams & Wilkins, 2005.

Q29-12: Image from Rubin E, Gorstein F, Rubin R, et al., eds. Rubin's Pathology: Clinicopathologic Foundations of Medicine. 4th Ed. Philadelphia: Lippincott Williams & Wilkins, 2005.

Q29-13: Image from Rubin E, Gorstein F, Rubin R, et al., eds. Rubin's Pathology: Clinicopathologic Foundations of Medicine. 4th Ed. Philadelphia: Lippincott Williams & Wilkins, 2005.

Q29-16: Image from Rubin E, Gorstein F, Rubin R, et al., eds. Rubin's Pathology: Clinicopathologic Foundations of Medicine. 4th Ed. Philadelphia: Lippincott Williams & Wilkins, 2005.

Q29-20: Image from Rubin E, Gorstein F, Rubin R, et al., eds. Rubin's Pathology: Clinicopathologic Foundations of Medicine. 4th Ed. Philadelphia: Lippincott Williams & Wilkins, 2005.

Q29-21: Image from Rubin E, Gorstein F, Rubin R, et al., eds. Rubin's Pathology: Clinicopathologic Foundations of Medicine. 4th Ed. Philadelphia: Lippincott Williams & Wilkins, 2005.

Chapter 30

Q30-1: Image from Rubin E, Gorstein F, Rubin R, et al., eds. Rubin's Pathology: Clinicopathologic Foundations of Medicine. 4th Ed. Philadelphia: Lippincott Williams & Wilkins, 2005.

Q30-2: Image from Rubin E, Gorstein F, Rubin R, et al., eds. Rubin's Pathology: Clinicopathologic Foundations of Medicine. 4th Ed. Philadelphia: Lippincott Williams & Wilkins, 2005.

Q30-4: Image from Rubin E, Gorstein F, Rubin R, et al., eds. Rubin's Pathology: Clinicopathologic Foundations of Medicine. 4th Ed. Philadelphia: Lippincott Williams & Wilkins, 2005.

Q30-6: Image from Rubin E, Gorstein F, Rubin R, et al., eds. Rubin's Pathology: Clinicopathologic Foundations of Medicine. 4th Ed. Philadelphia: Lippincott Williams & Wilkins, 2005.

Q30-9: Image from Rubin E, Gorstein F, Rubin R, et al., eds. Rubin's Pathology: Clinicopathologic Foundations of Medicine. 4th Ed. Philadelphia: Lippincott Williams & Wilkins, 2005.

Q30-11: Image from Rubin E, Gorstein F, Rubin R, et al., eds. Rubin's Pathology: Clinicopathologic Foundations of Medicine. 4th Ed. Philadelphia: Lippincott Williams & Wilkins, 2005.

Q30-13: Image from Rubin E, Gorstein F, Rubin R, et al., eds. Rubin's Pathology: Clinicopathologic Foundations of Medicine. 4th Ed. Philadelphia: Lippincott Williams & Wilkins, 2005.

Q30-14: Image from Rubin E, Gorstein F, Rubin R, et al., eds. Rubin's Pathology: Clinicopathologic Foundations of Medicine. 4th Ed. Philadelphia: Lippincott Williams & Wilkins, 2005.

Q30-15: Image from Rubin E, Gorstein F, Rubin R, et al., eds. Rubin's Pathology: Clinicopathologic Foundations of Medicine. 4th Ed. Philadelphia: Lippincott Williams & Wilkins, 2005.

Q30-16: Image from Rubin E, Gorstein F, Rubin R, et al., eds. Rubin's Pathology: Clinicopathologic Foundations of Medicine. 4th Ed. Philadelphia: Lippincott Williams & Wilkins, 2005.

Index